KT-103-306

HANDBOOK OF

Clinical Anesthesia

SIXTH EDITION

Paul G. Barash, MD
Professor, Department of Anesthesiology
Yale University School of Medicine
Attending Anesthesiologist
Yale-New Haven Hospital
New Haven, Connecticut

Bruce F. Cullen, MD
Emeritus Professor
Department of Anesthesiology
University of Washington
Seattle, Washington

Robert K. Stoelting, MD
Emeritus Professor and Past Chair
Department of Anesthesia
Indiana University School of Medicine
Indianapolis, Indiana

Michael K. Cahalan, MD
Professor and Chair
Department of Anesthesiology
The University of Utah School of Medicine
Salt Lake City, Utah

M. Christine Stock, MD
Professor and Chair
Department of Anesthesiology
Northwestern University Feinberg School of Medicine
Chicago, Illinois

 Wolters Kluwer | Lippincott Williams & Wilkins
Health
Philadelphia · Baltimore · New York · London
Buenos Aires · Hong Kong · Sydney · Tokyo

Acquisitions Editor: Brian Brown
Managing Editor: Nicole Dernoski
Marketing Manager: Angela Panetta
Production Editor: Bridgett Dougherty
Senior Manufacturing Manager: Benjamin Rivera
Design Coordinator: Stephen Druding
Compositor: Aptara, Inc.

6th Edition

Library of Congress Cataloging-in-Publication Data

Handbook of clinical anesthesia / edited by Paul G. Barash . . . [et al.]. — 6th ed.
  p. ; cm.
  Includes bibliographical references and index.
  ISBN-13: 978-0-7817-8948-6
  ISBN-10: 0-7817-8948-6
  1. Anesthesiology—Handbooks, manuals, etc. 2. Anesthesia—Handbooks, manuals,
etc. I. Barash, Paul G. II. Clinical anesthesia.
  [DNLM: 1. Anesthesia—Handbooks. 2. Anesthetics—Handbooks. WO 231 H236
2009]
  RD82.2.H35 2009
  617.9′6—dc22

                                                                          2008055183

LWW.COM

ROBERT K. STOELTING, MD
EDITOR EMERITUS, *CLINICAL ANESTHESIA*

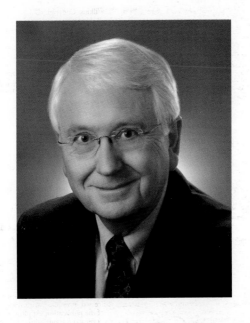

HIGHLY RESPECTED ANESTHESIOLOGIST,
DEDICATED EDUCATOR,
GIFTED AUTHOR AND EDITOR.

Welcome to the sixth edition of the *Handbook of Clinical Anesthesia*. Because the Handbook parallels the parent textbook, Clinical Anesthesia, extensive changes in the sixth edition of the text mandated similar changes to this volume. Two new chapters have been added to this edition, *Inflammation, Wound Healing and Infection*, as well as *Echocardiography*.

We would like to acknowledge the contributors to the textbook *Clinical Anesthesia*. Although the *Handbook of Clinical Anesthesia* is the product of the editors, its chapters were developed from the expert knowledge of the original contributors, reorganized and rewritten in a style necessary for a text of this scope. We would also like to thank Christopher Cambic, MD who proofread for details, as well as our administrative assistants—Gail Norup, Ruby Wilson, Deanna Walker, and Victoria Ramos—whose continued help has been a source of support. As always a special word of thanks is due to our colleagues at Lippincott Williams & Wilkins: Brian Brown, Executive Editor, Lisa McAllister, Publisher, Nicole Dernoski, Senior Managing Editor, and Bridgett Dougherty, Project Manager with the assistance of Chris Miller, Senior Project Manager, and Donna Kessler, Project Manager, Aptara. Their constructive comments during the process of writing and editing this book continue to demonstrate their commitment to medical education.

Paul G. Barash, MD
Bruce F. Cullen, MD
Robert K. Stoelting, MD
Michael K. Cahalan, MD
M. Christine Stock, MD

The authors would like to gratefully acknowledge the efforts of the contributors to the sixth edition of the textbook *Clinical Anesthesia*.

J. Jeffrey Andrews, MD
Shamsuddin Akhtar, MBBS
Michael L. Ault, MD, FCCP, FCCM
Douglas R. Bacon, MD
Paul G. Barash, MD
Honorio T. Benzon, MD
Christopher M. Bernards, MD
Arnold J. Berry, MD, MPH
David R. Bevan, MB
Barbara W. Brandom, MD
Ferne R. Braveman, MD, CM
Russell C. Brockwell, MD
Sorin J. Brull, MD
Michael K. Cahalan, MD
Levon M. Capan, MD
C. Richard Chapman, PhD
Amalia Cochran, MD
Barbara A. Coda, MD
Edmond Cohen, MD
Joseph P. Cravero, MD
Marie Csete, MD, PhD
Bruce F. Cullen, MD
Steven Deem, MD
Timothy R. Deer, MD
Stephen F. Dierdorf, MD
Karen B. Domino, MD, MPH
Francois Donati, MD, PhD, FRCPC
Michael B. Dorrough, MD
John C. Drummond, MD, FRCPC
Randal O. Dull, MD, PhD
Thomas J. Ebert, MD, PhD
Jan Ehrenwerth, MD
John H. Eichhorn, MD

James B. Eisenkraft, MD
John E. Ellis, MD
Matthew Eng, MD
Alex S. Evers, MD
Lynne R. Ferrari, MD
Scott M. Fishman, MD
Michael A. Fowler, MD, MBA
J. Sean Funston, MD
Steven I. Gayer, MD, MBA
Ronald George, MD, FRCP
Kathryn Glas, MD, FASE, MBA
Alexander W. Gotta, MD
Loreta Grecu, MD
Steven B. Greenberg, MD
Dhanesh K. Gupta, MD
Steven C. Hall, MD
Tara M. Hata, MD
Laurence M. Hausman, MD
Thomas K. Henthorn, MD
Simon C. Hillier, MB, ChB
Harriet W. Hopf, MD
Terese T. Horlocker, MD
Robert W. Hurley, MD, PhD
Adam K. Jacob, MD, MS
Joel O. Johnson, MD, PhD
Zeev N. Kain, MD, MBA
John P. Kampine, MD, PhD
Jonathan C. Katz, MD
Jonathan D. Katz, MD
Brian S. Kaufman, MD
M. Sean Kincaid, MD
Sandra L. Kopp, MD
Arthur M. Lam, MD, FRCPC
Thomas A. Lane, MD
Noel W. Lawson, MD

Wilton C. Levine, MD
Jerrold H. Levy, MD, FAHA
Adam D. Lichtman, MD
J. Lance Lichtor, MD
Yi Lin, MD, PhD
Spencer S. Liu, MD
David A. Lubarsky, MD, MBA
Stephen M. Macres, PharmD, MD
Srinivas Mantha, MD
Joseph P. Mathew, MD, MHSc
Michael S. Mazurek, MD
Kathryn E. McGoldrick, MD
Sanfold M. Miller, MD
Peter G. Moore, MD, BS, PhD, FANZCA
John R. Moyers, MD
Holly Muir, MD
Glenn S. Murphy, MD
Michael J. Murray, MD, PhD
Steve M. Neustein, MD
E. Andrew Ochroch, MD, MSCE
Babatunde O. Ogunnaike, MD
Charles W. Otto, MD, FCCM
Nathan Leon Pace, MD, Mstat
Paul S. Pagel, MD, PhD
Albert C. Perrino, Jr., MD
Charise Petrovitch, MD
Mihai V. Podgoreanu, MD, FASE
Wanda M. Popescu, MD
Karen L. Posner, PhD
Donald S. Prough, MD
Kevin T. Riutort, MD
J. David Roccoforte, MD
Michael F. Roizen, MD
G. Alec Rooke, MD, PhD
Stanley H. Rosenbaum, MD
Henry Rosenberg, MD, CPE
Meg A. Rosenblatt, MD

William R. Rosenblatt, MD
Richard W. Rosenquist, MD
Carl E. Rosow, MD, PhD
Nyamkhishig Sambuughin, PhD
Alan C. Santos, MD, MPH
Barbara M. Scavone, MD
Phillip G. Schmid, MD
Jeffrey J. Schwartz, MD
Harry A. Seifert, MD
Aarti Sharma, MD
Andrew Shaw, BSc, MBBS, FRCA, FCCM
Nikolaos J. Skubas, MD, FASE
Hugh M. Smith, MD, PhD
Karen J. Souter, BBS, FRCA
Bruce D. Spiess, MD, FAHA
Mark Stafford-Smith, MD, CM, FRCP, FASE
M. Christine Stock, MD
Robert K. Stoelting, MD
Karen J. Souter, BBS, FRCA
David F. Stowe, MD, PhD
Wariya Sukhupragarn, MD, FRCAT
Santhanam Suresh, MD
Christer H, Svensén, MD, PhD, DEAA, MBA
Stephen J. Thomas, MD
Miriam M. Treggiari, MD, PhD, MPH
Ban Tsui, BSc, MSc, MD, FRCPC
Jeffrey S. Vender, MD, FCCM, FCCP
J. Scott Walton, MD
Mark A. Warner, MD
Paul F. White, PhD, MD
Denise J. Wedel, MD
Charles W. Whitten, MD
Scott W. Wolf, MD
Cynthia A. Wong, MD
James R. Zaidan, MD, MBA

SECTION I ■ INTRODUCTION TO ANESTHESIOLOGY

SECTION II ■ SCIENTIFIC FOUNDATIONS OF ANESTHESIA

SECTION III ■ ANATOMY AND PHYSIOLOGY

SECTION IV ■ ANESTHETIC AGENTS, ADJUVANTS, AND DRUG INTERACTION

SECTION V ■ PREANESTHETIC EVALUATION AND PREPARATION

SECTION VI ■ ANESTHETIC MANAGEMENT

SECTION VII ■ ANESTHESIA FOR SURGICAL SUBSPECIALTIES

SECTION VIII ■ PERIOPERATIVE AND CONSULTATIVE SERVICES

■ APPENDICES

CHAPTER 1 ■ **THE HISTORY OF ANESTHESIA**

Although most human civilizations evolved some method for diminishing patient discomfort, anesthesia, in its modern and effective meaning, is a comparatively recent discovery with traceable origins dating back 160 years. (An epitaph on a monument to William T. G. Morton, one of the founders of anesthesia reads: "Before whom in all time Surgery was Agony.") (Jacob AK, Kopp SL, Bacon DR, Smith HM: The history of anesthesia. *Clinical Anesthesia.* Edited by Barash PG, Cullen BF, Stoelting RK, Cahalon MK; Stock MC. Philadelphia, Lippincott Williams and Wilkins, 2009, pp 1–26).

I. ANESTHESIA BEFORE ETHER

In addition to limitations in technical knowledge, cultural attitudes toward pain are often cited as reasons humans endured centuries of surgery without effective anesthesia.

A. Early Analgesics and Soporifics (Table 1-1)

B. Almost Discovery: Clarke, Long, and Wells
1. In January 1842, William E. Clarke, a medical student, may have given the first ether anesthetic in Rochester, NY, for a dental extraction.
2. Crawford Williamson Long administered ether for surgical anesthesia to James M. Venable on March 30, 1842, in Jefferson, GA, for the removal of a tumor on his neck. Long did not report his success until 1849 when ether anesthesia was already well known.
3. Horace Wells observed the "analgesic effects" of nitrous oxide when he attended a lecture exhibition by an itinerant "scientist," Gardner Quincy Colton. A few weeks later, in January 1845, Wells attempted a public demonstration in Boston at the Harvard Medical School, but the experience was judged a failure.

1

TABLE 1-1

EARLY ANALGESICS AND SOPORIFICS

Mandragora (soporific sponge)
Alcohol
Diethyl ether (known in the 16th century and perhaps as early as
    the 8th century)
Nitrous oxide (prepared by Joseph Priestly in 1773)

C. **Public Demonstration of Ether Anesthesia.** William
Thomas Morton Green was responsible for the first suc-
cessful public demonstration of ether anesthesia. This
demonstration, which took place in the Bullfinch
Amphitheater of the Massachusetts General Hospital on
October 16, 1846, is memorialized by the surgeon's
statement to his audience at the end of the procedure:
"Gentlemen, this is no humbug."

D. **Chloroform and Obstetrics**
1. James Young Simpson, a successful obstetrician of
Edinburgh, Scotland, was among the first to use ether
for the pain relief in obstetrics. He became dissatisfied
with ether and encouraged the use of chloroform.
2. Queen Victoria's endorsement of obstetric anesthesia
resulted in acceptance of the use of anesthesia in
labor.
3. John Snow took an interest in anesthetic practice
soon after the news of ether anesthesia reached Eng-
land in December 1846. Snow developed a mask that
closely resembles a modern facemask and also introduced a chloroform inhaler.

II. ANESTHESIA PRINCIPLES, EQUIPMENT, AND STANDARDS

A. **Control of the Airway**
1. Definitive control of the airway, a skill anesthesiologists now consider paramount, developed only after
many harrowing and apneic episodes spurred the
development of safer airway management techniques.
2. Joseph Clover, an Englishman, was the first person to
recommend the now universal practice of thrusting
the patient's jaw forward to overcome obstruction of
the upper airway by the tongue.

B. **Tracheal Intubation**
  1. The development of techniques and instruments for intubation ranks among the major advances in the history of anesthesiology.
  2. An American surgeon, Joseph O'Dwyer, designed a series of metal laryngeal tubes, which he inserted blindly between the vocal cords of children having diphtheritic crises.
  3. In 1895 in Berlin, Alfred Kirstein devised the first direct-vision laryngoscope.
  4. Before the introduction of muscle relaxants in the 1940s, intubation of the trachea could be challenging. This challenge was made somewhat easier, however, with the advent of laryngoscope blades specifically designed to increase visualization of the vocal cords.
  5. In 1926, Arthur Guedel began a series of experiments that led to the introduction of the cuffed tube.
  6. In 1953, single-lumen tubes were supplanted by double-lumen endobronchial tubes.
C. **Advanced Airway Devices.** Conventional laryngoscopes proved inadequate for patients with difficult airways. Dr. A. I. J. "Archie" Brain first recognized the principle of the laryngeal mask airway in 1981.
D. **Early Anesthesia Delivery Systems.** John Snow created ether inhalers, and Joseph Clover was the first to administer chloroform in known concentrations through the "Clover bag." Critical to increasing patient safety was the development of a machine capable of delivering calibrated amounts of gas and volatile anesthetics (also carbon dioxide absorption, vaporizers, and ventilators).
E. Two American surgeons, George W. Crile and Harvey Cushing, advocated systemic blood pressure monitoring during anesthesia. In 1902, Cushing applied the Riva Rocci cuff for blood pressure measurements to be recorded on an anesthesia record.
  1. The widespread use of electrocardiography, pulse oximetry, blood gas analysis, capnography, and neuromuscular blockade monitoring have reduced patient morbidity and mortality and revolutionized anesthesia practice.
  2. Breath-to-breath continuous monitoring and waveform display of carbon dioxide (infrared absorption) concentrations in the respired gases confirms endotracheal intubation (rules out accidental esophageal intubation).

F. **Safety Standards.** The introduction of safety features was coordinated by the American National Standards Institute Committee Z79, which was sponsored from 1956 until 1983 by the American Society of Anesthesiologists. Since 1983, representatives from industry, government, and health care professions have met as the Committee Z79 of the American Society for Testing and Materials. This organization establishes voluntary goals that may become accepted national standards for the safety of anesthesia equipment.

III. THE HISTORY OF ANESTHETIC AGENTS AND ADJUVANTS

A. **Inhaled Anesthetics.** Fluorinated hydrocarbons revolutionized inhalation anesthesia (halothane in 1956, methoxyflurane in 1960, enflurane and isoflurane in the 1970s, desflurane in 1992, and sevoflurane in 1994).

B. **Intravenous Anesthetics.** Thiopental was first administered to a patient at the University of Wisconsin in March 1934 followed by ketamine (1960s), etomidate, and most recently propofol.

C. **Local Anesthetics.** Amino esters (procaine in 1905, tetracaine) were commonly used for local infiltration and spinal anesthesia despite their low potency and high likelihood to cause allergic reactions. Lidocaine, an amino amide local anesthetic, was developed in 1944 and gained immediate popularity because of its potency, rapid onset, decreased incidence of allergic reactions, and overall effectiveness for all types of regional anesthetic blocks. Since the introduction of lidocaine, all local anesthetics developed and marketed (mepivacaine, bupivacaine, ropivacaine, levobupivacaine) have been of the amino amide variety.

D. **Opioids** are used routinely in the perioperative period, in the management of acute pain, and in a variety of terminal and chronic pain states. Meperidine, the first synthetic opioid, was developed in 1939 followed by fentanyl in 1960 and sufentanil, alfentanil, and remifentanil. Ketorolac, a nonsteroidal antiinflammatory drug (NSAID) approved for use in 1990, was the first parenteral NSAID indicated for postoperative pain.

E. **Muscle Relaxants** entered anesthesia practice nearly a century after inhalational anesthetics. Curare, the first known neuromuscular blocking agent, was originally used in hunting and tribal warfare by native peoples of South America. Clinical application had to await the introduction of tracheal intubation and controlled ventilation of the lungs. On January 23, 1942, Griffith and his resident, Enid Johnson, anesthetized and intubated the trachea of a young man before injecting curare early in the course of an appendectomy. Satisfactory abdominal relaxation was obtained, and the surgery proceeded without incident. Griffith and Johnson's report of the successful use of curare in a series consisting of 25 patients launched a revolution in anesthetic care. Succinylcholine was prepared by the Nobel laureate Daniel Bovet in 1949 and was in wide international use before historians noted that the drug had been synthesized and tested in the early 1900s. Recognition that atracurium and cis-atracurium undergo spontaneous degradation by Hoffmann elimination has defined a role for these muscle relaxants in patients with liver and renal insufficiency.

F. **Antiemetics.** Effective treatment of patients with postoperative nausea and vomiting (PONV) evolved relatively recently and has been driven by incentives to limit hospitalization expenses and improve patient satisfaction. The antiemetic effects of corticosteroids were first recognized by oncologists treating patients with intracranial edema from tumors. Recognition of the role of the serotonin 5-HT3 pathway in PONV has led to a unique class of drugs (including ondansetron in 1991) devoted only to addressing this particular problem.

IV. ANESTHESIA SUBSPECIALTIES

A. **Regional Anesthesia.** The term "spinal anesthesia" was coined in 1885 by a neurologist, Leonard Corning, although it is likely that he actually performed an epidural injection. In 1944, Edward Tuohy of the Mayo Clinic introduced the Tuohy needle to facilitate the use of continuous spinal techniques. In 1949, Martinez Curbelo of Havana, Cuba, used Tuohy's needle and a ureteral catheter to perform the first **continuous epidural anesthetic.** John J. Bonica's many contributions to anesthesiology during his periods of military, civilian, and academic service at the University of Washington included development of a multidisciplinary pain clinic and publication of the text *The Management of Pain.*

B. **Cardiovascular Anesthesia.** Many believe that the successful ligation of a 7-year-old girl's patent ductus arteriosus by Robert Gross in 1938 served as the landmark case for modern cardiac surgery. The first successful use of Gibbon's cardiopulmonary bypass machine in humans in May 1953 was a monumental advance in the surgical treatment of complex cardiac pathology. In 1967, J. Earl Waynards published one of the first articles on anesthetic management of patients undergoing surgery for coronary artery disease. Postoperative mechanical ventilation and surgical intensive care units appeared by the late 1960s. Transesophageal echocardiography helped to further define the subspecialty of cardiac anesthesia.

C. **Neuroanesthesia.** Although the introduction of agents such as thiopental, curare, and halothane advanced the practice of anesthesiology in general, the development of methods to measure brain electrical activity, cerebral blood flow, and metabolic rate put neuroanesthesia practice on a scientific foundation.

D. **Obstetric Anesthesia.** Social attitudes about pain associated with childbirth began to change in the 1860s, and women started demanding anesthesia for childbirth. Virginia Apgar's system for evaluating newborns, developed in 1953, demonstrated that there was a difference in the neonates of mothers who had been anesthetized. In the past decade, anesthesia-related deaths during cesarean sections under general anesthesia have become more likely than neuraxial anesthesia-related deaths, making regional anesthesia the method of choice. With the availability of safe and effective options for pain relief during labor and delivery, today's focus is improving the quality of the birth experience for expectant parents.

V. **PROFESSIONALISM AND ANESTHESIA PRACTICE**

A. **Organized Anesthesiology.** The first American medical anesthesia organization, the Long Island Society of Anesthetists, was founded by nine physicians on October 6, 1905. Members had annual dues of $1.00. One of the most noteworthy figures in the struggle to professionalize anesthesiology was Francis Hoffer McMechan. He became the editor of the first journal devoted to anesthesia, *Current Researches in Anesthesia and*

Analgesia, the precursor of *Anesthesia and Analgesia*, the oldest journal of the specialty. Ralph Waters and John Lundy, among others, participated in evolving organized anesthesia.

B. **Academic Anesthesia.** In 1927, Erwin Schmidt, a professor of surgery at the University of Wisconsin's medical school, encouraged Dean Charles Bardeen to recruit Dr. Ralph Waters for the first American academic position in anesthesia.

C. **Establishing a Society.** The New York Society of Anesthetists changed its name to the American Society of Anesthetists in 1936. Combined with the American Society of Regional Anesthesia, the American Board of Anesthesiology was organized as a subordinate board to the American Board of Surgery in 1938, and independence was granted in 1940. Ralph Waters was declared the first president of the newly named American Society of Anesthesiologists in 1945.

CHAPTER 2 ■ **SCOPE OF PRACTICE**

Medical practice, including its infrastructure and functional details, is changing and evolving rapidly in the United States (Eichhorn JH: Practice and operating room management. *Clinical Anesthesia*. Edited by Barash PG, Cullen BF, Stoelting RK, Cahalan MK, Stock MC. Philadelphia, Lippincott Williams & Wilkins, 2009, pp 27–56). Traditionally, anesthesia professionals were minimally involved in the management of the many components of their practice beyond the strictly medical elements.

I. ADMINISTRATIVE COMPONENTS OF ALL ANESTHESIOLOGY PRACTICES

A. Operational and Information Resources
1. The American Society of Anesthesiologists (ASA) provides extensive resource materials to its members regarding practice management (Table 2-1).
2. These documents are updated regularly by the ASA through its committees and House of Delegates.

B. Internet
1. A modern anesthesiology practice must use the information resources (journals, textbooks, electronic bulletin boards) provided by the Internet.
2. The Web site for the ASA is **asahq.org.**

C. The Credentialing Process and Clinical Privileges
1. The system of credentialing a health care professional and granting clinical privileges is motivated by the assumption that appropriate education, training, and experience, along with an absence of an excessive number of adverse patient outcomes, increase the likelihood that the health care professional will deliver high-quality care.
2. Models for credentialing anesthesiologists are offered by the ASA.

TABLE 2-1

PRACTICE MANAGEMENT MATERIALS PROVIDED BY THE
AMERICAN SOCIETY OF ANESTHESIOLOGISTS

The Organization of an Anesthesia Department
Guidelines for Delineation of Clinical Privileges in Anesthesiology
Guidelines for a Minimally Acceptable Program of Any
  Continuing Education Requirement
Guidelines for the Ethical Practice of Anesthesiology
Ethical Guidelines for the Anesthesia Care of Patients with Do-Not-
  Resuscitate Orders or Other Directives that Limit Treatment
Guidelines for Patient Care in Anesthesiology
Guidelines for Expert Witness Qualifications and Testimony
Guidelines for Delegation of Technical Anesthesia Functions for
  Nonphysician Personnel
The Anesthesia Care Team
Statement on Conflict of Interest
Statement on Economic Credentialing
Statement on Member's Right to Practice
Statement on Routine Preoperative Laboratory and Diagnostic
  Screening

INTRODUCTION

3. The **National Practitioner Data Bank** is a central repository of licensing and credentials information about physicians. The data bank is maintained by the federal government, and adverse events involving a physician (e.g., substance abuse, malpractice litigation, revocation or limitation of the physician's license) must be reported to it via the appropriate state board of medical registration.
4. An important issue in granting clinical privileges, especially in procedure-oriented specialties such as anesthesiology, is whether it is reasonable to grant "blanket" privileges (i.e., the right to do everything traditionally associated with the specialty).
5. Initial board certification after the year 2000 by the American Board of Anesthesiology is time limited and subject to periodic testing and recertification. This requirement encourages an ongoing process of continued medical education.

D. **Professional Staff Participation and Relationships**
  1. Medical staff activities are increasingly important in achieving a favorable accreditation status from The Joint Commission (JC).
  2. Anesthesiologists should be active participants in medical staff activities (Table 2-2).

TABLE 2-2

EXAMPLES OF ANESTHESIOLOGISTS AS PARTICIPANTS IN
MEDICAL STAFF ACTIVITIES

Credentialing
Peer review
Transfusion review
Operating room management
Medical direction of same-day surgery units
Medical direction of postanesthesia care units
Medical direction of intensive care units
Medical direction of pain management services and clinics

E. **Establishing Standards of Practice and Understanding
the "Standard of Care"**
1. American anesthesiology is one of the leaders in
establishing practice standards that are intended to
maximize the quality of patient care and help guide
anesthesiologists make difficult decisions, including
those about the risk–benefit and cost–benefit aspects
of specific practices (Table 2-3).
2. The standard of care is the conduct and skill of a prudent practitioner that can be expected at all times by
a reasonable patient.
   a. Failure to meet the standard of care is considered
   malpractice.
   b. Courts have traditionally relied on medical experts
   to give opinions regarding what the standard of
   care is and whether it has been met in an individual case.
3. Anesthesiologists have been very active in publishing
standards of care (Table 2-3).
   a. A practice guideline has some of the same elements
   as a standard of practice but is intended more to
   guide judgment, largely through algorithms.
   b. Practice guidelines serve as potential vehicles for
   helping to eliminate unnecessary procedures and to
   limit costs.
   c. Guidelines do not define the standard of care,
   although adherence to the outlined principles
   should provide the anesthesiologist with a reason-
   ably defensible position.
4. JC **standards** focus on credentialing and privileges,
verification that anesthesia services are of uniform

TABLE 2-3

MATERIALS PROVIDED BY THE AMERICAN SOCIETY
OF ANESTHESIOLOGISTS DESIGNED TO ESTABLISH
PRACTICE STANDARDS

Standards (Minimum Requirements for Sound Practice)
Basic Standards for Preanesthesia Care
Standards for Basic Anesthesia Monitoring
Standards for Postanesthesia Care
Guidelines (Recommendations for Patient Management)
Guidelines for Ambulatory Surgical Facilities
Guidelines for Critical Care in Anesthesiology
Guidelines for Nonoperating Room Anesthetizing Locations
Guidelines for Regional Anesthesia in Obstetrics
Practice Guidelines
Practice Guidelines for Acute Pain Management in the
  Perioperative Setting
Practice Guidelines for Management of the Difficult Airway
Practice Guidelines for Pulmonary Artery Catheterization
Practice Guidelines for Difficult Airway
Practice Parameters
Pain Management
Transesophageal Echocardiography
Sedation by Nonanesthesia Personnel
Preoperative Fasting
Avoidance of Peripheral Neuropathies
Fast-Track Management of Coronary Artery Bypass Graft Patients

quality, continuing education, and documentation of
preoperative and postoperative evaluations.
5. Another type of regulatory agency is the peer review
organization, whose objectives include issues related
to hospital admissions and quality of care.
F. **Policy and Procedure**
1. An important organizational aspect of an anesthesia
department is a policy and procedure manual.
2. This manual includes specific protocols for areas men-
tioned in the JC standards, including preanesthetic
evaluation, safety of the patient during anesthesia,
recording of all pertinent events during anesthesia,
and release of the patient from the postanesthesia care
unit (PACU).
3. A protocol for responding to an adverse event is useful (*Anesthesia Patient Safety Foundation Newsletter*,
2006:21:11, apsf.org).

G. **Meetings and Case Discussion**
   1. There must be regularly scheduled departmental meetings.
   2. The JC requires that there be at least monthly meetings at which risk management and quality improvement activities are documented and reported.
H. **Anesthesia Equipment and Equipment Maintenance.** Compared with human error, overt equipment failure rarely causes critical intraoperative incidents. The Anesthesia Patient Safety Foundation advocates that anesthesia departments develop a process to verify that all anesthesia professionals are trained to use new technology being introduced in the operating room (OR).
I. **Malpractice Insurance**
   1. **Occurrence** means that if the insurance policy was in force at the time of the occurrence of an incident resulting in a claim, the physician will be covered.
   2. **Claims made** provide coverage only for claims that are filed when the policy was in force. ("Tail coverage" is needed if the policy is not renewed annually.)
   3. A new approach in medical risk management and insurance is advocating immediate full disclosure to the victim or survivors. This shifts the culture of blame with punishment to a just culture with restitution.
J. **Response to an Adverse Event**
   1. Despite the decreased incidence of anesthesia catastrophes, even with the very best practice, it is statistically likely that an anesthesia professional will be involved in a major anesthesia accident at least once in his or her professional life.
   2. A movement to implement immediate disclosure and apology reflects as shift from the "culture of blame" with punishment to a "just culture" with restitution. Laudable as the policy of immediate full disclosure and apology may sound, it would be mandatory for the anesthesia professional to confer with the involved liability insurance carrier, the practice group, and the facility administration before pursuing this policy.

II. PRACTICE ESSENTIALS

A. **The "job market" for anesthesia professionals** is being influenced by the number of residents being trained, the geographic maldistribution of anesthesiologists, and marketplace forces as reflected by managed care organizations and the real and potential impact on the numbers of surgical procedures. By 2001, it was perceived that there was a shortage of anesthesia providers.

B. **Types of practice** include academic practice, private practice in the marketplace, private practice as an employee, practice for a management company, and practice as a hospital employee.

C. **Billing and collecting** may be based on calculations according to units and time, a single predetermined fee independent of time, or fees bundled with all physicians involved in the surgical procedure.
   1. Billing for specific procedures becomes irrelevant in systems with prospective "capitated" payments for large numbers of patients (a fixed amount per enrolled member per month).
   2. The federal government has issued a new regulation allowing individual states to "opt out" of the requirement that a nurse anesthetist be supervised by a physician to meet Medicare billing requirements.

D. **Antitrust Considerations**
   1. The law is concerned solely with the preservation of competition within a defined marketplace and the rights of consumers.
   2. The market is not threatened by the exclusion of one physician from the medical staff of a hospital.

E. **Exclusive service contracts** state that anesthesiologists seeking to practice must be members of the group holding the exclusive contract.
   1. In some instances, members of the group may be terminated by the medical staff without due process.
   2. Economic credentialing (which is opposed by the ASA) is defined as the use of economic criteria unrelated to quality of care or professional competency for granting and renewing hospital privileges.

F. **Hospital Subsidies.** Modern economic realities may necessitate anesthesiology practice groups to recognize that after overhead is paid, patient care revenue does not provide sufficient compensation to attract and retain the number and quality of staff members necessary. A direct cash subsidy from the hospital may be negotiated to augment practice revenue in order to maintain benefits while increasing the pay of staff members to a market-competitive level.

III. NEW PRACTICE ARRANGEMENTS

A. Even though the impact of managed care plans has waned somewhat, various iterations still exist and have ongoing impact on anesthesiology practice.

B. **Prospective Payments.** In this arrangement, each group of providers in the managed care organization receives a fixed amount per member per month and agrees, except in unusual circumstances ("carve-outs"), to provide care.

C. **Changing Paradigm.** There is an emerging trend for private contracting organizations to tie their payments for professional services to the government's Medicare rate for specific CPT-4 codes.

D. **Pay for performance** is the concept supported by commercial indemnity insurance carriers and the Center for Medicaid and Medicare Services to reduce health care costs by decreasing expensive complications of medical care.

IV. HIPPA

A. Implementation of the privacy rule of the Health Insurance Portability and Accountability Act (HIPAA) creates significant changes in how medical records and patient information are handled. Under HIPPA, patients' names may not be used on an "OR board" if there is any chance that anyone not directly involved in their care could see them.

B. **Electronic Medical Records (EMR).** Basic EMR implementation has been problematic for practices (e.g., expense, obvious savings, acceptable software), but true electronic anesthesia information management systems have been even more difficult to implement.

V. EXPANSION INTO PERIOPERATIVE MEDICINE, HOSPITAL CARE, AND HYPERBARIC MEDICINE

A. Formalized **preoperative screening clinics** operated and staffed by anesthesiologists may replace the historical practice of sending patients to primary care physicians or consultants for "preoperative clearance."

B. Anesthesiologists may become the coordinators of postoperative care, especially in the realm of providing comprehensive pain management.

VI. OPERATING ROOM MANAGEMENT

A. The current emphasis on cost containment and efficiency requires anesthesiologists to take an active role in eliminating dysfunctional aspects of OR practice (e.g., first-case morning start times).

   1. Anesthesiologists with insight, overview, and a unique perspective are best qualified to provide leadership in an OR.
   2. An important aspect of OR organization is materials management.

B. **Scheduling Cases**

   1. Anesthesiologists need to participate in scheduling of cases because the number of anesthesia professionals depends on the daily caseload, including "offsite" diagnostic areas.
   2. The majority of ORs use block scheduling (preassigned guaranteed OR time with an agreed cutoff time), open scheduling (first come, first serve), or a combination.
   3. **Computerization** will likely benefit every OR.

C. **Preoperative Clinics.** Use of an anesthesia preoperative evaluation clinic usually results in more efficient running of the OR and avoidance of unanticipated cancellations and delays.

D. **Anesthesiology Personnel Issues.** In light of the current and future shortage of anesthesia professionals, managing and maintaining a stable supply promises to dominate the OR landscape for years.

E. **Cost and Quality Issues**

   1. Health care accounts for approximately 14% of the US gross domestic product, and anesthesia (directly and indirectly) represents 3% to 5% of total health care costs.
   2. Anesthesia drug expenses represent a small portion of the total perioperative costs, but the great number of doses administered contributes substantially to the aggregate total cost to the institution.
      a. Reducing fresh gas flow from 5 to 2 L/min whenever possible would save approximately $100 million annually in the United States.
      b. More expensive techniques and drugs may reduce indirect costs (e.g., propofol is infusion more expensive but may decrease PACU time and reduce the patient's nausea and vomiting).

    c. For long surgical procedures, newer and more
expensive drugs may offer limited benefits over
older and less expensive longer acting alternatives.

    d. It is estimated that the 10 highest expenditure
drugs account for more than 80% of the anesthetic
drug costs at some institutions.

CHAPTER 3 ■ OCCUPATIONAL HEALTH

Anesthesia personnel spend long hours in an environment—the operating room (OR)—filled with many potential hazards, including vapors from chemicals, ionizing radiation, and infectious agents as well as psychological stress engendered by the high-stakes nature of the practice (Berry AJ, Katz JD: Occupational health. In *Clinical Anesthesia*. Edited by Barash PG, Cullen BF, Stoelting RK, Cahalan MK, Stock MC. Philadelphia: Lippincott Williams & Wilkins, 2009, pp 57–81).

I. PHYSICAL HAZARDS

A. Anesthetic Gases

1. Reports on the effects of chronic environmental exposure to anesthetics have included epidemiologic surveys, *in vitro* studies, cellular research, and studies in laboratory animals and humans. Areas addressed include the mortality rate and the incidence of fertility and spontaneous abortion, congenital malformations, cancer, hematopoietic diseases, liver disease, neurologic disease, and psychomotor and behavioral changes produced by exposure to anesthetics.

2. **Anesthetic Levels in the Operating Room.** Appropriate scavenging and adequate air exchange in the OR significantly lower levels of waste anesthetic gases.

3. **Epidemiologic studies** are difficult to interpret, and results often do not withstand scientific scrutiny.

4. **Reproductive outcomes** studies suggest that there is a slight increase in the risk of spontaneous abortion and congenital abnormalities in offspring of female physicians working in ORs. The routine use of scavenging has been implemented since the time of most of these studies.

   a. Retrospective surveys of large numbers of women who worked during pregnancy indicate that negative reproductive outcomes may be related to job-related conditions (e.g., increased work hours, hours worked while standing, occupational fatigue associated with preterm birth) rather than exposure to trace anesthetic gases.

b. Routine use of scavenging techniques has generally lowered environmental anesthetic levels in ORs and may make it difficult to prove any adverse effects using epidemiologic data.

5. **Neoplasms and Other Nonreproductive Diseases.** Overall, there appears to be some evidence that the OR environment produces a slight increase in the rate of spontaneous abortion and cancer in female anesthesiologists and nurses. Mortality risks from cancer and heart disease for anesthesiologists do not differ from those for other medical specialists.

6. **Laboratory Studies**

   a. Cellular effects. Nitrous oxide administered in clinically useful concentrations affects hematopoietic and neural cells by irreversibly oxidizing the cobalt atom of vitamin B_{12} from an active to inactive state. This inhibits methionine synthetase and prevents the conversion of methyltetrahydrofolate to tetrahydrofolate, which is required for DNA synthesis, assembly of myelin sheath, and methyl substitutions in neurotransmitters. Inhibition of methionine synthetase in individuals exposed to high concentrations of nitrous oxide may result in anemia and polyneuropathy, but chronic exposure to trace levels does not appear to produce these effects.

   b. Anesthetics are not mutagenic (carcinogenic) using the Ames bacterial assay. Analyses of sister chromatid exchanges or formation of micronucleated lymphocytes to assess for genotoxicity in association with anesthetic exposure have been negative.

   c. Anesthetists working where waste gas scavenging is not used have increased fractions of micronucleated lymphocytes compared with those practicing in ORs with scavenging; the significance of this is unclear.

7. **Reproductive Outcome.** Data from animals fail to confirm alterations in female or male fertility or reproduction with exposure to subanesthetic concentrations of currently used inhaled drugs.

TABLE 3-1

EXAMPLES OF RECOMMENDED THRESHOLD LIMITS FOR
OCCUPATIONAL EXPOSURE TO ANESTHETIC AGENTS*

Country	Nitrous Oxide	Enflurane	Isoflurane
United States (NIOSH)	25	2	2
United States (ACGIH)	50	75	Not determined
Great Britain	100	50	50
Norway	100	2	2
Sweden	100	10	10

*Time weighted average in parts per million.
ACGIH, American Conference on Governmental Industrial Hygienists;
NOSH, National Institute of Occupational Safety and Health.

INTRODUCTION

Other possible factors must also be considered, including stress, alterations in work schedule, and fatigue.

8. **Effects of Trace Anesthetic Levels on Psychomotor Skills.** Studies to clarify whether low concentrations of anesthetics alter psychomotor skills are inconclusive.

9. **Recommendations of the National Institute for Occupational Safety and Health (NIOSH)** (Table 3-1). Despite the use of scavenging devices, continued monitoring of anesthetic levels in the OR and routine attention to equipment maintenance are needed (Table 3-2).

10. **Anesthetic Levels in the Postanesthesia Care Unit**
    a. As patients awaken from general anesthesia, waste anesthetic gases are released into the postanesthesia care unit (PACU), especially if the patient's trachea is still intubated when he or she arrives in the PACU.
    b. NIOSH threshold limits for anesthetic gases can be obtained in the PACU by ensuring adequate room ventilation and fresh gas exchange and by discontinuing the anesthetic gases in sufficient time before leaving the OR.

B. **Chemicals**
   1. **Methylmethacrylate** concentrations in the OR (allowable exposure, 100 ppm) may be decreased by scavenging devices.
   2. **Allergic reactions** have been attributed to exposure of anesthesiologists to vapors of methylmethacrylate and inhaled anesthetics.

TABLE 3-2

SOURCES OF OPERATING ROOM CONTAMINATION

Anesthetic Techniques
Failure to turn off gas flow control vales at end of an anesthetic
Turning gas flow on before placing mask on patient
Poorly fitting masks (especially with induction of anesthesia)
Flushing the circuit
Filling of anesthesia vaporizers
Uncuffed or leaking tracheal tubes (pediatrics) or poorly fitting laryngeal mask airways
Pediatric circuits (Jackson-Rees version of Mapleson D system)
Sidestream sampling carbon dioxide and anesthetic gas analyzers

Anesthesia Machine Delivery System and Scavenging System
Open or closed system
Occlusion or malfunction of hospital disposal system
Maladjustment of hospital disposal system vacuum
Leaks
High-pressure hoses or connectors
Nitrous oxide tank mounting
O rings
CO_2 absorbent canisters
Low-pressure circuit

Other Sources
Cryosurgery units
Cardiopulmonary bypass circuits

---

3. **Latex sensitivity** has become a common source of allergic reactions among OR personnel (12.5 to 15.8% of anesthesiologists are sensitive to latex). Irritant or contact dermatitis from wearing latex-containing gloves accounts for about 80% of reactions to latex (Table 3-3). Use of powderless gloves limits exposure to ambient latex antigens.

C. **Radiation exposure** (fluoroscopic guidance procedures, electrophysiology laboratory) is a function of total exposure intensity and time, distance from the source of radiation, and use of shielding.

   1. Radiation exposure becomes minimal at a distance greater than 90 cm (36 inches) from the source.
   2. Pregnant workers should limit the dose to <500 mrem.

D. **Noise pollution** may approach unacceptable levels in the OR (75 to 90 dB is produced by ventilators, suction equipment, music, and conversation; safe noise exposure level for 8 hours is considered to be 90 dB).

TABLE 3-3

TYPES OF REACTIONS TO LATEX GLOVES

Reaction	Signs/Symptoms	Cause	Management
Irritant contact dermatitis	Scaling, drying, or cracking of skin	Direct skin irritation by gloves, powder, or soaps	Identify reaction, avoid irritant, possible use of glove liner, use of alternative product
Type IV delayed hypersensitivity	Itching, blistering, crusting (delayed 6 to 72 hr)	Chemical additives used in manufacturing (e.g., accelerators)	Identify chemical additive, possible use of glove liner
Type I immediate hypersensitivity		Proteins found in latex	Identify reaction; avoid latex-containing products; use of nonlatex or powder-free, low-protein gloves by coworkers
Localized contact urticaria	Itching and hives in the area of contact with latex (immediate)		Antihistamines, topical or systemic steroids
Generalized reaction	Runny nose, swollen eyes, generalized rash or hives, bronchospasm, anaphylaxis		Anaphylaxis protocol

E. **Human factors** that exist in the OR (configuration and placement of equipment [ergonomics], constant vigilance [mental fatigue], interpersonal relationships, and communication) remain the greatest potential sources contributing to patient morbidity and mortality. Production pressure is an organizational concern that has the potential to create an environment in which issues of productivity supersede those of safety.
   1. Poor communication can lead to conflict and compromised patient safety and has been identified as a root cause of 35% of anesthesia-related sentinel events.
   2. Successful resolution of conflict is a skill that can be learned.
F. **Work hours and night call** can contribute to fatigue and impaired performance of complex cognitive tasks such as monitoring and vigilance. Demands associated with night call have been identified as the most stressful aspect of anesthesia practice.
   1. Sleep deprivation and circadian disruption have deleterious effects on cognition, performance, mood, and health; acute sleep deprivation resembles alcohol intoxication.
   2. Complex cognitive tasks that are specific to anesthesiology (e.g., monitoring, accurate decision making) may be adversely affected by sleep deprivation.
   3. Residents in a sleep-deprived condition demonstrated progressive impairment of alertness and have longer response latency to vigilance probes using the anesthesia simulator, but there are no significant differences in the clinical management of the simulated patients between the rested and sleep-deprived groups.
   4. After a period of sleep deprivation, performance does not return to normal levels until 24 hours of rest and recovery has occurred.
   5. The Accreditation Council for Graduate Medical Education has set duty hours for residents. Although the residents' quality of life has generally improved, the effects on education, reduction in medical errors, and continuity of care are undetermined.
   6. Naps before the start of call as well as the use of caffeine to improve alertness during long shifts.

II. INFECTION HAZARDS

Anesthesia personnel are at risk for acquiring infections from both patients and other personnel (Table 3-4). Viral

TABLE 3-4

SOURCES OF INFECTION FROM PATIENTS

Respiratory Viruses
Influenza A or B (vaccination, amantadine, rimantadine, zanamivir, oseltamivir)
Avian influenza A (vaccination)
Respiratory syncytial virus

Herpes Viruses
Varicella-zoster virus (chickenpox or shingles; susceptible hospital personnel with exposure to the virus should not have direct patient contact from days 10 to 21 after exposure)
Herpes simplex (spread by direct contact with body fluids, such as during tracheal intubation)
Herpetic whitlow (consider limiting direct patient care because this virus can infect susceptible individuals; acyclovir may shorten the course of primary cutaneous infection)
Cytomegalovirus (the source is usually an infected infant or immuno-suppressed patient)
Rubella (vaccination is recommended for susceptible health care personnel)
Measles (rubeola) (vaccination is recommended for susceptible health care personnel)
Severe acute respiratory syndrome (SARS; emerging respiratory tract infection caused by coronavirus , high fever followed by headache and occasionally pneumonia and acute respiratory distress syndrome; prevent spread by isolation of infected patients)

Viral Hepatitis
Hepatitis A
Hepatitis B (significant risk for nonimmune health care personnel who have contact with blood and the possibility of needlesticks; vaccination is recommended for susceptible health care personnel)
Hepatitis C (leading cause of chronic liver disease often progressing to cirrhosis; risk of seroconversion after an infected needlestick injury is 1.8%)

Human Immunodeficiency Virus-1
The rate of seroconversion in health care workers sustaining a percutaneous exposure (needlestick injury) is about 0.3%, with conversion usually occurring within 6 to 12 weeks after exposure; the estimated risk of patient-transmitted infection to the anesthesiologist is between 0.001 and 0.129%; universal precautions should be used in managing known and high-risk patients (see Table 3-5)

Creutzfeldt-Jakob Disease
Tuberculosis (increased incidence in immigrants from countries with a high incidence of this disease and in alcoholics, medically underserved persons, immunosuppressed patients, and intravenous drug users)

infections are the greatest threat to health care workers and are most often spread by the respiratory route. Transmission of blood-borne pathogens (hepatitis virus, human immunodeficiency virus [HIV]) can be prevented by mechanical barriers or vaccination (hepatitis B). Hand washing between patients, appropriate use of gloves, and use of needleless or protected needle safety devices are the best protections for health care workers from the risks of contracting infections from patients.

A. **OSHA Standards, Universal Precautions, and Isolation Precautions**

1. Universal precautions for preventing transmission of blood-borne infections should be used for all patient contacts (Table 3-5).
2. General infection control practice recommends use of gloves when a health care worker comes in contact with patient mucous membranes or oral fluids, such as during tracheal intubation and pharyngeal suctioning.

TABLE 3-5

UNIVERSAL PRECAUTIONS

1. All needles, blades, and sharp instruments should be handled so as to prevent accidental injuries, and all of them should be considered potentially infected. Disposable sharp items should be placed in puncture-resistant containers located as close as is practical to the area where they are used. Needles should not be recapped, bent, broken, or removed from disposable syringes before they are placed in appropriate disposable containers.
2. Gloves should be worn when touching mucous membranes or open skin of all patients. When the possibility exists for exposure to blood, body fluid, or items soiled with these, gloves should be used. With some procedures such as endoscopy, during which aerosolization or splashes of blood or secretions are likely to occur, wearing of masks, eye coverings, and gowns is indicated. Gloves and body coverings should be removed and disposed of properly after patient contact.
3. Frequent hand washing, especially between patient contacts and after removal of gloves, should be encouraged. If hands are accidentally contaminated with blood or other body fluids, they should be washed as soon as possible.
4. Ventilation devices for resuscitation should be available at appropriate locations to prevent the need for emergency mouth-to-mouth resuscitation.
5. Health care workers who have exudative lesions or weeping dermatitis should not participate in direct patient care activities until the condition resolves.

B. **Viruses in Laser Plumes**
   1. Viable viruses have been found in plumes produced by laser vaporization of tissues that contain viruses.
   2. To protect OR personnel from exposure to the viral and chemical contents of laser plumes, it is recommended that the tubing from a smoke evacuator be held within 2.5 cm of the tissue being vaporized.

III. EMOTIONAL CONSIDERATIONS

A. **Stress** from working in the OR (similar to that experienced by air traffic controllers) may reflect an excessive workload, the necessity for making many difficult decisions, night duty, fatigue, increasing reliance on technology, interpersonal tensions, and concerns about liability and night call.

B. **Substance Use, Abuse, and Addiction**
   1. Substance abuse (particularly use of potent, short-acting opioids) is often considered an occupational hazard for anesthesiologists.
   2. Causative factors of substance abuse specific to anesthesiology include job stress, lack of external recognition, availability of addictive drugs (need to audit distribution of drugs within the OR), and a susceptible premorbid personality. Propofol abuse has been observed among residents.
   3. Potential consequences of substance abuse are multiple. When an anesthesiologist's professional conduct is impaired to the extent that it is apparent to his or her colleagues, the disease is approaching its end stage (i.e., death) (Table 3-6).
   4. Disciplinary action taken against a physician impaired by substance abuse must be reported to the National Practitioner Data Bank. Health care professionals are affected by chemical dependency (including alcohol abuse) at a rate roughly equivalent to that of the general population (8 to 12%).
   5. The risk of relapse is greatest when all of three factors (family history, major opioid abused, coexisting psychiatric disorder) are present.
   6. Controversy remains about the ultimate career path of anesthesiologists in recovery from chemical dependency. Because of contradictory data, no universal recommendation can be made about re-entry into the practice of anesthesiology after treatment. The

TABLE 3-6

SIGNS OF SUBSTANCE ABUSE AND ADDICTION

Social (Outside the Hospital)
Withdrawal from leisure activities, friends, and family
Uncharacteristic or inappropriate behavior in social settings
Impulsive behavior (overspending, gambling)
Domestic turmoil (separation from spouse, child abuse, sexual problems)
Change in behavior of spouse or children
Legal problems (arrested for driving while intoxicated)

Health
Deterioration in personal hygiene
Accidents
Numerous health complaints (frequent need for medical attention for unrelated illnesses)

Professional (In the Hospital)
Signing out ever increasing quantities of opioids
Sloppy and unreadable charting
Unusual changes in behavior (wide mood swings)
Preferring to work alone, declining relief, frequently relieving others, volunteering for additional cases and calls, staying in the hospital even when not on duty
Frequent requests for bathroom relief
Difficult to find between cases
Insisting on personally administering opioids in the PACU
Wearing long-sleeved gowns (to hide needle marks and combat subjective feeling of cold)

American Board of Anesthesiology has established a policy for candidates with a history of alcoholism or illegal use of drugs.

IV. THE AGING ANESTHESIOLOGIST

A. In contrast to other industries (e.g., commercial pilots are required to take regular medical examinations), little research has been directed toward challenges faced by older anesthesiologists.

B. An area of particular difficulty for anesthesiologists is maintaining the stamina required for long work shifts and night call.

V. MORTALITY AMONG ANESTHESIOLOGISTS

A. Studies have reported conflicting data regarding life expectancy among anesthesiologists, including a conclusion that the average age at death was the same as the national average.

1. Death from cancer is not increased among anesthesiologists compared with internists.
2. Increased risks for anesthesiologists result from drug-related death, suicide, HIV, and cerebrovascular disease.
3. The risk to anesthesiologists for drug-related deaths is highest in the first 5 years after graduation from medical school but remains increased the entire professional career.

B. **Suicide** is an occupational hazard for anesthesiologists, perhaps reflecting the high degree of stress associated with the care of anesthetized patients.

1. There is a close association between stressful life events and major depressive disorders. In susceptible individuals, feelings of an inability to cope resulting from stress-induced depression can lead to despair and suicide ideation.
2. A malpractice lawsuit or suspension of privileges may result in suicidal ideation.
3. Physicians whose privileges to practice medicine have been revoked for chemical dependence are at heightened risk for attempting suicide.

CHAPTER 4 ■ ANESTHETIC RISK, QUALITY IMPROVEMENT AND LIABILITY

In anesthesia, as in other areas of life, everything does not always go as planned. Undesirable outcomes may occur regardless of the quality of care provided. An anesthesia risk management program can work in conjunction with a program for quality improvement to minimize the liability risks of practice while ensuring the highest quality of care for patients (Posner KL, Domino KB: Anesthetic risk, quality improvement, and liability. In *Clinical Anesthesia*. Edited by Barash PG, Cullen BF, Stoelting RK, Cahalan MK, Stock MC. Philadelphia: Lippincott Williams & Wilkins, 2009, pp 82–92).

I. ANESTHESIA RISK

A. **Mortality and Major Morbidity Related to Anesthesia.** Estimates of anesthesia-related morbidity and mortality are difficult to quantify because of different methodologies, definitions of complications, lengths of follow-up, and evaluation of contribution of anesthesia care to patient outcomes (Table 4-1). It is generally accepted that anesthesia safety has improved over the past 50 years. However, several recent complications related to anesthesia have received increasing attention (Table 4-2).

II. RISK MANAGEMENT

A. **Conceptual Introduction.** Risk management and quality improvement programs work hand in hand in minimizing liability exposure while maximizing quality of patient care. Quality improvement (sometimes called patient safety) departments are responsible for providing the resources to provide safe, patient-centered, timely, efficient, effective, and equitable patient care.

B. **Risk Management.** Aspects of risk management most directly relevant to the liability exposure of

TABLE 4-1

RECENT ESTIMATES OF ANESTHESIA-RELATED DEATH

Time Period	Country	Data Sources and Methods	Anesthesia-Related Death
1989–1999	USA	Cardiac arrests within 24 hr of surgery (72,959 anesthetics) in a teaching hospital	0.55/10,000 anesthetics
1992–1994	USA	Suburban teaching hospital (37,924 anesthetics and 115 deaths)	0.79/10,000 anesthetics
1995–1997	USA	Urban teaching hospital (146,548 anesthetics and 232 deaths)	0.75/10,000 anesthetics
1995–1997	Holland	All deaths within 24 hr or patients who remained comatose 24 hr after surgery (869,483 anesthetics and 811 deaths)	1.4/10,000 anesthetics
1990–1995	Western Australia	Deaths within 48 hr or deaths in which anesthesia was considered a contributing factor	1/40,000 anesthetics
1994–1996	Australia	Deaths reported to the committee (8,500,000 anesthetics)	0.16/10,000 anesthetics
1992–2002	Japan	Deaths caused by life-threatening events in the operating room (3,855,384 anesthetics) in training hospitals	0.1/10,000 anesthetics
1994-1998	Japan	Questionnaires to training hospitals (2,363,038 anesthetics)	0.21/10,000 anesthetics
1989–1995	France	ASA 1–4 patients undergoing anesthesia (101,769 anesthetics and 24 cardiac arrests within 12 hr after anesthesia)	0.6/10,000 anesthetics
1994–1997	USA	Pediatric patients from 63 hospitals (1,089,200 anesthetics)	0.36/10,000 anesthetics

TABLE 4-2

COMPLICATIONS RELATED TO ANESTHESIA

Postoperative nerve injury
  Ulnar nerve injury
  Lower extremity neuropathy after surgery in the lithotomy
    position
  After neuraxial anesthesia (0.4–4.2/10,000 spinal anesthetics)
Awareness during general anesthesia (estimated to occur in 1–2
  per 1,000 patients in a tertiary care setting)
Eye injuries and visual deficits
  Corneal abrasion
  Ischemic optic neuropathy
  Central retinal artery occlusion
Dental injury (1/4,537 patients require intervention)
Postoperative cognitive dysfunction in elderly patients (cause
  unknown)

anesthesiologists include prevention of patient injury,
adherence to standards of care, documentation, and
patient relations.
  1. The key factors in the prevention of patient injury are
     vigilance, up-to-date knowledge, and adequate moni-
     toring. The website of the American Society of Anes-
     thesiologists (ASA) may be reviewed for any changes
     in ASA Standards of Practice as well as a review of
     ASA guidelines.
  2. Another risk management tool is the use of checklists
     before each case or at least daily in an attempt to
     reduce equipment-related problems.
C. **Informed consent** regarding anesthesia should be documented along with a note in the patient's chart that the
   risks of anesthesia and alternatives were discussed.
D. **Record Keeping.** The anesthesia record should be as
   accurate, complete, and as neat as possible. The use of
   automated records may be helpful in the defense of malpractice cases.
E. **What to Do After an Adverse Event**
  1. If a critical incident occurs during the conduct of an
     anesthetic, it is helpful to write a note in the patient's
     medical record describing the event, the drugs used,
     the time sequence, and who was present.
  2. If anesthetic complications occur, the anesthesiologist
     should be honest with both the patient and family
     about the cause. A formal apology should be issued if
     the unanticipated outcome is the result of an error or

system failure. Some states have laws mandating disclosure of serious adverse events to patients. (Disclosure discussions may be prohibited as evidence in malpractice litigation.)

3. Whenever an anesthetic complication becomes apparent after surgery, appropriate consultation should be obtained and the department or institutional risk management group should be notified. If the complication is likely to lead to prolonged hospitalization or permanent injury, the liability insurance carrier should be notified.

F. **Special Circumstances: "Do Not Attempt Resuscitation" and Jehovah's Witnesses.** Patients have well-established rights, and among them is the right to refuse specific treatments.

1. **Do Not Attempt Resuscitation (DNAR).** When a patient with DNAR status present for anesthesia care, it is important to discuss this with the patient or patient's surrogate to clarify the patient's intentions. In many hospitals, the institutional policy is to suspend the DNAR order during the perioperative period because the cause of cardiac arrest may be easily identified and treated during surgery.

2. **Jehovah's Witnesses.** The administration of blood or blood products may be refused because of a belief that the afterlife is forbidden if they receive blood.

3. As a general rule, physicians are not obligated to treat all patients who seek treatment in elective situations.

   a. Emergency medical care imposes greater constraints on the treating physician because there is limited to no opportunity to provide continuity of care in a life-threatening situation without the initial physician's continued involvement.

   b. Exceptions to patients' rights include parturients and adults who are the sole support of minor children. In these instances, it may be necessary to seek a court order to proceed with a refused medical therapy such as a blood transfusion.

G. **National Practitioner Data Bank** (Table 4-3)

III. QUALITY IMPROVEMENT AND PATIENT SAFETY IN ANESTHESIA

It is generally accepted that attention to quality improves patient safety and satisfaction with anesthesia care. There

TABLE 4-3

SOURCES OF INPUT FOR THE NATIONAL PRACTITIONER
DATA BANK

Medical malpractice payments (any payment made on behalf of a
  physician in response to a written complaint or claim)
License actions by medical boards
Professional review or clinical privilege actions taken by hospitals
  and other health care entities (professional societies)
Actions taken by the Drug Enforcement Agency
Medicare or Medicaid exclusions

may be an emphasis on patient safety and the prevention of
harm from medical care. Quality improvement programs
are generally guided by requirements of The Joint Commission, which accredits hospitals and health care
organizations.

A. **Structure, Process, and Outcome: The Building Blocks
   of Quality**
   1. Although quality of care is difficult to define, it is gen-
      erally accepted that it is composed of three components:
      structure (setting in which care is provided), process of
      care (preanesthetic evaluation plus continual attendance
      and monitoring during anesthesia), and outcome. A
      quality improvement program focuses on measuring
      and improving these basic components of care.
   2. **Continuous quality improvement (CQI)** focuses on
      system errors, which are controllable and solvable
      as opposed to random errors, which are difficult to
      prevent. A CQI program may focus on undesirable
      outcomes as a way of identifying opportunities for
      improvement in the structure and process of care.
      Peer review is critical to this process.

B. **Difficulty of Outcome Measurement in Anesthesia**
   1. Improvement in quality of care is often measured by a
      decrease in the rate of adverse outcomes.
   2. Adverse outcomes are rare in anesthesia, making
      measurement of improvement difficult. To complement
      outcome measurements, anesthesia CQI programs can
      focus on critical incidents (events that cause or have
      the potential to cause patient injury if not noticed or
      corrected in a timely manner [e.g., ventilator discon-
      nect]), sentinel events, and human errors [inevitable
      yet potentially preventable by appropriate system
      safeguards].

TABLE 4-4
THE JOINT COMMISSION PATIENT SAFETY GOALS FOR
ACCREDITED ORGANIZATIONS

Improved accuracy of patient identification
Improved effectiveness of communication among caregivers
(handoffs)
Improved safety of medication usage (e.g., anticoagulation therapy)
Reduction of health care–related infections
Improved recognition and response to changes in a patient's
condition

INTRODUCTION

C. **The Joint Commission's Requirement for Quality Improvement**
   1. Anesthesia care is an important function of patient care that has been identified by The Joint Commission. It is important that policies and procedures for administration of anesthesia be consistent in all locations within the hospital.
   2. The Joint Commission has adopted and annually updates patient safety goals for accredited organizations (Table 4-4).
   3. The Joint Commission's accreditation visits are unannounced and involve the inspector observing patient care to confirm that safe practices (e.g., timely administration of antibiotics, proper labeling of all syringes on the anesthesia cart) are routinely implemented.
   4. The Joint Commission requires that all *sentinel events* (i.e., unexpected occurrences involving death or serious physical or psychological injury) undergo root cause analysis.

D. **Pay for Performance**
   1. Conceptually, the goal is to provide monetary incentives for implementation of safe practices, measuring performance, and achieving performance goals (e.g., payment for quality rather than simply payment for services).
   2. The stimulus for pay for performance comes from the Leapfrog Group, the Institute for Healthcare Improvement, the Center for Medicare and Medicaid Services, and the National Quality Forum.
   3. Benchmarks as indicators for measurement and improvement may include "never events" (e.g., surgery on the wrong patient or site, unintentional retention of

a foreign body, patient death from a medication error, perioperative death of an ASA I patient).

IV. PROFESSIONAL LIABILITY

A. The Tort System

1. A tort may be loosely defined as a civil wrongdoing. **Negligence** is one type of tort. **Malpractice** refers to any professional misconduct, but its use in legal terms typically refers to professional negligence.

2. To be successful in a malpractice suit, the patient/plaintiff must prove four elements of negligence (Table 4-5).

B. Duty.
The anesthesiologist establishes a duty to the patient when a doctor–patient relationship exists. When the patient is seen before surgery and the anesthesiologist agrees to provide anesthesia care for the patient, a duty to the patient has been established. Because it would be impossible to delineate specific standards for all aspects of medical practices and all eventualities, the courts have created the concept of a *reasonable and prudent* physician. A general duty is obtaining informed consent that includes common risks, and in the case of regional anesthesia, risks that are rare but are of major consequence, including seizure, cardiac arrest, permanent neuropathy, and paralysis.

C. Breach of Duty.
In a malpractice action, expert witnesses review the medical records and determine whether the anesthesiologist acted in a reasonable manner in the specific situation and fulfilled his or her duty to the patient.

D. Causation.
Although the burden of proof of causation ordinarily falls on the patient/plaintiff, it may, under special circumstances, be shifted to the physician/defendant under the doctrine of *res ipsa loquitur* ("the thing speaks for itself") (Table 4-6).

TABLE 4-5

ELEMENTS REQUIRED TO PROVE MALPRACTICE

Duty (established when the patient is seen after surgery)
Breach of duty (often determined by expert witnesses)
Causation (the judge and jury determine if the breach of duty was the proximate cause of the injury)
Damages (breach of standard of care was the cause of damage)

TABLE 4-6

ELEMENTS NECESSARY TO PROVE *RES IPSA LOQUITUR*

The injury would not typically occur in the absence of negligence.
The injury was caused by something under the exclusive control
of the anesthesiologist.
The injury must not be attributable to any contribution on the
part of the patient.
The evidence for the explanation of events is more accessible to
the anesthesiologist than to the patient.

INTRODUCTION

E. **Damages** in a malpractice suit are characterized as **general damages** (pain and suffering as a direct result of the injury), **special damages** (medical expenses, lost income), and **punitive damages** (rarely invoked in malpractice suits). Determining the dollar amount of damages is the responsibility of the jury.

F. **Standard of Care**
1. Because medical malpractice usually involves issues beyond the comprehension of lay jurors and judges, the court establishes the standard of care in each case with the testimony of expert witnesses. Expert witnesses differ from factual witnesses mainly in that they may give opinions. The trial court judge has sole discretion in determining whether a witness may be qualified as an expert.
2. There is a tendency for experts to link severe injury with inappropriate care (a bias that bad outcomes mean bad care).
3. The essential difference between standards and guidelines is that guidelines *should be* adhered to and standards *must be* adhered to. The ASA publishes standards and guidelines for a variety of anesthesia-related activities.

G. **Causes of Anesthesia-Related Lawsuits**
1. Relatively few adverse outcomes end in a malpractice suit. It is estimated that <1 per 25 patient injuries result in malpractice litigation.
2. The leading causes of injuries for which suits are filed against anesthesiologists are death, nerve damage (spinal cord injury, peripheral nerve injury), and brain damage. The causes of death and brain damage most often reflect airway management problems. Nerve damage, especially to the ulnar nerve, often occurs

TABLE 4-7

STEPS TO TAKE WHEN NAMED IN A LAWSUIT

Do not discuss the case with others.
Never alter any records.
Gather all pertinent records.
Make notes relating to your recall of events.
Work closely with your attorney.

despite apparently adequate positioning. Chronic pain management is an increasing source of malpractice claims against anesthesiologists.

3. Anesthesiologists are more likely to be the target of lawsuits if an untoward outcome of a procedure occurs because the physician–patient relationship is often incomplete (e.g., the patient rarely chooses the anesthesiologist, the preoperative visit is brief, and a different anesthesiologist may administer the anesthesia).

H. **What to Do If Sued** (Table 4-7)

CHAPTER 5 ■ MECHANISMS OF ANESTHESIA AND CONSCIOUSNESS

Despite the importance of general anesthesia and more than 100 years of active research, the molecular mechanisms responsible for anesthetic action remain one of the unsolved mysteries of pharmacology (Evers AS, Crowder CM: Mechanisms of anesthesia and consciousness. In *Clinical Anesthesia*. Edited by Barash PG, Cullen BF, Stoelting RK, Cahalan MK, Stock MC. Philadelphia: Lippincott Williams & Wilkins, 2009, pp 93–114). Molecular and genetic tools are becoming available that should allow for major insights into anesthetic mechanisms in the next decade. A wide variety of structurally unrelated compounds (steroids to elemental xenon) are capable of producing anesthesia, suggesting that multiple molecular mechanisms may be operative.

I. WHAT IS ANESTHESIA?

A. The components of the anesthetic state include unconsciousness, amnesia, analgesia, immobility, and attenuation of autonomic nervous system responses to noxious stimulation.

B. Anesthesia is always defined by drug-induced changes in behavior or perception. As such, anesthesia can only be defined and measured in the intact organism.

C. Central to the mechanism of sleep is a set of hypothalamic nuclei that appear to form an awake/sleep switch mechanism.

1. The thalamus and cortex maintain wakefulness and consciousness through complex interactions that may involve intrinsic oscillators and widespread synaptic communication.

2. Awareness and consciousness are thought to emerge from communication between the prefrontal cortex and multiple cortical and subcortical areas that have distributed representations of perception.

37

II. HOW IS ANESTHESIA MEASURED?

A. To study the pharmacology of anesthetic action, a quantitative measurement of anesthetic potency is essential. This is provided in the concept of minimum alveolar concentration (MAC).

1. MAC is defined as the alveolar partial pressure (PA) of a gas (end-tidal concentration) at which 50% of humans will not move in response to a surgical skin incision (or in animals, in response to a noxious stimulus such as a tail clamp).

   a. MAC is the standard for determining the potency of volatile anesthetics.

   b. MAC is reproducible and constant over a wide range of species.

   c. The quantal nature of MAC (either anesthetized or not anesthetized with no partially anesthetized data point possible) makes it difficult to compare MAC measurements with concentration–response curves obtained *in vitro*.

2. A MAC equivalent for intravenous (IV) anesthetics is the plasma concentration of the drug required to prevent movement in response to a noxious stimulus in 50% of subjects.

3. The PA is an accurate reflection of the anesthetic concentration in the plasma and brain tissue at 37°C.

4. Because of the limitations of MAC, monitors that measure some correlate of anesthetic depth have been introduced into clinical practice. These monitors convert spontaneous electroencephalogram (EEG) waveforms into a single value that correlates with anesthetic depth for some general anesthetics.

   a. Anesthetic depth monitors may reduce the incidence of awareness during anesthesia (estimated incidence, 0.1 to 0.2%), reduce the amount of anesthetic used, and hasten emergence and recovery room discharge.

   b. It is controversial whether anesthetic depth monitors are superior to MAC, to standardized dosing of IV anesthetics, or to clinical indicators of anesthetic depth.

III. WHERE IN THE CENTRAL NERVOUS SYSTEM DO ANESTHETICS WORK?

A. Plausible sites of action of general anesthetics include the spinal cord, brainstem, and cerebral cortex. Peripheral sensory receptors are not important sites of anesthetic action.

B. Spinal Cord

1. The spinal cord is probably the site at which anesthetics act to inhibit purposeful responses to noxious stimulation (end point for determination of MAC).

2. Anesthetic actions at the spinal cord cannot explain either amnesia or unconsciousness.

C. Brainstem, Hypothalamic, and Thalamic Arousal Systems

1. It has long been speculated that the reticular activating system, a diffuse collection of brainstem neurons, is involved in the effects of general anesthetics on consciousness.

2. A role for the brainstem in anesthetic action is supported by changes in somatosensory evoked potentials (increased latency and decreased amplitude indicating that anesthetics inhibit information transfer through the brainstem).

3. Within the reticular formation is a set of pontine noradrenergic neurons (locus coeruleus) that innervates a number of targets in basal forebrain and cortex. It is likely that the tuberomammillary nucleus and associated pathways is a site of sedative action of anesthetics (propofol, barbiturates) that act on γ-aminobutyric acid (GABA) receptors.

4. Increasing evidence indicates that inhalational anesthetics can depress the excitability of thalamic neurons, thus blocking thalamocortical communication and potentially resulting in the loss of consciousness.

D. Cerebral Cortex. Anesthetics alter cortical electrical activity as evidenced by the consistent changes in surface EEG patterns recorded during anesthesia. Anesthetics produce a variety of effects on inhibitory transmission in the cortex.

IV. HOW DO ANESTHETICS INTERFERE WITH THE ELECTROPHYSIOLOGIC FUNCTION OF THE NERVOUS SYSTEM?

There are multiple mechanisms by which anesthetics may inhibit vital central nervous system (CNS) functions.

A. Pattern Generators. Evidence that clinical concentrations of anesthetics have effects on pattern-generating neuronal circuits in the CNS is provided by the observation that most anesthetics exert profound effects on the frequency

SCIENTIFIC FOUNDATIONS

and pattern of breathing (respiratory pattern generators in the brainstem).
B. **Neuronal Excitability.** Evidence indicates that anesthetics can hyperpolarize (i.e., create a more negative resting membrane potential) spinal motor neurons and cortical neurons.
C. **Synaptic function** is widely considered to be the most likely subcellular site of general anesthetic action. Neurotransmission across both excitatory and inhibitory synapses is markedly altered by general anesthetics.
   1. Enhancement of inhibitory transmission is observed with propofol, etomidate, and inhalational anesthetics.
   2. Clinical concentrations of general anesthetics can depress inhibitory postsynaptic potentials in the hippocampus and spinal cord.
D. **Presynaptic Effects.** Neurotransmitter release from glutamatergic synapses is inhibited by clinical concentrations of volatile anesthetics.
E. **Postsynaptic Effects.** A wide variety of anesthetics (barbiturates, etomidate, propofol, volatile anesthetics) affect synaptic function by enhancing the postsynaptic response to GABA.

V. ANESTHETIC ACTIONS ON ION CHANNELS

The notion that voltage-dependent sodium channels are insensitive to anesthetics may be incorrect.
A. **Anesthetic Effects on Voltage-Dependent Ion Channels.** A variety of ion channels can sense a change in membrane potential and respond by either opening or closing their pores.
   1. **Voltage-dependent calcium channels** serve to couple electrical activity to specific cellular functions, usually by opening to allow calcium to enter the cell and by activating calcium-dependent secretion of neurotransmitters into the synaptic cleft. Anesthetics inhibit these channels at concentrations estimated to be two to five times those necessary to produce anesthesia. This insensitivity makes these channels unlikely major targets of anesthetic action.
   2. **Potassium channels** include voltage-gated second messenger and ligand-activated inward rectifying channels. High concentrations of volatile and IV anesthetics are required to affect the function of voltage-gated

   potassium channels. Rectifying potassium channels are relatively insensitive to sevoflurane and barbiturates.
B. **Anesthetic Effects on Ligand-Gated Channels.** Selective effects of anesthetics on these channels may influence excitatory and inhibitory neurotransmission in the CNS.
C. **Glutamate-activated ion channels** include N-methyl-D-aspartate (NMDA) receptors to which ketamine (not other anesthetics) selectively binds, suggesting that this receptor may be the principal molecular target for the anesthetic actions of this drug.
D. **GABA-activated ion channels** mediate the postsynaptic response to GABA (the most important inhibitory neurotransmitter in the CNS) by selectively allowing chloride ions to enter and thereby hyperpolarizing neurons (inhibition).
   1. Data are most consistent with the idea that clinical concentrations of anesthetics produce a change in the conformation of $GABA_A$ receptors.
   2. Despite the similar effects of many anesthetics on $GABA_A$ receptor function, evidence suggests that various anesthetics do not act by binding to a single binding site on the channel protein.
E. **Anesthetic Effects on Background Potassium Ion Channels**
   1. Certain potassium channels (background or leak channels) are activated by both volatile and gaseous anesthetics.
   2. These channels tend to open at all voltages, producing a leak current that may regulate the excitability of neurons (their role in producing anesthesia is suggested by genetic evidence).

VI. WHAT IS THE CHEMICAL NATURE OF ANESTHETIC TARGET SITES?

A. **The Meyer-Overton Rule**
   1. Although there is a consensus that anesthetics act by affecting the function of ion channels, considerable controversy remains as to the molecular interactions underlying these functional effects.
   2. Because a wide variety of structurally unrelated compounds obey the Meyer-Overton rule (the potency of anesthetic gases is correlated to their solubility in olive oil), it has been reasoned that all anesthetics are likely to act at the same molecular site (unitary theory of anesthesia).

3. The anesthetic site is likely to be amphipathic (i.e., having both polar and nonpolar characteristics).
4. **Exceptions to the Meyer-Overton Rule**
   a. Halogenated compounds (e.g., flurothyl) exist that are structurally similar to the inhaled anesthetics but are convulsants rather than anesthetics.
   b. In the series of *n*-alkanols, anesthetic potency increases from methanol dodecanol, and all longer alkanols lack anesthetic properties (cutoff effect).
   c. Compounds that deviate from the Meyer-Overton rule suggest that anesthetic target sites are also defined by other properties, including size and shape.
   d. The fact that enantiomers of anesthetics differ in their potency as anesthetics argues against the Meyer-Overton rule and favors a protein-binding site.
5. **Pressure Reversal.** Evidence indicates that pressure reverses anesthesia by producing excitation that physiologically counteracts depression rather than by acting as an anesthetic antagonist at the anesthetic site of action.

B. **Lipid versus Protein Targets.** Anesthetics may interact with several possible molecular targets to produce their effects on the function of ion channels and other proteins. Anesthetics may dissolve in the lipid bilayer, causing physiochemical changes in the membrane structure that alter the ability of membrane proteins to undergo conformational changes important for their function. Alternatively, anesthetics may bind directly to proteins (either ion channel or modulatory proteins) to interfere with binding of a neurotransmitter or the ability of the protein to undergo conformational changes important for its function.

C. **Lipid Theories of Anesthesia**
1. The lipid theory of anesthesia postulates that anesthetics dissolve in lipid bilayers of biologic membranes and produce anesthesia when they reach a critical concentration in the membrane. (Membrane–gas solubility coefficients of anesthetic gases in pure lipids correlate with anesthetic potency.)
2. The magnitude of membrane perturbations produced by clinical concentrations of anesthetics is small and unlikely to disrupt nervous system function. As a result, most investigators do not consider membranes or lipids as the most likely targets of general anesthetics.

D. **Protein Theories of Anesthesia.** The Meyer-Overton rule may also be explained by the interaction of anesthetics with hydrophobic sites on protein. Direct interactions of anesthetic molecules with proteins would also provide explanations for exceptions from this rule because any protein-binding site is likely to be defined by properties such as size and shape in addition to its solvent properties.

E. **Evidence for Anesthetic Binding to Proteins.** A variety of physical techniques (e.g., nuclear magnetic resonance spectroscopy) have confirmed that anesthetic molecules can bind in the hydrophobic core of proteins and the size of the binding site can account for the cutoff effect.

F. Current evidence strongly supports proteins rather than lipids as the molecular targets for anesthetic action.

VII. HOW ARE THE EFFECTS OF ANESTHETICS ON MOLECULAR TARGETS LINKED TO ANESTHESIA IN THE INTACT ORGANISM?

A. It is likely that anesthetics affect the function of a number of ion channels and signaling proteins, probably via direct anesthetic–protein interactions. A number of approaches have been used to try to link anesthetic effects observed at a molecular level to anesthesia in intact animals.

B. **Pharmacologic Approaches**
   1. α_2-Agonists decrease halothane MAC but also have their own inherent CNS depressant effects.
   2. Development of a specific antagonist for anesthetics would provide a useful tool for linking anesthetic effects at the molecular level to anesthesia in the intact organism.
   3. Evidence is consistent with the conclusion that volatile anesthetics affect the function of a large number of important neuronal proteins and that no one target is likely to mediate all of the effects of these drugs.

C. **Genetic Approaches**
   1. In mammals, the most powerful genetic model organism is the mouse in which techniques have been developed to alter any gene of interest. The GABA$_A$ receptor has been extensively studied using mouse genetic techniques (e.g., gene knockouts, gene knockins).
   2. Results from both invertebrate and vertebrate genetics indicate that multiple proteins control volatile anesthetic sensitivity.

SCIENTIFIC FOUNDATIONS

      a. The NMDA glutamate receptor is a likely primary target of nitrous oxide.

      b. The $GABA_A$ receptor is the primary mediator for immobilization by etomidate, propofol, and pentobarbital.

VIII. CONCLUSIONS

A. Anesthetic actions cannot be localized to a specific anatomic site in the CNS; rather, different components of the anesthetic state may be mediated by actions at disparate sites.

B. Anesthetics preferentially affect synaptic function as opposed to action potential propagation.

C. At a molecular level, it is likely that anesthetic effects are mediated by direct protein–anesthetic interactions.

    1. Numerous proteins are involved, suggesting that the unitary theory of anesthesia is incorrect and that there are at least several mechanisms of anesthesia.

    2. Different anesthetic targets may mediate different components of the anesthetic state.

CHAPTER 6 ■ GENOMIC BASIS OF PERIOPERATIVE MEDICINE

Human biological diversity involves interindividual variability in morphology, behavior, physiology, development, susceptibility to disease, and response to stressful stimuli and drug therapy (*phenotypes*) (Podgoreanu MV, Mathew JP: Pharmacogenomics and proteomics. In *Clinical Anesthesia*. Edited by Barash PG, Cullen BF, Stoelting RK, Cahalan MK, Stock MC. Philadelphia: Lippincott Williams & Wilkins, 2009, pp 115–136). Phenotypic variation is determined, at least in part, by differences in the specific genetic makeup (*genotype*) of an individual.

I. GENETIC BASIS OF DISEASE

A. Many common diseases, such as atherosclerosis, coronary artery disease, hypertension, diabetes, cancer, and asthma and many individual responses to injury, drugs, and non-pharmacologic therapies are genetically complex, characteristically involving an interplay of many genetic variations in molecular and biochemical pathways.

B. The perioperative period represents a unique and extreme example of gene–environment interaction.

1. A hallmark of perioperative physiology is the striking variability in patient responses to the perturbations induced by events occurring in the operative period.

2. This translates into substantial interindividual variability in immediate perioperative adverse events (e.g., mortality, incidence, or severity of organ dysfunction), as well as long-term outcomes.

3. Genetic variation is partly responsible for the observed variability in outcomes.

C. With increasing evidence suggesting that genetic variation can significantly modulate the risk of adverse perioperative events, the emerging field of *perioperative genomics* aims to apply functional genomic approaches to discover underlying biological mechanisms.

1. These approaches explain why similar patients have such dramatically different outcomes after surgery. These outcomes are determined by a unique combination of environmental insults and postoperative phenotypes that characterize surgical and critically ill patient populations.
2. To integrate this new generation of genetic results into clinical practice, perioperative physicians need to understand the patterns of human genome variation, the methods of population-based genetic investigation, and the principles of gene and protein expression analysis.

II. OVERVIEW OF HUMAN GENETIC VARIATION

A. Although the human DNA sequence is 99.9% identical between individuals, the variations may greatly affect a person's disease susceptibility.

B. Rare genetic variants (*mutations*) are responsible for more than 1,500 monogenic disorders (e.g., hypertrophic cardiomyopathy, long-QT syndrome, sickle cell anemia, cystic fibrosis, familial hypercholesterolemia).

C. Most of the genetic diversity in the population is attributable to more widespread DNA sequence variations (*polymorphisms*), typically single nucleotide base substitutions (*single nucleotide polymorphisms* [SNPs]) (Fig. 6-1).

1. About 15 million SNPs are estimated to exist in the human genome, approximately once every 300 base pairs, located in genes as well as in the surrounding regions of the genome.
2. Polymorphisms may directly alter the amino acid sequence and therefore potentially alter protein function or alter regulatory DNA sequences that modulate protein expression.
3. Sets of nearby SNPs on a chromosome are inherited in blocks, referred to as *haplotypes*.

D. The year 2007 was marked by the realization that DNA differs from person to person much more than previously suspected.

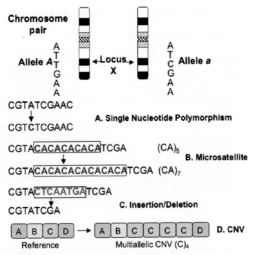

FIGURE 6-1. Categories of genetic polymorphisms. **A.** Single nucleotide polymorphisms (SNPs) can be silent or have functional consequences ranging from changes in amino acid sequence or premature termination of protein synthesis. **B.** Microsatellite polymorphism with varying number of dinucleotide (CA)n repeats. **C.** Insertion–deletion polymorphism. The locus is the location of a gene or genetic marker in the genome. Alleles are alternative forms of a gene or genetic marker. Genotype is the observed alleles for an individual at a genetic locus. Heterozygous means that two different alleles are present at a locus. Homozygous means that two identical alleles are present at a locus.

III. METHODOLOGIC APPROACHES TO STUDYING THE GENETIC ARCHITECTURE OF COMMON COMPLEX DISEASES

- A. Most ongoing research on complex disorders focuses on identifying genetic polymorphisms that enhance susceptibility to given conditions (e.g., candidate gene and genome scans used to identify polymorphisms affecting common diseases).
- B. **Linkage analysis** is used identify the chromosomal location of gene variants related to a given disease by studying the distribution of disease alleles in affected individuals throughout a pedigree. The nature of most complex diseases (especially for perioperative adverse events)

precludes the study of extended multigenerational family pedigrees.

C. **Genetic association studies** examine the frequency of specific genetic polymorphisms in a population-based sample of unrelated diseased individuals and appropriately matched unaffected controls. The fact that these studies do not require family-based sample collections is the main advantage of this approach over linkage analysis.

 1. Accumulating evidence from candidate gene association studies also suggests that specific genotypes are associated with a variety of organ-specific perioperative adverse outcomes (e.g., myocardial infarction [MI], neurocognitive dysfunction, renal compromise, vein graft restenosis, postoperative thrombosis, vascular reactivity, severe sepsis, transplant rejection, death).

 2. Replication of findings across different populations or related phenotypes remains the most reliable method of validating a true relationship between genetic polymorphisms and disease.

 3. The year 2007 marked the publication of adequately powered and successfully replicated *genome-wide association studies* that identified significant genetic contributors to the risk for common polygenic diseases (e.g., coronary artery disease, MI, types I and II diabetes, atrial fibrillation, obesity, asthma, common cancers, rheumatoid arthritis, Crohn's disease).

 4. Variants in or near *CDKN2A/B* (cyclin-dependent kinase inhibitor 2 A/B) have been shown to confer increased risk for both type II diabetes and MI, which may lead to a mechanistic explanation for the link between the two disorders.

IV. **LARGE-SCALE GENE AND PROTEIN EXPRESSION PROFILING: STATIC VERSUS DYNAMIC GENOMIC MARKERS OF PERIOPERATIVE OUTCOMES**

A. Genomic approaches are anchored in the concept of transcription of messenger RNA (mRNA) from a DNA template, followed by translation of RNA into protein (Fig 6-2).

B. Transcription is a key regulatory step that may eventually signal many other cascades of events.

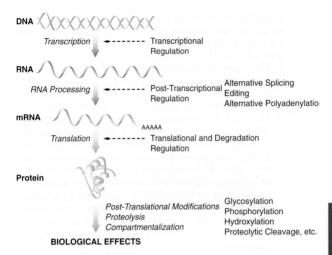

FIGURE 6-2. Central dogma of molecular biology. Protein expression involves two main processes, RNA synthesis (transcription) and protein synthesis (translation), with many intermediate regulatory steps.

1. Although the human genome contains only about 25,000 genes, functional variability at the protein level is far more diverse, resulting from extensive post-transcriptional, translational, and post-translational modifications.

2. It is believed that there are approximately 200,000 distinct proteins in humans, which are further modified post-translationally by phosphorylation, glycosylation, oxidation, and disulfide structures.

C. Increasing evidence suggests that variability in gene expression levels underlies complex diseases and is determined by regulatory DNA polymorphisms affecting transcription, splicing, and translation efficiency in a tissue- and stimulus-specific manner.

1. The main functional categories of genes identified as potentially involved in cardioprotective pathways include a host of transcription factors, proteins, and antioxidant genes.

2. Different gene programs appear to be activated in ischemic versus anesthetic preconditioning, resulting in two distinct cardioprotective phenotypes.

D. The *transcriptome* (the complete collection of transcribed elements of the genome) is not fully representative of the *proteome* (the complete complement of proteins encoded by the genome) because many transcripts are not targeted for translation, as evidenced recently by the concept of gene silencing by RNA interference.

1. Therefore, alternative splicing, a wide variety of post-translational modifications, and protein–protein interactions responsible for biological function would remain undetected by gene expression profiling.

2. This has led to the emergence of a new field, *proteomics*, which studies the sequence, modification, and function of many proteins in a biological system at a given time. Rather than focusing on "static" DNA, proteomic studies examine dynamic protein products with the goal of identifying proteins that undergo changes in abundance, modification, or localization in response to a particular disease state, trauma, stress, or therapeutic intervention.

3. Proteomics offers a more global and integrated view of biology, complementing other functional genomic approaches.

V. GENOMICS AND PERIOPERATIVE RISK PROFILING

A. More than 40 million patients undergo surgery annually in the United States at a cost that totals $450 billion. Each year, approximately 1 million patients sustain medical complications after surgery, resulting in costs of $25 billion annually.

1. Perioperative complications are significant, costly, variably reported, and often imprecisely detected and identified. There is a critical need for accurate, comprehensive perioperative outcome databases.

2. Presurgical risk profiling is inconsistent and deserves further attention, especially for noncardiac, nonvascular surgery and older patients.

3. It is becoming increasingly recognized that perioperative morbidity arises as a direct result of the environmental stress of surgery occurring on a landscape of susceptibility that is determined by an individual's clinical and genetic characteristics and may even occur in otherwise healthy individuals.

4. Understanding the role of allotypic variation in pro-inflammatory and pro-thrombotic pathways, the main pathophysiological mechanisms responsible for perioperative complications may contribute to the

development of target-specific therapies, thereby limiting the incidence of adverse events in high-risk patients.

B. **Genetic Susceptibility to Adverse Perioperative Cardiovascular Outcomes**
1. **Perioperative Myocardial Infarction.** Identifying patients at the highest risk of perioperative MI remains difficult.
    a. Genetic susceptibility to MI has been established.
    b. In the setting of cardiac surgery, postoperative MI involves three major converging pathophysiological processes, including systemic and local inflammation, "vulnerable" blood, and neuroendocrine stress
2. **Inflammation Variability and Perioperative Myocardial Outcomes.** Inflammatory gene polymorphisms that are independently predictive of postoperative MI after cardiac surgery with cardiopulmonary bypass have been identified.
3. **Coagulation Variability and Perioperative Myocardial Outcomes.** In addition to inflammatory activation, the host response to surgery is also characterized by an increase in fibrinogen concentration, platelet adhesiveness, and plasminogen activator inhibitor-1 production.
    a. Perioperative thrombotic outcomes after cardiac surgery (e.g., coronary graft thrombosis, MI, stroke, pulmonary embolism) represent one extreme on a continuum of coagulation dysfunction, with coagulopathy at the other end of the spectrum.
    b. Evidence suggests genetic variability modulates the activation of each of these mechanistic pathways, reflecting a significant heritability of the prothrombotic state.
4. **Genetic Variability and Perioperative Vascular Reactivity**
    a. Perioperative stress responses are also characterized by sympathetic nervous system activation, known to play a role in the pathophysiology of postoperative MI.
    b. Patients with coronary artery disease and specific adrenergic receptor genetic polymorphisms may be particularly susceptible to catecholamine toxicity and cardiac complications.
5. **Perioperative Atrial Fibrillation.** New-onset perioperative atrial fibrillation (AF) remains a common complication of cardiac and major noncardiac thoracic surgical procedures (incidence, 27 to 40%)

and is associated with increased morbidity, longer hospital lengths of stay, increased rehospitalization, increased health care costs, and reduced survival.

    a. Heritable forms of AF occur in the ambulatory nonsurgical population.

    b. A role for inflammation for perioperative AF is suggested by baseline C-reactive protein levels in male patients and exaggerated postoperative leukocytosis, which both predict perioperative AF; postoperative administration of nonsteroidal antiinflammatory drugs shows a protective effect.

  6. Cardiac Allograft Rejection. Identification of peripheral blood gene- and protein-based biomarkers to noninvasively monitor, diagnose, and predict perioperative cardiac allograft rejection is an area of rapid scientific growth.

  7. Genetic Variability and Postoperative Event-Free Survival. Increasing evidence suggests that the *ACE* gene polymorphism may influence complications after coronary artery bypass graft (CABG) surgery, with carriers of the *D* allele having higher mortality and restenosis rates after CABG surgery compared with carriers of the *I* allele.

C. Genetic Susceptibility to Adverse Perioperative Neurologic Outcomes

  1. Despite advances in surgical and anesthetic techniques, significant neurologic morbidity continues to occur after cardiac surgery, ranging in severity from coma and focal stroke (incidence, 1 to 3%) to more subtle cognitive deficits (incidence, ≤69%), with a substantial impact on the risk of perioperative death, quality of life, and resource utilization.

  2. The pathophysiology of perioperative neurologic injury is thought to involve complex interactions between primary pathways associated with atherosclerosis and thrombosis and secondary response pathways such as inflammation, vascular reactivity, and direct cellular injury.

    a. Many functional genetic variants have been reported in each of these mechanistic pathways involved in modulating the magnitude and the response to neurologic injury, which may have implications in chronic as well as acute perioperative neurocognitive outcomes. Specific pathways are associated with the development of postoperative complications such as postoperative cognitive dysfunction.

   b. There is a significant association between the apolipoprotein E genotype and adverse cerebral outcomes in patients undergoing cardiac surgery. The incidence of postoperative delirium after major noncardiac surgery in elderly and critically ill patients is increased in carriers of this genotype.

   c. Platelet activation may be important in the pathophysiology of adverse neurologic sequelae. The implications for perioperative medicine include identifying populations at risk that might benefit not only from an improved informed consent, stratification, and resource allocation but also from targeted antiinflammatory strategies.

D. **Genetic Susceptibility to Adverse Perioperative Renal Outcomes**

   1. Acute renal dysfunction is a common, serious complication of cardiac surgery. About 8 to 15% of patients develop moderate renal injury (peak creatinine increase of >1.0 mg/dL), and up to 5% of them develop renal failure requiring dialysis. Acute renal failure is independently associated with in-hospital mortality rates exceeding 60% in patients requiring dialysis.

   2. Studies have demonstrated that inheritance of genetic polymorphisms are associated with acute kidney injury after CABG surgery.

VI. PHARMACOGENOMICS AND ANESTHESIA

A. The term *pharmacogenomics* is used to describe how inherited variations in genes modulating drug actions are related to interindividual variability in drug response.

   1. Such variability in drug action may be *pharmacokinetic* or *pharmacodynamic* (Fig. 6-3).

      a. *Pharmacokinetic variability* refers to variability in a drug's absorption, distribution, metabolism, and excretion that mediates its efficacy and toxicity. The molecules involved in these processes include drug-metabolizing enzymes (e.g., members of the cytochrome P450 or CYP superfamily) and drug transport molecules that mediate drug uptake into and efflux from intracellular sites.

      b. *Pharmacodynamic variability* refers to variable drug effects despite equivalent drug delivery to molecular sites of action. This may reflect variability in the function of the molecular target of the drug or in the

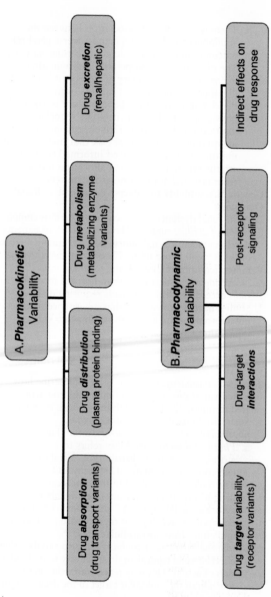

FIGURE 6-3. Pharmacogenomic determinants of individual drug response operate by pharmacokinetic and pharmacodynamic mechanisms.

pathophysiological context in which the drug interacts with its receptor–target (affinity, coupling,
expression).
B. **Pseudocholinesterase Deficiency.** Individuals with an
atypical form of pseudocholinesterase resulting in a
markedly reduced rate of drug metabolism are at risk for
excessive neuromuscular blockade and prolonged apnea.
More than 20 variants have since been identified in the
butyrylcholinesterase gene. Therefore, pharmacogenetic
testing is currently not recommended in the population
at large but only as an explanation for an adverse event.
C. **Genetics of Malignant Hyperthermia**
1. Malignant hyperthermia (MH) is a rare autosomal
dominant genetic disease of skeletal muscle calcium
metabolism that is triggered by administration of a
volatile anesthetic agent or succinylcholine in susceptible individuals.
2. MH susceptibility was initially linked to the ryanodine
receptor (*RYR1*) gene locus on chromosome 19q, but it
is becoming increasingly apparent that MH susceptibility results from a complex interaction between multiple
genes and environmental factors (e.g., environmental
toxins).
3. Because of the polygenic determinism and variable penetrance, direct DNA testing in the general population
for susceptibility to MH is currently not recommended.
In contrast, testing in individuals from families with
affected individuals has the potential to greatly reduce
mortality and morbidity.
D. **Genetic Variability and Response to Anesthetic Agents**
1. Anesthetic potency, defined by the minimum alveolar
concentration (MAC) of an inhaled anesthetic that
abolishes purposeful movement in response to a noxious stimulus, varies among individuals, with a coefficient of variation (the ratio of standard deviation to
the mean) of approximately 10%.
2. Evidence of a genetic basis for increased anesthetic
requirements is suggested by the observation that desflurane requirements are increased in subjects with red
hair versus those with dark hair.
E. **Genetic Variability and Response to Anesthetic Agents**
1. Similar to the observed variability in anesthetic potency,
the response to painful stimuli and analgesic manipulations varies among individuals.
2. Increasing evidence suggests that pain behavior in
response to noxious stimuli and its modulation by the

central nervous system in response to drug administration or environmental stress, as well as the development of persistent pain conditions through pain amplification, are strongly influenced by genetic factors.

F. **Genetic Variability in Response to Other Drugs Used Perioperatively**
   1. A wide variety of drugs used in the perioperative period display significant pharmacokinetic or pharmacodynamic variability that is genetically modulated (Table 6-1).
   2. The most commonly cited categories of drugs involved in adverse drug reactions include cardiovascular, antibiotic, psychiatric, and analgesic medications, and each category has a known genetic basis for increased risk of adverse reactions.
   3. Genetic variation in drug targets (receptors) can have profound effect on drug efficacy.
      a. Carriers of susceptibility alleles have no manifest QT-interval prolongation or family history of sudden death until a QT-prolonging drug challenge is superimposed.
      b. Predisposition to QT-interval prolongation (considered a surrogate for risk of life-threatening ventricular arrhythmias) has been responsible for more withdrawals of drug from the market than any other category of adverse event.

G. Pharmacogenomics is emerging as an additional modifying component to anesthesia along with age, gender, comorbidities, and medication usage. Specific testing and treatment guidelines allowing clinicians to appropriately modify drug utilization (e.g., adjust doses or change drugs) already exist for a few compounds and will likely be expanded to all relevant therapeutic compounds, together with identification of novel therapeutic targets.

VI. GENOMICS AND CRITICAL CARE

A. **Genetic Variability in Response to Injury**
   1. Systemic injury (including trauma and surgical stress), shock, and infection trigger physiological responses of fever, tachycardia, tachypnea, and leukocytosis that collectively define the systemic inflammatory response syndrome.
   2. A new paradigm in critical care medicine states that outcomes of critical illness are determined by the interplay

TABLE 6-1

EXAMPLES OF GENETIC POLYMORPHISMS INVOLVED IN VARIABLE RESPONSES TO DRUGS USED IN THE PERIOPERATIVE PERIOD

Drug Class	Gene Name (Gene Symbol)	Effect of Polymorphism
Pharmacokinetic Variability		
β-blockers	Cytochrome P450 2D6 (*CYP2D6*)	Enhanced drug effect
Codeine, dextromethorphan	(*CYP2D6*)	Decreased drug effect
Calcium channel blockers	Cytochrome P450 3A4 (*CYP3A4*)	Uncertain
Alfentanil	*CYP3A4*	Enhanced drug response
Angiotensin II receptor type 1 blockers	Cytochrome P450 2C9 (*CYP2C9*)	Enhanced blood pressure response
Warfarin	*CYP2C9*	Enhanced anticoagulant effect, risk of bleeding
Phenytoin	*CYP2C9*	Enhanced drug effect
ACE inhibitors	Angiotensin I converting enzyme (*ACE*)	Blood pressure response
Procainamide	N-acetyltransferase 2 (*NAT2*)	Enhanced drug effect
Succinylcholine	Butyrylcholinesterase (*BCHE*)	Enhanced drug effect
Digoxin	P-glycoprotein (*ABCB1, MDR1*)	Increased bioavailability
Pharmacodynamic Variability		
Beta-blockers	$β_1$ and $β_2$ adrenergic receptors (*ADRB1, ADRB2*)	Blood pressure and heart rate response, airway responsiveness to $β_2$-agonists
QT-prolonging drugs (antiarrhythmics, cisapride, erythromycin)	Sodium and potassium ion channels (*SCN5A, KCNH2, KCNE2, KCNQ1*)	Long Q-T syndrome, risk of *torsade de pointes*
Aspirin, glycoprotein IIb/IIIa inhibitors	Glycoprotein IIIa subunit of platelet glycoprotein IIb/IIIa (*ITGB3*)	Variability in antiplatelet effects
Phenylephrine	Endothelial nitric oxide synthase (*NOS3*)	Blood pressure response

between the *injury* and *repair* processes triggered by the initial insults.

  a. Negative outcomes are the combined result of direct tissue injury, the side effects of resulting repair processes, and secondary injury mechanisms leading to suboptimal repair.

  b. This concept forms the basis of the new PIRO (predisposition, infection or insult, response, organ dysfunction) staging system in critical illness.

  c. Genomic factors play a role along this continuum, from inflammatory gene variants and modulators of pathogen–host interaction to microbial genomics and rapid detection assays that identify pathogens to biomarkers differentiating infection from inflammation to dynamic measures of cellular responses to insult, apoptosis, cytopathic hypoxia, and cell stress.

  3. The large interindividual variability in the magnitude of response to injury, including activation of inflammatory and coagulation cascades, apoptosis, and fibrosis, suggests the involvement of genetic regulatory factors.

B. **Functional Genomics of Injury**

  1. At a cellular level, injurious stimuli trigger adaptive stress responses determined by quantitative and qualitative changes in interdigitating cascades of biological pathways interacting in complex, often redundant ways. As a result, numerous clinical trials attempting to block single inflammatory mediators have been largely unsuccessful.

  2. Organ injury may be defined by patterns of altered gene and protein synthesis.

VII. FUTURE DIRECTIONS

A. **Systems Biology Approach to Perioperative Medicine: The "Perioptome."** Systems biology is a conceptual framework within which scientists attempt to correlate massive amounts of apparently unrelated data into a single unifying explanation.

B. **Targeted Therapeutic Applications: The "5 Ps" of Perioperative Medicine and Pain Management**

  1. Genomic and proteomic approaches are rapidly becoming platforms for all aspects of drug discovery and development, from target identification and validation to individualization of drug therapy.

2. The human genome contains about 25,000 genes encoding for approximately 200,000 proteins, which represent potential drug targets.

C. **Ethical Considerations**
   1. Although one of the aims of the Human Genome Project is to improve therapy through genome-based prediction, the birth of personal genomics opens up a Pandora's box of ethical issues, including privacy and the risk for discrimination against individuals who are genetically predisposed to medical disorders.
   2. Another ethical concern is the transferability of genetic tests across ethnic groups, particularly in the prediction of adverse drug responses.
      a. Most polymorphisms associated with variability in drug response show significant differences in allele frequencies among populations and racial groups.
      b. The patterns of linkage disequilibrium are markedly different between ethnic groups, which may lead to spurious findings when markers, instead of causal variants, are used in diagnostic tests extrapolated across populations.
   3. With the goal of personalized medicine being the prediction of risk and treatment of disease on the basis of an individual's genetic profile, some have argued that biologic consideration of race will become obsolete.

VIII. CONCLUSIONS

A. The Human Genome Project has revolutionized all aspects of medicine, allowing us to assess the impact of genetic variability on disease taxonomy, characterization, and outcome and of individual responses to various drugs and injuries.

B. Mechanistically, information gleaned through genomic approaches is already unraveling long-standing mysteries behind general anesthetic action and adverse responses to drugs used during surgery.

C. Using currently available high-throughput molecular technologies, genetic profiling of drug-metabolizing enzymes, carrier proteins, and receptors will enable personalized choice of drugs and dosage regimens tailored to suit a patient's pharmacogenetic profile. At that point, perioperative physicians will have far more robust information to use in designing the most appropriate and safest anesthetic plan for a given patient.

SCIENTIFIC FOUNDATIONS

CHAPTER 7 ■ PHARMACOLOGIC PRINCIPLES

Anesthetic drugs are administered with the goal of rapidly establishing and maintaining a therapeutic effect while minimizing undesired side effects (Gupta DK, Henthorn TK: Pharmacologic principles. In *Clinical Anesthesia*. Edited by Barash PG, Cullen BF, Stoelting RK, Cahalan MK, Stock MC. Philadelphia: Lippincott Williams and Wilkins, 2009, pp 137–164).

I. PHARMACOKINETIC PRINCIPLES: DRUG ABSORPTION AND ROUTES OF ADMINISTRATION

A. **Transfer of Drugs Across Membranes.** Even the simplest drug that is directly administered into the blood to exert its action must move across at least one cell membrane to its site of action.

1. Because biologic membranes are lipid bilayers composed of a lipophilic core sandwiched between two hydrophilic layers, only small lipophilic drugs can passively diffuse across the membrane down its concentration gradient.

2. For water-soluble drugs to passively diffuse across the membrane down its concentration gradient, transmembrane proteins that form a hydrophilic channel are required.

B. **Intravenous (IV) administration** results in rapid increases in drug concentration. Although this can lead to a very rapid onset of drug effect, for drugs that have a low *therapeutic index* (the ratio of the IV dose that produces a toxic effect in 50% of the population to the IV dose that produces a therapeutic effect in 50% of the population), rapid overshoot of the desired plasma concentration can potentially result in immediate and severe side effects.

1. **Bioavailability** is the **relative amount** of a drug dose that reaches the systemic circulation unchanged and the **rate** at which this occurs. For most intravenously administered drugs, the absolute bioavailability of drug available is close to unity, and the rate is nearly instantaneous.
2. The pulmonary endothelium can slow the rate at which intravenously administered drugs reach the systemic circulation if distribution into the alveolar endothelium is extensive such as occurs with the pulmonary uptake of fentanyl. The pulmonary endothelium also contains enzymes that may metabolize intravenously administered drugs (propofol) on first pass and reduce their absolute bioavailability.

C. **Oral administration** is not used significantly in anesthetic practice because of the limited and variable rate of bioavailability.
   1. Because of this extensive **first-pass metabolism,** the oral dose of most drugs must be significantly higher to generate a therapeutic plasma concentration.
   2. Highly lipophilic drugs that can maintain a high contact time with nasal or oral (sublingual) mucosa can be absorbed without needing to traverse the gastrointestinal (GI) tract. Sublingual administration of drug has the additional advantage over GI absorption in that absorbed drug directly enters the systemic venous circulation, so it is able to bypass the metabolically active intestinal mucosa and the hepatic first-pass metabolism.

D. **Transcutaneous Administration.** A few lipophilic drugs (e.g., scopolamine, nitroglycerin, fentanyl) have been manufactured in formulations that are sufficient to allow penetration of intact skin.

E. **Intramuscular and Subcutaneous Administration.** Absorption of drugs from the depots in the subcutaneous tissue or in muscle tissue directly depends on the drug formulation and the blood flow to the depot.

F. **Intrathecal, Epidural, and Perineural Injection.** The major downside to these three techniques is the relative expertise required to perform regional anesthetics relative to oral, IV, and inhalational drug administration.

G. **Inhalational Administration.** The large surface area of the pulmonary alveoli available for exchange with the large volumetric flow of blood found in the pulmonary capillaries makes inhalational administration an extremely attractive method (approximates IV administration) by which to administer drugs.

II. DRUG DISTRIBUTION

The relative distribution of cardiac output among organ vascular beds determines the speed at which organs are exposed to drug. The highly perfused core circulatory components (the brain, lungs, heart, and kidneys) receive the highest relative distribution of cardiac output and therefore are the initial organs to reach equilibrium with plasma drug concentrations. Drug transfer to the less well-perfused, intermediate-volume muscle tissue may take hours to approach equilibrium, and drug transfer to the poorly perfused, large cellular volumes of adipose tissue does not equilibrate for days.

A. Redistribution

1. As soon as the concentration of drug in the brain tissue is higher than the plasma concentration of drug, a reversal of the drug concentration gradient takes place so that the lipophilic drug readily diffuses back into the blood and is redistributed to the other tissues that are still taking up drug.
2. Although single, moderate doses of highly lipophilic drugs have very short central nervous system (CNS) durations of action because of redistribution of drug from the CNS to the blood and other less well-perfused tissues, repeated injections of a drug allow the rapid establishment of significant peripheral tissue concentrations.

III. DRUG ELIMINATION

Drug elimination is the pharmacokinetic term that describes all the processes that remove a drug from the body. Although the liver and the kidneys are considered the major organs of drug elimination, drug metabolism can occur at many other locations that contain active drug metabolizing enzymes (e.g., the pulmonary vasculature, red blood cells), and drugs can be excreted unchanged from other organs (e.g., the lungs).

A. Elimination clearance (drug clearance) is the theoretical volume of blood from which drug is completely and irreversibly removed in a unit of time.

B. **Biotransformation Reactions.** Most drugs that are
   excreted unchanged from the body are hydrophilic and
   therefore readily passed into urine or stool. Drugs that
   are not sufficiently hydrophilic to be able to be excreted
   unchanged require modification (enzymatic reactions)
   into more hydrophilic, excretable compounds.
   1. **Phase I reactions** may hydrolyze, oxidize, or reduce
      the parent compound.
      a. **Cytochrome P450 enzymes** (CYPs) are a superfam-
         ily of constitutive and inducible enzymes that cat-
         alyze most phase I biotransformations. CYP3A4 is
         the single most important enzyme, accounting for
         40% to 45% of all CYP-mediated drug metabo-
         lism.
      b. CYPs are incorporated into the smooth endoplas-
         mic reticulum of hepatocytes and the membranes
         of the upper intestinal enterocytes in high concen-
         trations (Table 7-1).

TABLE 7-1

SUBSTRATES FOR CYP ISOENZYMES ENCOUNTERED
IN ANESTHESIOLOGY

CYP3A4	CYP2D6	CYP2C9	CYP2C19
Acetaminophen	Captopril	Diclofenac	Diazepam
Alfentanil	Codeine	Ibuprofen	Omeprazole
Alprazolam	Hydrocodone	Indomethacin	Propranolol
Bupivacaine	Metoprolol		Warfarin
Cisapride	Ondansetron		
Codeine	Propranolol		
Diazepam	Timolol		
Digitoxin	Captopril		
Diltiazem	Codeine		
Fentanyl	Hydrocodone		
Lidocaine			
Methadone			
Midazolam			
Nicardipine			
Nifedipine			
Omeprazole			
Ropivacaine			
Statins			
Sufentanil			
Verapamil			
Warfarin			

SCIENTIFIC FOUNDATIONS

2. **Phase II reactions** are known as *conjugation* or *synthetic reactions.* Similar to the cytochrome P450 system, the enzymes that catalyze phase II reactions are inducible.
3. **Genetic Variations in Drug Metabolism.** Drug metabolism varies substantially among individuals because of variability in the genes controlling the numerous enzymes responsible for biotransformation.
4. **Chronologic Variations in Drug Metabolism.** The activity and capacity of the CYP enzymes increase from subnormal levels in the fetal and neonatal period to reach normal levels at about 1 year of age. Neonates have a limited ability to perform phase II conjugation reactions, but after normalizing phase II activity over the initial year of life, advanced age does not affect the capacity to perform phase II reactions.

C. **Renal Drug Clearance.** The primary role of the kidneys in drug elimination is to excrete into urine the unchanged hydrophilic drugs and the hepatic derived metabolites from phase I and II reactions of lipophilic drugs. In patients with acute and chronic causes of decreased renal function, including age, low cardiac output states, and hepatorenal syndrome, drug dosing must be altered to avoid accumulation of parent compounds and potentially toxic metabolites (Table 7-2).

D. **Hepatic Drug Clearance.** Drug elimination by the liver depends on the intrinsic ability of the liver to metabolize the drug and the amount of drug available to diffuse into the liver (hepatic blood flow) (Table 7-3).

TABLE 7-2

DRUGS WITH SIGNIFICANT RENAL EXCRETION ENCOUNTERED IN ANESTHESIOLOGY

Aminoglycosides	Nor-meperidine
Atenolol	Pancuronium
Cephalosporins	Penicillins
Digoxin	Procainamide
Edrophonium	Pyridostigmine
Nadolol	Quinolones
Neostigmine	Rocuronium

TABLE 7-3

CLASSIFICATION OF DRUGS ENCOUNTERED IN ANESTHESIOLOGY
ACCORDING TO HEPATIC EXTRACTION RATIOS

Low	Intermediate	High
Diazepam	Alfentanil	Alprenolol
Lorazepam	Methohexital	Bupivacaine
Methadone	Midazolam	Diltiazem
Phenytoin	Vecuronium	Fentanyl
Rocuronium		Ketamine
Theophylline		Lidocaine
Thiopental		Meperidine
		Metoprolol
		Morphine
		Naloxone
		Nifedipine
		Propofol
		Propranolol
		Sufentanil

IV. PHARMACOKINETIC MODELS

The concentration of drug at its tissue site or sites of action
is the fundamental determinant of a drug's pharmacologic
effects.

A. Physiologic vs. Compartment Models

1. Awakening after a single dose of thiopental is primarily a result of redistribution of thiopental from the
   brain to the muscle with little contribution by distribution to less well-perfused tissues or drug metabolism;
   this fundamental concept of redistribution applies to
   all lipophilic drugs.
2. Drug concentrations in the blood are used to define
   the relationship between dose and the time course of
   changes in the drug concentration.

B. Pharmacokinetic Concepts

1. **Rate Constants and Half-Lives.** The disposition of
   most drugs follows first-order kinetics. A first-order
   kinetic process is one in which a constant fraction of
   the drug is removed during a finite period of time
   regardless of the drug's amount or concentration.
   Rather than using rate constants, the rapidity of

TABLE 7-4

HALF-LIVES AND PERCENTAGE OF DRUG REMOVED

Number of Half-Lives	Percentage of Drug Removed	Percentage of Drug Remaining
0	100	0
1	50	50
2	25	75
3	12.5	87.5
4	6.25	93.75
5	3.125	96.875

pharmacokinetic processes is often described with half-lives, which is the time required for the concentration to change by a factor of 2. After five half-lives, the process is almost 97% complete (Table 7-4). For practical purposes, this is essentially 100%, so there is a negligible amount of drug remaining in the body.

2. **Volume of distribution** quantifies the extent of drug distribution (overall capacity of tissues versus the capacity of blood for that drug). If a drug is extensively distributed, then the concentration will be lower relative to the amount of drug present, which equates to a larger volume of distribution. The apparent volume of distribution is a numeric index of the extent of drug distribution that does not have any relationship to the actual volume of any tissue or group of tissues. In general, lipophilic drugs have larger volumes of distribution than hydrophilic drugs.

3. **Elimination half-life** is the time during which the amount of drug in the body decreases by 50%. Although elimination of drug from the body begins the moment the drug is delivered to the organs of elimination, the rapid termination of effect of a bolus of an IV agent is attributable to redistribution of drug from the brain to the blood and subsequently other tissue (muscle). Therefore, the effects of most anesthetics have waned long before even one elimination half-life has been completed. Thus, the elimination half-life has limited utility in anesthetic practice.

C. **Effect of Hepatic or Renal Disease on Pharmacokinetic Parameters.** Diverse pathophysiologic changes preclude precise prediction of the pharmacokinetics of a given drug in individual patients with hepatic or renal disease.

1. When hepatic drug clearance is reduced, repeated bolus dosing or continuous infusion of such drugs as benzodiazepines, opioids, and barbiturates may result in excessive accumulation of drug as well as excessive and prolonged pharmacologic effects.

2. Because recovery from small doses of drugs such as thiopental and fentanyl is largely the result of redistribution, recovery from conservative doses is minimally affected by reductions in elimination clearance.

V. COMPARTMENTAL PHARMACOKINETIC MODELS

A. **One-Compartment Model.** Although the one-compartment model is an oversimplification for most drugs, it does serve to illustrate the basic relationships among clearance, volume of distribution, and the elimination half-life (Fig. 7-1).

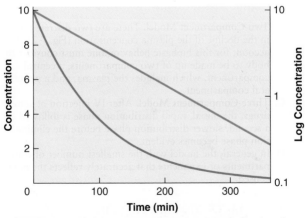

FIGURE 7-1. The plasma concentration versus time profile plotted on both linear (*dashed line*, left *y*-axis) and logarithmic (*dotted line*, right *y*-axis) scales for a hypothetical drug exhibiting one-compartment, first-order pharmacokinetics.

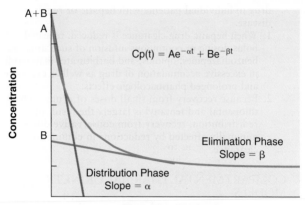

Time After IV Injection

FIGURE 7-2. The logarithmic plasma concentration versus time profile for a hypothetical drug exhibiting two-compartment, first-order pharmacokinetics. Note that the distribution phase has a slope that is significantly larger than that of the elimination phase, indicating that the process of distribution is not only more rapid than elimination of the drug from the body but that it is also responsible for the majority of the decline in plasma concentration in the several minutes after drug administration.

B. **Two-Compartment Model.** There are two discrete phases in the decline of the plasma concentration (Fig. 7-2). To account for this biphasic behavior, one must consider the body to be made up of two compartments, a central compartment, which includes the plasma, and a peripheral compartment.

C. **Three-Compartment Model.** After IV injection of some drugs, the initial, rapid distribution phase is followed by a second, slower distribution phase before the elimination phase becomes evident.

D. In general, the model with the smallest number of compartments or exponents that accurately reflects the data is used.

VI. PHARMACODYNAMIC PRINCIPLES

Pharmacodynamic studies focus on the quantitative analysis of the relationship between the drug concentration in the blood and the resultant effects of the drug on physiologic processes.

VII. DRUG–RECEPTOR INTERACTIONS

Most pharmacologic agents produce their physiologic effects by binding to a drug-specific receptor, which brings about a change in cellular function. The majority of pharmacologic receptors are cell membrane–bound proteins, although some receptors are located in the cytoplasm or the nucleoplasm of the cell.

A. **Desensitization and Downregulation of Receptors.** Receptors are dynamic cellular components that adapt to their environment. Prolonged exposure of a receptor to its agonist leads to desensitization; subsequent doses of the agonist produce lower maximal effects.

B. **Agonists, Partial Agonists, and Antagonists.** Drugs that bind to receptors and produce an effect are called *agonists*. *Partial agonists* are drugs that are not capable of producing the maximal effect, even at very high concentrations. Compounds that bind to receptors without producing any changes in cellular function are referred to as *antagonists*. *Competitive antagonists* bind reversibly to receptors, and their blocking effect can be overcome by high concentrations of an agonist (competition). *Noncompetitive antagonists* bind irreversibly to receptors.

C. **Dose–response relationships** determine the relationship between increasing doses of a drug and the ensuing changes in pharmacologic effects (Fig. 7-3).

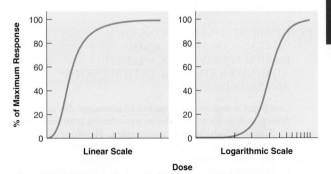

FIGURE 7-3. Schematic curve of the effect of a drug plotted against dose. In the *left panel*, the response data are plotted against the dose data on a linear scale. In the *right panel*, the same response data are plotted against the dose data on a logarithmic scale, yielding a sigmoid dose–response curve that is linear between 20% and 80% of the maximal effect.

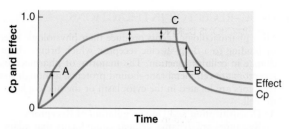

FIGURE 7-4. The changes in plasma drug concentration and pharmacologic effect during and after an intravenous infusion. Cp = plasma concentration.

    D. **Concentration–Response Relationships** (Fig. 7-4). The magnitude of the pharmacologic effect is a function of the amount of drug present at the site of action, so increasing the dose increases the peak effect. Larger doses have a more rapid onset of action because pharmacologically active concentrations at the site of action occur sooner. Increasing the dose also increases the duration of action because pharmacologically effective concentrations are maintained for a longer time.

VIII. DRUG INTERACTIONS

    Ten or more drugs may be given for a relatively routine anesthetic (Table 7-5).

IX. CLINICAL APPLICATIONS OF PHARMACOKINETIC AND PHARMACODYNAMICS TO THE ADMINISTRATION OF INTRAVENOUS ANESTHETICS

    Computer simulation is required to meaningfully interpret dosing and to accurately devise new dosing regimens.

    A. **Rise to Steady-State Concentration.** The drug concentration versus time profile for the rise to steady state is the mirror image of its elimination profile.

    B. **Infusion Dosing Schemes.** Based on a one-compartment pharmacokinetic model, a stable steady-state plasma concentration (*Cp, ss*) can be maintained by administering an infusion at a rate that is proportional to the elimination of drug from the body.

TABLE 7-5

DRUG INTERACTIONS DURING THE PERIOPERATIVE PERIOD

Opioid to decrease volatile anesthetic requirements
Mixing acidic drugs (thiopental) with basic drugs (opioids, muscle relaxant), resulting in a precipitate
Absorption of drugs (nitroglycerin, fentanyl) by plastics
Drugs that alter absorption by impact on gastric pH (ranitidine) or rate of gastric emptying (metoclopramide)
Vasoconstrictors are added to local anesthetic solutions to prolong their duration of action at the site of injection and to decrease the risk of systemic toxicity from rapid absorption.
Drugs that inhibit or induce the enzymes that catalyze biotransformation reactions can affect clearance of other concomitantly administered drugs (e.g., phenytoin shortens the duration of action of the nondepolarizing neuromuscular junction blocking agents). Pharmacodynamic interactions in which drugs interact directly or indirectly at the same receptors (opioid antagonists directly displace opioids from opiate receptors) may also occur.

C. **Isoconcentration Nomogram.** To make the calculations of the various infusion rates required to maintain a target plasma concentration for a drug that follows multi-compartment pharmacokinetics, a clinician needs access to a basic computer and the software to perform the appropriate simulations.

D. **Context-Sensitive Decrement Times.** During an infusion, drug is taken up by the inert peripheral tissues. After drug delivery is terminated, recovery occurs when the effect site concentration decreases below a threshold concentration for producing a pharmacologic effect.

E. **Target-Controlled Infusions.** By linking a computer with the appropriate pharmacokinetic model to an infusion pump, it is possible for the physician to enter the desired target plasma concentration of a drug and for the computer to nearly instantaneously calculate the appropriate infusion scheme to achieve this concentration target in a matter of seconds.

F. **Time to Maximum Effect Compartment Concentration (TMAX).** By simultaneously modeling the plasma drug concentration versus time data (pharmacokinetics) and the measured drug effect (pharmacodynamics), an estimate of the drug transfer rate constant between plasma and the putative effect site can be estimated.

G. **Volume of Distribution at Peak Effect.** It is possible to calculate a bolus dose that will attain the estimated effect site concentration at TMAX without overshoot in the effect site.

H. **Front-end pharmacokinetics** refers to the intravascular mixing, pulmonary uptake, and recirculation events that occur in the first few minutes during and after IV drug administration. These kinetic events and the drug concentration versus time profile that results are important because the peak effect of rapidly acting drugs occurs during this temporal window.

I. **Closed-Loop Infusions.** When a valid and nearly continuous measure of drug effect is available, drug delivery can be automatically titrated by feedback control. Such systems have been used experimentally for control of blood pressure, oxygen delivery, blood glucose, neuromuscular blockade, and depth of anesthesia.

1. Closed-loop systems for anesthesia are the most difficult systems to design and implement because the precise definition of anesthesia remains elusive, as does a robust monitor for anesthetic depth.

2. Because modification of consciousness must accompany anesthesia, processed electroencephalographic (EEG) parameters that correlate with level of consciousness, such as the bispectral index, EEG entropy, and auditory evoked potentials, make it possible to undertake closed-loop control of anesthesia.

J. **Response Surface Models of Drug–Drug Interactions.** During the course of an operation, the level of anesthetic drug administered is adjusted to ensure amnesia to ongoing events, provide immobility to noxious stimulation, and blunt the sympathetic response to noxious stimulation. To limit side effects, an opioid and a sedative–hypnotic are often administered together (synergistic for most pharmacologic effects).

CHAPTER 8 ■ ELECTRICAL AND FIRE SAFETY

The myriad electronic devices in the modern operating room greatly improve patient care and safety but also subject patients and operating room personnel to increased risks (Ehrenwerth J, Seifert HA: Electrical and fire safety. In *Clinical Anesthesia*. Edited by Barash PG, Cullen BF, Stoelting RK, Cahalan MK, Stock MC. Philadelphia: Lippincott Williams and Wilkins, 2009, pp 165–191).

I. PRINCIPLES OF ELECTRICITY

A basic principle of electricity is known as Ohm's law and is represented by the equation $E = I \times R$ (electromotive force in volts = current in amperes times resistance in ohms). Ohm's law forms the basis for the physiologic equation in which the blood pressure is equal to the cardiac output times the systemic vascular resistance ($BP = CO \times SVR$). Electrical power is measured as watts (voltage × amperage). The amount of electrical work done (watt-second or joule) is a common designation for electrical energy expended. (Energy produced by a defibrillator is measured in joules.)

A. **Direct and Alternating Currents.** The flow of electrons (current) through a conductor is characterized as direct current (electron flow is always in the same direction) or alternating current (electron flow reverses direction at a regular interval).

B. **Impedance** is the sum of forces that oppose electron movement in an alternating current circuit.

C. **Capacitance** is the ability of a capacitor (two parallel conductors separated by an insulator) to store charge.
   1. In a direct current circuit, the charged capacitor plates (battery) do not result in current flow unless a resistance is connected between the two plates and the capacitor is discharged.

2. Stray capacitance is capacitance that is not designed into the system but is incidental to the construction of the equipment. (All alternating current operating equipment produces stray capacitance even while turned off.)

II. ELECTRICAL SHOCK HAZARDS

A. Alternating and Direct Currents
1. Whenever an individual contacts an external source of electricity, an electrical shock is possible. (It requires approximately three times as much direct current as alternating current to cause ventricular fibrillation [VF].)
2. A short circuit occurs when there is zero impedance with a high current flow.

B. Source of Shocks
1. Electrical accidents or shocks occur when a person becomes part of or completes an electrical circuit (Fig. 8-1).
2. Damage from electrical current is caused by disruption of normal electrical function of cells (skeletal muscle

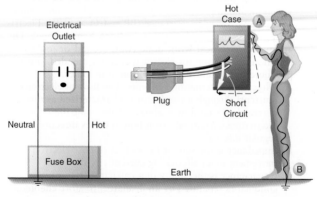

FIGURE 8-1. When a faulty piece of equipment without an equipment ground wire is plugged into an electrical outlet not containing a ground wire, the instrument case becomes energized ("hot"). If an individual touches the case (**A**), he or she will receive a shock (*dashed line* depicts path of electrical current) because he or she is standing on the ground (**B**) and completes the circuit.

contracture, VF) or dissipation of electrical energy (burn).

3. The severity of an electrical shock is determined by the amount of current and the duration of current flow.

   a. Macroshock describes large amounts of current flow that can cause harm or death.

   b. Microshock describes small amounts of current flow and applies only to electrically susceptible patients (those with an external conduit that is in direct contact with the heart, such as a pacing wire or saline-filled central venous pressure [CVP] catheter) in whom even minute amounts of current (1 mA, which is the threshold of perception) may cause VF.

4. Very high-frequency current does not excite contractile tissue and does not cause cardiac dysrhythmias.

C. **Grounding.** To fully understand electrical shock hazards and their prevention, one must have a thorough knowledge of the concepts of grounding. In electrical terminology, grounding is applied to electrical power and equipment.

III. ELECTRICAL POWER: GROUNDED

A. Electrical utilities universally provide power to homes that are grounded. (By convention, the earth ground potential is zero.)

B. Electrical shock is an inherent danger of grounded power systems. (An individual standing on ground or in contact with an object that is referenced to the ground needs only one additional contact point to complete the circuit.)

C. Modern wiring systems have added a third wire (a low-resistance pathway through which the current can flow to ground) to decrease the severity of potential electrical shocks (Fig. 8-2).

IV. ELECTRICAL POWER: UNGROUNDED

A. The numerous electronic devices, along with power cords and puddles of saline-filled solutions on the floor, tend to make the operating room an electrically hazardous environment for both patients and personnel.

B. In an attempt to decrease the risk of electrical shock, the power supplied to most operating rooms is ungrounded (i.e., current is isolated from the ground).

SCIENTIFIC FOUNDATIONS

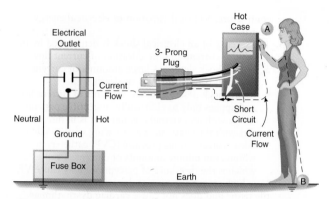

FIGURE 8-2. When a faulty piece of equipment containing an equipment ground wire is properly connected to an electrical outlet with grounding protection, the electrical current (*dashed line*) will preferentially flow down the low-resistance ground wire. An individual touching the instrument case (**A**) and standing on the ground (**B**) still completes the circuit; however, only a small part of the current flows through the individual.

C. Supplying ungrounded power to the operating room requires the use of an isolation transformer (Fig. 8-3).
   1. The isolated power system provides protection from macroshock (Fig. 8-4).
   2. A faulty piece of equipment plugged into an isolated power system does not present a shock hazard.

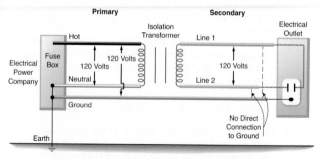

FIGURE 8-3. In the operating room, the isolation transformer converts the grounded power on the primary side to an ungrounded power system on the secondary side of the transformer. There is no direct connection from the power on the secondary side to ground. The equipment ground wire, however, is still present.

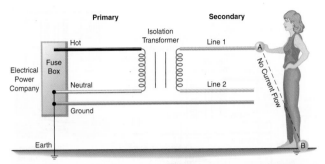

FIGURE 8-4. A safety feature of the isolated power system is illustrated. An individual contacting one side of the isolated power system (**A**) and standing on the ground (**B**) will not receive a shock. In this instance, the individual is not contacting the circuit at two points and thus is not completing the circuit.

V. THE LINE ISOLATION MONITOR

A. The line isolation monitor is a device that continuously monitors the integrity of the isolated power system (i.e., it measures the impedance to ground on each side of the isolated power system).

B. If a faulty piece of equipment is connected to the isolated power system, it will, in effect, change the system to a conventional grounded system, yet the faulty piece of equipment will continue to function normally.

   1. The meter of the line isolation monitor indicates the amount of leakage in the system resulting from any device plugged into the isolated power system.

   2. Visual and audible alarms are triggered if the isolation from the ground has been degraded beyond a predetermined limit (Fig. 8-5).

C. If the line isolation monitor alarm is triggered, the first step is to determine if it is a true fault.

   1. If the gauge reads between 2 and 5 mA, there probably is too much electrical equipment plugged into the circuit. (All alternating current-operated devices have some capacitance and associated leakage current.)

   2. If the gauge reads above 5 mA, it is likely that a faulty piece of equipment is present in the operating room. This equipment may be identified by unplugging each piece of equipment until the alarm is silenced.

SCIENTIFIC FOUNDATIONS

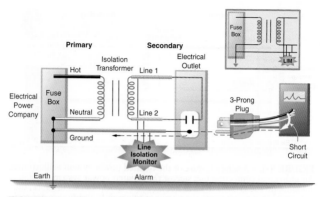

FIGURE 8-5. When a faulty piece of equipment is plugged into the isolated power system, it decreases the impedance from line 1 or line 2 to ground. This is detected by the line isolation monitor, which sounds an alarm. The faulty piece of equipment does not present a shock hazard but converts the isolated power system into a grounded power system.

    3. If the faulty piece of equipment is not essential, it should be removed from the operating room for repair. If it is a vital piece of life support equipment, it can be safely used, but no other piece of electrical equipment should be connected during the remainder of the case or until the faulty piece of equipment can be removed.

    4. The line isolation monitor is not designed to provide protection from microshock.

VI. GROUND FAULT CIRCUIT INTERRUPTER

  A. The ground fault circuit interrupter (circuit breaker) is used to prevent individuals from receiving an electrical shock in a grounded power system. (It monitors both sides of the circuit for equality of current flow, and if a difference is detected, the power is immediately interrupted.)

  B. The disadvantage of using a ground fault circuit interrupter in the operating room is that it interrupts the power without warning. A defective piece of equipment can no longer be used, which might be a problem if it were necessary for life support.

VII. DOUBLE ISOLATION

This applies to equipment that has a two-prong plug (infusion pumps) and is permissible to use in the operating room with an isolated power system.

VIII. MICROSHOCK

A. In an electrically susceptible patient (one who has a direct external connection to the heart such as a CVP catheter or transvenous pacing wires), VF can be produced by a current that is below the threshold of human perception (1 mA).

B. The stray capacitance that is part of any alternating current–powered electrical instrument may result in significant amounts of charge build-up on the case of the instrument.

1. An individual who simultaneously touches the case of this instrument and an electrically susceptible patient may unknowingly cause a discharge to the patient that results in VF.

2. An intact equipment ground wire provides a low-resistance pathway for leakage current and constitutes the major source of protection against microshock in electrically susceptible patients.

3. The anesthesiologist should never simultaneously touch an electrical device and a saline-filled CVP catheter or external pacing wires. Rubber gloves should be worn.

4. Modern patient monitors are designed to electrically isolate all direct patient connections from the power supply of the monitor by placing a very high impedance between the patient and the device (this limits the amount of internal leakage through the patient connection to <0.01 mA).

C. The objective of electrical safety is to make it difficult for electrical current to pass through people. Patients and anesthesiologists should be isolated from the ground as much as possible.

1. The isolation transformer is used to convert grounded power to ungrounded power. The line isolation monitor warns that isolation of the power from the ground has been lost in the event that a defective piece of equipment has been plugged into one of the isolated circuit outlets.

2. All equipment that is plugged into the isolated power system has an equipment ground wire that provides an alternative low-resistance pathway enabling potentially dangerous currents (macroshock) to flow to the ground. The ground wire also dissipates leakage currents and protects against microshock in electrically susceptible patients.

3. All electrical equipment must undergo routine maintenance, service, and inspection to ensure that it conforms to designated electrical safety standards. Records of the routine maintenance service must be kept.

4. Electrical power cords should be located overhead or placed in areas of low traffic because they are subject to being crushed if they are left on the floor.

5. Multiple-plug extension boxes should not be left on the floor where they can come in contact with electrolyte solutions.

IX. ELECTROSURGERY

A. The electrosurgical unit (ESU), invented by Professor William T. Bovie, operates by generating high-frequency currents (radiofrequency range). Heat is generated whenever a current passes through a resistance. By concentrating the energy at the tip of the "Bovie pencil," the surgeon can accomplish either therapeutic cutting or coagulation.

1. High-frequency currents have a low tissue penetration and do not excite contractile cells. (Direct contact with the heart does not cause VF.)

2. High-frequency electrical energy generated by the ESU interferes with signals from physiologic monitors.

B. The ESU cannot be safely operated unless the energy is properly routed from the unit through the patient and back to the unit via a large surface area dispersive electrode (often erroneously referred to as the "ground plate") (Fig. 8-6).

1. Because the area of the return plate is large, the current density is low, and no harmful heat or tissue destruction occurs.

2. If the return plate is improperly applied to the patient or if the cord connecting the return plate to the ESU is broken, the high-frequency electrical current will seek an alternate return path (electroencephalographic leads, temperature probe), possibly resulting in a serious burn

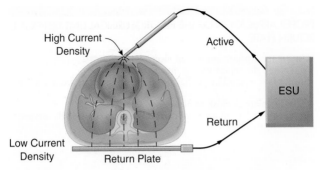

FIGURE 8-6. A properly applied electrosurgical unit (ESU) return plate. The current density at the return plate is low, resulting in no danger to the patient.

to the patient at this return site because high-current density generates heat (Fig. 8-7).

3. In most modern ESUs, the power supply is isolated from the ground to protect the patient from burns by eliminating alternate return pathways. The isolated ESU does not protect the patient from burns if the return electrode does not make proper contact with the patient.

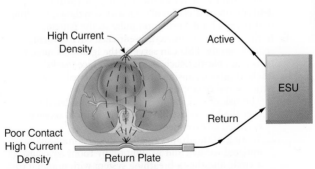

FIGURE 8-7. An improperly applied electrosurgical unit (ESU) return plate. Poor contact with the return plate results in a high current density (heat) and a possible burn to the patient.

SCIENTIFIC FOUNDATIONS

TABLE 8-1

PROPER APPLICATION OF THE ELECTROSURGICAL UNIT DISPERSIVE RETURN PLATE

Use an appropriate amount of electrolyte gel.
Make sure the return wire is intact.
Ensure that electrolyte gel has not dried on the plate from a prior use.
Place the plate as close as possible to operative site.
If the patient has an artificial cardiac pacemaker, place the plate below the thorax.

4. The most important factor in preventing patient burns from the ESU is proper application of the return plate (Table 8-1).
5. The need for higher than normal settings should initiate an inspection of the return plate and cable.
C. In a bipolar ESU, the current passes only between the two blades of a pair of forceps.
   1. Because the active and return electrodes are the two blades of the forceps, it is not necessary to attach another dispersive electrode to the patient.
   2. The bipolar ESU generates less power than the unipolar ESU and is mainly used for ophthalmic and neurologic surgery.
D. The use of a unipolar ESU (also electroconvulsive therapy) may cause electrical interference, which may be interpreted by an automatic implantable cardioverter-defibrillator as a ventricular tachydysrhythmia, resulting in delivery of a defibrillation pulse to the patient.
E. In the presence of an oxygen-enriched environment, a spark from the ESU can serve as the ignition source for fuels (e.g., plastics such as anesthesia face masks, tracheal tubes), causing fires with associated injuries to patients and operating room personnel.
   1. The risk of surgical fires should be considered whenever the ESU is used in close proximity to oxygen-enriched environments.
   2. Tenting of the drapes to allow dispersion of any accumulated oxygen and its dilution by room air or use of a circle anesthesia breathing system with minimal to no leak of gases around the anesthesia mask will decrease the risk of ignition from a spark generated by an ESU.

F. **Conductive flooring** is not necessary in anesthetizing areas where flammable anesthetics are not used.

X. ENVIRONMENTAL HAZARDS

A. Potential hazards in the operating room include electrical shock to the patient and operating room personnel and the presence of cables and power cords to electrical equipment and monitoring devices (ceiling mounts).

B. Modern monitoring devices include an isolated patient input from the power supply of the device.

C. All health care facilities are required to have a source of emergency power (electrical generators; battery-operated light sources, including laryngoscopes).

XI. ELECTROMAGNETIC INTERFERENCE

A. Wireless communication devices (cellular telephones, cordless telephones, walkie-talkies) emit electromagnetic interference (EMI).

B. There is concern that EMI may interfere with implanted pacemakers or various types of monitoring devices in critical care areas.

1. Cellular telephones should be kept at least 15 cm from a pacemaker.

2. Cellular telephones do not seem to interfere with automatic implantable cardioverter-defibrillators.

XII. CONSTRUCTION OF NEW OPERATING ROOMS

A. The National Fire Protection Association standards for health care facilities no longer require isolated power systems or line isolation monitors in areas designated for use of only nonflammable anesthetics.

B. The decision to install isolated power is determined by whether the operating room is a wet location (presence of blood, fluid, saline solutions) and, if so, whether an interruptible power supply is acceptable,

1. When power interruption is acceptable, a ground fault circuit interrupter is permitted as a protective means.

2. When power interruption would be unacceptable, an isolated power system and a line isolation monitor are preferred.

SCIENTIFIC FOUNDATIONS

XIII. FIRE SAFETY

A. Fires in the operating room are just as much a danger today as they were 100 years ago when patients were anesthetized with flammable anesthetic agents (Table 8-2). However, in contrast to situations during the era of flammable anesthetics, today there appears to be a lack of awareness of the potential for operating room fires (Table 8-3).

B. Dangers of fires are burns to patients and operating room personnel and release of toxic compounds (e.g., carbon monoxide, ammonia, hydrogen chloride, cyanide) when plastics burn.

1. Laser-resistant endotracheal tubes may act as a blowtorch type of flame, resulting in severe injury to the trachea and lungs.

2. Leakage of gases around an uncuffed tube in the presence of the ESU can ignite flammable endotracheal tubes. The risk can be minimized by keeping the inspired oxygen concentration as low as possible.

3. In critically ill patients requiring high concentrations of oxygen during a surgical tracheostomy, it may be prudent not to use the ESU.

TABLE 8-2

THE FIRE TRIAD: ELEMENTS NECESSARY FOR A FIRE TO START

Heat (Ignition Source)
Electrical surgical unit
Lasers
Electrical tools
Fiberoptic light cords

Fuel
Prep agents (alcohol)
Paper drapes
Hair
Alimentary gases
Ointments
Anesthesia equipment (e.g., breathing circuit hoses, masks, endotracheal tubes, laryngeal mask airways, volatile anesthetics, carbon dioxide absorbents)

Oxidizer
Air
Oxygen
Nitrous oxide

TABLE 8-3

RECOMMENDATIONS FOR THE PREVENTION AND MANAGEMENT OF OPERATING ROOM FIRES

Preparation
Determine if a high-risk situation exists.
The team determines how to prevent and manage fires.
Each person is given a task (e.g., remove endotracheal tube, disconnect circuit).
Display fire management protocol.
Ensure that fire management equipment is readily available.

Prevention
The anesthesiologist collaborates with the team throughout the procedure to minimize an oxidizer-enriched environment near the ignition source.
Surgical drapes are configured properly to avoid build-up of oxidizer.
Allow flammable skin preps to dry before draping.
Moisten gauze and sponges that are near an ignition source.
Notify the surgeon if an oxidizer and the ignition source are in close proximity.
Keep oxygen concentrations as low as clinically possible.
Avoid nitrous oxide.
Allow increases in time for the oxidizer to dissipate.

Management
Look for early warning signs of a fire (e.g., pop, flash, smoke).
Stop the procedure; each team member immediately carries out his or her assigned task.

Airway Fire
Simultaneously remove the endotracheal tube and stop gas delivery or disconnect the circuit.
Pour saline into the airway.
Remove burning materials.
Mask ventilate, assess the injury, consider bronchoscopy, and reintubate the patient's trachea.

Fire on the Patient
Turn off gases.
Remove drapes and burning materials.
Extinguish flames with water, saline, or a fire extinguisher.
Assess the patient's status, devise a care plan, and assess for smoke inhalation.

Failure to Extinguish
Use a carbon dioxide fire extinguisher.
Activate the fire alarm.
Consider evacuation of the room (close the door and do not reopen).
Turn off medical gases to the room.

SCIENTIFIC FOUNDATIONS

(continued)

TABLE 8-3

RECOMMENDATIONS FOR THE PREVENTION AND MANAGEMENT OF OPERATING ROOM FIRES *(Continued)*

Risk Management
Preserve the scene.
Notify the hospital risk manager.
Follow local regulatory reporting requirements.
Treat the fire as an adverse event.
Conduct fire drills.

Adapted from American Society of Anesthesiologists: Practice advisory for the prevention and management of operating room fires: A Report by the American Society of Anesthesiologists Task Force on Operating Room Fires. *Anesthesiology* 2008; 108:786–801.

4. Diffusion of nitrous oxide into the abdomen may create a fire hazard during laparoscopic surgery; carbon dioxide will not support combustion.

C. Fires on the patient are most likely during surgery in and around the head and neck where the patient is receiving monitored anesthesia care and supplemental oxygen (facemask or nasal cannulae).

1. Oxygen should be treated as a drug and administered to provide optimum benefits (e.g., titrated to the desired level).

2. Tenting the drapes and using adhesive sticky drape that seals the operative site from the oxygen flow reduce the risk of a fire.

3. Pooling of prep solutions may result in alcohol vapors that are flammable.

D. Desiccated carbon dioxide absorbents in the presence of volatile anesthetics (especially sevoflurane) may result in an exothermic reaction. (Fires may occur involving the breathing circuit.)

E. If a fire occurs, the first step is to interrupt the fire triad by removing one of the components. This is best accomplished by removing the oxidizer (Table 8-3).

1. Disconnecting a burning endotracheal tube from the anesthetic circuit usually results in extinguishing the fire. (It is not recommended to remove a burning endotracheal tube because doing so may cause even greater harm to the patient.)

2. When the endotracheal tube fire has been extinguished, it is safe to remove the tracheal tube

and inspect the patient's airway by bronchoscopy followed by reintubation.
3. If the fire is on the patient, extinguishing it with a basin of saline is a rapid and effective intervention.
   a. Paper drapes are impervious to water, so throwing water or saline on them is likely to be ineffective.
   b. After removing the burning drapes from the patient, the flame should be extinguished with a fire extinguisher.
F. Prep solutions with alcohol should be dry before surgery begins.

CHAPTER 9 ■ EXPERIMENTAL DESIGN AND STATISTICS

Practitioners of scientific medicine must be able to read the language of science to independently assess and interpret the scientific literature and the increasing emphasis on statistical methods (Pace NL: Experimental design and statistics. In *Clinical Anesthesia*. Edited by Barash PG, Cullen BF, Stoelting RK, Cahalan MK, Stock MC. Philadelphia: Lippincott Williams & Wilkins, 2009, pp 192–206).

I. DESIGN OF RESEARCH STUDIES

A **case report** engenders interest and the desire to experiment but does not provide sufficient evidence to advance scientific medicine.

A. **Sampling**
   1. A **sample** is a subset of a **target population** that is intended to allow the researcher to generalize the results of the small sample to the entire population. The elements of experimental design are intended to prevent and minimize the possibility of bias.
   2. The best hope for a representative sample of the population would be realized if every subject in the population had the same chance of being in the experiment (**random sampling**). However, most clinical anesthesia studies are limited to using patients who are available (**convenience sampling**).

B. **Control groups** may be self-control or parallel control groups versus historical control groups. (Studies using historical controls are more likely than those using self-controls or parallel controls to show a benefit from a new therapy.)

C. **Random allocation of treatment groups** is helpful to avoid research bias in entering patients into specific study groups. Random allocation is most commonly accomplished by computer-generated random numbers.

D. **Blinding** refers to masking from the view of both the patient and experimenter the experimental group to which the subject has been assigned.
  1. In a single-blind study, the patient is unaware of the treatment given. (Patient expectations from a treatment could influence results.)
  2. In a double-blind study, the subject and the data collector are unaware of the treatment group. This is the best way to test a new therapy.
E. **Types of Research Design**
  1. **Longitudinal studies** evaluate changes over time using research subjects chosen **prospectively** (cohort) or **retrospectively** (case-control). Retrospective studies are a primary tool of epidemiology.
  2. **Cross-sectional studies** evaluate changes at a certain point in time.

II. DATA AND DESCRIPTIVE STATISTICS

A. Statistics is a method for working with sets of numbers (X and Y) and determining if the values are different. Statistical methods are necessary because there are sources of variation in any data set, including random biologic variation and measurement error. These errors make it difficult to avoid bias and to be precise.
B. **Data Structure.** Properly assigning a variable to the correct data type is essential for choosing the correct statistical technique (Table 9-1).
C. **Descriptive statistics** are intended to describe the sample of numbers obtained and to characterize the population from which the sample was obtained. The two summary statistics most frequently used are the **central location** and **spread** or **variability** (Table 9-2).

III. HYPOTHESES AND PARAMETERS

A. **Hypothesis Formulation**
  1. The researcher starts the work with some intuitive feel for the phenomenon to be studied (biologic hypothesis).
  2. The biologic hypothesis becomes a statistical hypothesis during research planning.
B. **Logic of Proof**
  1. If sample values are sufficiently unlikely to have occurred by chance (alpha [p] < 0.05), the **null**

TABLE 9-1
DATA TYPES

Data Types	Definition	Examples
Interval		
Discrete	Data measured with an integer-only scale	Parity Number of teeth
Continuous	Data measured with a constant scale interval	Blood pressure Temperature
Categorical		
Dichotomous	Binary data	Mortality Gender
Nominal	Qualitative data that cannot be ordered or ranked	Eye color Drug category
Ordinal	Data are ordered, ranked, or measured without a constant scale interval	ASA physical status score Pain score

ASA = American Society of Anesthesiologists.

     hypothesis (which assumes there is no difference) is rejected.
2. Because statistics deal with probabilities rather than certainties, there is a chance that decisions made concerning the null hypothesis are erroneous.
    a. **A type I (alpha) error** is wrongly rejecting the null hypothesis (false-positive). The smaller the chosen alpha, the smaller the risk of a type I error.
    b. **A type II (beta) error** is failing to reject the null hypothesis (false-negative). Variability in the

TABLE 9-2
DESCRIPTIVE STATISTICS

Central Location for Interval Variables
Arithmetic mean (average of the numbers in the data set)
Median (middle most number or number that divides the samples into two equal parts; not affected by very high or low numbers)
Mode (number in a sample that appears most frequently)

Spread or Variability
Standard deviation (SD; approximates the spread of the sample data; 1 SD encompasses roughly 68% of the sample and population members, and 3 SDs encompass 99%)

Confidence Intervals
Standard error of the mean (approximates the precision with which the population center is known)

TABLE 9-3

INFORMATION NECESSARY TO ACCEPT OR REJECT THE
NULL HYPOTHESIS

Confirm that experimental data conform to the assumptions of
the intended statistical test.
Choose a significance level (alpha).
Calculate the test statistic.
Determine the degree(s) of freedom.
Find the critical value for the chosen alpha and the degree(s) of
freedom from the appropriate theoretical probability
distribution.
If the test statistic exceeds the critical value, reject the null
hypothesis.
If the test statistic does not exceed the critical value, do not reject
the null hypothesis.

population increases the chance of type II error.
Increasing the number of subjects (which is very
important in research design for controlled clinical
trials), raising the alpha value, and dealing with
large differences between two conditions decrease
the chances of a type II error.

C. **Inferential Statistics.** The testing of hypotheses or significance testing is the main focus of inferential statistics
(Table 9-3).

IV. STATISTICAL TESTS AND MODELS

A. General guidelines relate the variable type and the experimental design to the choice of statistical test (Table 9-4).

B. **t Test.** The Student's *t* test is used to compare the values
of the means of two populations. The **paired *t* test** is
used when each subject serves as his or her own control
(before and after measurements in the same patient
decrease variability and increase statistical power). An
unpaired *t* test is used when measurements are taken on
two groups of subjects.

C. **Analysis of Variance**
   1. The most versatile approach for handling
      comparisons of means among more than two groups
      is called the **analysis of variance** (ANOVA).
   2. For parametric statistics (*t* tests and ANOVA), it is
      assumed that the populations follow the normal
      distribution.

TABLE 9-4

GUIDELINES FOR WHICH STATISTICAL TEST TO USE

Variable Type	One-Sample Tests	Two-Sample Tests	Multiple-Sample T
Dichotomous or nominal	Binomial distribution	Chi-square test, Fisher's exact test	Chi-square test
Ordinal	Chi-square test	Chi-square test, nonparametric tests	Chi-square test, nonparametric tests
Continuous or discrete	z or t distribution	Unpaired t test, paired t test, nonparametric tests	ANOVA, nonparametric analysis of variance

ANOVA = analysis of variance.

D. **Robustness and nonparametric tests can** be used when there is concern that the populations do not follow a normal distribution.

E. **Systematic Reviews and Meta-Analyses.** To answer the experimental question, data are obtained from controlled trials (usually randomized) in the medical literature rather than from newly conducted clinical trials.
   1. The American Society of Anesthesiologists has developed a process for the creation of practice parameters that include a variant form of systematic reviews.

F. **Linear Regression.** Often the goal of the experiment is to predict the value of one characteristic from knowledge of another characteristic using **regression analysis.**

G. **Interpretation of Results**
   1. Scientific studies do not end with the statistical test. (Statistical significance does not always equate with biologic relevance.)
   2. Even small, clinically unimportant differences between groups can be detected if the sample size is sufficiently large. If the sample size is small, there is a greater chance that confounding variables may explain any difference.
   3. If the experimental groups in a properly designed study are given three or more doses of a drug, the reader should expect to observe a steadily increasing or decreasing dose–response relationship.

TABLE 9-5

STRENGTH OF EVIDENCE (INCREASING ORDER)
CONCERNING EFFICACY

Case report
Retrospective study
Prospective study with historical controls
Randomized and controlled clinical trial
Series of randomized and controlled clinical trials

4. In comparing alternative therapies, the confidence
that a claim for a superior therapy is true depends on
the study design (Table 9-5).

V. CONCLUSIONS

A. **Guidelines for Reading Journal Articles**
1. Clinicians with limited time should select journal
articles to read that are relevant (determined by the
specifics of one's anesthetic practice) and credible
(function of the merits of the research methods).
2. Although the statistical knowledge of most physicians
is limited, these skills of critical appraisal of the literature can be learned and can greatly increase the efficiency and benefit of journal reading.
B. **Statistics and Anesthesia.** Understanding the principles
of experimental design can prevent premature
acceptance of new therapies from faulty studies.

SCIENTIFIC FOUNDATIONS

CHAPTER 10 ■ CARDIOVASCULAR ANATOMY AND PHYSIOLOGY

I. **INTRODUCTION** (Kampine JP, Stowe DF, Pagel PS: Heart and peripheral circulation. In *Clinical Anesthesia*. Edited by Barash PG, Cullen BF, Stoelting RK, Cahalan MK, Stock MC. Philadelphia: Lippincott Williams and Wilkins, 2009, pp 207–232).

A. **Functional Anatomy of the Heart**

1. Synchronous contraction of the left ventricular (LV) muscles shortens the long axis of the heart, decreases the circumference of the LV, and lifts the apex toward the anterior chest wall. This action produces the familiar palpable point of maximum impulse, which is normally located in the fifth or sixth intercostal space in the mid-clavicular line.

2. The pulmonary circulation is a low-pressure, low-resistance system into which the right ventricle (RV) transfers blood.

3. During contraction, LV pressure increases from end-diastolic values of 10 to 12 mm Hg to a peak pressure of 120 to 140 mm Hg during systole. The peak pressures generated by the LV reflect the requirement to circulate blood through the high resistance systemic circulation.

4. Efficient pumping action of the heart requires two pairs of unidirectional valves. One pair is located at the outlets of the RV and LV (pulmonic and aortic valves, respectively). The atrioventricular (AV) valves separating the atria from the ventricles are the tricuspid and mitral valve on the right and left sides of the heart, respectively.

5. The RV and LV are the major cardiac pumping chambers, but the atria play a critically important supporting roles. The atria function as reservoirs, conduits,

and contractile chambers and facilitate the transition between continuous, low-pressure venous to phasic, high-pressure arterial blood flow. When atrial contraction is absent or ineffective (e.g., in atrial failure, atrial fibrillation or flutter), the heart may be capable of compensating for the loss of the atrial contractile function and continue to function effectively under resting conditions.

B. **The Cardiac Cycle**

1. LV systole is commonly divided into the isovolumic contraction, rapid ejection, and slower ejection phases. Closure of both the tricuspid and mitral valves occurs when RV and LV pressures exceed corresponding atrial pressure and cause the source of the first heart sound (Fig. 10-1).

2. The normal LV end-diastolic volume is about 120 mL. The average ejected stroke volume is 80 mL, and the normal ejection fraction (EF) is approximately 67%. A decrease in EF below 40% is typically observed when the myocardium is affected by ischemia, infarction, or cardiomyopathic disease processes.

3. Disease processes known to reduce LV compliance (myocardial ischemia, pressure-overload hypertrophy) attenuate early filling and increase the importance of atrial systole to overall LV filling.

4. Diastolic dysfunction may independently cause heart failure, even in the presence of relatively normal contractile function. This "heart failure with normal systolic function" has been increasingly recognized as a major underlying cause of congestive heart failure.

C. **Determinants of Cardiac Output**

1. Cardiac output is the product of heart rate and stroke volume and may be normalized to the body surface area (cardiac index).

2. Cardiac output is a function of preload, afterload, myocardial contractility (inotropic state), and heart rate.

3. Systemic vascular resistance (the ratio of driving pressure to cardiac output) is the most commonly used nonparametric expression of peripheral resistance and is primarily affected by autonomic nervous system activity.

ANATOMY AND PHYSIOLOGY

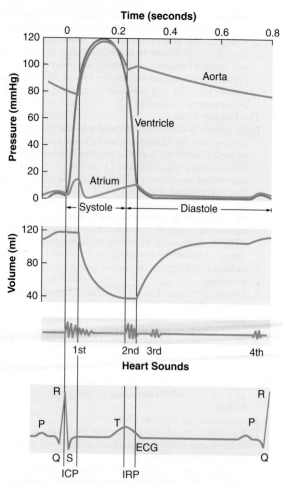

FIGURE 10-1.   Mechanical and electrical events of the cardiac cycle showing also the ventricular volume curve and the heart sounds. Note the isovolumic contraction (ICP) and the relaxation period (IRP) during which there is no change in ventricular volume because all valves are closed. The ventricle decreases in volume as it ejects its contents into the aorta. During the first third of systolic ejection (the rapid ejection period), the curve of emptying is steep. ECG = electrocardiogram.

4. The inotropic state is the intrinsic force of myocardial contraction independent of changes in preload, afterload, or heart rate.

5. The primary determinant of myocardial oxygen consumption is heart rate because the more frequently the heart performs pressure-volume work, the more oxygen must be consumed. At high heart rates, particularly in patients with heart disease, there may not be adequate diastolic filling time to maintain cardiac output and coronary artery perfusion (which is highly dependent on the duration of diastole). Such events may cause acute myocardial ischemia or infarction.

D. **Measures of Cardiac Function**

1. Clinical indicators of contractile performance include cardiac output, EF, fractional shortening or area change of the LV short axis, and LV systolic wall thickening.

2. These indices of contractility are dependent on heart rate, preload, and afterload but nevertheless may be measured with reasonable reliability using echocardiographic techniques and remain useful indices of contractile performance.

II. CELLULAR AND MOLECULAR BIOLOGY OF CARDIAC MUSCLE FUNCTION

A. **Ultrastructure of the Cardiac Myocyte.** The heart contracts and relaxes nearly 3 billion times during an average lifetime (heart rate, 70 bpm; life expectancy, 75 years). A review of cardiac myocyte ultrastructure provides important insights into how the heart accomplishes this astonishing performance.

B. **Proteins of the Contractile Apparatus.** Myosin, actin, tropomyosin, and the three-protein troponin complex make up the six major components of the contractile apparatus.

C. **Calcium–Myofilament Interaction.** Binding of calcium to troponin C precipitates a series of conformational changes in the troponin–tropomyosin complex that lead to the exposure of the myosin-binding site on the actin molecule.

D. **Myosin–Actin Contraction Biochemistry.** The biochemistry of cardiac muscle contraction is most often described using a simplified four-component model (Fig. 10-2).

ANATOMY AND PHYSIOLOGY

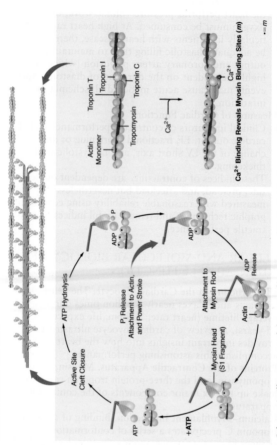

FIGURE 10-2. Schematic illustration of the actin filaments and its individual monomers and active myosin binding sites (m; *left panel*). The myosin head is dissociated from actin by binding with adenosine triphosphate (ATP). Subsequent ATP hydrolysis and release of inorganic phosphate (Pi) "cocks" the head group into a tension-generating configuration. Attachment of the myosin head to actin allows the head to apply tension to the myosin rod and the actin filament. The *right panel* illustrates calcium binding to troponin C, which causes its affinity for actin. As a result in a conformational shift in tropomyosin position (see text), seven sites on actin monomers are revealed. ADP = adenosine diphosphate.

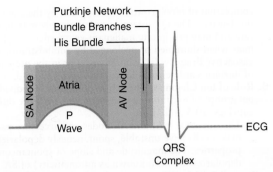

FIGURE 10-3. Major waves (P, QRS, and T) of the electrocardiogram are indicated as well as the timing of the activation of some of the key conductive structures. AV = atrioventricular; SA = sinoatrial.

III. ELECTRICAL PROPERTIES OF THE HEART

A. **The clinical electrocardiogram** (ECG) consists of a regular series of deflections from the isoelectric line. The first deflection of the ECG is the P-wave. (Figs. 10-3 and 10-4). (Einthoven, who developed the system, began his depiction of the ECG in the middle of the alphabet.) The QT interval is the duration between the onset of ventricular depolarization (indicated by the QRS complex) and

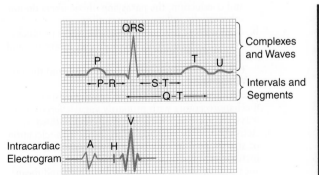

FIGURE 10-4. *Top*: Electrocardiogram (ECG) recorded from the body surface. *Bottom*: Intracardiac ECG.

completion of repolarization (as signified by the end of the T-wave). The QT interval varies inversely with heart rate and may precipitate malignant ventricular arrhythmias when shortened or prolonged by administration of vasoactive drugs (volatile anesthetics) or in the presence of intrinsic cardiac pathology (prolonged QT syndrome).

B. **Role of Ion Channels.** The action potentials of individual groups of excitable cardiac myocytes are quite different (Figs. 10-5 and 10-6).

1. The sinoatrial (SA) and AV nodes and accessory pacemaker cells have unstable, spontaneously depolarizing properties. The magnitude and slope of spontaneous depolarization (also known as automaticity) of SA node cells are important in the regulation of heart rate and are dependent on sympathetic and vagal (parasympathetic) neural innervation and activity.

2. The SA node pacemaker may be displaced by a latent pacemaker elsewhere in the heart during myocardial ischemia because of primary suppression of the SA node or because of spontaneous discharge of a latent pacemaker at a higher intrinsic rate.

IV. NEURAL INNERVATION OF THE HEART AND BLOOD VESSELS

A. **Baroreflex Regulation of Blood Pressure**

1. The heart is innervated by the parasympathetic and sympathetic nervous systems.

   a. Aside from their effects on heart rate, excitability, and conduction, the parasympathetic fibers do not substantially influence contractility.

   b. Activation of cardiac sympathetic fibers produces positive chronotropic, dromotropic, inotropic, and lusitropic effects (increases in heart rate, conduction velocity, myocardial contractility, and the rate of myofibrillar relaxation).

2. The afferent innervation of the heart consists of mechanoreceptors with primarily vagal afferent pathways and receptors with spinal afferent pathways.

3. Activation of the ventricular receptors by nociception or stretch, such as may occur in response to a sudden increase in ventricular volume, causes a vagal depressor response with a decrease in heart rate and mean arterial pressure (MAP; Bezold-Jarisch reflex).

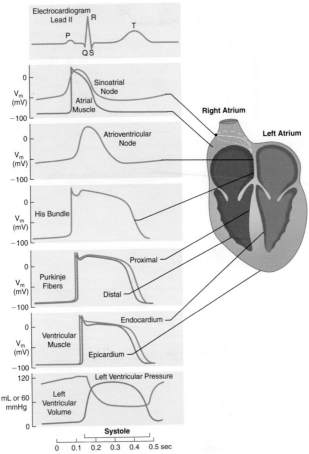

FIGURE 10-5. Cardiac action potentials throughout the conductance system from the sinoatrial (SA) node through the ventricular muscle during one cardiac cycle. Note the automatic pacemaker activity (slow, spontaneous depolarization) of the SA and atrioventricular (AV) nodal cells and the lack of spontaneous activity of atrial, Purkinje, and ventricular muscle cells. ECG = electrocardiogram; LV = left ventricle.

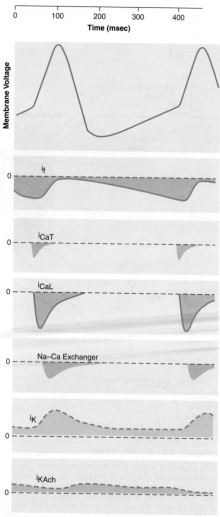

FIGURE 10-6. Changes in four ionic currents responsible for action potential (AP) depolarization and repolarization in a sinoatrial (SA) nodal pacemaker cell. Two are increasing inward currents (ii and iCa), and two are decreasing outward currents (delayed rectifier [iK] and inward rectifier [iK1]).

B. **Other Cardiovascular Reflexes.** Other reflexogenic areas within the cardiovascular system regulate hemodynamics through arterial chemoreceptors and the central nervous system (CNS) response to ischemia.

1. In addition to the baroreceptor responses, severe hypotension also causes arterial vaso- and venoconstriction in response to brainstem hypoxia. This CNS ischemic response may be activated when MAP is reduced below 50 mm Hg.

2. Somatic pain increases heart rate and MAP by activation of sympathetic efferent nerves. In contrast, visceral pain or distention of a hollow viscus (small intestine, bladder) may produce reflex vagal bradycardia and hypotension.

3. The oculocardiac reflex is activated by pressure on the ocular globe and causes pronounced bradycardia and hypotension by activation of vagal nerve fibers innervating the SA node.

4. The Valsalva maneuver consists of forced expiration against a closed glottis. This maneuver reduces venous return to the right heart, decreases cardiac output and MAP, and increases heart rate.

V. THE CORONARY CIRCULATION

A. **Anatomy of the Coronary Arterial and Venous Systems.** The heart is the only organ that furnishes its own blood supply (Fig. 10-7).

B. **Coronary Microcirculation.** As in other capillary beds, the coronary capillaries are the sites for exchange of O_2 and CO_2 and for the movement of larger molecules across the endothelial cell lining, where it is devoid of vascular smooth muscle.

C. **Mechanics of Coronary Blood Flow**

1. Blood supply to the LV is directly dependent on the difference between the aortic pressure and LV end-diastolic pressure (coronary perfusion pressure) and inversely related to the vascular resistance to flow, which varies to the fourth power of the radius of the vessel (Poiseuille's law). Two other determinants of coronary flow are vessel length and viscosity of the blood, but these factors are generally constant.

2. Resting coronary blood flow in adults is approximately 250 mL/min (1 mL/g), representing approximately 5% of the cardiac output.

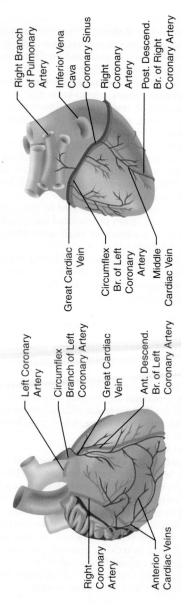

FIGURE 10-7. The anterior view (*left*) shows the right coronary and left anterior descending arteries. The posterior view (*right*) shows the left circumflex and posterior descending arteries. Note that the right coronary or left circumflex artery may form the latter artery. The anterior cardiac veins from the right ventricle and the coronary sinus, which primarily drain the left ventricle, empty into the right atrium.

3. Aortic pressure is slightly less than LV pressure during systole. As a result, blood flow in the LV subendocardium occurs only during diastole (Fig. 10-8). Coronary blood flow is also compromised when aortic diastolic pressure is reduced (severe aortic insufficiency).

4. In contrast to left coronary blood flow, right coronary artery flow is continuous throughout the cardiac cycle because the lower pressure in the RV compared with the LV causes substantially less extravascular compression (Fig. 10-8).

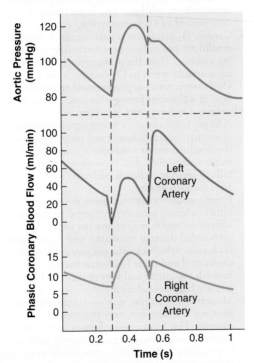

FIGURE 10-8. Schematic representation of blood flow in the left and right coronary arteries during phases of the cardiac cycle. Note that most left coronary flow occurs during diastole, and right coronary flow (and coronary sinus flow) occurs mostly during late systole and early diastole.

D. **Regulation of Coronary Blood Flow.** The two major determinants of coronary blood flow (perfusion pressure and vascular resistance) vary substantially during the cardiac cycle. However, metabolic factors are the major physiologic determinants of coronary vascular tone and hence myocardial perfusion.

E. **Oxygen Delivery and Demand**
   1. The heart normally extracts between 75% and 80% of arterial O_2 content, by far the greatest O_2 extraction of all organs.
   2. The majority of O_2 demand is derived from the increase in LV pressure during isovolumic contraction.
   3. An increase in myocardial contractility enhances O_2 consumption, but heart rate is the primary determinant of O_2 consumption.
   4. Cardiac O_2 extraction is near maximal under resting conditions and cannot be substantially increased during exercise. Thus, the primary mechanism by which myocardium meets its O_2 demand is through enhanced O_2 delivery, which is proportional to coronary blood flow at a constant hemoglobin concentration.

F. **Myocardial Ischemia and Infarction**
   1. A large, acute coronary artery occlusion produces acute myocardial ischemia and often contributes to the development of a malignant ventricular arrhythmia because blood flow through coronary collaterals fails to provide sufficient perfusion to the ischemic zone (sudden death).
   2. If the coronary artery occlusion develops more slowly (atherosclerotic plaques), collateral formation in the watershed region may reduce the degree of myocardial damage associated with acute coronary occlusion. Atherosclerotic plaques are composed of cholesterol and other lipids that become deposited beneath the intima and fibrous tissue, which also frequently becomes calcified.
   3. Myocardial infarction may also occur without evidence of major coronary thromboses, emboli, or stenosis. This form of infarction is caused by excessive metabolic demands resulting from severe LV hypertrophy (critical aortic stenosis) or vasoactive drug ingestion (amphetamines, cocaine) or may also result from coronary artery vasospasm.
   4. Despite past arguments to the contrary, the vast majority of experimental and clinical evidence

collected to date indicates that volatile anesthetics do not cause coronary artery steal unless profound hypotension (<50 mm Hg) is present. Volatile anesthetics are not potent vasodilators, unlike drugs such as adenosine and sodium nitroprusside that are known to produce coronary artery steal.

VI. THE PULMONARY CIRCULATION

A. **Comparison with the Systemic Circulation.** The pulmonary circulation receives the blood pumped by the RV. Total pulmonary blood flow is equivalent to cardiac output. There are major differences in hemodynamics between the systemic and pulmonary circulations (Fig. 10-9).

B. **Regional Differences in Perfusion and V/Q Matching** (Fig 10-10).

C. **Hypoxic Pulmonary Vasoconstriction.** Pulmonary arteriolar vasoconstriction triggered by hypoxia shunts blood flow away from poorly to well-ventilated regions of the lung, thereby improving arterial O_2 saturation.

D. **Physiologic Modulation of the Pulmonary Circulation.** The blood volume stored in the pulmonary circulation is substantial (≥900 mL), and when combined with the blood volume contained within the heart and proximal great vessels, this pulmonary blood volume provides a crucial, rapidly available source of reserve intravascular volume during acute, massive hemorrhage.

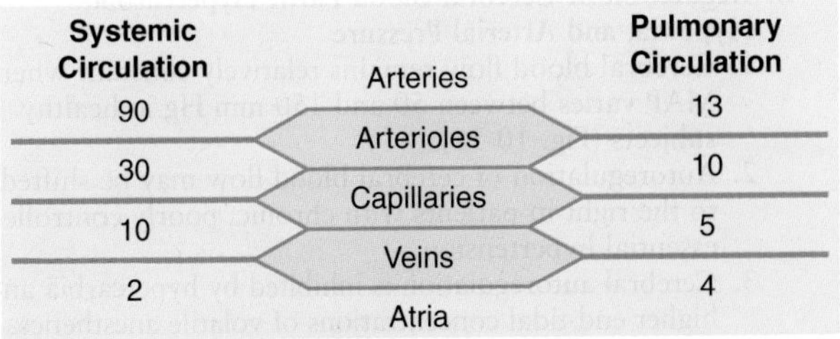

Systemic Circulation		Pulmonary Circulation
	Arteries	
90		13
	Arterioles	
30		10
	Capillaries	
10		5
	Veins	
2		4
	Atria	

FIGURE 10-9. Comparison of pressure gradients (in mm Hg) along the high-pressure systemic and low-pressure pulmonary circulation.

Percentage of Lung Volume Studied		Alveolar Ventilation (l./min.)	Pulmonary Blood Flow (l./min.)	Ventilation Perfusion Ratio
25		1.0	0.6	1.7
36		1.8	2.0	0.9
39		2.3	3.4	0.7
100	Total	5.1	6.0	0.85

FIGURE 10-10. Relative ventilation and perfusion (V/Q) distribution in different areas of the lungs (upright position). The *left side* shows the percentage distribution of the total lung volume, and the *right side* shows the alveolar ventilation, pulmonary blood flow, and V/Q ratio of each horizontal slice of lung volume. Note that the upper zone is relative over-ventilated and the lower zone is relatively overperfused.

VII. THE CEREBRAL CIRCULATION

A. Anatomy and Cerebral Autoregulation

1. Blood flow to the brain is provided through the internal carotid and vertebral arteries. The vertebral arteries join to form the basilar artery, which (along with branches of the internal carotid arteries) forms the circle of Willis.

2. The brain is approximately 2% of total body weight, yet this organ receives approximately 15% of cardiac output. This remarkably large cerebral blood flow (45 to 55 mL/100 g/min) reflects the high metabolic rate of the brain. Cerebral blood flow and metabolic rate are closely linked and are approximately four times greater in gray compared with white matter.

B. Regulation of Cerebral Blood Flow: Hypercarbia, Hypoxia, and Arterial Pressure

1. Cerebral blood flow remains relatively constant when MAP varies between 50 and 150 mm Hg in healthy subjects (Fig. 10-11).

2. Autoregulation of cerebral blood flow may be shifted to the right in patients with chronic, poorly controlled essential hypertension.

3. Cerebral autoregulation is inhibited by hypercarbia and higher end-tidal concentrations of volatile anesthetics.

4. Arterial carbon dioxide partial pressure ($PaCO_2$) is a major regulator of cerebral blood flow within the

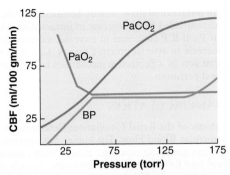

FIGURE 10-11. Cerebral blood flow (CBF) is autoregulated (relatively unchanged) as mean systemic blood pressure increases between 50 to 150 mm Hg. However, CBF is nearly linearly increased with an increase in arterial carbon dioxide partial pressure ($PaCO_2$) and increased if arterial oxygen partial pressure (PaO_2) decreases below 50 mm Hg.

physiologic range of arterial CO_2 tensions. Cerebral blood flow linearly increases 1 to 2 mL/100 g/min for each 1–mm Hg increase in $PaCO_2$ (Fig 10-11).

  a. Alterations in cerebral blood flow produced by changes in $PaCO_2$ are not sustained because bicarbonate is eventually transported out of the brain extracellular fluid, thereby returning pH to a normal value.

  b. In contrast to the effects of respiratory acidosis on cerebral blood flow, the actions of metabolic acidosis are more gradual because the blood–brain barrier is relatively impermeable to H^+.

5. Hypoxia-induced increases in cerebral blood flow occur at PaO_2 values below 60 mm Hg (Fig. 10-11).

6. Neural control of the cerebral circulation plays a relatively minor role in regulation of cerebral blood flow despite the extensive sympathetic nervous system innervation of cerebral blood vessels.

C. **Effects of Increased Intracranial Pressure**

  1. Along with the brain, the cerebral circulation is entirely constrained within the rigid cranial cavity. This unique anatomic arrangement implies that increases in cerebral blood flow must be matched by comparable increases in venous flow from the skull because the volume of blood and extracellular fluid within the brain is relatively constant.

ANATOMY AND PHYSIOLOGY

2. An intracranial mass (tumor, hematoma) is inevitably accompanied by an increase in intracranial pressure (ICP). If ICP continues to increase, a compensatory increase in arterial pressure occurs (Cushing's reflex) that acts as a protective mechanism to maintain cerebral perfusion.

VIII. RENAL CIRCULATION

A. **Anatomy of the Renal Circulation: Determinants of Glomerular Blood Flow.** The kidney has approximately 1 million glomeruli that filter plasma from circulating blood into Bowman's capsule surrounding each glomerulus capillary tuft. The entire glomerular capillary tuft is enveloped by Bowman's capsule, which collects the glomerular filtrate and transports it to the renal tubules, where urine is concentrated.

B. **Renal Hemodynamics**
   1. The MAP in the glomerular capillaries is normally between 50 and 60 mm Hg, which favors the outward filtration of plasma water along the entire length of the capillary loop. Renal blood flow is approximately 20% of cardiac output and is heavily balanced toward perfusion of the renal cortex.
   2. Renal blood flow is very important for the delivery of the large volumes of blood to the glomeruli required for ultrafiltration.
   3. Renal blood flow remains relatively constant between MAP of 75 and 170 mm Hg but becomes pressure dependent beyond this range of autoregulation.
   4. Alterations in afferent arteriole resistance autoregulate glomerular filtration rate by constricting the diameter of afferent arterioles in response to increases in driving pressure.

IX. THE SPLANCHNIC AND HEPATIC CIRCULATION

A. **Regulation of Gastrointestinal Blood Flow**
   1. The intestinal circulation is weakly autoregulated compared with the cerebral, coronary, and renal vascular beds. Intestinal autoregulation appears to be primarily metabolic in origin.
   2. Pronounced sympathetic stimulation during acute hypovolemia produces gastrointestinal arterial

constriction and venoconstriction, thereby shifting blood from a large vascular capacitance bed into the central circulation.

B. **Regulation of Hepatic Blood Flow**
   1. The liver receives approximately 25% of total cardiac output, 75% of which is derived from the portal vein that contains venous blood from the gastrointestinal tract, spleen, and pancreas. The remaining 25% of hepatic blood flow is provided by the hepatic artery, which supplies the majority of O_2 to the liver.
   2. Blood flow in the portal venous and hepatic arterial systems tends to vary reciprocally, but these respective hepatic blood supplies do not fully interact. Thus, a reduction of blood flow in the portal vein may not be fully compensated by an increase in hepatic arterial flow.
   3. The hepatic arterial system (but not the portal venous system) is autoregulated.
   4. The liver contains about 15% of the total blood volume of the body and is an important volume reservoir that may be rapidly mobilized in response to sympathetic nervous system activation during acute hypovolemia.

CHAPTER 11 ■ **RESPIRATORY FUNCTION**

Anesthesiologists directly manipulate pulmonary function, so it is important to have a thorough knowledge of pulmonary physiology for the safe conduct of anesthesia (Ault ML, Stock MC: Respiratory function. In *Clinical Anesthesia*. Edited by Barash PG, Cullen BF, Stoelting RK, Cahalan MK, Stock MC. Philadelphia: Lippincott Williams & Wilkins, 2009, pp 233–255).

I. FUNCTIONAL ANATOMY OF THE LUNGS

A. Muscles of Ventilation
1. The muscles of ventilation are endurance muscles that are adversely affected by poor nutrition, chronic obstructive pulmonary disease (COPD), and increased airway resistance.
2. The primary ventilatory muscle is the diaphragm with minor contributions from the intercostal muscles. The muscles of the abdominal wall are important for expulsive efforts such as coughing.

B. Lung Structures
1. The visceral and parietal pleura are in constant contact, creating a potential intrapleural space in which pressure decreases when the diaphragm descends and the rib cage expands.
2. The lung parenchyma is subdivided into three airway categories based on functional lung anatomy (Table 11-1).
   a. Large airways with diameters of above 2 mm create 90% of total airway resistance.
   b. The number of alveoli increases progressively with age, starting at about 24 million at birth and reaching the final adult count of 300 million by age 8 or 9 years. There is an estimated 70 m^2 of surface area for gas exchange.

TABLE 11-1

FUNCTIONAL AIRWAY DIVISIONS

Type	Function	Structure
Conductive	Bulk gas movement	Trachea to terminal bronchioles
Transitional	Bulk gas movement Limited gas exchange	Respiratory bronchioles Alveolar ducts
Respiratory	Gas exchange	Alveoli Alveolar sacs

    c. The adult trachea is 10 to 12 cm long with an outside diameter of about 20 mm. The cricoid cartilage corresponds to the level of the sixth cervical vertebral body. Both ends of the trachea are attached to mobile structures, and in adults, the carina can move an average of 3.8 cm with flexion and extension of the neck. (This is important in intubated patients.) In children, tracheal tube movement is even more critical because displacement of even 1 cm can move the tube out of the trachea or below the carina.

    d. In adults, the right mainstem bronchus leaves the trachea at approximately 25 degrees from the vertical tracheal axis; the angle of the left mainstem bronchus is approximately 45 degrees. (Therefore, accidental endobronchial intubation or aspiration is more likely to occur on the right side.) In children younger than age 3 years, the angles created by the right and left mainstem bronchi are approximately equal.

    e. The right mainstem bronchus is approximately 2.5 cm long before its initial branching; the left mainstem bronchus is about 4.5 cm. In 2% to 3% of adults, the right upper lobe bronchus opens into the trachea above the carina, which is important to know during placement of a double-lumen tube.

3. **Respiratory Airways and the Alveolar–Capillary Membrane**

    a. The alveolar–capillary membrane is important for transport of alveolar gases (O_2, CO_2) and metabolism of circulating substances.

      b. Type I alveolar cells provide the extensive surface for gas exchange, and these cells are susceptible to injury (e.g., acute respiratory distress syndrome).

      c. Type III alveolar cells are macrophages. They provide protection against infection and participate in the lung inflammatory response.

    4. Pulmonary Vascular Systems

      a. Two major circulatory systems supply blood to the lungs: the pulmonary (which supplies gas exchange and metabolic needs of the alveolar parenchyma) and the bronchial (which supplies O_2 to the conductive airways and pulmonary vessels) vascular networks.

      b. Anatomic connections between the bronchial and pulmonary venous circulations create an absolute shunt of about 2% of the cardiac output ("normal or physiologic shunt").

II. LUNG MECHANICS

Lung movement is entirely passive and responds to forces external to the lungs. (During spontaneous ventilation, the external forces are produced by ventilatory muscles.)

A. Elastic Work

    1. The lung's natural tendency is to collapse (elastic recoil) such that normal expiration at rest is passive.

    2. Surface tension at an air–fluid interface is responsible for keeping alveoli open. (During inspiration, surface tension increases, ensuring that gas tends to flow from larger to smaller alveoli, thereby preventing collapse.)

    3. **Esophageal pressure** is a reflection of the intrapleural pressure and allows an estimation of the patient's work of breathing (i.e., elastic work and resistive work to overcome resistance to gas flow in the airway).

    4. Patients with low lung compliance typically breathe with smaller tidal volumes at more rapid rates. Patients with diseases that increase lung compliance (e.g., gas trapping caused by asthma or COPD) must use the ventilatory muscles to actively exhale.

B. **Resistance to Gas Flow.** Both laminar and turbulent flow exist within the respiratory tract.
   1. **Laminar flow** is not audible and is influenced only by viscosity. Helium has a low density, but its viscosity is close to that of air.
   2. **Turbulent flow** is audible and is almost invariably present when high resistance to gas flow is problematic. (Helium will improve flow.)
C. **Increased Airway Resistance**
   1. The normal response to increased inspiratory resistance is increased inspiratory muscle effort.
   2. The normal response to increased expiratory resistance is use of accessory muscles to force gas from the lungs. Patients who chronically use accessory muscles to exhale are at risk for ventilatory muscle fatigue if they experience an acute increase in ventilatory work, most commonly precipitated by pneumonia or heart failure.
   3. An increased $PaCO_2$ in the setting of increased airway resistance may signal that the patient's compensatory mechanisms are nearly exhausted.
D. **Physiologic Changes in Respiratory Function Associated with Aging** (Table 11-2). Despite changes, the respiratory system is able to maintain adequate gas exchange at rest and during exertion throughout life with only modest decrements in PaO_2 and no change in $PaCO_2$.

TABLE 11-2

PHYSIOLOGIC CHANGES IN RESPIRATORY FUNCTION
ASSOCIATED WITH AGING

Dilation of alveoli
Enlargement of airspaces
Decrease in exchange surface area
Loss of supporting tissue
Decreased lung recoil
Increased functional residual capacity
Decreased chest compliance (increased work of breathing)
Decreased respiratory muscle strength (nutrition, cardiac index)
Decreased expiratory flow rates
Blunted respiratory response to hypoxemia and hypercapnia
  (manifests during heart failure, airway obstruction, pneumonia)

ANATOMY AND PHYSIOLOGY

III. CONTROL OF VENTILATION

Mechanisms that control ventilation are complex, requiring integration of many parts of the central and peripheral nervous systems (Fig. 11-1).

A. **Terminology.** The terms *breathing* (the act of inspiring and exhaling), *ventilation* (movement of gas into and out of the lungs), and *respiration* (occurs when energy is released from organic molecules) are often used interchangeably. Breathing requires energy utilization for muscle work. When spontaneous, ventilation requires energy for muscle work and thus is breathing.

B. **Generation of a Ventilatory Pattern** (Table 11-3)
   1. The medulla oblongata contains the most basic ventilatory control centers in the brain.
   2. The pontine centers process information that originates in the medulla.

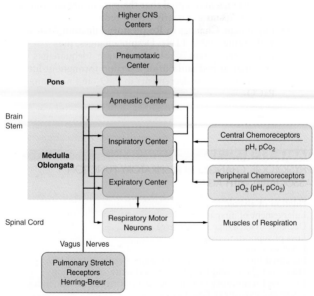

FIGURE 11-1. Diagram of central nervous system respiratory centers, neurofeedback circuits, primary neurohumoral sensory inputs, and mechanical outputs.

TABLE 11-3

DEFINITIONS OF RESPIRATORY TERMS

Term	Definition
Eupnea	Continuous inspiratory and expiratory movement without interruption
Apnea	Cessation of ventilatory effort at passive end-expiration
Apneusis	Cessation of ventilatory effort at end-inspiration
Apneustic ventilation	Apneusis with periodic expiratory spasms
Biot's ventilation	Ventilatory gasps interposed between periods of apnea (agonal ventilation)

   3. The reticular activating system in the midbrain increases the rate and amplitude of ventilation.

   4. The cerebral cortex can affect the breathing pattern.

C. **Reflex Control of Ventilation**

   1. Reflexes that directly influence the ventilatory pattern (swallowing, coughing, vomiting) usually do so to prevent airway obstruction.

   2. The Hering-Breuer reflex (apnea during sustained lung distention) is only weakly present in humans.

D. **Chemical Control of Ventilation**

   1. Peripheral chemoreceptors include the carotid bodies (ventilatory effects characterized by increased breathing rate and tidal volume) and aortic bodies (circulatory effects characterized by bradycardia and hypertension).

     a. Both carotid and aortic bodies are stimulated by decreased PaO_2 (<60 mm Hg) but not by arterial hemoglobin saturation with O_2, arterial O_2 concentration (anemia), or $PaCO_2$.

     b. Patients who depend on hypoxic ventilatory drive have PaO_2 values around 60 mm Hg.

     c. Potent inhaled anesthetics depress hypoxic ventilatory responses by depressing the carotid body response to hypoxemia.

   2. **Central Chemoreceptors**

     a. Approximately 80% of the ventilatory response to inhaled CO_2 originates in the central medullary centers.

ANATOMY AND PHYSIOLOGY

      b. The chemosensitive areas of the medullary ventilatory centers are exquisitely sensitive to the extracellular fluid hydrogen ion concentration. (CO_2 indirectly determines this concentration by reacting with water to form carbonic acid.)

      c. Increased $PaCO_2$ is a more potent stimulus (increased breathing rate and tidal volume within 60 to 120 seconds) to ventilation than is metabolic acidosis. (CO_2 but not hydrogen ions can easily cross the blood–brain barrier.)

      d. Normalization of the cerebrospinal fluid pH (active transport of bicarbonate ions) over time results in a decline in ventilation despite persistent increases in the $PaCO_2$. The reverse sequence occurs when acute ascent to altitude initially stimulates ventilation, leading to an abrupt decrease in $PaCO_2$.

E. Breath-Holding

    1. The rate of increase in $PaCO_2$ in awake, preoxygenated adults with normal lungs who hold their breath without previous hyperventilation is 7 mm Hg in the first 10 seconds, 2 mm Hg in the next 10 seconds, and 6 mm Hg thereafter.

    2. The rate of increase in $PaCO_2$ in apneic anesthetized patients is 12 mm Hg during the first minute and 3.5 mm Hg for every subsequent minute. This reflects a decreased metabolic rate and CO_2 production in the anesthetized compared with awake patients.

    3. Hyperventilation is rarely followed by an apneic period in awake humans despite a decreased $PaCO_2$. In contrast, even mild hyperventilation during general anesthesia produces apnea.

F. Quantitative Aspects of Chemical Control of Breathing (Fig. 11-2)

    1. The CO_2 response curve approaches linearity at $PaCO_2$ values between 20 and 80 mm Hg (>100 mm Hg, CO_2 acts as a ventilatory depressant).

    2. The slope of the CO_2 response curve is considered to represent CO_2 sensitivity (normally 0.5–0.7 L/min/mm Hg CO_2).

    3. The apneic threshold occurs at a $PaCO_2$ of about 32 mm Hg.

    4. Various events cause a shift in the position or change in the slope of the CO_2 response curve (Table 11-4).

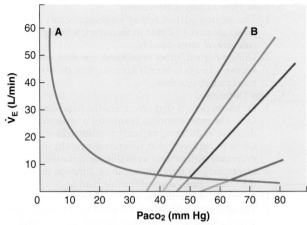

FIGURE 11-2. CO_2–ventilatory response curves. *Curve A* is generated by varying minute ventilation ($\dot{V}_E$) and measuring changes $PaCO_2$. *Curve B* is the classic CO_2–ventilatory response curve that is generated by varying the $PaCO_2$ and measuring the resultant $\dot{V}_E$. The slope of the curve defines sensitivity to the ventilatory-stimulating effects of CO_2. Volatile anesthetics and opioids shift the curve to the right and eventually depress the slope (*dashed lines*).

IV. OXYGEN AND CARBON DIOXIDE TRANSPORT

A. The movement of gas across the alveolar–capillary membrane depends on the integrity of the pulmonary and cardiac systems.

TABLE 11-4

CLINICAL STATES ASSOCIATED WITH CHANGES IN THE VENTILATORY RESPONSE TO CARBON DIOXIDE

Left Shift or Increased Slope
Hyperventilation (increased minute ventilation resulting in decreased $PaCO_2$ and respiratory alkalosis)
Arterial hypoxemia
Metabolic acidosis
Central causes (drugs [salicylates], intracranial hypertension, cirrhosis, anxiety)

Right Shift or Decreased Slope
Physiologic sleep ($PaCO_2$ increases up to 10 mm Hg)
Metabolic alkalosis
Denervation of peripheral chemoreceptors
Opioids (decreased breathing rate and increased tidal volume)
Volatile anesthetics

B. **Bulk Flow of Gas (Convection)**
   1. The greatest part of airway resistance occurs in the larger airways (>2 mm in diameter), where gas molecules travel more quickly.
   2. During normal, quiet ventilation, gas flow within convective airways is mainly laminar, thus decreasing resistance to gas flow.

C. **Gas Diffusion**
   1. Diffusion defects that create arterial hypoxemia are rare. The most common reason for a measured decrease in diffusing capacity is mismatching of ventilation to perfusion that functionally results in a decreased surface area available for diffusion.
   2. Hypercarbia is never the result of diffusion defects. (CO_2 is 20 times more diffusible than O_2.)

D. **Distribution of Ventilation and Perfusion**
   1. The efficiency with which O_2 and CO_2 exchange at the alveolar–capillary membrane depends on the matching of capillary perfusion and alveolar ventilation.
   2. **Distribution of blood flow** within the lungs is mainly gravity dependent, depending on the relationship between pulmonary artery pressure, alveolar pressure, and pulmonary venous pressure (Fig. 11-3).
   3. **Distribution of ventilation** is preferentially directed to more dependent areas of the lung.
   4. The ideal matching of ventilation to perfusion (V/Q = 1) is believed to occur at approximately the level of the third rib. Above this level, ventilation

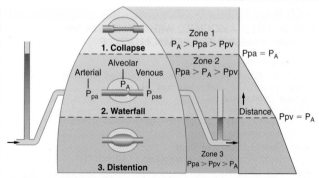

FIGURE 11-3. Distribution of blood flow in the isolated lung. P_A = alveolar pressure; Ppa = pulmonary artery pressure; Ppv = pulmonary venous pressure.

occurs slightly in excess of perfusion; below this level, the ratio becomes less than 1 (Fig. 11-4).

    a. Hypoxic pulmonary vasoconstriction decreases blood flow to unventilated (hypoxic) alveoli in an attempt to maintain a desirable V/Q ratio.

    b. Whereas increases in dead space ventilation primarily affect CO_2 elimination and have little effect on arterial oxygenation, physiologic shunt primarily affects arterial oxygenation with little effect on CO_2 elimination.

E. Physiologic Dead Space

    1. Anatomic dead space (2 mL/kg) accounts for the majority of dead space ventilation and is attributable

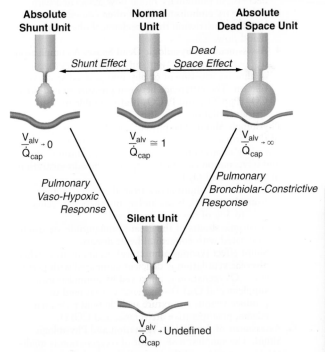

FIGURE 11-4. Continuation of ventilation-to-perfusion relationships. Gas exchange is maximally effective in normal lung units and only partially effective in shunt and dead space units. It is totally absent in silent units, absolute shunt, and dead space units.

ANATOMY AND PHYSIOLOGY

to ventilation of structures that do not participate in oxygenation (oronasopharynx to the terminal and respiratory bronchioles). Clinical conditions that modify anatomic dead space include tracheal intubation, tracheostomy, and large lengths of ventilatory tubing between the tracheal tube and the ventilator Y-piece.

2. **Alveolar dead space** arises from ventilation of alveoli where there is little or no perfusion.

3. **Increases in physiologic dead space** are most often caused by increases in alveolar dead space (decreased cardiac output as may occur with decreased venous return after institution of positive pressure ventilation of the lungs, pulmonary embolism, and COPD). A decrease in pulmonary blood flow associated with pulmonary embolism is more often caused by reflex bronchoconstriction than mechanical obstruction to blood flow.

4. **Assessment of Physiologic Dead Space.** A comparison of the minute ventilation and $PaCO_2$ allows a gross qualitative assessment of physiologic dead space ventilation. The difference between pressure of end-tidal CO_2 ($P_{ET}CO_2$) and $PaCO_2$ is attributable to dead space ventilation.

F. **Physiologic Shunt.** The physiologic shunt is the portion of the cardiac output that returns to the left heart without being exposed to ventilated alveoli. (Absolute shunt and oxygenation cannot be improved by administration of supplemental O_2.)

1. An anatomic shunt arises from the venous return from the pleural, bronchiolar, and thebesian veins (2% to 5% of the cardiac output).

2. Anatomic shunts of the greatest magnitude are usually associated with congenital heart disease.

3. **Shunt effect (venous admixture)** occurs in areas where alveolar ventilation is deficient compared with perfusion. (Oxygenation is improved by administration of supplemental O_2.) Disease entities that tend to produce venous admixture include mild pulmonary edema, postoperative atelectasis, and COPD.

G. **Assessment of Arterial Oxygenation and Physiologic Shunt.** The simplest assessment of oxygenation is qualitative comparison of the patient's inspired O_2 concentration and resulting PaO_2. (Venous admixture magnifies the effect of a small shunt.)

H. **Physiologic shunt calculation** includes the contribution of mixed venous blood, which may be extremely desaturated in critically ill patients owing to low cardiac output, anemia, arterial hypoxemia, and increased metabolic O_2 requirements. This calculation is the best estimate of how well the lungs can oxygenate the arterial blood.

V. PULMONARY FUNCTION TESTING (Table 11-5) (Fig. 11-5)

A. **Lung Volumes and Capacities** (Fig. 11-6)

B. **Flow-Volume Loops.** Imaging techniques (e.g., magnetic resonance imaging) provide more precise and useful information in the diagnosis of upper airway and extrathoracic obstruction and have replaced use of flow-volume loops.

C. **Carbon Monoxide Diffusing Capacity**
   1. Whereas decreased hemoglobin concentration decreases the carbon monoxide diffusing capacity (DLCO), an increased P_ACO_2 increases the DLCO.
   2. DLCO is deceased by alveolar fibrosis associated with O_2 toxicity and pulmonary edema.

D. **Preoperative Pulmonary Assessment** (Table 11-6)
   1. Specific measurements of lung function do not predict postoperative complications.
   2. History of smoking (>40 pack years), COPD, asthma, cough, and exercise intolerance (<one flight of stairs) are more predictive of postoperative complications.
   3. Baseline pulmonary function data are reserved for patients with severely impaired preoperative

TABLE 11-5

PULMONARY FUNCTION TESTS IN RESTRICTIVE AND OBSTRUCTIVE LUNG DISEASE

Measurement	Restrictive Disease	Obstructive Disease
FVC	Decreased	Normal to slightly decreased
FEV_1	Decreased	Normal to slightly decreased
FEV_1/FVC	Normal	Decreased
$FEF_{25-75\%}$	Normal	Decreased
FRC	Decreased	Normal to slightly increased
FRC	Decreased	Normal to slightly increased

FVC = forced vital capacity; FEV_1 = forced exhaled volume in 1 second; $FEF_{25-75\%}$ = forced expiratory flow between 25% and 75% of total exhaled volume; FRC = functional residual capacity; TLC = total lung capacity.

ANATOMY AND PHYSIOLOGY

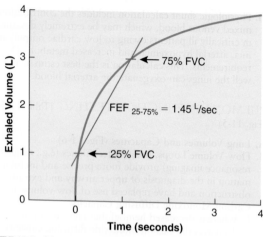

FIGURE 11-5. The spirogram depicts a 4-L forced vital capacity (FVC) on which the points representing 25% and 75% FVC are marked. The slope of the line connecting the points is the forced expiratory flow (FEF; 25% to 75%).

pulmonary function (e.g., those with quadriplegia or myasthenia), so assessment of weaning from mechanical ventilation or tracheal extubation may be guided by preoperative values.

4. Arterial blood gases are not indicated unless patient's history suggests hypoxemia or CO_2 retention (identify reversible disease or to define severity as a baseline).

5. Defining baseline PaO_2 and $PaCO_2$ is important if it is anticipated that a patient with severe COPD will require postoperative mechanical ventilation (Table 11-7).

VI. ANESTHESIA AND OBSTRUCTIVE PULMONARY DISEASE

A. Patients with marked obstructive pulmonary disease are at increased risk for intraoperative (reflex bronchoconstriction during direct laryngoscopy and tracheal intubation) and postoperative complications.

1. Patients with asthma and COPD may benefit from preoperative bronchodilator therapy.

2. Controlled ventilation of the lungs at less than 10 breaths/min should prevent hypercarbia,

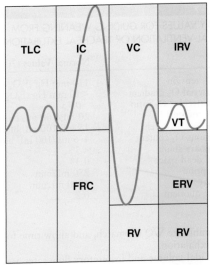

FIGURE 11-6. Lung volumes and capacities. The *darkest bar* depicts the four basic lung volumes that sum to create total lung capacity (TLC). ERV = expiratory reserve volume; FRC = functional residual capacity; IC = inspiratory capacity; IRV = inspiratory reserve volume; RV = residual volume; VC = vital capacity; VT = tidal volume.

TABLE 11-6

PREOPERATIVE PULMONARY ASSESSMENT

Anticipate impaired pulmonary function in specific patients and situations
Chronic lung disease
Smoking history
Persistent cough or wheezing
Morbid obesity
Requirement for one-lung anesthesia or lung resection
Neuromuscular disease

History determines the need for testing (exercise tolerance)
Chest radiography
Arterial blood gases
Screening spirometry (identify patients who will benefit from preoperative therapy; provide baseline before lung resection)

ANATOMY AND PHYSIOLOGY

TABLE 11-7

RESPIRATORY VALUES FOR GUIDING WEANING FROM
MECHANICAL VENTILATION OR TRACHEAL EXTUBATION

Parameter	Normal Values (70-kg Adult)
Alveolar O_2 tension	110 mm Hg (F_IO_2 0.21)
Alveolar-arterial O_2 gradient	<10 mm Hg (F_IO_2)
Arterial-to-alveolar O_2 ratio	>0.75
Arterial O_2 content	20 mL/100 mL blood
Mixed venous O_2 content	15 mL/100 mL blood
Arterial-venous O_2 content	4–6 mL/100 mL blood
Intrapulmonary shunt	<5%
Physiologic dead space	0.33
O_2 consumption	250 mL/min
O_2 transport	1000 mL/min
Respiratory quotient	0.8

     minimize V/Q mismatch, and allow time for
     exhalation.
   3. Tidal volume and inspiratory flow rates are adjusted
     to keep peak airway pressure below 40 cm H_2O.
  B. Tracheal extubation as soon as possible after the end of
    the operation is desirable in an attempt to decrease the
    risk of iatrogenic infection.

VII. ANESTHESIA AND RESTRICTIVE PULMONARY DISEASE

  A. These patients typically breathe rapidly and shallowly
    because more pressure is required to expand stiff lungs.
  B. Positive end-expiratory pressure increases the functional
    residual capacity and reverses arterial hypoxemia.
   1. High peak airway pressures may be required to expand
     stiffened lungs, but large tidal volumes are avoided
     because of the risk of barotrauma and volutrauma.
   2. Arterial hypoxemia can develop rapidly (as during
     apnea for tracheal intubation or transportation from
     the operating room), reflecting the limited O_2 stores in
     the lungs because of the decreased functional residual
     capacity.
   3. General anesthesia further decreases the functional
     residual capacity that persists into the postoperative
     period (this is offset with positive airway pressure).
  C. The most important aspect of postoperative pulmonary
    care is getting the patient out of bed, preferably walking.

VIII. EFFECTS OF CIGARETTE SMOKING ON PULMONARY FUNCTION (Table 11-8)

A. Cessation of smoking for 12 to 24 hours is sufficient to decrease carboxyhemoglobin levels to near normal but does not predictably influence the incidence of postoperative pulmonary complications.
   1. Normalization of mucociliary function requires 2 to 3 weeks of abstinence from smoking during which time sputum increases.
   2. Smokers who decrease but do not stop cigarette consumption (change their smoking technique) continue to acquire the same amount of nicotine, and it is unlikely that postoperative pulmonary complications will be altered.
B. Patients who smoke should be advised to stop smoking 2 months before elective operations to maximize the effect of smoking cessation or for at least 4 weeks to gain some benefit from mucociliary function.
C. Smoking is one of the main risk factors associated with postoperative morbidity (pneumonia).

IX. POSTOPERATIVE PULMONARY FUNCTION

A. **Postoperative Pulmonary Function**
   1. Changes in pulmonary function that occur after surgery are primarily restrictive (gauged by a decrease in functional residual capacity).

TABLE 11-8

EFFECTS OF SMOKING

Decreased ciliary motility
Increased sputum production
Increased airway reactivity
Development of obstructive pulmonary disease
Ventilation-to-perfusion mismatch (venous admixture and arterial hypoxemia)
Gas trapping
Increased minute ventilation
Barrel chest deformity
Decreased lung compliance (exhale forcibly to prevent gas trapping)
Increased carboxyhemoglobin concentration (normal <1%; may be 8% to 10% in smokers)

ANATOMY AND PHYSIOLOGY

TABLE 11-9

RELATION OF OPERATIVE SITE TO POSTOPERATIVE DECREASES IN
FUNCTIONAL RESIDUAL CAPACITY

Operative Site	Decrease in Functional Residual Capacity (%)
Nonlaparoscopic upper abdominal surgery	40–50*
Lower abdominal and thoracic surgery	30
Intracranial	15–20
Peripheral vascular	15–20

*In the presence of conventional postoperative analgesic techniques.

   2. The operative site is the single most important deter-
      minant of postoperative pulmonary restriction and
      pulmonary complications (Table 11-9).
B. **Postoperative Pulmonary Complications**
   1. Atelectasis and pneumonia, as reflected by changes in the
      color and quantity of sputum, oral temperature above
      38°C, and a new infiltrate seen on chest radiography, are
      the two most common postoperative complications.
   2. The risk of postoperative pulmonary complications
      can be minimized by ensuring the absence of active
      pulmonary infection and use of therapeutic
      bronchodilation if reactive airway disease is
      associated with increased airway resistance.
   3. Strategies to decrease the risk of postoperative
      pulmonary complications include the use of lung-
      expanding therapies, choice of analgesia, and
      cessation of smoking.
      a. Stir-up regimens (e.g., walking) are as effective as
         incentive spirometry.
      b. After median sternotomy, functional residual capac-
         ity does not return to normal for several weeks
         regardless of postoperative pulmonary therapy.
      c. The most important aspect of postoperative pul-
         monary care is getting the patient out of bed,
         preferably walking.
      d. Postoperative analgesia influences the risk of post-
         operative pulmonary complications (epidural anal-
         gesia, especially for abdominal and thoracic opera-
         tions, decreases the risk).

CHAPTER 12 ■ IMMUNE FUNCTION AND ALLERGIC RESPONSE

Allergic reactions during anesthesia represent an important cause of perioperative complications (Levy JH: Immune function and allergic response. In *Clinical Anesthesia*. Edited by Barash PG, Cullen BF, Stoelting RK, Cahalan MK, Stock MC. Philadelphia: Lippincott Williams & Wilkins, 2009, pp 256–270). Anesthesiologists routinely manage patients during the perioperative period, during which exposure to foreign substances (drugs, including injected anesthetics, antibiotics, neuromuscular blocking drugs, protamine, blood products) and environmental antigens (latex) occurs.

I. BASIC IMMUNOLOGIC PRINCIPLES

Host defense systems can be divided into cellular (T-cell lymphocytes) and humoral (antibodies, complement, cytokines) elements.

A. **Antigens** are molecules capable of stimulating an immune response (antibody production or lymphocyte stimulation) (Table 12-1).

B. **Thymus-Derived Lymphocytes and Bursa-Derived Lymphocytes**

1. **Thymus-derived (T-cell) lymphocytes** contain receptors that are activated by binding with antigens and subsequently secrete mediators that regulate the immune response (e.g., acquired immunodeficiency syndrome is caused by infection of helper T lymphocytes with a retrovirus known as the immunodeficiency virus).

2. **Bursa-derived (B-cell) lymphocytes** differentiate into plasma cells that synthesize antibodies.

C. **Antibodies** are specific proteins (immunoglobulins) that can recognize and bind to a specific antigen (see Table 12-1). Antibodies function as specific receptor molecules for immune cells and proteins.

TABLE 12-1

BIOLOGIC CHARACTERISTICS OF IMMUNOGLOBULINS

	IgG	IgM	IgA	IgE	IgD
Molecular weight	160,000	900,000	170,000	188,000	184,000
Serum concentration (mg/dL)	6–14	0.5–1.5	1–3	$<0.5 \times 10^3$	<0.1
Complement activation	All but IgG4	+	–	–	–
Placental transfer	+	–	–	–	–
Serum half-time (days)	23	5	6	1–5	2–8
Cell binding	Mast cells, neutrophils, lymphocytes, mononuclear cells, platelets	Lymphocytes	Mast cells, basophils, lymphocytes	Neutrophils, lymphocytes	

D. **Effector Cells and Proteins of the Immune Response Cells** (Table 12-2)
1. Monocytes, neutrophils (polymorphonuclear leukocytes), and eosinophils are effector cells that migrate into areas of inflammation in response to chemotactic factors.
2. **Opsonization** is deposition of antibody or complement fragments on surfaces of foreign cells with subsequent facilitation of the process that allows the effector cells to destroy the foreign cell.

TABLE 12-2

CELLS THAT PARTICIPATE IN THE IMMUNE RESPONSE

Macrophages (ingest antigens)
Polymorphonuclear leukocytes (neutrophils; first cells to appear in an acute inflammatory reaction)
Eosinophils (function unknown)
Basophils (granulocytes in blood; cell surfaces contain IgE receptors)
Mast cells (located in perivascular spaces of skin, lungs, and intestine; cell surfaces contain IgE receptors)

TABLE 12-3

SYMPTOMS PRODUCED BY RELEASE OF CYTOKINES

Fever
Hypotension
Myocardial depression
Catabolism

E. **Proteins**
  1. **Cytokines and Interleukins**
    a. Cytokines (**interleukin-1, tumor necrosis factor**) are inflammatory cell activators that are synthesized by macrophages to act as secondary messengers that activate endothelial cells and white blood cells (produce an inflammatory response) (Table 12-3).
    b. T-cell lymphocytes produce interleukins.
  2. **Complement**
    a. The primary humoral response to antigen and antibody binding is activation of the complement system (about 20 different proteins that are activated by antigen–antibody interactions, plasmin, and endotoxins).
    b. A series of inhibitors regulates the complement system (e.g., angioneurotic edema, which may be activated by surgery manifesting as laryngeal obstruction, is caused by a deficiency of an inhibitor of the C1 complement system).
F. **Effects of Anesthesia on Immune Function.** Anesthesia and surgery depress both T- and B-cell responsiveness as well as nonspecific host resistance mechanisms, including phagocytosis. The significance, if any, of these responses is not known. (It is probably of minor importance compared with the hormonal aspects of the stress response.)

II. **HYPERSENSITIVITY RESPONSES (ALLERGY)** (Table 12-4 and Fig. 12-1)

A. **Intraoperative Allergic Reactions**
  1. More than 90% of the allergic reactions evoked by drugs administered intravenously occur within 3 minutes of administration. (It is estimated that allergic reactions occur once in every 5000 to 25,000 anesthetics administered.)
  2. The only manifestation of an intraoperative allergic reaction may be **refractory hypotension** (Table 12-5 and Fig. 12-2).

ANATOMY AND PHYSIOLOGY

TABLE 12-4

CLASSIFICATION OF HYPERSENSITIVITY

Type I Reaction: Immediate-type hypersensitivity reaction (anaphylaxis) with release of chemical mediators (see Table 12-6) from mast cells and basophils in response to binding of IgE antibodies to the surfaces of these cells
Type II Reaction: Mediated by IgG or IgM antibodies directed against antigens on surfaces of foreign cells (e.g., ABO incompatibility reactions)
Type III Reaction: Antigen–antibody complexes that form insoluble complexes that deposit in the microvasculature (e.g., poststreptococcal infections)
Type IV Reaction: Delayed hypersensitivity reaction of cell-mediated immunity (e.g., tissue rejection, tuberculin immunity)

III. ANAPHYLACTIC REACTIONS

   A. **IgE-Mediated Pathophysiology.** Antigen binding to IgE antibodies, which reflects prior exposure to the antigen, initiates anaphylaxis. The antigen binds by bridging two immunospecific antibodies located on the surfaces of mast cells and basophils, resulting in the release of **histamine** and other chemicals.
   B. **Chemical Mediators of Anaphylaxis** (Table 12-6)
   C. **Recognition of Anaphylaxis** (see Table 12-5)
      1. Individuals vary greatly in their manifestations and course of anaphylaxis (spectrum ranges from minor clinical significance to death).

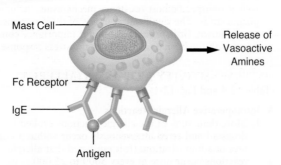

FIGURE 12-1. Type I immediate hypersensitivity reactions (anaphylaxis) involve IgE antibodies binding to mast cells or basophils at the Fc receptors. On encountering immunospecific antigens, the IgE becomes cross-linked, inducing degranulation, intracellular activation, and release of chemical mediators.

TABLE 12-5

RECOGNITION OF ANAPHYLAXIS DURING REGIONAL AND
GENERAL ANESTHESIA

System	Symptoms	Signs
Respiratory	Dyspnea	Coughing
		Wheezing
		Sneezing
		Laryngeal edema
		Decreased pulmonary compliance
		Fulminant pulmonary edema
		Acute respiratory failure
Cardiovascular	Dizziness	Disorientation
	Malaise	Diaphoresis
	Retrosternal discomfort	Hypotension
		Tachycardia
		Cardiac dysrhythmias
		Decreased systemic resistance
		Pulmonary hypertension
		Cardiac arrest
Cutaneous	Itching	Urticaria
	Burning	Flushing
	Tingling	Periorbital edema
		Perioral edema

2. The enigma of anaphylaxis lies in the unpredictability of its occurrence, the severity of the attack, and the lack of a prior patient allergic history.

D. **Nonimmunologic Release of Histamine**
   1. Many diverse molecules administered during the perioperative period release histamine in a dose-dependent, nonimmunologic fashion (Table 12-7).
   2. Nonimmunologic histamine release differs from antigen-mediated histamine release in that histamine appears to be the only mediator released.
   3. When administered at clinically recommended doses, aminosteroid muscle relaxants (e.g., rocuronium) have minimal effects on histamine release.
   4. **Antihistamine pretreatment** does not inhibit histamine release but instead competes with histamine at the receptor and attenuates the resulting physiologic effects.

E. **Treatment Plan.** The treatment plan is the same for life-threatening anaphylactic or anaphylactoid reactions. All patients who have experienced life-threatening allergic reactions should be admitted to the hospital for 24 hours of monitoring because manifestations may recur even after successful treatment.

ANATOMY AND PHYSIOLOGY

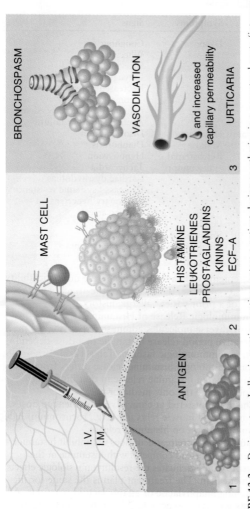

FIGURE 12-2. During a type I allergic reaction, antigen enters a patient during anesthesia via a parenteral route (intravenous [IV] or intramuscular [IM]) (*panel 1*). The antigen bridges two IgE antibodies on the surface of mast cells or basophils, causing degranulation (*panel 2*). The released chemical mediators produce the characteristic clinical symptoms of an allergic reaction (*panel 3*). ECF = extracellular fluid.

TABLE 12-6

CHEMICAL MEDIATORS OF ANAPHYLAXIS

Histamine
Peptide mediators
Eosinophilic chemotactic factor
Neutrophilic chemotactic factor
Arachidonic acid metabolites (leukotrienes and prostaglandins are
    synthesized after mast cell activation from arachidonic acid
    metabolism of phospholipid cell membranes)
Kinins
Platelet-activating factor
Tryptase

F. **Initial Therapy** (Table 12-8)
  1. **Epinephrine** is the drug of choice for resuscitation of
     patients experiencing an allergic reaction (α-Adrener-
     gic effects reverse hypotension, and β-adrenergic stim-
     ulation produces bronchodilation and inhibits contin-
     ued release of chemical mediators.)
  2. Arterial blood gases should be monitored during
     resuscitation.
  3. Up to 40% of intravascular fluid volume may be
     translocated into the interstitial space during an allergic
     reaction.
G. **Secondary Treatment** (see Table 12-8)
  1. **Bronchodilators.** Inhaled β-adrenergic agents, including
     inhaled albuterol and terbutaline, are indicated
     if bronchospasm is a major feature. Inhaled ipratropium
     may be especially useful for treatment of bronchospasm.
  2. **Airway Evaluation.** If there is any evidence of upper
     airway edema (e.g., facial edema, absence of air leak
     when the tracheal tube cuff is deflated), direct laryn-
     goscopic examination should be performed before the
     trachea is extubated.

TABLE 12-7

DRUGS CAPABLE OF NONIMMUNOLOGIC HISTAMINE RELEASE

Antibiotics (vancomycin)
Basic compounds (protamine)
Hyperosmotic agents
Nondepolarizing skeletal muscle relaxants (atracurium >
    pancuronium, vecuronium, and rocuronium)
Opioids (morphine)
Possibly thiobarbiturates

ANATOMY AND PHYSIOLOGY

TABLE 12-8

MANAGEMENT OF ANAPHYLAXIS DURING GENERAL ANESTHESIA

Initial Therapy
Stop administration of antigen
Maintain upper airway and administer 100% oxygen
Discontinue all anesthetic drugs
Initiate intravascular volume expansion (2–4 L of crystalloid or colloid solution in the presence of hypotension)
Administer epinephrine (5–10 μg IV with hypotension and titrate as needed; 0.1–1.0 mg IV with cardiovascular collapse)

Secondary Treatment
Antihistamines (0.5–1 mg/kg diphenhydramine IV)
Catecholamine infusions (starting doses: epinephrine, 4–8 μg/min; norepinephrine, 4–8 μg/min; isoproterenol, 0.5 to 1 μg/min as continuous infusion and titrated to effect)
Albuterol (4–8 puffs by metered-dose inhaler)
Corticosteroids (cortisol, 250–1000 mg; methylprednisolone, 1–2 g, especially if complement activation is suspected)
Bicarbonate
Airway evaluation before extubation
Refractory hypotension (vasopressin to treat refractory vasodilatory shock, 0.01 U/min)

3. **Refractory Hypotension.** Vasopressin may attenuate pathologic refractory vasodilation. Monitoring, including echocardiography, is a consideration in patients with refractory hypotension to better evaluate cardiac function or hypovolemia.

IV. **PERIOPERATIVE MANAGEMENT OF THE PATIENT WITH ALLERGIES**

Allergic drug reactions account for 6% to 10% of all adverse drug reactions. It is estimated that 5% of adults in the United States are allergic to one or more drugs.

A. **Immunologic Mechanisms of Drug Allergy**

1. Most drugs administered to patients by anesthesiologists have been reported to produce allergic reactions (Table 12-9).

2. Muscle relaxants are the drugs that are most commonly responsible for evoking intraoperative allergic reactions. (Cross-sensitivity is present between succinylcholine and nondepolarizing muscle relaxants.)

3. Unexplained intraoperative cardiovascular collapse has been attributed to anaphylaxis triggered by latex (natural rubber). Patients with **spina bifida** have an increased incidence of allergy to latex. Symptoms

TABLE 12-9

DRUGS IMPLICATED IN ALLERGIC REACTIONS
DURING ANESTHESIA

Anesthetic Drugs
Muscle relaxants (cross-sensitivity among all drugs is possible)
Induction drugs (barbiturates, propofol)
Local anesthetics (para-aminobenzoic acid ester drugs)
Opioids

Other Drugs
Antibiotics (cephalosporins, penicillin, vancomycin)
Blood products (whole blood, packed cells, platelets, fresh-frozen
  plasma, fibrinogen, gamma globulin)
Aprotinin
Methylmethacrylate
Protamine
Radiocontrast dye
Latex (natural rubber)
Drug preservatives/additives
Colloid volume expanders
Vascular graft material

    caused by latex allergy may not occur until several
    minutes after exposure and thus may be erroneously
    attributed to other causes.

  4. Life-threatening allergic reactions are more likely to
    occur in patients with a history of allergy, atopy, or
    asthma. Because the incidence of allergic reactions is
    so rare, even this history does not mandate further
    evaluation or pharmacologic pretreatment.

B. **Evaluation of Patients with Allergic Reactions.** Identify-
    ing the drug responsible for a suspected allergic reaction
    depends on circumstantial evidence indicating the tem-
    poral sequence of drug administration.

  1. Direct challenge of a patient with a test dose of the
    suspected offending drug is potentially hazardous and
    not recommended.

  2. A small test dose of drug given during anesthesia
    more accurately reflects a **pharmacologic test dose**
    and has nothing to do with immunologic dosages.

  3. The demonstration of drug-specific antibodies is gen-
    erally accepted as evidence that the patient may be at
    risk for anaphylaxis if the drug is administered.

C. **Testing for Allergy**

  1. After an allergic reaction, it is important to identify the
    offending allergen in order to prevent readministration.

ANATOMY AND PHYSIOLOGY

TABLE 12-10

TESTS FOR DRUG ALLERGY

Leukocyte histamine release (incubate patient's leukocytes with
the drug in question and measure histamine release as a marker
for basophil activation)
Radioallergosorbent test (RAST; commercially available antigens
[few anesthetic drugs are available] are incubated with the
patient's plasma for detection of specific IgE antibodies)
Enzyme-linked immunosorbent assay (ELISA; measures antigen-
specific antibodies; similar to the RAST test)
Intradermal testing (histamine release from mast cells causes
vasodilation [flare] and localized edema)

(Patients often have simultaneously received multiple
different drugs with or without preservatives.)
2. *In vitro* tests are available for anesthetic drugs (Table
12-10).
D. **Agents Implicated in Allergic Reactions.** Any agent a
patient received as an injection, infusion, or environmental
antigen has the potential to produce an allergic reaction.
E. **Latex Allergy.** Health care workers and children with
spina bifida and urogenital abnormalities are at
increased risk for latex allergy. Patients who are allergic
to bananas, avocados, and kiwis may also cross-react
with latex. It is a daunting task to create a latex-free
environment for care of sensitized patients. (These
patients should wear Medic Alert bracelets.)
F. **Muscle Relaxants** possess molecular features that make
them potential allergens.
1. Prick tests are often used for authenticating
neuromuscular blocking drugs as causes of allergic
reactions. There is the potential for cross-sensitivity
between muscle relaxants because of similarity of the
active site (quaternary ammonium molecule).
2. An alternative muscle relaxant cannot be chosen without some degree of immunologic testing.

V. SUMMARY

A spectrum of unpredictable life-threatening allergic reactions to any drug may occur in the perioperative period. A
high index of suspicion, prompt recognition, and appropriate
and aggressive therapy can help avoid a disastrous outcome.

CHAPTER 13 ■ INFLAMMATION, WOUND HEALING AND INFECTION

Despite major advances in the management of patients undergoing surgery (e.g., aseptic technique, prophylactic antibiotics) and advances in surgical approaches (e.g., laparoscopic surgery), surgical wound infection and wound failure remain common complications of surgery (Hopf W, Chapman CR, Cochran A, et al: Inflammation, wound healing and infection. In *Clinical Anesthesia*. Edited by Barash PG, Cullen BF, Stoelting RK, Cahalan MK, Stock MC. Philadelphia: Lippincott Williams & Wilkins, 2009, pp 271–289). Along with aseptic technique and prophylactic antibiotics, maintaining perfusion and oxygenation of surgical wounds is paramount.

I. INFECTION CONTROL

A. Hand Hygiene (Table 13-1)

1. Perhaps the most crucial component of infection prevention is frequent and effective hand hygiene. (In 1847, Ignaz Semmelweis instituted the use of hand washing between patient examinations.)

2. Despite our current knowledge of the germ theory, hand hygiene remains an inexplicably neglected component of infection control.

3. Even "clean" activities such as taking a patient's pulse or applying monitors can lead to hand contamination.

4. A number of products are available for hand hygiene. The ideal agent kills a broad spectrum of microbes, has antimicrobial activity that persists for at least 6 hours after application, is simple to use, and has few side effects.

   a. Plain (not antiseptic) soap and water are generally the least effective at reducing hand contamination. Soap and water are, however, the most effective at

TABLE 13-1

HAND HYGIENE TECHNIQUE

Decontaminating hands with an alcohol-based hand rub:
Apply the recommended volume of product to the palm of one
hand.
Rub the hands together, covering all surfaces of the hands and
fingers until the hands are dry.

When washing hands with soap and water:
Wet the hands first with water.
Apply an amount of product recommended by the manufacturer
to the hands.
Rub the hands together vigorously for at least 15 seconds,
covering all surfaces of the hands and fingers.
Rinse the hands with water and dry thoroughly them with a
disposable towel.
Use a towel to turn off the faucet.
Avoid using hot water because repeated exposure to hot water
may increase the risk of dermatitis.

*Liquid, bar, leaflet, or powdered forms of plain soap are
acceptable when washing hands with a non-antimicrobial soap
and water.*
When bar soap is used, soap racks that facilitate drainage and
small bars of soap should be used.

      removing spores (*Clostridium difficile* or *Bacillus
      anthracis*).
  b. Antiseptics containing 60% to 95% ethanol with
     a water base are germicidal and effective against
     gram-positive and gram-negative bacteria and
     lipophilic viruses (herpes simplex, human im-
     munodeficiency, influenza, respiratory syncytial,
     vaccinia viruses, hepatitis B and C viruses).
  c. Chlorhexidine is a cationic bisbiguanide that is
     germicidal against gram-positive bacteria and
     lipophilic viruses. It has substantial persistence on
     the skin, and the Centers for Disease Control and
     Prevention has identified it as the topical agent of
     choice for skin preparation in central venous
     catheter insertion. Chlorhexidine may cause severe
     corneal damage after direct contact with the eye,
     ototoxicity after direct contact with the inner or
     middle ear, and neurotoxicity after direct contact
     with the brain or meninges.
  d. Iodine and iodophors (iodine with a polymer
     carrier) are bactericidal against gram-positive,

gram-negative, and some spore-forming bacteria. Allergies to this class of topical agent are common.
   e. Wearing gloves does not reduce the need for hand hygiene. Hand hygiene should be practiced both before putting on gloves and immediately after removal.
5. Wearing rings does not increase overall bacterial levels measured on the hands of health care workers. Therefore, it remains unclear whether transmission of infection could be reduced by prohibiting health care workers from wearing rings.

B. **Antisepsis**
   1. Masks have long been advocated as preventing surgical site infection (SSI); however, data suggest that wearing a head cover is useful for preventing SSIs but wearing a mask is not.
   2. Masks do serve the purpose of protecting the health care provider, particularly when combined with eye protection, and thus should most likely be used during tracheal intubation and at other times when protection from body fluids is appropriate.
   3. Most postoperative surgical infections are caused by flora that are endogenous to the patient; environmental and airborne contaminants may also play a causative role.
   4. An important but frequently overlooked consideration is the role that traffic patterns into an operating room can play in patient exposure to airborne organisms. Current recommended practices are that traffic patterns should limit the flow of people through an operating room that is in use and that no more people than necessary should be in an operating room during a procedure.
   5. Gowning, gloving, careful aseptic technique, and use of a wide sterile field should be routine for placement of central venous lines.
   6. Epidural abscess formation is an extremely rare but potentially catastrophic complication of neuraxial anesthesia and epidural catheter placement. The most important consideration is preventing contamination of the needle and catheter.
      a. Hand washing, skin preparation, and draping and maintenance of a sterile field should be used.
      b. Gowning and wearing a mask, however, are unlikely to reduce the risk of infection.

ANATOMY AND PHYSIOLOGY

      c. Epidurals should probably be avoided in patients known or suspected to have bacteremia or should be deferred until after appropriate antibiotics have been administered.

C. **Antibiotic Prophylaxis** (Tables 13-2 and 13-3)

  1. Antibiotic prophylaxis is standard for surgeries in which there is more than a minimum risk of infection.

  2. Recommendations published in 2004 by the National Surgical Infection Prevention Project emphasize timing and choice of appropriate agents.

      a. The agent selected for antibiotic prophylaxis must cover the most likely spectrum of bacteria presented in the surgical field.

      b. The most commonly used antibiotic for surgical prophylaxis is cefazolin, a first-generation cephalosporin, because the potential pathogens for the vast majority of surgeries are gram-positive cocci from the skin.

  3. The exact timing for the administration of the antibiotic depends on the pharmacology and half-life of the drug. Ideally, administration of the prophylaxis should be within 30 minutes to 1 hour of incision. In general, it is considered acceptable if the infusion is started before incision. When a tourniquet is used, the infusion must be complete before inflation of the tourniquet.

      a. Administration of antibiotics is uncomplicated when the drug can be given as a bolus dose (e.g., cephalosporins) or as an infusion over a few minutes (e.g., clindamycin) and thus provides tissue levels within minutes.

      b. For drugs such as vancomycin that require infusion over an hour, coordination of administration is more complex.

      c. Depending on half-life, antibiotics should be repeated during long operations or operations with large blood loss. (Cefazolin is normally dosed every 8 hours, but the dose should be repeated every 4 hours intraoperatively.)

      d. Prophylactic antibiotics should be discontinued by 24 hours after surgery because prolonging the course of prophylactic antibiotics does not reduce the risk of infection but does increase the risk of adverse consequences of antibiotic administration.

TABLE 13-2

GUIDELINES FOR PROPHYLACTIC ANTIBIOTICS IN ADULT PATIENTS

Hip and Knee Arthroplasty, Extradural Spine Surgery, Cardiothoracic, Vascular Surgery, and Kidney Transplantation

Drug	Dose	Timing	Additional Dose
Cefazolin	<80 kg: 1 g ≥80 kg: 2 g	<60 min before incision as a bolus over 3–5 min; with bolus dose, tissue levels are adequate in a few minutes	Every 4 hours Exclude kidney transplants

Neurosurgery (Cranial and Intradural Spine)

Drug	Dose	Timing	Additional Dose
Ceftriaxone	<80 kg: 1 g	<60 min before incision as a bolus over 3–5 min	Every 12 hours

Liver Transplantation

Drug	Dose	Timing	Additional Dose
Ceftriaxone	<80 kg: 1 g ≥80 kg: 2 g	<60 min before incision as a bolus over 3–5 min	Every 12 hours

Liver Transplantation: β-Lactam Allergy

Drug	Dose	Timing	Additional Dose
Vancomycin	1 g	Start infusion on arrival in the operating room (after monitors are attached); infuse over 30–60 min	Every 12 hours
Clindamycin	<100 kg: 600 mg	<60 min before incision as infusion over 10–15 min	Every 6 hours

Colon Surgery

Drug	Dose	Timing	Additional Dose
Cefotetan	<80 kg: 1 g ≥80 kg: 2 g	<60 min before incision as a bolus over 3–5 min	Every 6 hours

Colon Surgery: β-Lactam Allergy

Drug	Dose	Timing	Additional Dose
Ciprofloxacin and	400 mg	<60 min before incision as infusion over 30 min	Every 6 hours
Metronidazole	500 mg		

(continued)

TABLE 13-2

GUIDELINES FOR PROPHYLACTIC ANTIBIOTICS IN ADULT PATIENTS (CONTINUED)

Drug	Dose	Timing	Additional Dose
Vaginal and Abdominal Hysterectomy			
Cefazolin or Cefotetan (if bowel involved)	<80 kg: 1 g ≥80 kg: 2 g	<60 min before incision as a bolus over 3–5 min	Every 4 hours Every 6 hours
Vaginal and Abdominal Hysterectomy: β-Lactam Allergy			
Ciprofloxacin and Metronidazole or	400 mg 500 mg	<60 min before incision as infusion over 30 min	Every 6 hours
Clindamycin and Gentamicin	600 mg 1.5 mg/kg	<60 min before incision as infusion over 10–15 minutes	Every 6 hours

Always confirm with surgeons at the time-out or earlier; in some cases, the surgeon may wish to delay antibiotics until after culture.

Make sure the dose has been given before tourniquet is inflated.

An additional intraoperative dose should also be given in circumstances of significant blood loss.

Used with permission from the University of California, San Francisco Department of Anesthesia and Perioperative Care.

TABLE 13-3

GUIDELINES FOR PROPHYLACTIC ANTIBIOTICS IN PEDIATRIC PATIENTS

Drug	Dose
Cefazolin	20–30 mg/kg
Ceftriaxone	25 mg/kg
Cefotetan	20–30 mg/kg
Cefuroxime	50 mg/kg
Vancomycin	15 mg/kg (as an infusion over 30–60 min)
Gentamicin	2 mg/kg
Clindamycin	15 mg/kg
Metronidazole	10 mg/kg
Ciprofloxacin	Not recommended

4. Methicillin-resistant *Staphylococcus aureus* (MRSA) is becoming a more common pathogen. Hand hygiene is among the most effective means of preventing develop-

ment of MRSA because when used properly, alcohol-based gel kills more than 99.9% of all transient pathogens, including MRSA. There does not appear to be a justification for using antibiotics effective against MRSA for prophylaxis in most clinical settings.

5. Anesthesiologists should work in consultation with surgeons to use guidelines determined by the local infection control committee to take initiative for administering prophylactic antibiotics.

II. MECHANISMS OF WOUND REPAIR

A. Many factors may impair wound healing (Table 13-4).
B. **Initial Response to Injury**
   1. Wound healing has traditionally been described in four separate phases: hemostasis, inflammation, proliferation, and remodeling. Each phase is composed of complex interactions between host cells, contaminants, cytokines, and other chemical mediators that, when functioning properly, lead to repair of injury. These processes are highly conserved across species, indicating the critical importance of the inflammatory response that directs the process of cellular and tissue repair.
   2. In wounds, local blood supply is compromised at the same time that metabolic demand is increased. (The wound environment becomes hypoxic and acidotic.) Hypoxia acts as a stimulus to repair but also leads to poor healing and increased susceptibility to infection.

TABLE 13-4
FACTORS THAT MAY IMPAIR WOUND HEALING
Oxygen supply to the wound (most important element)
Systemic Factors
Medical comorbidities
Nutrition
Sympathetic nervous system activation
Age
Local Environmental Factors
Bacterial load
Degree of inflammation
Moisture content
Oxygen tension
Vascular perfusion

ANATOMY AND PHYSIOLOGY

C. **Resistance to Infection**
  1. After a disruption of the normal skin barrier, successful wound healing requires the ability to clear foreign material and resist infection. Neutrophils provide nonspecific immunity and prevent infection. In the absence of infection, neutrophils disappear by about 48 hours after surgery.
  2. Resistance to infection is critically impaired by hypoxia and wound healing becomes more efficient as PO_2 increases even to very high levels (500–1,000 mm Hg as produced by hyperbaric oxygenation).
D. **Proliferation.** The proliferative phase (granulation and epithelization) normally begins approximately 4 days after injury, concurrent with a waning of the inflammatory phase.
E. **Neovascularization** in wounds proceeds both by angiogenesis (vessel growth via budding from existing vessels) and vasculogenesis.
F. **Collagen and Extracellular Matrix Deposition**
  1. New blood vessels grow into the matrix that is produced by fibroblasts.
  2. Wound strength, which results from collagen deposition, is highly vulnerable to wound hypoxia.
G. **Epithelization** is characterized by replication and migration of epithelial cells across the skin edges in response to growth factors. Topical oxygen applied in a manner that does not dry out epithelial cells has been advocated as a method of increasing the rate of epithelization.
H. **Maturation and Remodeling**
  1. The final phase of wound repair is maturation, which involves ongoing remodeling of the granulation tissue and increasing wound tensile strength.
  2. Contraction is inhibited by the use of high doses of corticosteroids (even steroids given several days after injury have this effect). In wounds in which contraction is detrimental, this effect can be beneficial.
  3. Some wounds heal to excess. Hypertrophic scar (most common after burn injury) and keloids are common forms of abnormal scar tissue caused by abnormal responses to healing. Keloids likely have a genetic predisposition.

III. WOUND PERFUSION AND OXYGENATION

A. Complications of wounds include failure to heal, infection, and excessive scarring or contracture.

B. All surgical procedures lead to some degree of contamination that must be controlled by local host defenses. The initial hours after contamination represent a decisive period during which inadequate local defenses may allow an infection to become established.

1. Normally, wounds on the extremities and trunk heal more slowly than those on the face. The major difference in these wounds is the degree of tissue perfusion and thus the wound tissue oxygen tension.

2. Ischemic or hypoxic tissue is highly susceptible to infection and heals poorly, if at all. A high PO_2 is needed to force oxygen into injured and healing tissues, particularly in subcutaneous tissue, fascia, tendon, and bone, the tissues at highest risk for poor healing.

   a. In surgical patients, the rate of wound infections is inversely proportional and collagen deposition is directly proportional to postoperative subcutaneous wound tissue oxygen tension.

   b. High oxygen tensions (>100 mm Hg) can be reached in wounds, but only if perfusion is rapid and arterial PO_2 is high. Oxygen-carrying capacity (hemoglobin concentration) is not particularly important to wound healing, provided that perfusion is normal.

   c. Peripheral vasoconstriction, which results from central sympathetic control of subcutaneous vascular tone, is probably the most frequent and clinically the most important impediment to wound oxygenation (Table 13-5).

   d. Prevention or correction of hypothermia and blood volume deficit decreases wound infections and increases collagen deposition in patients undergoing major abdominal surgery.

   e. Preoperative systemic (forced air warmer) or local warming decrease wound infections.

   f. Delivery of antibiotics also depends on perfusion.

IV. PATIENT MANAGEMENT

A. **Preoperative Preparation** (Table 13-6)

B. **Intraoperative Management** (Table 13-7)

TABLE 13-5

CAUSES OF SYMPATHETICALLY INDUCED PERIPHERAL
VASOCONSTRICTION

Hypothermia (anesthetic drugs, exposure to cold, redistribution
  of body heat from core to the periphery)
Pain
Fear
Blood volume deficit
Pharmacologic agents
  Nicotine
  β-Adrenergic antagonists
  α-1 Agonists

1. Careful surgical technique is fundamental to optimal
   wound healing.
2. Delicate handling of the tissue, adequate hemostasis,
   and surgeon experience lead to healthier wounds.

C. **Volume Management**
  1. Surgical stress results in increased intravenous fluid
     requirements.
  2. The major complications associated with
     hypervolemia include pulmonary edema, congestive
     heart failure, edema of the gut with prolonged ileus,
     and possibly an increase in cardiac arrhythmias.
  3. Aside from hemodynamic instability, the major com-
     plications of hypovolemia include decreased
     oxygenation of surgical wounds (which predisposes
     to wound infection), decreased collagen formation,
     impaired wound healing, and increased wound
     breakdown.
  4. Intraoperative transesophageal echocardiography has
     been advocated as a more useful monitor of intraop-
     erative volume status than pulmonary artery
     catheters.

TABLE 13-6

PREOPERATIVE CHECKLIST

Assess and optimize cardiopulmonary function (correct
  hypotension).
Treat vasoconstriction (blood volume, pain, anxiety).
Assess recent nutrition and treat as appropriate.
Treat existing infection (clean and treat skin infections).
Improve or maintain blood sugar control.

TABLE 13-7

INTRAOPERATIVE MANAGEMENT

Administer appropriate prophylactic antibiotics at the start of any
procedure in which infection is highly probable or has
potentially disastrous consequences. Antibiotic levels should be
maintained during long operations.
Keep patients warm.
Observe gentle surgical technique with minimal use of ties and
cautery.
Keep wounds moist.
Use antibiotic irrigation in contaminated cases.
Elevate PaO_2.
Use delayed closure for heavily contaminated wounds.
Use appropriate sutures (and skin tapes).
Use appropriate dressings.

From Hunt T: Fundamentals of wound management in surgery, Wound Healing:
Disorders of Repair. South Plainfield, NJ, Chirugecom, Inc, 1976, with permission.

     5. Current recommendations include replacing fluid
losses based on standard guidelines for the type of
surgery, replacement of blood loss, and replacement
of other ongoing fluid losses (Table 13-8).
   D. **Postoperative Management** (Table 13-9)
     1. Wounds are most vulnerable in the early hours after
surgery. Although antibiotics lose their effectiveness
after the first few hours, oxygen-mediated natural
wound immunity lasts longer.

TABLE 13-8

STANDARD VOLUME MANAGEMENT GUIDELINES FOR
SURGICAL PATIENTS

*Fluid Requirement = Deficit + Maintenance (baseline plus
replacement) + Estimated blood Loss (and other sensible fluid
losses)*
Deficit = Maintenance (1.5 mL/kg) × hours NPO
Adjust for fever, high nasogastric output, bowel preps
Replace estimated blood loss with 3:1 crystalloid and 1:1 with
colloid

Maintenance Requirements for Different Surgeries
Superficial surgical trauma (peripheral surgery): 1–2 mL/kg/hr
Minimal surgical trauma (head and neck, hernia, knee surgery):
3–4 mL/kg/hr
Moderate surgical trauma (major surgery without exposed
abdominal contents): 5–6 mL/kg/hr
Severe surgical trauma (major abdominal with exposed abdominal
contents): 8–10 mL/kg/hr

ANATOMY AND PHYSIOLOGY

TABLE 13-9

POSTOPERATIVE MANAGEMENT

Keep the patient warm.
Provide analgesia to keep the patient comfortable, if not pain free.
Patient report and the ability to move freely are the best signs of
   adequate pain relief.
Only use one more doses of antibiotic unless an infection is
   present or contamination continues.
Keep up with third-space losses (fever increases fluid losses).
Assess perfusion and react to abnormalities.
Avoid diuresis until pain is gone and the patient is warm.
Assess losses (including thermal losses) if the wound is open.
Assess the need for parenteral or enteral nutrition and respond.
Continue to control hypertension and hyperglycemia.

From Hunt T: Fundamentals of wound management in surgery, Wound Healing:
Disorders of Repair. South Plainfield, NJ, Chirugecom, Inc, 1976, with permission.

2. Even a short period of vasoconstriction during the
   first day after surgery is sufficient to reduce oxygen
   supply and increase the risk of infection. Correction
   and prevention of vasoconstriction in the first 24 to
   48 hours after surgery has significant beneficial
   effects.

3. Strict glycemic control is also important, although the
   best method to achieve this in the non-intensive care
   unit setting has not yet been established.

4. Local perfusion is not assured until patients have a
   normal blood volume, are warm and pain free, and
   are receiving no vasoconstrictive drugs.

   a. Warming should continue until patients are thor-
      oughly awake and active and can maintain their
      own thermal balance.

   b. Low output may indicate decreased renal perfu-
      sion, but normal or even high urine output has
      little correlation to wound or tissue PO_2.

   c. Physical examination (capillary return, eye turgor,
      warm and dry skin) of the patient is a better guide
      to hypovolemia and vasoconstriction.

   d. Vasoconstrictive drugs (nicotine, beta-blockers)
      should be avoided.

   e. Maintenance of tissue PO_2 requires attention to
      pulmonary function after surgery. Administration
      of supplemental oxygen via a face mask or nasal
      cannulae may increase safety in patients receiving
      systemic opioids. Pain control also appears

important because it favorably influences both pulmonary function and vascular tone.

V. SUMMARY

A. During surgery, appropriate antibiotic use, prevention of vasoconstriction through volume and warming, and maintenance of a high PaO_2 (300–500 mm Hg) are key.

B. After surgery, the focus should remain on prevention of vasoconstriction through pain relief, warming, and adequate volume administration in the postanesthesia care unit.

CHAPTER 14 ■ FLUIDS, ELECTROLYTES AND ACID–BASE PHYSIOLOGY

As a consequence of underlying diseases and therapeutic manipulations, surgical patients may develop potentially harmful disorders of acid-base equilibrium, intravascular and extravascular volume, and serum electrolytes (Prough DS, Funston JS, Svensen CH, Wolf SW: Acid-base, fluids and electrolytes. In *Clinical Anesthesia*. Edited by Barash PG, Cullen BF, Stoelting RK, Cahalan MK, Stock MC. Philadelphia: Lippincott Williams & Wilkins, 2009, pp 290–325). Precise management of acid–base status, fluids, and electrolytes may limit perioperative morbidity and mortality.

I. ACID–BASE INTERPRETATION AND TREATMENT

Management of acid–base disturbances requires an understanding of the four simple acid–base disorders (metabolic alkalosis, metabolic acidosis, respiratory alkalosis, and respiratory acidosis) as well as combinations of more complex disturbances.

A. **Overview of Acid–Base Equilibrium.** Conventionally, acid–base equilibrium is described using the Henderson-Hasselbalch equation (Fig. 14-1). Because the concentration of bicarbonate is largely regulated by the kidneys but CO_2 is controlled by the lungs, acid–base interpretation has emphasized examining disorders in terms of metabolic disturbances (bicarbonate primarily increased or decreased) and respiratory disturbances ($PaCO_2$ primarily increased or decreased).

1. The negative logarithm of the hydrogen ion concentration is described as the pH. A pH of 7.4 corresponds to a hydrogen ion concentration of 40 nmol/L.

2. From a pH of 7.2 to 7.5, the curve of hydrogen ion concentration is relatively linear, and for each change of 0.01 pH unit from 7.4, the hydrogen ion concentration

$$pH = 6.1 + \log [HCO_3]/0.03 \times Paco_2$$

FIGURE 14-1.   Henderson-Hasselbalch equation.

can be estimated to increase (pH >7.4) or decrease (pH >7.4) by 1 nmol/L.

B. **Metabolic alkalosis** (pH >7.45 and bicarbonate >27 mEq/L) is the most common acid-base abnormality in critically ill patients (Tables 14-1 and 14-2).
   1. Metabolic alkalosis exerts multiple physiologic effects (Table 14-3).
   2. Recognition of hyperbicarbonatemia justifies arterial blood gas (ABG) analysis and should alert the anesthesiologist to the possibility that the patient has hypovolemia or hypokalemia.
   3. Treatment of metabolic alkalosis (Table 14-4).
C. **Metabolic Acidosis** (pH <7.35 and bicarbonate <21 mEq/L)
   1. Two types of metabolic acidosis occur based on whether the calculated anion gap is normal or increased (Table 14-5). The commonly measured cation

TABLE 14-1

GENERATION OF METABOLIC ALKALOSIS

Generation	Examples
Loss of Acid from the Extracellular Space	
Loss of gastric fluid (HCl)	Vomiting
Acid loss in urine, increased distal sodium delivery in the presence of hyperaldosteronism	Primary aldosteronism plus diuretic
Acid shifts into cells	Potassium deficiency
Loss of acid into stool	Congenital chloride-losing diarrhea
Excessive Bicarbonate Loads	
Absolute	
Oral or parenteral bicarbonate	Milk alkali syndrome
Metabolic conversion of the salts of organic acids to bicarbonate	Lactate, acetate, or citrate administration
Relative	Sodium bicarbonate dialysis
Posthypercapnic States	Correction (mechanical ventilatory support) of chronic hypercapnia

TABLE 14-2
FACTORS THAT MAINTAIN METABOLIC ALKALOSIS

Factor	Proposed Mechanism
Decreased GFR	Increases fractional bicarbonate reabsorption and prevents elevated plasma bicarbonate concentrations from exceeding Tm
Volume contraction	Stimulates proximal tubular bicarbonate reabsorption
Hypokalemia	Decreases GFR and increases proximal tubular bicarbonate reabsorption
	Stimulates sodium-independent/potassium-dependent (low) secretion in cortical collecting tubules
Hypochloremia*	Increases renin
	Decreases distal chloride delivery
Passive backflux of bicarbonate	Creates a favorable concentration gradient for passive bicarbonate movement from proximal tubular lumen to blood
Aldosterone	Increases sodium-dependent proton secretion in cortical collecting tubules and sodium-independent proton secretion in cortical collecting tubules and medullary collecting tubules

*Animal models.
GFR = glomerular filtrate rate.

TABLE 14-3
PHYSIOLOGIC EFFECTS PRODUCED BY METABOLIC ALKALOSIS

Hypokalemia (potentiates effects of digoxin; evokes ventricular cardiac dysrhythmias)

Decreased serum ionized calcium concentration

Compensatory hypoventilation (may be exaggerated in patients with chronic obstructive pulmonary disease or those who have received opioids; compensatory hypoventilation rarely results in $PaCO_2$ >55 mm Hg)

Arterial hypoxemia (reflects effect of compensatory hypoventilation)

Increased bronchial tone (may contribute to atelectasis)

Leftward shift of oxyhemoglobin dissociation curve (oxygen less available to tissues)

Decreased cardiac output

Cardiovascular depression and cardiac dysrhythmias (result of inadvertent iatrogenic respiratory alkalosis to pre-existing metabolic alkalosis during anesthetic management)

TABLE 14-4

TABLE 14-4
TREATMENT OF METABOLIC ALKALOSIS

Etiologic Therapy
Expand intravascular fluid volume (intraoperative fluid management with 0.9% saline; lactated Ringer's solution provides an additional substrate for generation of bicarbonate).
Administer potassium.
Avoid iatrogenic hyperventilation of the patient's lungs.

Nonetiologic Therapy
Administer acetazolamide (causes renal bicarbonate wasting).
Administer hydrogen (ammonium chloride, arginine hydrochloride, hydrochloric acid [must be injected into a central vein]).

    (sodium) usually exceeds the total concentration of anions (chloride, bicarbonate) by 9 to 13 mEq/L.
2. Metabolic acidosis exerts multiple physiologic effects (Table 14-6).
3. Anesthetic implications of metabolic acidosis are proportional to the severity of the underlying process (Table 14-7).
4. Treatment of metabolic acidosis consists of the treatment of the primary pathophysiologic process (hypoperfusion, arterial hypoxemia), and if pH is severely depressed, administration of sodium bicarbonate (Table 14-8). Current opinion is that sodium bicarbonate should rarely be used to treat acidemia induced by metabolic acidosis because it does not improve the cardiovascular response to catecholamines and does decrease plasma ionized calcium.

TABLE 14-5
DIFFERENTIAL DIAGNOSIS OF METABOLIC ACIDOSIS

Normal Anion Gap
Renal tubular acidosis
Diarrhea
Carbonic anhydrase administration
Early renal failure
Saline administration

Elevated Anion Gap (>13 mEq/L)
Uremia
Ketoacidosis
Lactic acidosis
Toxins (methanol, ethylene glycol, salicylates)

TABLE 14-6

PHYSIOLOGIC EFFECTS PRODUCED BY METABOLIC ACIDOSIS

Decreased myocardial contractility
Increased pulmonary vascular resistance
Decreased systemic vascular resistance
Impaired response of the cardiovascular system to endogenous
    and exogenous catecholamines
Compensatory hyperventilation

D. **Respiratory alkalosis** (pH >7.45 and $PaCO_2$ <35 mm Hg)
    results from an increase in minute ventilation that is greater
    than that required to excrete metabolic CO_2 production.
    1. The development of spontaneous respiratory alkalosis
        in a previously normocarbic patient requires prompt
        evaluation (Table 14-9).
    2. Respiratory alkalosis exerts multiple physiologic
        effects (Table 14-10).
    3. Treatment of respiratory alkalosis per se is often not
        required. The most important steps are recognition
        and treatment of the underlying cause (e.g., arterial
        hypoxemia, hypoperfusion-induced lactic acidosis).
    4. Preoperative recognition of chronic hyperventilation
        necessitates intraoperative maintenance of a similar
        $PaCO_2$.
E. **Respiratory acidosis** (pH, 7.35; $PaCO_2$ >45 mm Hg)
    occurs because of a decrease in minute ventilation and
    or an increase in production of metabolic CO_2.
    1. Respiratory acidosis may be acute (absence of renal
        bicarbonate retention) or chronic (renal retention of
        bicarbonate returns the pH to near normal).
    2. Respiratory acidosis occurs because of a decrease in
        minute ventilation or an increase in CO_2 production
        (Table 14-11).

TABLE 14-7

ANESTHETIC IMPLICATIONS OF METABOLIC ACIDOSIS

Monitor arterial blood gases and pH
Possible exaggerated hypotensive responses to drugs and positive-
    pressure ventilation of the patient's lungs (reflects hypovolemia)
Consider monitoring with an intra-arterial catheter and
    pulmonary artery catheter
Maintain previous degree of compensatory hyperventilation

TABLE 14-8

CALCULATION OF SODIUM BICARBONATE DOSE

$$\text{Sodium Bicarbonate (mEq/L)} = \frac{\text{weight (kg)} \times 0.3 \times (24 \text{ mEq/L [actual bicarbonate]})}{2}$$

TABLE 14-9

CAUSES OF RESPIRATORY ALKALOSIS

Hyperventilation syndrome (diagnosis of exclusion; most often encountered in the emergency department)
Iatrogenic hyperventilation
Pain
Anxiety
Arterial hypoxemia
Central nervous system disease
Systemic sepsis

TABLE 14-10

PHYSIOLOGIC EFFECTS PRODUCED BY RESPIRATORY ALKALOSIS

Hypokalemia (potentiates toxicity of digoxin)
Hypocalcemia
Cardiac dysrhythmias
Bronchoconstriction
Hypotension
Decreased cerebral blood flow (returns to normal over 8 to 24 hours corresponding to the return of cerebrospinal fluid pH to normal)

TABLE 14-11

CAUSES OF RESPIRATORY ACIDOSIS

Decreased Alveolar Ventilation
Central nervous system depression (opioids, general anesthetics)
Peripheral skeletal muscle weakness (neuromuscular blockers, myasthenia gravis)
Chronic obstructive pulmonary disease
Acute respiratory failure

Increased Carbon Dioxide Production
Hypermetabolic states
Sepsis
Fever
Multiple trauma
Malignant hyperthermia
Hyperalimentation

ANATOMY AND PHYSIOLOGY

3. Patients with chronic hypercarbia caused by intrinsic pulmonary disease require careful preoperative evaluation (ABG and pH determinations), anesthetic management (direct arterial blood pressure monitoring and frequent ABG measurements), and postoperative care (pain control, often with neuraxial opioids, and mechanical support of ventilation).

   a. Administration of opioids and sedatives, even in low doses, may cause hazardous depression of ventilation.

   b. Intraoperatively, a patient with chronic hypercapnia should be ventilated to maintain a normal pH. (An abrupt increase in alveolar ventilation may produce profound alkalemia because renal excretion of bicarbonate is slow.)

4. Treatment of acute respiratory acidosis is elimination of the causative factor (opioids, muscle relaxants) and mechanical support of ventilation as needed. Chronic respiratory acidosis is rarely managed with mechanical ventilation but rather with efforts to improve pulmonary function in order to permit more effective elimination of CO_2.

F. In patients requiring mechanical ventilation for respiratory failure, ventilation with a lung-protective strategy may result in hypercapnia, which in turn can be managed with alkalinization.

II. PRACTICAL APPROACH TO ACID–BASE INTERPRETATION

Rapid interpretation of a patient's acid–base status involves integration of data provided by ABG, pH, and electrolyte measurements and history. After obtaining these data, a stepwise approach facilitates interpretation (Table 14-12).

A. The pH status usually indicates the primary process (acidosis or alkalosis).

B. If the $PaCO_2$ and the pH change reciprocally but the magnitude of the pH and bicarbonate changes is not consistent with a simple acute respiratory disturbance, a chronic respiratory or metabolic problem (>24 hr) should be considered. (pH becomes nearly normal as the body compensates.)

C. If neither an acute nor chronic respiratory change could have resulted in the ABG measurements, then a metabolic disturbance must be present.

TABLE 14-12

SEQUENTIAL APPROACH TO ACID–BASE INTERPRETATION

Is the pH life threatening, requiring immediate intervention?
Does the pH reflect a primary acidosis or alkalosis?
Could the arterial blood gas and pH readings represent an acute change in $PaCO_2$?
If there is no evidence of an acute change in $PaCO_2$, is there evidence of a chronic respiratory disturbance or of an acute metabolic disturbance?
Are appropriate compensatory changes present?
Is an anion gap present?
Do the clinical data fit the acid–base picture?

    D. Whereas compensation in response to metabolic disturbances is prompt via changes in $PaCO_2$, renal compensation for respiratory disturbances is slower.

    E. Failure to consider the presence or absence of an increased anion gap results in an erroneous diagnosis and failure to initiate appropriate treatment. Correct assessment of the anion gap requires correction for hypoalbuminemia.

III. PHYSIOLOGY OF FLUID MANAGEMENT

    A. **Body Fluid Compartments.** Accurate replacement of fluid deficits necessitates an understanding of the distribution spaces of water, sodium, and colloid. Total body water approximates 60% of total body weight (42 L in a 70-kg adult). Total body water consists of intracellular fluid (ICF; 28 L) and extracellular fluid (ECF; 14 L). Plasma volume is about 3 L, and red blood cell volume is about 2 L. Whereas sodium is present principally in the ECF (140 mEq/L), potassium is present principally in the ICF (150 mEq/L). Albumin is the most important oncotically active constituent of ECF (4 g/dL).

    B. **Distribution of Infused Fluids.** Conventionally, clinical prediction of plasma volume expansion after fluid infusion assumes that body fluid spaces are static. However, infused fluid does not simply equilibrate throughout an assumed distribution volume but is added to a highly regulated system that attempts to maintain intravascular, interstitial, and intracellular volume. Kinetic modes of intravenous (IV) fluid therapy allow clinicians to more

ANATOMY AND PHYSIOLOGY

accurately predict the time course of volume changes
produced by infusions of fluids of various compositions.

C. **Regulation of ECF volume** is influenced by aldosterone
(enhances sodium reabsorption), antidiuretic hormone
(enhances water reabsorption), and atrial natriuretic
peptide (enhances sodium and water excretion).

IV. FLUID REPLACEMENT THERAPY

A. **Maintenance Requirements for Water, Sodium, and Potassium.** In healthy adults, sufficient water is required to balance gastrointestinal losses (100–200 mL/day), insensible losses (500–1000 mL/day representing respiratory and cutaneous losses), and urinary losses (1000 mL/day)

1. Water maintenance requirements are often calculated on the basis of body weight. For a 70-kg adult, the daily water maintenance requirement is about 2500 mL (Table 14-13).

2. Renal sodium conservation is highly efficient, such that the average daily maintenance requirement in an adult is about 75 mEq.

3. The average daily maintenance requirement of potassium is about 40 mEq. Physiologic diuresis induces an obligate potassium loss of at least 10 mEq for every 1000 mL of urine.

4. Electrolytes such as chloride, calcium, and magnesium do not require short-term replacement, although they must be supplied during chronic IV fluid maintenance.

B. **Dextrose.** Addition of glucose to maintenance fluid solutions is indicated only in patients considered to be at risk for developing hypoglycemia (infants, patients on insulin therapy). Otherwise, the normal hyperglycemic response to surgical stress is sufficient to prevent hypoglycemia. Iatrogenic hyperglycemia can limit the effectiveness of fluid resuscitation by inducing an osmotic diuresis.

TABLE 14-13

MAINTENANCE WATER REQUIREMENTS

Weight	mL/kg/hr	mL/kg/day
1–10 kg	4	100
11–20 kg	2	50
>20 kg	1	20

C. **Surgical Fluid Requirements**
   1. **Water and Electrolyte Composition of Fluid Losses.**
      Surgical patients require replacement of plasma volume and ECF secondary to hemorrhage and tissue manipulation (third-space loss). Lactated Ringer's solution is often selected for replacement of third-space losses as well as for gastrointestinal secretions.
   2. **Influence of Perioperative Fluid Infusion Rates on Clinical Outcomes.** Conventionally, intraoperative fluid management included replacement of fluids assumed to accumulate extravascularly in surgically manipulated tissues. Until recently, perioperative clinical practice included, in addition to maintenance fluids and blood loss, 4 to 6 mL/kg/hr for procedures involving minimal tissue trauma, 6 to 8 mL/kg/hr for those involving moderate trauma, and 8 to 12 mL/kg/hr for those involving extreme trauma. Yet perioperative fluid management may be linked to minor and major morbidity.
      a. Fluid restriction appears to be less well tolerated than liberal fluid administration in patients undergoing surgery of a limited scope (e.g., knee arthroscopy).
      b. In patients undergoing major intraabdominal surgery, restrictive fluid administration is associated with combinations of positive and negative effects.
      c. Critically ill patients with acute lung injury may benefit from conservative fluid replacement without an increased incidence of renal failure.

V. **COLLOIDS, CRYSTALLOID, AND HYPERTONIC SOLUTIONS**

   A. **Physiology and Pharmacology.** IV fluids vary in oncotic pressure, osmolarity, and tonicity. When the capillary membrane is intact, fluids containing colloid, such as albumin or hydroxyethyl starch, preferentially expand plasma volume rather than ICF volume.
   B. **Clinical Implications of Choices between Alternative Fluids.** Despite the relative advantages and disadvantages, no evidence supports the superiority of either colloid-containing or crystalloid-containing solutions (Table 14-14).

TABLE 14-14

POSSIBLE ADVANTAGES AND DISADVANTAGES OF COLLOID
VERSUS CRYSTALLOID INTRAVENOUS FLUIDS

	Advantages	Disadvantages
Colloid	Smaller volume infused	Greater cost
	Prolonged increase in plasma volume	Coagulopathy (dextran > hetastarch)
	Greater peripheral edema	Pulmonary edema (capillary leak states)
	Less cerebral edema	Decreased glomerular filtration rate
		Osmotic diuresis (low-molecular-weight dextran)
Crystalloid	Lower cost	Transient hemodynamic improvement
	Greater urinary flow	Peripheral edema (protein dilution)
	Replaces interstitial fluid	Pulmonary edema (protein dilution plus high pulmonary artery occlusion pressure)

1. Despite a commonly held opinion, the risk of pulmonary edema seems to be independent of the selection of a crystalloid- or colloid-containing solution.
2. Colloid-induced expansion of the plasma volume redistributes slowly, such that diuretic therapy is often required if pulmonary edema develops.
3. There appears to be no important clinical difference in pulmonary function after administration of crystalloid or colloid solutions in the absence of hypervolemia.

C. **Implications of Crystalloid and Colloid Infusions on Intracranial Pressure.** Despite a clinical notion, the risk of increased intracranial pressure seems to be independent of the selection of a crystalloid- or colloid-containing solution.

D. **Clinical Implications of Hypertonic Fluid Administration.** Hypertonic and hyperoncotic fluids seem most likely to be effective in the treatment of hypovolemic patients who have decreased intracranial compliance.

TABLE 14-15

CONDITIONS ASSOCIATED WITH DEFICITS IN BLOOD VOLUME
AND EXTRACELLULAR FLUID VOLUME

Trauma
Pancreatitis
Burns
Bowel obstruction
Sepsis
Chronic systemic hypertension
Chronic diuretic use
Prolonged gastrointestinal losses

VI. FLUID STATUS: ASSESSMENT AND MONITORING

A. **Conventional Clinical Assessment.** The preoperative clinical assessment of blood volume and ECF volume begins with the recognition of conditions in which deficits are likely to occur (Table 14-15).

1. Physical signs of hypovolemia are insensitive and nonspecific (Table 14-16). A normal blood pressure reading may represent relative hypotension in an elderly or chronically hypertensive patient. Conversely, substantial hypovolemia may occur despite an apparently normal blood pressure and heart rate.

   a. Elderly patients may demonstrate orthostatic hypotension despite a normal blood volume.

   b. Young, healthy subjects can tolerate an acute blood loss equivalent to 20% of their blood volume while exhibiting only postural tachycardia and variable postural hypotension.

   c. Orthostatic changes in central venous pressure, coupled with assessment of the response to fluid infusion, may represent a useful test of the adequacy of blood volume.

TABLE 14-16

SIGNS AND SYMPTOMS OF HYPOVOLEMIA

Oliguria (rule out renal failure, stress-induced endocrine response)
Hypotension in the supine position (implies blood volume deficit
 >30%)
Positive tilt test result (increase in heart rate [>20 bpm] and
 decrease in systolic blood pressure [>20 mm Hg] when patient
 assumes the standing position)

TABLE 14-17

LABORATORY EVIDENCE OF HYPOVOLEMIA

Hemoconcentration (hematocrit is a poor indicator of blood volume)
Azotemia (may be influenced by events unrelated to blood volume)
Low urine sodium concentration (<20 mEq for every 1000 mL of urine)
Metabolic alkalosis
Metabolic acidosis (reflects organ hypoperfusion)

2. Laboratory data may suggest hypovolemia or ECF volume depletion (Table 14-17).
   a. Hematocrit is a poor indicator of blood volume because it is influenced by the time elapsed since hemorrhage and the volume of asanguineous fluid replacement. Hematocrit is virtually unchanged by acute hemorrhage; later, hemodilution occurs as fluids are administered or as fluid shifts from the interstitial to the intravascular space. If the intravascular fluid volume has been restored, hematocrit measurement will more accurately reflect red blood cell mass and can be used to guide transfusion.
   b. Blood urea nitrogen and serum creatinine levels may be increased if hypovolemia is sufficiently prolonged. (Both measurements may also be influenced by events unrelated to blood volume.) Although hypovolemia does not cause metabolic alkalosis, ECF volume depletion is a potent stimulus for the maintenance of metabolic alkalosis.
B. **Intraoperative Clinical Assessment.** Visual estimation, as seen on operative sponges and drapes, is the simplest technique for quantifying intraoperative blood loss.
   1. Adequacy of intraoperative blood volume replacement cannot be ascertained by any single modality (Table 14-18).

TABLE 14-18

CLINICAL INDICATORS OF THE ADEQUACY OF INTRAOPERATIVE BLOOD VOLUME REPLACEMENT

Heart rate (tachycardia is insensitive and nonspecific)
Blood pressure
Central venous pressure
Urinary output
Arterial oxygenation and pH

2. Preservation of the blood pressure accompanied by a central venous pressure of 6 to 12 mm Hg in the presence of a volatile anesthetic suggests an adequate blood volume.
   a. During profound hypovolemia, indirect measurement of blood pressure may significantly underestimate true blood pressure, emphasizing the potential value of direct blood pressure measurements in selected patients.
   b. An additional advantage of direct arterial pressure monitoring may be recognition of increased systolic blood pressure variation accompanying positive pressure ventilation in the presence of hypovolemia.
3. Urinary output usually decreases precipitously (<0.5 mL/kg/hr) in the presence of moderate to severe hypovolemia.

C. **Oxygen Delivery as a Goal of Management.** No intraoperative monitor is sufficiently sensitive or specific to detect hypoperfusion in all patients. In high-risk surgical patients, systemic oxygen delivery of 600 mL/m^2/min or above (equivalent to a cardiac index of 3 L/m^2/min and a hemoglobin concentration equivalent to 14 g/dL) may result in improved outcome.

VII. ELECTROLYTES

A. **Physiologic Role of Electrolytes** (Table 14-19).
B. **Sodium.** Disorders of sodium concentration (hyponatremia, hypernatremia) usually result from relative excesses or deficits of water. Regulation of the quantity and concentration of electrolytes is accomplished primarily by the endocrine and renal systems.
   1. **Hyponatremia** (<130 mEq/L) is the most common electrolyte disturbance in hospitalized patients (postoperative, acute intracranial disease) and is usually caused by excess total body water.
      a. Signs and symptoms of hyponatremia depend on the rate at which the plasma sodium concentration decreases and the severity of the decrease (Table 14-20).
      b. The cerebral salt-wasting syndrome appears to be mediated by brain natriuretic peptide; the secretion of antidiuretic hormone is appropriate.
      c. Many patients develop hyponatremia as a result of the syndrome of inappropriate antidiuretic

TABLE 14-19

PHYSIOLOGIC ROLE OF ELECTROLYTES

Electrolyte	Physiologic Role
Sodium	Osmolarity
	Extracellular fluid volume
	Action potential
Potassium	Transmembrane potential
	Action potential
Calcium	Excitation–contraction
	Neurotransmission
	Enzyme function
	Cardiac pacemaker activity
	Cardiac action potential
	Bone structure
Phosphorus	Stores energy (adenosine triphosphate)
	Component of second messengers (cyclic adenosine monophosphate)
	Component of cell membranes (phospholipids)
Magnesium	Enzyme cofactor (sodium-potassium pump)
	Controls potassium movement into cells
	Membrane excitability
	Bone structure

       hormone secretion (SIADH). The cornerstone of SIADH management is free water restriction and elimination of precipitating causes (Table 14-21).

    d. Inappropriately rapid correction of hyponatremia may result in abrupt brain dehydration (osmotic demyelination syndrome is most likely when hyponatremia has persisted >48 hours).

TABLE 14-20

SIGNS AND SYMPTOMS OF HYPONATREMIA

Neurologic
Altered consciousness (sedation to coma)
Seizures
Cerebral edema

Gastrointestinal
Loss of appetite
Nausea and vomiting

Muscular
Cramps
Weakness

TABLE 14-21

PRECIPITATING CAUSES OF INAPPROPRIATE ANTIDIURETIC
HORMONE SECRETION

Hypovolemia
Pulmonary disease
Central nervous system trauma
Endocrine dysfunction
Drugs that mimic antidiuretic hormone

2. **Hypernatremia** (>150 mEq/L) is usually the result of
    decreased total body water.
    a. Signs and symptoms of hypernatremia most likely
       reflect the effect of dehydration on neurons and the
       presence of hypoperfusion caused by hypovolemia
       (Table 14-22). When hypernatremia develops
       abruptly, the associated sudden brain shrinkage
       may stretch and disrupt cerebral vessels, leading to
       subdural hematoma, subarachnoid hemorrhage,
       and venous thrombosis.
    b. Postoperative neurosurgical patients who have
       undergone pituitary surgery are at particular risk
       of developing transient or prolonged diabetes
       insipidus, leading to hypernatremia.
    c. **Treatment** of hypernatremia is influenced by the
       clinical assessment of ECF volume (Table 14-23).
 C. Potassium
    1. **Hypokalemia** (<3.0 mEq/L) may result from acute
       redistribution of potassium from the extracellular to
       the ICF (total body potassium concentration is

TABLE 14-22

SIGNS AND SYMPTOMS OF HYPERNATREMIA

Neurologic
Thirst
Weakness
Hyperreflexia
Seizures
Intracranial hemorrhage

Cardiovascular
Hypovolemia

Renal
Polyuria or oliguria
Renal insufficiency

ANATOMY AND PHYSIOLOGY

TABLE 14-23

TREATMENT OF HYPERNATREMIA

Sodium Depletion (Hypovolemia)
Correct hypovolemia (0.9% saline).
Correct hypernatremia (hypotonic fluids).

Sodium Overload (Hypervolemia)
Enhance sodium removal (loop diuretics, dialysis).
Replace water deficit (hypotonic fluids).

Normal Total Body Sodium (Euvolemia)
Replace water deficit (hypotonic fluids).
Control diabetes insipidus (desmopressin, vasopressin, chlorpropamide).
Control nephrogenic diabetes insipidus (restrict sodium and water intake, thiazide diuretics).

normal) or from chronic depletion of total body potassium. With chronic potassium loss, the ratio of intracellular to extracellular potassium remains relatively constant, but acute redistribution of potassium substantially changes the resting potential difference across cell membranes.

a. Plasma potassium concentration poorly reflects total body potassium, and hypokalemia may occur with high, normal, or low total body potassium. The plasma potassium concentration (98% of potassium is intracellular) correlates poorly with total body potassium stores. Total body potassium approximates 50 to 55 mEq/kg. As a guideline, a chronic decrease in serum potassium of 1 mEq/L corresponds to a total body deficit of about 200 to 300 mEq.

b. Signs and symptoms of hypokalemia reflect the diffuse effects of potassium on cell membranes and excitable tissues (Table 14-24).

c. Cardiac rhythm disturbances are among the most dangerous complications of hypokalemia. Although no clear threshold has been defined for a level of hypokalemia below which safe conduct of anesthesia is compromised, serum potassium concentrations below 3.5 mEq/L may be associated with an increased incidence of perioperative dysrhythmias (atrial fibrillation or flutter in cardiac surgical patients).

TABLE 14-24

SIGNS AND SYMPTOMS OF HYPOKALEMIA

Cardiovascular
Cardiac dysrhythmias (premature ventricular contractions)
ECG changes (widened QRS segment, S-T segment depression,
  first-degree AV heart block)
Potentiates digitalis toxicity
Postural hypotension

Neuromuscular
Skeletal muscle weakness (hypoventilation)
Hyporeflexia
Confusion

Renal
Polyuria
Concentrating defect

Metabolic
Glucose intolerance
Potentiation of hypercalcemia and hypomagnesemia

AV = atrioventricular; ECG = electrocardiograph.

    d. Potassium depletion may induce defects in renal
       concentrating ability, resulting in polyuria.
    e. Hypokalemia causes skeletal muscle weakness and,
       when severe, may even cause paralysis.
    f. Treatment of hypokalemia consists of potassium
       repletion, correction of alkalosis, and discontinua-
       tion of offending drugs (diuretics, aminoglycosides)
       (Table 14-25). Hypokalemia secondary only to
       acute redistribution may not require treatment. Oral
       potassium chloride (chloride deficiency may limit
       the ability of the kidneys to conserve potassium) is
       preferable to IV replacement if total body potassium

TABLE 14-25

TREATMENT OF HYPOKALEMIA

Correct Precipitating Factors (alkalosis, hypomagnesemia, drugs)

Mild Hypokalemia (>2.0 mEq/L)
Infuse potassium chloride ≤10 mEq/hr IV.

Severe Hypokalemia (<2.0 mEq/L, ECG changes, intense skeletal
  muscle weakness)
Infuse potassium chloride ≤40 mEq/hr IV.
Continuously monitor the ECG.

ECG = electrocardiograph; IV = intravenous.

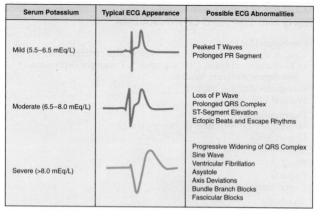

Serum Potassium	Typical ECG Appearance	Possible ECG Abnormalities
Mild (5.5–6.5 mEq/L)		Peaked T Waves Prolonged PR Segment
Moderate (6.5–8.0 mEq/L)		Loss of P Wave Prolonged QRS Complex ST-Segment Elevation Ectopic Beats and Escape Rhythms
Severe (>8.0 mEq/L)		Progressive Widening of QRS Complex Sine Wave Ventricular Fibrillation Asystole Axis Deviations Bundle Branch Blocks Fascicular Blocks

FIGURE 14-2.   Electrocardiographic (ECG) changes that may accompany progressive increases in serum potassium concentrations.

stores are decreased. IV potassium replacement at a rate of greater than 20 mEq/hr should be continuously monitored with electrocardiography (ECG).

2. **Hyperkalemia** (>5 mEq/L) is most often caused by renal insufficiency or drugs that limit potassium excretion (nonsteroidal antiinflammatory drugs, angiotensin-converting enzyme inhibitors, cyclosporine, potassium-sparing diuretics). The most lethal manifestations of hyperkalemia involve the cardiac conducting system (Fig. 14-2). Overall, ECG is an insensitive and nonspecific method of detecting hyperkalemia.

   a. Signs and symptoms of hyperkalemia primarily involve the central nervous and cardiovascular systems (Table 14-26).

TABLE 14-26

SIGNS AND SYMPTOMS OF HYPERKALEMIA

Cardiovascular
Cardiac dysrhythmias (heart block)
ECG changes (widened QRS segment, tall peaked T waves, atrial asystole, prolongation of P-R interval)

Neuromuscular
Skeletal muscle weakness
Paresthesias
Confusion

ECG = electrocardiograph.

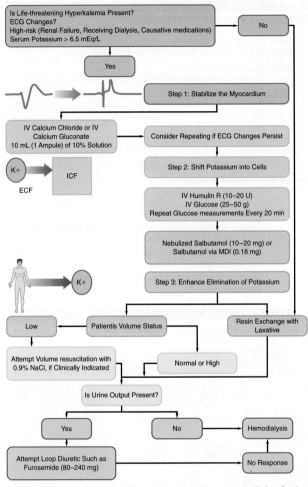

FIGURE 14-3. Treatment of hyperkalemia. ECF = extracellular fluid; ECG = electrocardiogram; ICF = intracellular fluid; IV = intravenous.

b. Treatment of hyperkalemia is designed to eliminate the cause, reverse membrane hyperexcitability, and remove potassium from the body (Fig. 14-3 and Table 14-27).

TABLE 14-27

TREATMENT OF SEVERE HYPERKALEMIA*

Reverse Membrane Effects
Calcium (10% calcium chloride IV over 10 min)

Transfer Potassium Into Cells
Glucose (D10W) and regular insulin (5–10 U regular insulin for every 25–50 g of glucose)
Sodium bicarbonate (50–100 mEq over 5 to 10)
β-2 agonists

Remove Potassium from Body
Diuretics (proximal or loop)
Potassium-exchange resins
Hemodialysis (removes 25–50 mEq/hr)

*>7 mEq/L, ECG changes.
ECG = electrocardiograph.

> D. Calcium
> 1. **Hypocalcemia** (ionized calcium <4.0 mg/dL) occurs as a result of parathyroid hormone deficiency (surgical parathyroid gland damage or removal, burns, sepsis) or because of calcium chelation or precipitation (hyperphosphatemia, as from cell lysis secondary to chemotherapy).

TABLE 14-28

SIGNS AND SYMPTOMS OF HYPOCALCEMIA

Cardiovascular
Cardiac dysrhythmias
ECG changes (prolongation of the Q-T interval, T-wave inversion)
Hypotension
Congestive heart failure

Neuromuscular
Skeletal muscle spasm
Tetany
Skeletal muscle weakness
Seizures

Pulmonary
Laryngospasm
Bronchospasm
Hypoventilation

Psychiatric
Anxiety
Dementia
Depression

ECG = electrocardiograph.

TABLE 14-29

TREATMENT OF HYPOCALCEMIA

Administer calcium.
10 mL of 10% calcium gluconate IV over 10 min followed by a
  continuous infusion of 500 to 1000 mg of calcium orally every
  6 hr.
Administer vitamin D.
Monitor ECG.

ECG = electrocardiograph; IV = intravenous; PO = per os.

       a. The hallmark of hypocalcemia is increased neuronal
          membrane irritability and tetany (Table 14-28).
       b. Decreased total serum calcium concentration occurs
          in as many as 80% of critically ill and postsurgical
          patients, but few patients develop ionized hypocal-
          cemia (multiple trauma, after cardiopulmonary
          bypass, massive transfusion [citrate]).
       c. Treatment of hypocalcemia (Table 14-29).
    2. Hypercalcemia (ionized calcium >5.2 mg/dL) occurs
      when calcium enters the ECF more rapidly than the
      kidneys can excrete the excess. Clinically, hypercalcemia
      most commonly results from an excess of bone resorp-
      tion over bone formation, usually secondary to malig-
      nant disease, hyperparathyroidism, or immobilization.
      a. Signs and symptoms (Table 14-30).

TABLE 14-30

SIGNS AND SYMPTOMS OF HYPERCALCEMIA

Cardiovascular
Hypertension
Heart block
Digitalis sensitivity

Neuromuscular
Skeletal muscle weakness
Hyporeflexia
Sedation to coma

Renal
Nephrolithiasis
Polyuria (renal tubular concentration defect)
Azotemia

Gastrointestinal
Peptic ulcer disease
Pancreatitis
Anorexia

ANATOMY AND PHYSIOLOGY

TABLE 14-31

SIGNS AND SYMPTOMS OF HYPOMAGNESEMIA

Cardiovascular
Coronary vasospasm
Cardiac dysrhythmias (especially after myocardial infarction or
  after cardiopulmonary bypass)
Refractory ventricular fibrillation
Congestive heart failure

Neuromuscular
Neuronal irritability (tetany)
Skeletal muscle weakness
Sedation
Seizures

Miscellaneous
Dysphagia
Anorexia
Nausea
Hypokalemia (magnesium-induced potassium wasting)
Hypocalcemia (magnesium-induced suppression of parathyroid
  hormone secretion)

     b. Treatment of hypercalcemia in the perioperative
        period includes saline infusion and administration
        of furosemide to enhance calcium excretion (urine
        output should be maintained at 200–300 mL/hr).
   E. Magnesium is principally intracellular and is necessary
     for enzymatic reactions.
     1. Hypomagnesemia (<1.8 mg/dL) is common in
        critically ill patients, most likely reflecting nasogastric
        suctioning and an inability of the renal tubules to
        conserve magnesium. Hypomagnesemia can aggravate
        digoxin toxicity and congestive heart failure.
        a. Signs and symptoms (Table 14-31).
        b. Treatment of hypomagnesemia (Table 14-32).
           During magnesium repletion, the patellar reflexes

TABLE 14-32

TREATMENT OF HYPOMAGNESEMIA

Administer magnesium.*
Administer IV magnesium 8 to 16 mEq over 1 hr followed by 2 to
  4 mEq/hr.
Administer IM magnesium 10 mEq every 4 to 6 hr.

*$MgSO_4$ 1 g = 8 mEq; $MgCl_2$ 1 g = 10 mEq.
IM = intramuscular; IV = intravenous.

TABLE 14-33

SIGNS AND SYMPTOMS OF HYPERMAGNESEMIA

Plasma Magnesium Concentration (mg/dL)	
Normal	1.8–2.5
Therapeutic range (pre-eclampsia)	5–8
Hypotension	3–5
Deep tendon hyporeflexia	5
Somnolence	7–12
Deep tendon areflexia	7–12
Hypoventilation	>12
Heart block	>12
Cardiac arrest	>12

should be monitored frequently and magnesium withheld if the reflexes become suppressed. During IV infusion of magnesium, it is important to continuously monitor the ECG to detect cardiotoxicity.

2. **Hypermagnesemia** (>2.5 mg/dL) is usually iatrogenic (e.g., treatment of pregnancy-induced hypertension or premature labor).

   a. Signs and symptoms (Table 14-33).

   b. Hypermagnesemia antagonizes the release and effect of acetylcholine at the neuromuscular junction, manifesting as potentiation of the action of nondepolarizing muscle relaxants.

   c. Treatment of neuromuscular and cardiac toxicity produced by hypermagnesemia can be promptly but transiently antagonized by 5 to 10 mEq IV of calcium. Urinary excretion of magnesium can be increased by expanding the ECF volume and inducing diuresis with a combination of furosemide and saline. In emergency situations and in patients with renal failure, magnesium may be removed by dialysis.

CHAPTER 15 ■ AUTONOMIC NERVOUS SYSTEM

Anesthesiology is the practice of autonomic nervous system (ANS) medicine (Johnson JO, Grecu L, Lawson NW: Autonomic nervous system. In *Clinical Anesthesia*. Edited by Barash PG, Cullen BF, Stoelting RK, Cahalan MK, Stock MC. Philadelphia: Lippincott Williams & Wilkins, 2009, pp 326–368). Data recorded on the anesthesia record often reflect ANS function and homeostasis. Drugs used during anesthesia as well as painful stimulation and disease states frequently produce ANS-related side effects.

I. FUNCTIONAL ANATOMY

The ANS is divided into the sympathetic nervous system (SNS; adrenergic system) and the parasympathetic nervous system (PNS; cholinergic system) (Fig. 15-1). The SNS and PNS produce complementary effects on the activity of various organ systems (Table 15-1).

A. **Central Autonomic Organization.** The principal site of ANS integration (blood pressure control, temperature regulation, stress responses) is the hypothalamus. Vital centers for hemodynamic and ventilatory control are located in the medulla oblongata and pons. ANS hyperreflexia is an example of spinal cord mediation of ANS reflexes without integration of function from higher inhibitory centers.

B. **Peripheral Autonomic Nervous System Organization** (Fig. 15-2)
   1. The cell body of the preganglionic neuron originates in the central nervous system (CNS) and synapses in an autonomic ganglion. (The adrenal medulla is an exception.) Preganglionic fibers are myelinated (rapid conducting).

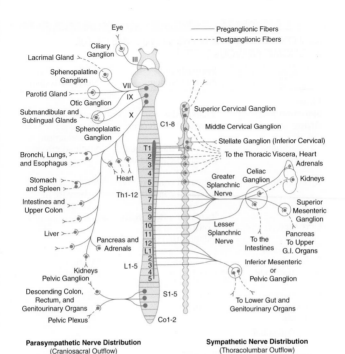

FIGURE 15-1. Schematic distribution of the craniosacral (parasympathetic) and thoracolumbar (sympathetic) nervous systems. Parasympathetic preganglionic fibers pass directly to the organ that is innervated (with discrete and limited effects). Activation of the sympathetic fibers produces a more diffuse physiologic response. GI = gastrointestinal.

2. Postganglionic neurons arise from the autonomic ganglia and are distributed to effector organs. Postganglionic fibers are unmyelinated (slow conducting).
   a. The 22 pairs of SNS (paravertebral) ganglia are located closer to the spinal cord than to the innervated organ.
   b. The PNS ganglia are located in or near the innervated organ.
3. Whereas activation of the SNS produces a diffuse physiologic response (mass reflex), activation of the PNS produces more discrete responses. For example, vagal stimulation may produce bradycardia with no effect on intestinal motility.

ANATOMY AND PHYSIOLOGY

TABLE 15-1

HOMEOSTATIC BALANCE BETWEEN DIVISIONS OF THE
AUTONOMIC NERVOUS SYSTEM

	Sympathetic Nervous System	Parasympathetic Nervous System
Heart		
Sinoatrial node	Tachycardia	Bradycardia
Atrioventricular node	Increased conduction	Decreased conduction
His-Purkinje system	Increased automaticity Increased conduction velocity	Minimal effect
Myocardium	Increased contractility Increased conduction velocity Increased automaticity	Minimal decrease in contractility
Coronary vessels	Constriction (α_1) Dilation (β_1)	
Blood Vessels		
Skin and mucosa	Constriction	Dilation
Skeletal muscle	Constriction (α_1) > dilation (β)	Dilation
Pulmonary	Constriction	Dilation
Bronchial Smooth Muscle	Relaxation	Contraction
Gastrointestinal Tract		
Gallbladder	Relaxation	Contraction
Gut motility and secretions	Decreased	Increased
Bladder		
Detrusor	Relaxation	Contraction
Trigone	Contraction	Relaxation
Glands (nasal, lacrimal, salivary, pancreatic)	Vasoconstriction and reduced secretion	Stimulation of secretions
Sweat Glands	Diaphoresis (cholinergic)	No effect
Apocrine Glands	Thick and odiferous secretions	No effect
Eyes		
Pupil	Mydriasis	Miosis
Ciliary	Relaxation for far vision	Contraction for near vision

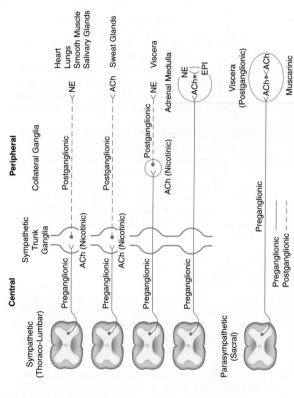

FIGURE 15-2. Schematic diagram of the efferent autonomic nervous system. Ach = acetylcholine.

C. **Autonomic Innervation**
   1. **Heart.** SNS and PNS innervation of the heart (via the stellate ganglion) influences heart rate (chronotropism), strength of contraction (inotropism), and coronary blood flow.
      a. The PNS cardiac vagal fibers are distributed mainly to the sinoatrial (SA) and atrioventricular (AV) nodes, such that the main effect of cardiac vagal stimulation is chronotropic. (Strong vagal stimulation can arrest SA node firing and block impulse conduction to the ventricles.)
      b. The SNS has the same supraventricular distribution as the PNS but with stronger distribution to the ventricles. (Normal SNS tone maintains contractility about 20% above that in the absence of SNS stimulation.)
   2. **Peripheral circulation.** The SNS is the most important regulator of the peripheral circulation. Basal ANS tone maintains arteriolar diameter at about 50% of maximum, thus permitting the potential for further vasoconstriction or vasodilation. By functioning as a reservoir for about 80% of the blood volume, small changes in venous capacitance produced by SNS-mediated venoconstriction produce large changes in venous return.

II. AUTONOMIC NERVOUS SYSTEM TRANSMISSION

A. Transmission of impulses across the nerve terminal junctional sites (synaptic cleft) of the peripheral ANS occurs through the mediation of liberated chemicals (neurotransmitters). These neurotransmitters interact with a receptor on the end organ to evoke a biologic response.

B. **Parasympathetic Nervous System Neurotransmission**
   1. **Acetylcholine (ACh)** is the neurotransmitter at preganglionic nerve endings of the SNS and PNS and at postganglionic nerve endings of the PNS.
   2. The ability of a receptor to modulate the function of an effector organ depends on rapid recovery to its baseline state after stimulation. ACh removal occurs by rapid hydrolysis by acetylcholinesterase (true cholinesterase). Pseudocholinesterase (plasma

cholinesterase) is not physiologically significant in the termination (hydrolysis) of ACh action.

C. **Sympathetic Nervous System Neurotransmission**
1. Norepinephrine is the neurotransmitter at postganglionic nerve endings of the SNS (except in the sweat glands, where ACh is the neurotransmitter).
    a. Adenosine triphosphate (ATP) is released with norepinephrine and thus functions as a co-neurotransmitter.
    b. Epinephrine is the principal hormone released by chromaffin cells (which function as postganglionic SNS neurons) into the circulation to function as a neurotransmitter hormone.
2. **Catecholamines: The First Messenger**
    a. Endogenous catecholamines are dopamine (neurotransmitter in the CNS), norepinephrine, and epinephrine. A catecholamine (including synthetic catecholamines) is any compound with a catechol nucleus (benzene ring with two adjacent hydroxyl groups) and an amine-containing side chain (Fig. 15-3).
    b. The effects of endogenous or synthetic catecholamines on adrenergic receptors can be indirect (little intrinsic activity but stimulate release of stored neurotransmitter) and direct.
3. **Inactivation** of catecholamines is by reuptake back into presynaptic nerve terminals by extraneuronal uptake, diffusion, and metabolism.

III. RECEPTORS

Receptors appear to be protein macromolecules on cell membranes, which when activated by an agonist (ACh or norepinephrine) lead to a response by an effector cell. An antagonist is a substance that attaches to the receptor (prevents access of an agonist) but does not elicit a response by the effector cell.

A. **Cholinergic receptors** are subdivided into muscarinic (postganglionic nerve endings) and nicotinic (autonomic ganglia, neuromuscular junction) receptors. ACh is the neurotransmitter at cholinergic receptors. Atropine is a specific antagonist at muscarinic receptors.

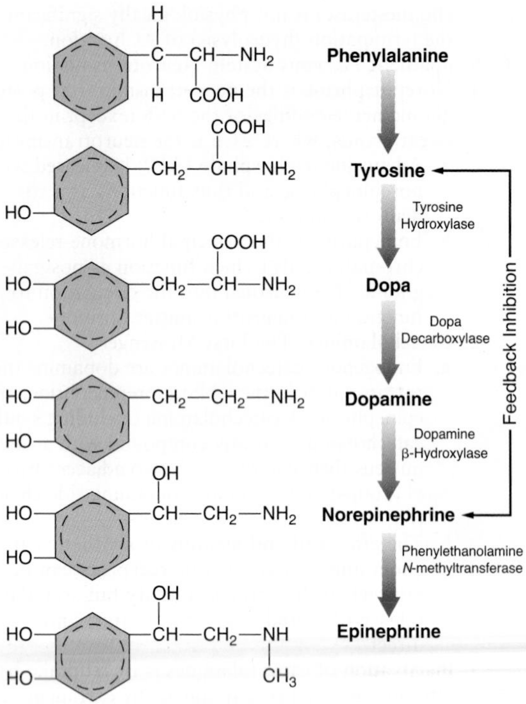

FIGURE 15-3. Synthesis of catecholamines.

B. **Adrenergic receptors** are subdivided into α, β, and dopaminergic, with subtypes for each category (Table 15-2).

1. **α-Adrenergic Receptors in the Cardiovascular System**

a. **Coronary arteries.** Postsynaptic α_2 receptors predominate in the large epicardial conductance vessels. (They contribute about 5% to total coronary artery resistance, which is why phenylephrine has little influence on resistance to blood flow in coronary arteries.) Postsynaptic α_2 receptors predominate in small coronary artery resistance vessels. The density of α_2 receptors in the coronary arteries increases in response to myocardial ischemia.

TABLE 15-2

ADRENERGIC RECEPTORS AND ORDER OF POTENCY OF AGONISTS AND ANTAGONISTS

Receptor	Potency	Agonists	Antagonists	Location	Action
α_1	++++	Norepinephrine	Phenoxybenzamine*	Smooth muscle (vascular, iris, radial, pilomotor, uterus, trigone, GI and bladder sphincters)	Contraction
	+++	Epinephrine	Phentolamine*		Vasoconstriction
	++	Dopamine	Ergot alkaloids*		
	+	Isoproterenol	Prazosin	Brain	Neurotransmission
			Tolazoline*	Smooth muscle (GI)	Relaxation
			Labetalol*	Heart	Glycogenolysis
				Adrenergic nerve endings	Inhibition of norepinephrine release
α_2	++++	Clonidine	Yohimbine		
	+++	Norepinephrine	Piperoxan	Presynaptic (CNS)	Aggregation
	+++	Epinephrine	Phentolamine*	Platelets	Granule release
	++	Norepinephrine	Phenoxybenzamine*		
	+	Phenylephrine	Tolazoline*	Adipose tissue	Inhibition of lipolysis
			Labetalol*		Inhibition of insulin release
				Endocrine pancreas	Inhibition of renin release
				Kidney	
				Brain	Neurotransmission

(continued)

183

TABLE 15-2
ADRENERGIC RECEPTORS AND ORDER OF POTENCY OF AGONISTS AND ANTAGONISTS (Continued)

Receptor	Potency	Agonists	Antagonists	Location	Action
β_1	++++	Isoproterenol*	Acebutolol	Heart	Increased heart rate Increased contractility Increased conduction velocity
	+++ ++	Epinephrine Norepinephrine	Practolol Propranolol*		Coronary vasodilation
	+	Dopamine	Alprenolol* Metoprolol Esmolol	Adipose tissue	Lipolysis
β_2	++++	Isoproterenol	Propranolol*	Liver	Glycogenolysis Gluconeogenesis
	+++	Epinephrine Norepinephrine	Butoxamine Alprenolol Esmolol	Skeletal muscle	Glycogenolysis Lactate release
	+	Dopamine			Relaxation
			Nadolol Timolol Labetalol	Smooth muscle Vascular smooth muscle Renal Mesentery	Vasodilation
Dopamine$_1$	++++ ++ +	Fenoldopam Dopamine Epinephrine Metoclopramide	Haloperidol Droperidol Phenothiazines		
Dopamine$_2$	++ +	Dopamine Bromocriptine	Domperidone	Presynaptic-adrenergic nerve endings	Inhibition of norepinephrine release

*Nonselective.
CNS = central nervous system; GI = gastrointestinal.

    b. **Peripheral Vessels.** Presynaptic α_2-vascular receptors mediate vasodilation, and postsynaptic α_1- and α_2-vascular receptors mediate vasoconstriction. Postsynaptic α_2-vascular receptors predominate on the venous side of the circulation. Actions attributed to postsynaptic α_2 receptors include arterial and venous vasoconstriction, platelet aggregation, inhibition of insulin release, inhibition of bowel motility, and inhibition of antidiuretic hormone release.

2. **α Receptors in the Kidneys.** The α_1 receptors dominate in the renal vasculature (vasoconstriction modulates renal blood flow), and the α_2 receptors predominate in the renal tubules, especially the loops of Henle (which stimulate water and sodium excretion).

3. **β Receptors in the Cardiovascular System**

    a. **Myocardium.** Postsynaptic β_1 receptors and presynaptic β_2 receptors probably play similar roles in the regulation of heart rate and myocardial contractility. Increased circulating catecholamine levels associated with congestive heart failure result in down-regulation of β_1 receptors with relative sparing of β_2 and α_1 receptors. (β_2 and α_1 receptors increasingly mediate the inotropic response to catecholamines during cardiac failure.)

    b. **Peripheral Vessels.** Postsynaptic vascular β receptors are predominantly β_2.

4. **β Receptors in the Kidneys.** β_1 receptors are more prominent than β receptors in the kidneys, and their activation results in renin release.

C. **Adrenergic Receptor Numbers and Sensitivity**

1. Receptors are dynamically regulated by a variety of conditions (ambient concentrations of catecholamines and drugs and genetic factors), resulting in altered responses to catecholamines and ANS stimulation.

2. Alteration in the number or density of receptors is referred to as up-regulation or down-regulation. Chronic treatment with clonidine or propranolol results in up-regulation and a withdrawal syndrome if the drug is acutely discontinued.

IV. AUTONOMIC NERVOUS SYSTEM REFLEXES AND INTERACTIONS

The ANS has been compared to a computer circuit (sensor, afferent pathway, CNS integration, efferent pathway).

A. **Baroreceptors** located in the carotid sinus and aortic arch react to alterations in stretch caused by changes in blood pressure (Fig. 15-4). Volatile anesthetics interfere with baroreceptor function; thus, anesthetic-induced decreases in blood pressure may not evoke changes in heart rate. Compliance of stretch receptors and their sensitivity may be altered by carotid sinus atherosclerosis. (Carotid artery disease may be a source of hypertension rather than a result.)

B. **Venous baroreceptors** located in the right atrium and great veins produce an increased heart rate when the right atrium is stretched by increased filling pressure

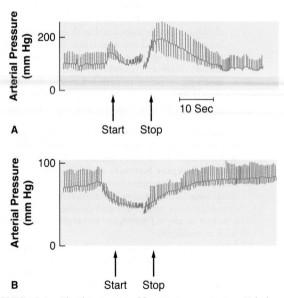

FIGURE 15-4. Blood pressure and heart rate response to a Valsalva maneuver (**A**, normal; **B**, abnormal in a patient with cervical quadriplegia).

(Bainbridge reflex). Slowing of the heart rate during spinal anesthesia may reflect activation of venous baroreceptors as a result of decreased venous return.

V. CLINICAL AUTONOMIC NERVOUS SYSTEM PHARMACOLOGY

Drugs that modify ANS activity can be classified by their site of action and the mechanism of action or pathology (antihypertensives) for which they are administered.

A. **Cholinergic Drugs. Muscarinic agonists** act at sites in the body where ACh is the neurotransmitter.

1. **Indirect Cholinomimetics.** Anticholinesterases (neostigmine, pyridostigmine, edrophonium) inhibit activity of acetylcholinesterase, which normally destroys ACh by hydrolysis. As a result of this inhibition, ACh accumulates at muscarinic and nicotinic receptors. Simultaneous administration of an anticholinergic drug protects patients against undesired muscarinic effects (bradycardia, salivation, bronchospasm, intestinal hypermotility) without preventing the nicotinic effects of ACh (reversal of nondepolarizing muscle relaxants).

B. **Cholinergic Drugs. Muscarinic antagonist** refers to a specific drug action for which the term *anticholinergic* is often used (any drug that interferes with the action of ACh as a transmitter). Anticholinergic drugs (atropine, scopolamine, glycopyrrolate) interfere with the muscarinic actions of ACh by competitive inhibition of cholinergic postganglionic nerves.

1. There are marked variations in sensitivity to anticholinergic drugs at different muscarinic sites.

2. **Central anticholinergic syndrome** is characterized by symptoms that range from sedation to delirium, presumably reflecting inhibition of muscarinic receptors in the CNS by anticholinergics (this is unlikely with glycopyrrolate, which cannot easily cross the blood–brain barrier). Treatment is with physostigmine. Its tertiary amine structure allows it to cross the blood–brain barrier rapidly; other anticholinesterases are quaternary ammonium compounds that lack the lipid solubility necessary to gain prompt entrance into the CNS.

C. **Sympathomimetic Drugs.** Catecholamines and sympathomimetic drugs continue to be the pharmacologic mainstay of cardiovascular support for the low-flow state (Table 15-3). It is necessary to become familiar with only a few drugs to manage most clinical situations (Table 15-4). **Low-output syndrome** is present when an individual has abnormalities of the heart, blood volume, or blood flow distribution. When low-output syndrome is present for more than 1 hour, it usually reflects all three abnormalities.

1. Septic shock is the most common distributive abnormality, and volume repletion is an important initial consideration. Treatment of cardiogenic shock requires multiple autonomic interventions.
2. **Adverse Effects.** Side effects of α agonists most often reflect excessive α- or β-receptor activity.

D. **Adrenergic Agonists**

1. **Phenylephrine** is considered a pure α agonist that produces greater venoconstriction than arterial constriction. As a result, venous return and blood pressure are increased.

   a. **Side Effects.** Excessive vasoconstriction produced by phenylephrine can elicit baroreceptor-mediated bradycardia with associated decreases in cardiac output. Increased systemic vascular resistance may further contribute to decreases in cardiac output and increases in myocardial oxygen requirements.

   b. **Clinical Uses.** Phenylephrine is administered as a single dose (50–100 μg intravenously [IV]) to treat anesthetic-induced decreases in blood pressure and hypotension during cardiopulmonary bypass and as a continuous infusion to maintain perfusion pressure during cerebral and peripheral vascular procedures. Use of phenylephrine to maintain perfusion pressures during cerebral and peripheral vascular procedures must be done cautiously because it may evoke myocardial ischemia in susceptible patients.

2. **Norepinephrine** and methoxamine produce similar dose-related hemodynamic effects characterized by greater α than β effects.

   a. Vasoconstriction increases systemic blood pressure but may also decrease tissue blood flow (especially renal blood flow) and increase myocardial oxygen requirements.

TABLE 15-3

DOSES AND PRINCIPAL SITES OF ACTION OF ADRENERGIC AGONISTS

Agent	Bolus (IV)	Continuous Infusion	α_1	α_2	β_1	β_2	Dopamine$_1$	Dopamine$_2$
Phenylephrine	50–100 μg	0.15 μg/kg/min (10 mg in 250 mL, 40 μg/mL)	+++++	?	+/−	0	0	
Norepinephrine		0.1 μg/kg/min (4 mL in 250 mL, 16 μg/mL)	+++++	+++++	+++	0	0	
Epinephrine	2–8 μg* 0.3– 0.5 μg†	0.015 μg/kg/min (1 mL in 250 mL, 4 μg/mL)	+++++	+++	+++++	++	0	
Ephedrine	5–10 mg		++ + to		+++ +++	++ ++	0	
Dopamine		2–10 μg/kg/min (200 mg in 250 mL, 800 μg/mL)	+++++	? ?	++++	++	+++	?
Dobutamine		2–30 μg/kg/min (250 mg in 250 mL, 1000 μg/mL)	0 to +	?	++++	++	0	
Isoproterenol	4 μg	0.015 μg/kg/min (0.15 μg/kg/min to desired effect for third-degree heart block) 1 mg in 250 mL, 4 μg/mL	0	0	+++++	+++++	0	

*Dose to treat hypotension.
†Dose to treat cardiac arrest.

189

TABLE 15-4

HEMODYNAMIC EFFECTS OF ADRENERGIC AGONISTS

Drug	Heart Rate	Cardiac Output	Systemic Vascular Resistance	Venous Return	Renal Blood Flow
Phenylephrine	Decreased	Decreased	Increased	Increased	Decreased
Norepinephrine	Decreased	Decreased	Increased	Increased	Decreased
Epinephrine	Increased	Increased	Increased	Increased	Decreased
Ephedrine	Increased	Increased	Increased	Increased	Unpredictable
Dopamine	No change	Increased	Decreased to no change	Increased	Increased
Dobutamine	Increased	Increased	Decreased to no change	Unpredictable	Increased to no change
Isoproterenol	Increased	Increased	Decreased	Decreased	Increased to no change

    b. Continuous infusion of norepinephrine (which must be through a centrally placed IV catheter) to maintain systolic blood pressure above 90 mm Hg requires invasive monitoring and attention to fluid management.

    c. In clinical conditions characterized by a low perfusion pressure and high flow (vasodilation) and maldistribution of flow, norepinephrine has been shown to improve renal and splanchnic blood flow by increasing perfusion pressure provided the patient has been volume resuscitated.

3. **Epinephrine.** Whereas the α effects of epinephrine predominate in renal and cutaneous vasculature to decrease blood flow, the β effects increase blood flow to skeletal muscles.

    a. Side Effects. Cardiac dysrhythmias are a hazard of excess β stimulation.

    b. Clinical Uses. Epinephrine is administered to treat asthma (0.3–0.5 mg subcutaneously), treat cardiac arrest or life-threatening allergic reactions (0.3–0.5 mg IV), produce hemostasis (1:200,000 or 5 µg/mL injected subcutaneously or submucosally), prolong regional anesthesia (0.2 mg added to local anesthetic solutions for spinal block or as a 1:200,000 concentration for epidural block), or provide a bloodless arthroscopic field by large-volume infusions of dilute epinephrine-containing solutions (1:200,000). (Unpredictable absorption of epinephrine, especially in denuded cancellous bone, may result in overdose and acute heart failure, pulmonary edema, cardiac dysrhythmias, and cardiac arrest in otherwise healthy patients.)

4. **Ephedrine** produces cardiovascular effects that resemble those produced by epinephrine; however, its potency is greatly decreased, although its duration of action is about 10 times longer than that of epinephrine. Venoconstriction is greater than arterial constriction; thus, venous return and cardiac output are improved. A β effect increases heart rate and further facilitates cardiac output. The α and β effects of ephedrine result in a modest and predictable increase in blood pressure.

   a. **Side Effects.** Tachycardia and cardiac dysrhythmias are possible but less likely to occur than after administration of epinephrine.
   b. **Clinical Uses.** Ephedrine is the most commonly used vasopressor (5–10 mg IV) to treat decreases in blood pressure produced by anesthesia (especially regional blocks) and is considered the drug of choice in obstetrics because uterine blood flow directly parallels ephedrine-induced increases in blood pressure. It is appropriate to administer ephedrine as a temporizing measure to restore perfusion pressure while the underlying cause of hypotension is corrected.

5. **Isoproterenol** is a nonspecific β-agonist that lacks α-agonist effects. Whereas cardiac output is increased by virtue of increases in heart rate as well as increased myocardial contractility, decreases in systemic vascular resistance contribute to decreased afterload.
   a. **Side Effects.** Myocardial ischemia may be evoked in vulnerable patients (increased myocardial oxygen requirements caused by tachycardia and increased myocardial contractility paralleled by decreased coronary oxygen delivery because of decreased diastolic blood pressure). Increases in cardiac output may be diverted to nonvital tissues such as skeletal muscles.
   b. **Clinical Uses.** Isoproterenol is most often administered as a continuous IV infusion for the treatment of congestive heart failure associated with bradycardia, asthma, or pulmonary hypertension. This catecholamine acts as a chemical cardiac pacemaker in the presence of complete heart block.

6. **Dobutamine** is a synthetic catecholamine derived from isoproterenol that acts directly on β_1 receptors and does not cause norepinephrine release or stimulation of dopamine receptors. Weak α_1-agonist effects of dobutamine may be unmasked by β-blockade. Dobutamine produces a positive inotropic effect with minimal effects on heart rate and systemic vascular resistance (an advantage over isoproterenol).
   a. **Side Effects.** Increases in automaticity of the SA node and increases in conduction of cardiac impulses through the AV node and ventricles

may occur, emphasizing the need for caution in administering this drug to patients with atrial fibrillation or other tachydysrhythmias. Dobutamine may increase heart rate more than epinephrine for a given increase in cardiac output.

   b. **Clinical Uses.** Dobutamine is most often administered (2–30 μg/kg/min IV) for its inotropic effects in patients with poor myocardial contractility, such as after cardiopulmonary bypass.

7. **Dopamine** is an agonist at dopaminergic (0.5–2.0 μg/kg/min IV), β (2 to 10 μg/kg/min IV), and α (>10 μg/kg/min IV) receptors. Infusion rates above 10 μg/kg/min IV may produce sufficient vasoconstriction to offset desirable dopaminergic (increases renal blood flow) and β (increased cardiac output) receptor stimulation. The concept of "renal dose" dopamine (0.5–2.0 μg/kg/min IV) is considered outdated. Despite the apparent dose–response dependency of dopamine, a wide variability of individual responses has been observed.

   a. **Side Effects.** Tachycardia and cardiac dysrhythmias occur infrequently. Extravasation of dopamine can produce gangrene. Pulmonary artery pressure may be increased, detracting from the use of dopamine in patients with right-sided heart failure. Insulin secretion is inhibited, explaining the common occurrence of hyperglycemia during infusion of dopamine.

   b. **Clinical Uses.** Dopamine is most often administered as a continuous IV infusion (2–10 μg/kg/min) for its inotropic and diuretic effects in patients with poor myocardial contractility, such as after cardiopulmonary bypass.

8. **Combination therapy** is most often with dopamine and dobutamine in an attempt to maximize positive inotropic effect with less vasoconstriction.

E. **Fenoldopam** is a selective dopamine$_1$ agonist with no α or β activity compared with dopamine.

F. **Clonidine** is a centrally acting selective partial α_2 agonist. It is an antihypertensive drug by virtue of its ability to decrease central sympathetic outflow.

1. **Side Effects.** Sedation, bradycardia, and dry mouth from sympatholytics are common. Abrupt

discontinuation of clonidine, as before surgery, may result in rebound hypertension, especially if the daily dose is above 1.2 mg. This hypertension may be confused with a response to emergence from anesthesia, but it is typically delayed for about 18 hours. Transdermal administration of clonidine is an alternative to the oral route because an IV preparation is not available. Life-threatening hypertension after withdrawal may be treated with nitroprusside.

2. **Clinical Uses.** In addition to its antihypertensive effect, clonidine administered preoperatively (5 μg/kg orally) attenuates SNS reflex responses, such as those associated with direct laryngoscopy or surgical stimulation, and greatly decreases anesthetic requirements ($\geq$40%) for volatile drugs or opioids. When placed in the subarachnoid or epidural space, this drug produces analgesia that may be accompanied by sedation and bradycardia but not depression of ventilation.

G. **Dexmedetomidine** is a more selective α_2 agonist than clonidine. A stereoselective ability to interact with receptors resulting in decreased anesthetic requirements is evidence for an "anesthetic receptor."

1. This drug produces excellent sedation (no depression of ventilation but upper airway obstruction may occur), produces analgesia, reduces blood pressure and heart rate (promotes hemodynamic stability), and greatly decreases plasma catecholamines.

2. The loading infusion of 1 μg/kg is administered over 10 minutes in a monitored setting.

VI. NONADRENERGIC SYMPATHOMIMETIC AGENTS

A. **Vasopressin** (and its congener, desmopressin) are exogenous preparations of the endogenous antidiuretic hormone.

1. Clinical uses of vasopressin have included treatment of diabetes and as an adjunct to treatment of gastrointestinal (GI) bleeding and esophageal varices.

2. New clinical indications for vasopressin include support of patients with septic shock and cardiac

arrest (40 IU in 40 mL IV) secondary to ventricular fibrillation or pulseless ventricular tachycardia. Advanced Cardiac Life Support (ACLS) guidelines recommend vasopressin in place of the first or second dose of epinephrine during treatment of pulseless arrest.

B. **Adenosine** is an endogenous byproduct of ATP and has negative chronotropic effects on the SA node as well as negative dromotropic effects on the AV node when administered IV. The principal clinical use of adenosine is termination of paroxysmal supraventricular tachycardia (6 mg IV [100–150 µg/kg IV for pediatric patients]).

C. **Phosphodiesterase inhibitors** do not rely on stimulation of α or β receptors. These drugs combine positive inotropism with vasodilator activity by selectively inhibiting phosphodiesterase.
   1. **Milrinone** is a more potent phosphodiesterase inhibitor that lacks effects on platelets and may be useful for short-term IV therapy of congestive heart failure.

D. **Digitalis Glycosides.** Digoxin is administered principally to treat congestive heart failure and control supraventricular tachydysrhythmias such as atrial fibrillation. A therapeutic effect occurs within 10 minutes (0.25–1.0 mg IV for adults). Signs of digitalis toxicity (cardiac dysrhythmias, GI disturbances) must be inquired about when evaluating patients preoperatively. Digitalis toxicity is enhanced by hypokalemia or injection of calcium. Iatrogenic hyperventilation of the lungs with associated hypokalemia should be avoided during anesthesia. Most recommend continuation of digitalis therapy in the perioperative period, especially when the drug is being administered for heart rate control. Prophylactic preoperative administration of digitalis preparation is controversial but may be of unique value in elderly patients undergoing thoracic surgery.

VII. SYMPATHOLYTIC DRUGS

A. **α Antagonists** produce orthostatic hypotension, tachycardia, and miosis.
   1. **Phentolamine** is a nonselective and competitive antagonist at α_1 and α_2 receptors that is typically

administered (2–5 mg IV) until adequate control of blood pressure is achieved. Tachycardia reflects continued presynaptic release of norepinephrine owing to α_2-receptor blockade.

2. **Prazosin** is a selective postsynaptic α_1 antagonist that leaves intact the negative feedback mechanism for norepinephrine release that is mediated by presynaptic α_2 activity. This drug is useful in the preoperative preparation of patients with pheochromocytoma.

B. **β Antagonists** are distinguished by differing pharmacokinetic and pharmacodynamic characteristics (Table 15-5).

1. An important class of drugs is beta-blockers, which are indicated for the treatment of coronary artery disease, hypertension, heart failure, and tachyarrhythmias. They have a primary role in treatment of patients after myocardial infarction (MI). Beta-blockers decrease mortality in patients with heart failure caused by left ventricular systolic dysfunction. They also reduce the incidence of perioperative MI and may be useful perioperatively in high-risk patients undergoing vascular and other high-risk surgical procedures.

2. Selective beta blockade (**cardioselective**) implies greater safety in the treatment of patients with obstructive pulmonary disease, diabetes mellitus, and peripheral vascular disease because β_2-agonist effects (bronchodilation, vasodilation) are presumably maintained. The clinical significance of membrane-stabilizing activity (a local anesthetic effect on myocardial cells at high doses) and intrinsic sympathomimetic activity (partial β-agonist activity at low doses) has not been documented. Because of their selectivity, the use of beta-blockers has extended to include treatment of congestive heart failure.

3. **Propranolol** is a nonselective β antagonist that may be administered in single IV doses of 0.1 to 0.5 mg (maximum dose, ~2 mg) to slow heart rate during anesthesia. Additive negative inotropic or chronotropic effects with inhaled or injected anesthetics are likely to occur but have not been a significant clinical problem.

4. **Timolol** is administered as a topical preparation for the treatment of glaucoma. There may be sufficient

TABLE 15-5

PHARMACOKINETICS OF β ANTAGONISTS

Drug	Relative β_1 Selectivity	Membrane Stabilizing Activity	Intrinsic Sympathomimetic Activity	Elimination Half-Time (hr)	Lipid Solubility	Route of Elimination
Propranolol	0	+	0	3–4	+++	Hepatic
Metoprolol	++	0	0	3–4	+	Hepatic
Atenolol	++	0	0	6–9	0	Renal
Esmolol	++	0	0	0.16	?	Plasma esterase
Timolol	0	0	0	4–5	+	Hepatic Renal

systemic absorption to cause bradycardia and hypotension that are resistant to reversal with atropine.

5. **Mixed Antagonists**
   a. **Labetalol** produces selective α_1- and nonselective β-antagonist effects. Administered as a single dose (0.05–0.15 mg/kg IV over 2 minutes), this drug is useful in controlling hypertension and tachycardia in response to painful stimulation during general anesthesia. Although the magnitude is less than with β antagonists, worsening of congestive heart failure or appearance of bronchospasm may occur after administration of labetalol.

VIII. CALCIUM CHANNEL BLOCKERS

Interact with cell membranes to interfere with movement of calcium into cells through ion-specific channels (known as slow channels because their transition among the resting, activated, and inactivated states is delayed compared with fast sodium channels). Calcium channel blockers are a heterogeneous group of drugs with dissimilar structures and different electrophysiologic and pharmacologic properties. These drugs are most useful for the treatment of supraventricular tachydysrhythmias and coronary artery vasospasm (Table 15-6).

TABLE 15-6

COMPARATIVE EFFECTS OF CALCIUM CHANNEL BLOCKERS

	Verapamil	Nifedipine	Diltiazem
Dose			
IV (μg/kg)	75–150	5–15	75–150
PO (mg every 8 hr)	80–160	10–20	60–90
Negative inotropy	+	0	0/+
Negative chronotropy	+	0	0/+
Negative dromotropy	++++	0	+++
Coronary artery vasodilation	++	++++	+++
Systemic vasodilation	++	++++	++
Bronchodilation	0/+	0/+	
Elimination half-time (hr)	2–7	4–5	4
Route of elimination	Renal	Renal	Hepatic

IV = intravenous; PO = per os.

A. **Verapamil** is the drug of choice for termination of supraventricular dysrhythmias, and it is also effective in slowing the heart rate in patients with atrial fibrillation and atrial flutter. There is a dose-dependent increase in the P-R interval on the electrocardiogram and a delay in conduction of cardiac impulses through the AV node.

1. Caution must be exercised when treating patients with Wolff-Parkinson-White syndrome because verapamil may increase conduction velocity in the accessory tract.

2. Unlike β antagonists, verapamil does not increase airway resistance in patients with obstructive pulmonary disease.

B. **Nifedipine** is more effective than nitroglycerin for treatment of angina pectoris caused by coronary artery vasospasm.

1. Vasodilation results in compensatory tachycardia, and cardiac output may increase as a result of afterload reduction.

2. Administration of nifedipine is useful during anesthesia when there is evidence of myocardial ischemia associated with hypertension.

C. **Diltiazem** is an effective coronary artery vasodilatory but a poor peripheral vasodilator; it may produce bradycardia.

D. **Nicardipine** produces vasodilation of coronary arterioles without altering activity of the sinus node or conduction of cardiac impulses through the AV node.

E. **Nimodipine** is a highly lipophilic drug that produces somewhat selective vasodilation of cerebral arteries, resulting in a favorable effect on the severity of neurologic deficits caused by cerebral vasospasm after subarachnoid hemorrhage.

F. **Calcium Channel Blockers and Anesthesia.** These drugs may exhibit additive myocardial depressant effects with volatile anesthetics, which may also interfere with inward calcium movement. Opioids do not seem to alter the response to calcium channel blockers. Calcium channel blockers seem to augment the effects of both depolarizing and nondepolarizing muscle relaxants in a manner similar to those of "mycin" antibiotics.

ANATOMY AND PHYSIOLOGY

IX. ANGIOTENSIN-CONVERTING ENZYME INHIBITORS

A. Inhibitors of angiotensin-converting enzyme (captopril, enalapril, lisinopril) prevent the conversion of angiotensin I to angiotensin II. These drugs are effective in the treatment of congestive heart failure and essential hypertension as well as renovascular and malignant hypertension.

B. Side effects are minor, with the principal cardiovascular effect being decreasing systemic vascular resistance.

X. VASODILATORS

Vasodilators decrease blood pressure by dose-related direct effects on vascular smooth muscle independent of α or β receptors (Table 15-7). These drugs may evoke baroreceptor-mediated increases in heart rate. Combination with a β-antagonist may be necessary to offset this reflex tachycardia (maintain heart rate <100 bpm).

A. **Hydralazine** (5–10 mg IV every 10 to 20 minutes) is useful to control perioperative hypertension.

TABLE 15-7

DOSES AND SITES OF ACTION OF VASODILATORS

Drug	Bolus (Adult, IV)	Continuous Infusion (Adult, IV)	Site of Action	Onset	Duration
Hydralazine	5–10 mg		Arterial	15–20 min	4–6 hr
Nitroprusside	50–100 μg	0.25–5 μg/kg/min (50 mg in 250 mL, 200 μg/mL)	Arterial Venous	1–2 min	2–5 min
Nitroglycerin		0.25–3 μg/kg/min (50 mg in 250 mL, 200 μg/mL)	Venous Arterial	2–5 min	3–5 min

B. **Nitroprusside** is administered as a continuous infusion (0.25–0.5 µg/kg/min IV) using an infusion pump and continuous monitoring of blood pressure. The dose is increased slowly as needed to control hypertension or to produce controlled hypotension. Rarely is more than 3 to 5 µg/kg/min of nitroprusside required in an anesthetized patient. Acute hypertensive responses can be treated with single IV doses of 50 to 100 µg.

1. The hypotensive effect of nitroprusside reflects direct relaxation of arterial and venous smooth muscle, causing decreases in preload and afterload. Hypotensive effects of nitroprusside are potentiated by volatile anesthetics and blood loss.

2. **Side Effects.** The ferrous iron of nitroprusside reacts with sulfhydryl groups in red blood cells and releases cyanide, which is reduced to thiocyanate in the liver. High doses of nitroprusside (>10 µg/kg/min IV) may result in cyanide toxicity. There is no evidence that renal or hepatic diseases increase the likelihood of cyanide toxicity.

   a. **Diagnosis.** Tachyphylaxis, increased venous oxygen tension, and metabolic acidosis signal the development of cyanide toxicity (cyanide binds to cytochrome oxidase, causing cellular hypoxia) and the need to discontinue the infusion of nitroprusside immediately.

   b. **Treatment** of cyanide toxicity is with sodium thiosulfate (150 mg/kg IV in 50 mL of water) administered over 15 minutes to speed the conversion of cyanide to thiocyanate.

C. **Nitroglycerin** is administered as a continuous infusion (0.25–3.0 µg/kg/min IV) to treat myocardial ischemia. Its predominant action is on venules, causing increased venous capacitance and decreased venous return.

1. Control of hypertension with nitroglycerin is less reliable than with nitroprusside, emphasizing the minimal effect of this drug on arterial smooth muscle.

2. Unlike nitroprusside, nitroglycerin poses no risk of cyanide toxicity. For this reason, nitroglycerin may be chosen over nitroprusside to control hypertension associated with pregnancy-induced hypertension.

D. **Nesiritide** is a recombinant form of human B-type natriuretic peptide that produces beneficial hemodynamic effects by venous and arterial vasodilation, including coronary vasodilation.

CHAPTER 16 ■ HEMOSTASIS AND TRANSFUSION MEDICINE

Anesthesia providers may be involved in as many as 8.3 million donor unit exposures per year in the United States, so it is important that anesthesiologists understand the principles of transfusion medicine (Drummond JC, Petrovich CT, Lane TA: Hemotherapy and hemostasis. In *Clinical Anesthesia*. Edited by Barash PG, Cullen BF, Stoelting RK, Cahalan MK, Stock MC. Philadelphia: Lippincott Williams and Wilkins, 2009, pp 369–410).

I. RISKS OF BLOOD PRODUCT ADMINISTRATION

The three leading causes of transfusion-related death in the United States are transfusion-related acute lung injury (TRALI), ABO incompatibility, and sepsis caused by bacterial contamination.

A. **Infectious Risks Associated with Blood Product Administration** (Tables 16-1 and 16-2)

B. **Non-Infectious Risks Associated with Blood Product Administration** (Table 16-3)

1. **Immunologically mediated transfusion reactions** can occur as a result of the presence of antibodies that are either constitutive (anti-A, anti-B) or that have been formed as a result of prior exposure to donor erythrocytes (RBCs), white blood cells (WBCs), platelets, or proteins.

   a. **Acute hemolytic transfusion reactions** against foreign RBCs often manifest as hemolysis of the donor RBCs, leading to acute renal failure, disseminated intravascular coagulation (DIC), and death. Hypotension, hemoglobinuria, and diffuse bleeding may be the only clues that a hemolytic transfusion reaction has occurred during anesthesia. If a

TABLE 16-1

INFECTIOUS RISKS ASSOCIATED WITH BLOOD PRODUCT
ADMINISTRATION

Hepatitis A, B, C, D, and E
Human T-cell lymphotropic viruses (HTLV-1, HTLV-2),
Human immunodeficiency viruses 1 and 2
Cytomegalovirus
West Nile virus
Parasitic diseases (malaria, Chagas' disease)
Bacterial contamination of blood components
Prion-related diseases (Creutzfeldt Jacob disease and variant
  Creutzfeldt Jacob disease)
Contaminating bacteria
Parasites (malaria)

reaction is suspected, the transfusion should be
stopped and the identity of the patient and labeling
of the blood rechecked. Management has three
main objectives—maintenance of systemic blood
pressure, preservation of renal function, and prevention of DIC.

TABLE 16-2

ESTIMATES OF THE RATE (PER DONOR EXPOSURE) OF
TRANSFUSION-TRANSMITTED INFECTIOUS DISEASE IN
NORTH AMERICA

Disease	Rate
Hepatitis B (HBV)	1/269,000
Hepatitis C (HCV)	1/1,600,000
Human immunodeficiency virus (HIV)	1/1,780,000
Human T-cell lymphotrophic virus (HTLV)	1/2,900,000
West Nile virus (WNV)	Indeterminate/very low
Cytomegalovirus (CMV)	
Non-leukoreduced random donor	7%
Leukoreduced random donor	2%–4%
CMV seronegative donor	1%–2%
Epstein-Barr virus (EBV)	0.5%
Bacterial sepsis	
Platelets (apheresis, culture tested)	1/50,000
Platelets (whole blood derived, surrogate tested)	1/33,000

ANATOMY AND PHYSIOLOGY

TABLE 16-3	
THE NON-INFECTIOUS ADVERSE REACTIONS ASSOCIATED WITH BLOOD PRODUCT ADMINISTRATION	

Adverse Reaction	Comment/Incidence
Immunologically Mediated Transfusion Reactions	
Acute hemolytic transfusion reactions	Acute renal failure; 2% mortality
Delayed hemolytic transfusion reactions	Evidence by 7 to 14 days; one in 2000 to 2500 transfusions
Reactions to Donor Proteins	
Minor allergic reactions	Urticarial reactions; 0.5% to 4% of all transfusions
Anaphylactoid reactions	Dyspnea, bronchospasm, angioedema, hypotension
WBC-Related Transfusion Reactions	
Febrile reactions	Temperature increase within 4 hours
TRALI	Noncardiogenic pulmonary edema; ≤5% mortality
GVHD	Pancytopenia
TRIM	Inflammatory response induced by transfusion
Transfusion-Induced Inflammatory Response	Inflammatory response induced by transfusion
Leukoreduction	Decreased alloimmunization or platelet refractoriness, prevention of febrile reactions, reduction of CMV transmission, decreased inflammatory mediator

CMV = cytomegalovirus; DIC = disseminated intravascular coagulation; GVHD = graft-versus-host disease; TRALI = transfusion-related acute lung injury; TRIM = transfusion-related immunomodulation; WBC = white blood cell.

  b. **Delayed hemolytic transfusion reactions** should be suspected when a low-grade fever accompanied by increased bilirubin and an unexplained decrease in hematocrit (Hct) occurs 7 to 14 days after a transfusion.

 2. **Reactions to donor proteins** (minor allergic reactions) cause urticarial reactions in 0.5% of all transfusions. Patients with mild symptoms can be treated with diphenhydramine. Infrequently, a more severe form of allergic reaction involving anaphylaxis occurs in which the patient experiences dyspnea,

TABLE 16-4

DIAGNOSTIC CRITERIA FOR TRANSFUSION-RELATED
ACUTE LUNG INJURY

Acute onset of arterial hypoxemia (within 6 hours after
  transfusion)
Bilateral infiltrates on chest radiography
Absence of evidence of left atrial hypertension
Absence of other temporally related causes of acute lung injury

bronchospasm, hypotension, laryngeal edema, chest
pain, and shock. (This may occur when patients with
hereditary IgA deficiency who have been sensitized by
previous transfusions or pregnancy are exposed to
blood with "foreign" IgA protein.)

3. **WBC-related transfusion reactions** (febrile reactions)
   may occur as a result of antibody attack on donor
   leukocytes. The febrile response occurs in about 1% of
   all RBC transfusions. Typically, the patient experiences
   a temperature increase of more than 1°C within 4 hours
   of a blood transfusion and defervesces within 48 hours.
4. **Transfusion-Related Acute Lung Injury** (Table 16-4)
5. **Graft-versus-host disease (GVHD)** occurs when viable
   donor lymphocytes are transfused into immunocompro-
   mised patients. The donor lymphocytes may become
   engrafted, proliferate, and establish an immune
   response against the recipient. GVHD typically
   progresses rapidly to pancytopenia, and the fatality rate
   is very high. GVHD has been reported only after the
   transfusion of cellular blood components. It has not
   occurred after transfusion of fresh-frozen plasma (FFP),
   cryoprecipitate, or frozen RBCs. Irradiation remains the
   only effective means of preventing GVHD.
6. **Transfusion-Related Immunomodulation.** Alteration
   of immune function has been associated with
   allogenic transfusion. Transfused WBCs are thought
   to be the mediators of the immunity-attenuating
   effects. Transfusion also induces an inflammatory
   response in the recipient.
7. **Leukoreduction** is application of techniques for leukocyte depletion of donor blood products based on the
   suspicion that transfused leukocytes are the mediators
   of the immunity-attenuating effects of transfusions.
C. **Other Non-Infectious Risks Associated with Transfusion**
   (Table 16-5)

ANATOMY AND PHYSIOLOGY

TABLE 16-5

CONSEQUENCES OF MASSIVE BLOOD TRANSFUSIONS

Hypothermia (slows coagulation and causes sequestration of platelets)
Volume overload
Dilutional coagulopathy (manifests as deficiencies of platelets and clotting factors)
Decreases in 2,3-diphosphoglycerate (2,3-DPG) (left shifting of the oxyhemoglobin dissociation curve)
Metabolic acidosis
Hyperkalemia
Citrate intoxication

II. BLOOD PRODUCTS AND TRANSFUSION THRESHOLDS

A. **Red Blood Cells.** The contemporary transfusion trigger for general medical-surgical patients is a Hct of 21% and a hemoglobin (Hb) of 7.0 g/dL (Table 16-6). The Practice Guidelines for Blood Component Therapy developed by the American Society of Anesthesiologists state that "red blood cell transfusion is rarely indicated when the hemoglobin concentration is greater than 10 g/dL and is almost always indicated when it is less than 6 g/dL." Ultimately, the decision to transfuse RBCs should be made based on the clinical judgment that the oxygen-carrying capacity of the blood must be increased.

B. **Compensatory Mechanisms During Anemia** (Table 16-7)

C. **Isovolemic Anemia vs. Acute Blood Loss.** With acute blood loss, hypovolemia induces stimulation of the sympathetic nervous system, leading to vasoconstriction and tachycardia. In chronically anemic patients, cardiac output increases as the Hb decreases to approximately 7 to 8 g/dL.

D. **Platelets** (Table 16-8). One platelet unit typically increases the platelet count by 5 to 10,000/mL^3. However, the increase must be verified by platelet count, especially in patients who may have been alloimmunized by frequent platelet administration.

E. **Fresh-Frozen Plasma** (Table 16-9). Empiric administration of 2 U of FFP or thawed plasma with every 5 U of packed RBCs is commonly used when massive transfusion is anticipated or ongoing. Normal coagulation can be achieved with clotting factor levels of 20% to 30% of

TABLE 16-6

CONDITIONS THAT MAY DECREASE TOLERANCE FOR ANEMIA
AND INFLUENCE THE RED BLOOD CELL TRANSFUSION THRESHOLD

Increased oxygen demand
  Hyperthermia
  Hyperthyroidism
  Sepsis
  Pregnancy
Limited ability to increase cardiac output
Coronary artery disease
  Myocardial dysfunction (infarction, cardiomyopathy)
  β-adrenergic blockade
  Inability to redistribute cardiac output
Low SVR states
  Sepsis
  Post-cardiopulmonary bypass
  Occlusive vascular disease (cerebral, coronary)
Left shift of the O_2 Hb curve
  Alkalosis
  Hypothermia
Abnormal hemoglobins
  Presence of recently transfused Hb (decreased 2,3 DPG)
  HbS (sickle cell disease)
Acute anemia (limited 2,3-DPG compensation)
Impaired oxygenation
  Pulmonary disease
  High altitude
Ongoing or imminent blood loss
  Traumatic or surgical bleeding
  Placenta previa or accreta, abruption, uterine atony
  Clinical coagulopathy

Hb = hemoglobin; SVR = systemic vascular resistance.

normal. (These levels can be achieved by administration
of 10 to 15 mL/kg of FFP.)

   F. **Cryoprecipitate** contains factor VIII, the von Willebrand
factor (vWF), fibrinogen, fibronectin, and factor XIII
(Table 16-10).

TABLE 16-7

COMPENSATORY MECHANISMS THAT MAINTAIN OXYGEN
DELIVERY DURING ISOVOLEMIC HEMODILUTION

Increased cardiac output
Redistribution of cardiac output
Increased oxygen extraction
Changes in oxygen–hemoglobin affinity

TABLE 16-8

INDICATIONS FOR THE ADMINISTRATION OF PLATELETS

Indication	Platelet Count (/mL^3)
Non-bleeding patients without other abnormalities of hemostasis	10,000
Lumbar puncture, epidural anesthesia, central line placement, endoscopy with biopsy, liver biopsy or laparotomy in patients without other abnormalities of hemostasis	50,000
Intended procedures in which closed cavity bleeding might be especially hazardous (e.g., neurosurgery)	100,000
To maintain platelets during ongoing bleeding and transfusion	Not less than 50,000
To maintain platelets during DIC with ongoing bleeding	Not less than 50,000

DIC = disseminated intravascular coagulation.

III. BLOOD CONSERVATION STRATEGIES (Table 16-11)

IV. JEHOVAH'S WITNESSES accept neither administration of homologous blood products nor readministration of autologous products that have left the circulation. (This is at the individual's personal discretion, and many Jehovah's

TABLE 16-9

INDICATIONS FOR ADMINISTRATION OF FRESH-FROZEN PLASMA

Correction of multiple coagulation factor deficiencies (DIC with evidence of microvascular bleeding and PT or aPTT >1.5 times normal)

Correction of microvascular bleeding during massive transfusion (>1 blood volume) when PT and aPTT cannot be obtained in a timely manner

Urgent reversal of warfarin therapy (prothrombin complex concentrate [II, VII, IX, X] is an alternative)

Correction of single coagulation factor deficiencies for which specific concentrates are not available (e.g., factor V)

aPTT = activated partial thromboplastin time; DIC = disseminated intravascular coagulation; PT = prothrombin time.

TABLE 16-10

INDICATIONS FOR THE ADMINISTRATION OF CRYOPRECIPITATE

Microvascular bleeding when there is a disproportionate decrease
in fibrinogen (DIC and massive transfusion) with fibrinogen
below 80 to 100 mg/dL (FFP is the first-line component for the
factor depletion associated with massive transfusion)
Bleeding caused by uremia that is unresponsive to DDAVP
Presurgical prophylaxis or treatment of bleeding in patients with
hemophilia A and vWD
Presurgical prophylaxis or treatment of bleeding in patients with
congenital dysfibrinogenemias
Factor XIII deficiency

DIC = disseminated intravascular coagulation; FFP = fresh-frozen plasma;
vWD = von Willebrand disease.

Witnesses do accept procedures that maintain
extracorporeal blood in continuity with the circulation.)

V. COLLECTION AND PREPARATION OF BLOOD PRODUCTS FOR TRANSFUSION

A. **RBCs** for transfusion are first collected in bags containing
citrate–phosphate–dextrose–adenine or citrate–phosphate–
dextrose solution. The citrate chelates the calcium present
in the blood and prevents coagulation. **Packed RBCs** are
prepared by centrifugation (Hct ~70% to 75%; contains
50–70 mL of residual plasma in a total volume of 250–275
mL and has a shelf life of 35 days). The administration of
1 U of packed RBCs increases the Hb of a 70-kg adult by
approximately 1g/dL and the Hct by approximately 3%.

TABLE 16-11

BLOOD CONSERVATION TECHNIQUES

Preoperative autologous donation (hip replacement, scoliosis
surgery)
Acute normovolemic hemodilution
Intraoperative blood salvage (cell savers, risk of air embolism)
Postoperative blood salvage
Pharmacologic agents
  Erythropoietin
  Blood substitutes (hemoglobin and non–hemoglobin-based
    oxygen-carrying solutions)
  DDAVP
  Antifibrinolytics

ANATOMY AND PHYSIOLOGY

TABLE 16-12

MAJOR RBC SURFACE ANTIGEN INCIDENCE IN THE
US POPULATION

Group	Whites (%)	Blacks (%)
O	45	49
A	40	27
B	11	20
AB	4	4
Rh (D)	85	92

B. **Compatibility testing** involves three separate procedures.
1. **ABO** and **Rhesus Typing** (Table 16-12)
2. **The antibody screen** (indirect Coomb's test) is performed to identify recipient antibodies against RBC antigens. The likelihood that the antibody screen will miss a potentially dangerous antibody has been estimated to be no more than one in 10,000.
3. **The Cross-Match**, in which donor RBCs are mixed with recipient serum, requires about 45 minutes and is carried out in three phases: the immediate, incubation, and antiglobulin phases.
   a. The immediate phase requires only 1 to 5 minutes and detects ABO incompatibilities. Determining the ABO blood group type and Rh status alone yields the probability that the transfusion will be compatible in 99.8% of instances.
   b. The second phase, the incubation phase, requires 30 to 45 minutes and detects antibodies primarily in the Rh system.
   c. The third phase (antiglobulin phase crossmatch or the indirect antiglobulin test) is performed only on blood yielding a positive antibody screen and takes 60 to 90 minutes.
C. **Type and screen orders** are used preoperatively for surgical cases in which it is unlikely that the blood will actually be transfused. The ABO, Rh status of the patient is determined, and the antibody screen is performed. If the antibody screen result is negative, type-specific uncrossmatched blood will result in a hemolytic reaction in fewer than 1 in 50,000 U.
D. **Emergency Transfusions** (Table 16-13)
E. **Platelets**
1. One unit of platelets will increase the platelet count of a 70-kg recipient by 5 to $10,000/mL^3$.

TABLE 16-13

PREFERRED ORDER FOR SELECTING BLOOD IN THE ABSENCE OF COMPATIBILITY TESTING

Type-specific, partially crossmatched blood
Uncrossmatched blood (urgent situations when blood is needed before compatibility testing can be completed):
Group O red blood cells until there is time to complete ABO and Rh testing
Rh-negative blood is preferable if the patient's Rh type is unknown or if the patient is a woman of childbearing age
Non–group O patients who have received group O red cells approximating one patient blood volume (10–12 U) during the period of acute blood loss should not be switched back to their own ABO group unless testing has been performed to confirm that significant titers of anti-A or anti-B antibodies are not present

    2. Platelets bear both ABO and human leukocyte antigens. ABO compatibility is ideal (but not required) because incompatibility shortens the life span of the platelet. Platelets do not carry the Rh antigen.

    3. Platelets should be administered through a 170-μfilter.

  F. **FFP and Thawed Plasma.** Plasma is separated from the RBC component of whole blood by centrifugation. To preserve the two labile clotting factors (V and VIII), it is frozen promptly and thawed only immediately before administration. FFP must be ABO compatible.

VI. THE HEMOSTATIC MECHANISM

  A. Normal "hemostasis" involves a series of physiologic checks and balances that ensure that blood remains in an invariably liquid state as it circulates throughout the body, but as soon as the vascular network is violated, it transforms rapidly to a solid state (coagulation). Coagulation must inevitably be complemented by processes for eliminating clot that is no longer needed for hemostasis (fibrinolysis).

  B. **The Nomenclature of Coagulation** (Table 16-14)

  C. **The Coagulation Mechanism.** The classical dual-cascade (intrinsic and extrinsic pathway) model of coagulation is now recognized to be an inadequate representation of in vivo coagulation (this fails to explain several clinical phenomena). Although the classical theories may

ANATOMY AND PHYSIOLOGY

TABLE 16-14

FACTOR NOMENCLATURE AND HALF-LIVES

Factor	Synonyms	*in vivo* Half-Life (hr)
I	Fibrinogen	100–150
II	Prothrombin	50–80
III	Tissue thromboplastin, tissue factor	
IV	Calcium ion	
V	Proaccelerin, labile factor	24
VII	SPCA, stable factor	6
VIII	AHF	12
vWF	von Willebrand factor	24
IX	Christmas factor	24
X	Stuart Power factor, Stuart factor, autoprothrombin	25–60
XI	PTA	40–80
XII	Hageman factor	50–70
XIII	FSF	150
Prekallikrein	Fletcher factor	35
HMW kininogen	Fitzgerald, Flaujeac, or Williams factor; contact activation cofactor	150

AHF = antihemophilic factor; FSF = fibrin stabilizing factor; PTA = plasma thromboplastin antecedent; SPCA = serum prothrombin conversion accelerator.

provide a model for *in vitro* coagulation tests, they fail to incorporate the central role of cell-based surfaces in the *in vivo* coagulation process (which has three stages).

1. **Activation** of the coagulation process begins when a breach in the vascular endothelium exposes blood to the membrane-bound protein, tissue factor.
2. **Amplification** of coagulation includes activation of adjacent platelets and factors V, VIII, and IX. The net result of this amplification stage is the availability of activated platelets and activated factors V, VIII, and IX.
3. **Propagation** is characterized by an explosive generation of thrombin.

D. **Additional Principles of Coagulation** (Table 16-15)

E. **Fibrinolysis** leads to the dissolution of fibrin clots and recanalizes vessels that have been occluded by thrombosis.

TABLE 16-15

CHARACTERISTICS OF COAGULATION

Most clotting factors circulate in an inactive form
Most clotting factors are synthesized by the liver
Factor VIII is a large two-molecule complex (vWF and coagulant
  factor VIII)
Absence of vWF causes two hemostatic abnormalities
  A defect in primary hemostasis because of a failure of platelet
    adhesion to the sites of vascular injury
  Clinical hemophilia A because of an absence of circulating factor
    VIII:C
Synthesis of the vWF occurs in endothelial cells and
  megakaryocytes. Four clotting factors are vitamin K dependent
  Clotting factors, II, VII, IX, and X require vitamin K for
    completion of their synthesis in the liver
  Warfarin administration displaces vitamin K, and the vitamin
    K–dependent factors are not carboxylated
  Factor VII has the shortest half-life and is the first clotting factor
    to disappear from the circulation when a patient prescribed
    warfarin begins to develop vitamin K deficiency
Factors V and VIII (labile factors) have short storage half-lives
  (Massive transfusion with stored blood leads to a dilutional
  coagulopathy because of diminished activity of factors V
  and VI)

vWF = von Willebrand factor.

1. **The Formation of Plasmin.** Fibrinolysis involves primarily the production of plasmin, an active fibrinolytic enzyme. Plasmin is formed by the conversion of plasminogen to plasmin. Plasminogen circulates, and when it comes into contact with fibrin, binds to it. After it is bound to the fibrin surface, plasminogen is converted to plasmin by tissue plasminogen activator. When plasmin is released into the bloodstream, it is immediately neutralized by $\alpha2$-antiplasmin.

2. **Fibrin degradation products** (FDPs), or fibrin split products (FSPs), are removed from the blood by the liver, kidney, and reticuloendothelial system. If the FDPs are produced at a rate that exceeds their normal clearance, they accumulate. In high concentrations, FDPs impair platelet function, inhibit thrombin, and prevent cross-linking of fibrin strands.

F. **Control of Coagulation: Checks and Balances.** Coagulation must be precisely regulated to prevent uncontrolled clotting (i.e., DIC). The first line of defense is the intact vascular endothelium, which has antithrombotic properties. In addition, clotting factors circulate in an inactive form.

VII. LABORATORY EVALUATION OF THE HEMOSTATIC MECHANISM

A. **Laboratory Evaluation of Primary Hemostasis.**
1. **Platelet count** (which does not reflect platelet activity) is the first test ordered in the evaluation of primary hemostasis. Normal platelet counts range between 50,000 and 440,000/mL^3, and counts below 150,000/mL^3 are defined as thrombocytopenia. Spontaneous bleeding is unlikely in patients with platelet counts above 10,000 to 20,000/mL^3. With counts from 40,000 to 70,000/mL^3, surgery-induced bleeding may be severe.
2. **Bleeding time** is an accepted clinical test of platelet function. Both poor platelet function and thrombocytopenia may prolong the bleeding time (normal range, 2–9 minutes). Even though bleeding time reliably becomes progressively prolonged as platelet count falls below 80,000/mL^3, no convincing data confirm that bleeding time is a reliable predictor of the bleeding that will occur in association with surgical procedures.

B. **Laboratory Evaluation of Coagulation**
1. **Prothrombin Time (PT) and the Partial Thromboplastin Time (PTT).** In 1936, when Quick introduced the PT to clinical medicine, sufficient "thromboplastin" was used to yield a clotting time of approximately 12 seconds. Under these circumstances, even patients lacking factors VIII or IX showed normal clotting times. However, when "dilute" thromboplastin (or a "partial" thromboplastin) was used in lieu of the "12-second reagent," individuals with hemophilia showed much longer clotting times than did healthy control subjects. The two different pathways could be tested individually simply by varying the amount and type of thromboplastin added to blood.
2. **Prothrombin time** evaluates the coagulation sequence initiated by tissue factor (TF) and leads to the formation of fibrin without the participation of factors VIII or IX (classical extrinsic pathway).

    a. Normal PT is 10 to 12 seconds. PT is prolonged if deficiencies, abnormalities, or inhibitors of factors VII, X, V, II, or I are present.

    b. When prothrombin levels are only 10% of normal, the increase in PT may be only 2 seconds. PT is not prolonged until the fibrinogen level is below 100 mg/dL.

    c. A prolonged PT is most likely to represent a deficiency or abnormality of factor VII. Because factor VII has the shortest half-life of the clotting factors synthesized in the liver, it is the clotting factor that first becomes deficient with liver disease, vitamin K deficiency, or Warfarin therapy.

3. **International Normalized Ratio (INR).** A difficulty with the PT test is that many different thromboplastin reagents are used. This results in wide variation in normal values, which makes comparison of PT results between laboratories difficult. The INR was introduced to circumvent this difficulty.

4. **Activated partial thromboplastin time** (aPTT) assesses the function of the classical intrinsic (time to fibrin strand formation) and final common pathways. It entails the addition of a "partial thromboplastin" and calcium to citrated plasma.

    a. Normal aPTT values are between 25 and 35 seconds.

    b. The aPTT is most sensitive to deficiencies of factors VIII and IX, but as is the case with the PT, levels of these factors must be reduced to approximately 30% of normal values before the test is prolonged. Heparin prolongs the aPTT, but with high levels also prolongs PT. As with the PT, the level of fibrinogen must also be reduced to 100 mg/dL before the aPTT is prolonged.

5. **Activated clotting time** (ACT) is similar to the aPTT in that it tests the ability of blood to clot in a test tube and it depends on factors that are all "intrinsic" to blood (the classical intrinsic pathway of coagulation).

    a. The automated ACT is widely used to monitor heparin therapy in the operating room. Normal values range from 90 to 120 seconds.

    b. The ACT is far less sensitive than the aPTT to factor deficiencies in the classical intrinsic coagulation pathway.

6. **Thrombin time** (TT) is a measure of the ability of thrombin to convert fibrinogen to fibrin. The TT is prolonged when an inadequate amount of fibrinogen (<100 mg/dL) is present or when the fibrinogen molecules that are present are abnormal (dysfibrinogenemia as in advanced liver disease). The normal TT is below 30 seconds.

7. **Reptilase Time.** When the TT is prolonged, the reptilase time can be used to differentiate between the effects of heparin and FDPs. A prolonged TT and a normal reptilase time suggest the presence of heparin. Prolongation of both TT and reptilase time occur in the presence of FDPs or when fibrinogen level is low. The normal reptilase time is 14 to 21 seconds.

8. The **anti-Ax activity assay** is used to monitor the effects of low-molecular-weight inhibitors and unfractionated heparin.

9. **Fibrinogen Level.** Normal values are between 160 and 350 mg/dL (<100 mg/dL may be inadequate to produce a clot). Fibrinogen is rapidly depleted during DIC. A marked increase in fibrinogen may occur in response to stress, including surgery and trauma (hypercoagulable state).

C. **Evaluation of Fibrinolysis: FDP and D-Dimer.** FDPs are increased in any state of accelerated fibrinolysis (e.g., advanced liver disease, cardiopulmonary bypass, administration of exogenous thrombolytics [streptokinase], DIC). D-dimer is specific to conditions in which extensive lysis of the cross-linked fibrin of mature thrombus is occurring, in particular DIC but also deep vein thrombosis and pulmonary embolism.

D. **The thromboelastogram** provides a measure of the mechanical properties of evolving clot as a function of time. A principal advantage of this test is that the processes it measures require the integrated action of all the elements of the hemostatic process: platelet aggregation, coagulation, and fibrinolysis.

E. **Interpretation of Tests of the Hemostatic Mechanism** (Table 16-16)

1. The most commonly ordered coagulation tests are the platelet count, PT, aPTT, and occasionally bleeding time. Coagulation defects that appear most often are revealed as abnormal values of PT or aPTT.

2. When a greater disruption of the hemostatic mechanism is suspected, further tests, including fibrinogen,

TABLE 16-16

INTERPRETATION OF COAGULATION TESTS

Platelet Count	Bleeding Time	aPTT	PT	TT	Fibrinogen	FDPs	Possible Causes	Examples
D	N or D	N	N	N	N	N	Decreased production, sequestration Increased consumption Immune destruction	Radiation, chemotherapy Tissue damage Heparin
N	I	N	N	N	N	N	Platelet destruction	Drugs (ASA, NSAIDs), uremia, mild von Willebrand's disease
N	I	I	N	N	N	N	Severe vWF deficiency	von Willebrand's disease
N	N	I	N	N	N	N	Factor deficiency Factor inhibition Antiphospholipid antibody	Hemophilia A or B Low-dose heparin Lupus anticoagulant
N	N	N	I	N	N	N	Factor VII deficiency	Early liver disease Early vitamin K deficiency Early Warfarin therapy

(continued)

TABLE 16-16

INTERPRETATION OF COAGULATION TESTS (Continued)

Platelet Count	Bleeding Time	aPTT	PT	TT	Fibrinogen	FDPs	Possible Causes	Examples
N	N	I	I	I	N	N	Multiple factor deficiencies	Late vitamin K deficiency Late Warfarin deficiency Heparin therapy* Massive transfusion
D	I	I	I	I	I	D	Dilution of factors and platelets	
D	I	I	I	I	D	I	Hypercoagulable state with or without decreased production of clotting factors	DIC† Advanced liver disease

*Bleeding time may also be prolonged in association with a marked aPTT increase.

†DIC may be distinguished by the presence of D-dimers.

aPTT = activated plasma partial thromboplastin time; ASA = aspirin; D = decreased; DIC = disseminated intravascular coagulation; FDP = fibrin degradation product; I = increased; N = normal; NSAID = nonsteroidal antiinflammatory drug; PT = prothrombin time; TT = thrombin time; vWF = von Willebrand factor.

TABLE 16-17

COMMON COAGULATION PROFILES

Platelet count decreased (normal aPTT and PT)
  Decreased platelet production
  Consumption of platelets
  Sequestration of platelets
Prolonged BT (normal platelet count, aPTT, PT)
  Antiplatelet drug ingestion (NSAIDs, ASA)
  Uremia
  vWD
  Heparin
Prolonged PT (normal platelet count and aPTT)
  Vitamin K deficiency
  Warfarin administration
  Early liver dysfunction
  Factor VII deficiency
  Acquired coagulation factor inhibitors
Prolonged PT, aPTT, and TT (normal platelet count)
  Heparin
  Dysfibrinogenemia

aPTT = activated plasma partial thromboplastin time; ASA = aspirin;
nonsteroidal antiinflammatory drug; PT = prothrombin time; TT = thrombin
time; vWF = von Willebrand factor.

    TT, and assays for fibrin degradation products and
    the D-dimer, may be ordered.
  F. **Common Coagulation Profiles** (Table 16-17). The inter-
    pretation of coagulation tests may be difficult because
    patients who develop a bleeding diathesis in the periop-
    erative period may have more than one bleeding disor-
    der (e.g., DIC and coagulopathy caused by massive
    transfusion) and may also have a surgical cause for
    bleeding.

VIII. DISORDERS OF HEMOSTASIS: DIAGNOSIS AND TREATMENT (Table 16-18)

The preoperative history is invaluable in the identification
of disorders of hemostasis. Abnormalities of primary
hemostasis, usually caused by reduced platelet number or
function, are revealed by evidence of "superficial" (skin and
mucosal) bleeding, including easy bruising, petechiae,
prolonged bleeding from minor skin lacerations, recurrent
epistaxis, and menorrhagia. Coagulation abnormalities are

ANATOMY AND PHYSIOLOGY

TABLE 16-18

CLASSIFICATION AND TREATMENT OF DISORDERS
OF HEMOSTASIS

Classification
Abnormal bleeding
Abnormal clotting
Involve platelets
Involve clotting factors
Presence of absence of inhibitors (FDPs)
Hereditary
Acquired

Treatment
Hemostatic agents (platelets or clotting factors)
Pharmacologic agents (desmopressin, antiplatelet drugs, vitamin
  K, Warfarin, heparin, aprotinin, antifibrinolytic agents,
  protamine, fibrinolytics)

FDP = fibrin degradation product.

associated with "deep" bleeding events, including
hemarthroses or hematomas after blunt trauma.
  A. **Hereditary Disorders of Hemostasis** (Table 16-19)
  B. **Acquired Disorders of Hemostasis** (Table 16-20)
    1. It is helpful to classify bleeding disorders according to
      which of the three hemostatic processes are involved:

TABLE 16-19

HEREDITARY DISORDERS OF HEMOSTASIS

von Willebrand's disease
  Most common hereditary bleeding disorder (approximately 1%
    of the general population has the disorder, although it is
    overtly symptomatic in only about 10% of those afflicted)
  Result of abnormal synthesis of the vWF that is important for
    binding of platelets to sites of vascular injury and for
    coagulation
  Diagnosis is based on history (abnormal bleeding from mucosal
    surfaces)
  Platelet count, aPTT, and PT may be normal
  Treatment is DDAVP and factor concentrate
Hemophilia A (deficient or functionally defective factor VIII:C)
Hemophilia B (Christmas disease; deficiency or abnormality of
  factors IX)
Hemophilia C (deficiency or abnormality of factor XI)

aPTT = activated plasma partial thromboplastin time;
PT = prothrombin time; vWF = von Willebrand factor.

TABLE 16-20

ACQUIRED DISORDERS OF HEMOSTASIS

Acquired Disorders of Platelets
Thrombocytopenia
Uremia
Agents (inhibit platelet aggregation)
  COX inhibitors (aspirin is the prototype)
  COX-2 inhibitors reduce prostacyclin generation by vascular
    endothelial cells and tilt the natural balance toward platelet
    aggregation (increased rate of myocardial ischemic events)
  Dipyridamole
  ADP receptor antagonists (ticlopidine, clopidogrel)
  GP IIb/IIIa receptor antagonists (management of acute coronary
    syndromes)
  Herbal medications (ginkgo, ginseng, garlic, ginger) and vitamins
    (vitamin E)
Myeloproliferative and myelodysplastic syndromes

**Acquired Disorders of Clotting Factors (including anticoagulant
therapy)**
Vitamin K deficiency (prolongation of PT)
Warfarin therapy (competes with vitamin K for the carboxylation
  binding sites; administered for prevention of DVT and PE and to
  patients with AF and patients with prosthetic heart valves)

Heparin Therapy (inhibits coagulation principally through its
  interaction with one of the body's natural anticoagulant
  proteins, antithrombin III)
LMWH
Heparin-induced thrombocytopenia or thrombosis (relatively
  uncommon with LMWH)
Heparin in cardiopulmonary bypass (protamine is titrated against
  ACT for heparin reversal)
Inhibitors of Xa (fondaparinux, idraparinux)

**Acquired Combined Disorders of Platelets and Clotting Factors
with Increased Fibrinolysis**
Liver disease

Disseminated Intravascular Coagulation
Diagnosis (increased PT, aPTT, thrombocytopenia, decreased
  fibrinogen level, presence of FDPs and D-dimer)
Treatment should focus on management of the underlying
  condition (septicemia, evacuation of the uterus, correction of
  hypovolemia, acidosis, and hypoxemia)

ACT = activated clotting time; ADP = adenosine diphosphate;
AF = atrial fibrillation; aPTT = activated plasma partial thromboplastin time;
COX = cyclo-oxygenase; DVT = deep venous thrombosis; FDP = fibrin
degradation product; GP = glycoprotein; LMWH = low-molecular-weight
heparin; PE = pulmonary embolism; PT = prothrombin time.

ANATOMY AND PHYSIOLOGY

primary hemostasis (platelet disorders), coagulation (clotting factor disorders), fibrinolysis (production of inhibitors such as FDPs), or some combination of the three.

2. It is useful to use the results of coagulation tests to determine whether the clinical problem involves primary hemostasis (decreased platelet count, increased bleeding time), coagulation (prolonged PT and aPTT, decreased factor levels), fibrinolysis (increased FDPs, increased D-dimer) or some combination of the three.

C. **Heparin in Cardiopulmonary Bypass.** A common practice is to maintain ACT at 480 to 500 seconds for the duration of bypass.

D. **Direct thrombin inhibitors** are used during cardiopulmonary bypass when heparin is contraindicated. With the exception of bivalirudin, there is no antidote.

CHAPTER 17 ■ INHALED ANESTHETICS

The popularity of inhaled anesthetics for establishing general anesthesia is based on their ease of administration (via inhalation) and the ability to monitor their effects (clinical signs and end-tidal concentrations) (Fig. 17-1) (Ebert TJ, Schmid PG: Inhaled anesthetics. In *Clinical Anesthesia.* Edited by Barash PG, Cullen BF, Stoelting RK, Cahalan MK, Stock MC. Philadelphia: Lippincott Williams & Wilkins, 2009, pp 411–443). The most popular potent inhaled anesthetics used in adult surgical procedures are sevoflurane, desflurane, and isoflurane (Fig. 17-1). Sevoflurane is the most commonly used inhaled anesthetic for pediatric patients.

I. PHARMACOKINETIC PRINCIPLES

A. **Drug pharmacology** is classically divided into pharmacodynamics (what the body does to a drug) and pharmacokinetics (what the drug does to the body). Drug pharmacokinetics has four phases: absorption (uptake), distribution, metabolism, and excretion (elimination).

B. **Unique Features of Inhaled Anesthetics**
   1. **Speed, Gas State, and Route of Administration.** The inhaled anesthetics are among the most rapidly acting drugs in existence, and when administering a general anesthetic, this speed provides a margin of safety and also means efficiency.
   2. Technically, nitrous oxide and xenon are the only true gases; the other inhaled anesthetics are vapors of volatile liquids (for simplicity, all of them are referred to as gases).
   3. A unique advantage of anesthetic gases is the ability to deliver them to the bloodstream via the patient's lungs.

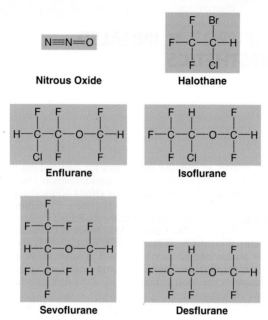

FIGURE 17-1. Chemical structure of inhaled anesthetics. Whereas halothane (no longer commercially available) is an alkane, all the other volatile anesthetics are ether derivatives. Isoflurane, enflurane, and desflurane are methyl ethyl ether derivatives, and sevoflurane is a methyl isopropyl ether. Isoflurane and enflurane are isomers, and desflurane differs from isoflurane in the substitution of a fluorine for a chlorine atom.

- C. **Physical Characteristics of Inhaled Anesthetics** (Tables 17-1 and 17-2)
    1. The goal of delivering inhaled anesthetics is to produce the anesthetic state by establishing a specific concentration (partial pressure) in the central nervous system (CNS). This is achieved by establishing the desired partial pressure in the lungs that ultimately equilibrates with the brain and spinal cord.
    2. At equilibrium, the CNS partial pressure equals the blood partial pressure, which equals alveolar partial pressure.

TABLE 17-1

PHYSIOCHEMICAL PROPERTIES OF VOLATILE ANESTHETICS

	Sevoflurane	Desflurane	Isoflurane	Enflurane	Halothane	Nitrous Oxide
Boiling point (°C)	59	24	49	57	50	−88
Vapor pressure at 20°C (mm Hg)	157	669	238	172	243	38,770
Molecular weight (g)	200	168	184	184	197	44
Oil:gas partition coefficient	47	19	91	97	224	1.4
Blood:gas partition coefficient	0.65	0.42	1.46	1.9	2.50	0.46
Brain:blood solubility	1.7	1.3	1.6	1.4	1.9	1.1
Fat:blood solubility	47.5	27.2	44.9	36	51.1	2.3
Muscle:blood solubility	3.1	2.0	2.9	1.7	3.4	1.2
MAC in oxygen, 30–60 yr at 37°C, PB760 (%)	1.8	6.6	1.17	1.63	0.75	104
MAC in 60% to 70% nitrous oxide	0.66	2.38	0.56	0.57	0.29	
MAC, >65 yr (%)	1.45	5.17	1.0	1.55	0.64	
Preservative	No	Yes	No	No	Thymol	No
Stable in moist carbon dioxide absorbents	No	Yes	Yes	Yes	No	Yes
Flammability (%) (in and 30% oxygen)	10	17	7	5.8	4.8	
Recovered as metabolites (%)	2–5	0.02	0.2	2.4	20	

MAC = minimum alveolar concentration.

225

TABLE 17-2

TISSUE GROUPS AND PHARMACOKINETICS

Group	% Body Mass	% Cardiac Output	Perfusion (mL/min/100 g)
Vessel rich	10	75	75
Muscle	50	19	3
Fat	20	6	3

D. **Anesthetic Transfer: Machine to Central Nervous System** (Table 17-3)
E. **Uptake and Distribution**
  1. F_A/F_I. A common way to assess anesthetic uptake is to follow the ratio of the alveolar anesthetic concentration (F_A) to the inspired anesthetic concentration (F_I) over time (F_A/F_I) (Fig. 17-2).

TABLE 17-3

FACTORS THAT INCREASE OR DECREASE THE RATE OF INCREASE OF ALVEOLAR ANESTHETIC CONCENTRATION (F_A)/INSPIRED ANESTHETIC CONCENTRATION (F_I)

Increase	Decrease	
Low blood solubility	High blood solubility	The lower the blood:gas solubility, the faster the increase in F_A/F_I
Low cardiac output	High cardiac output	The lower the cardiac output, the faster the increase in the F_A/F_I
High minute ventilation	Low minute ventilation	The higher the minute ventilation, the faster the increase in F_A/F_I
High pulmonary arterial to venous partial pressure	Low pulmonary arterial to venous partial pressure	At the beginning of induction, the pulmonary to venous blood partial pressure gradient is zero, but it increases rapidly, and F_A/F_I increases rapidly. Later during induction and maintenance, the pulmonary venous blood partial pressure increases more slowly, so F_A/F_I increases more slowly

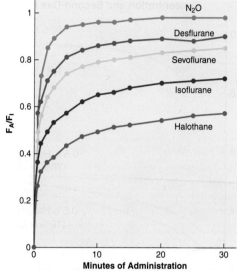

FIGURE 17-2. The increase in the alveolar anesthetic concentration (F_A) toward the inspired anesthetic concentration (F_I) is most rapid with the least-soluble anesthetics (nitrous oxide, desflurane, and sevoflurane) and intermediate with the more soluble anesthetics (isoflurane and halothane). After 10 to 15 minutes of administration (about three time constants), the slope of the curve decreases reflecting saturation of vessel-rich group tissues and subsequent decreased uptake of the inhaled anesthetic.

2. **Distribution (Tissue Uptake).** Factors that increase or decrease the rate of increase of F_A/F_I determine the speed of induction of anesthesia (Fig. 17-2 and Table 17-3).
3. **Metabolism** plays little role in opposing induction but may have some significance in determining the rate of recovery.

F. **Overpressurization and Concentration Effect**
   1. Overpressurization (delivering a higher F_I than the F_A actually desired for the patient) is analogous to an intravenous bolus and thus speeds the induction of anesthesia.
   2. Concentration effect (the greater the F_I of an inhaled anesthetic, the more rapid the rate of increase of the F_A/F_I) is a method used to speed the induction of anesthesia (Fig. 17-3).

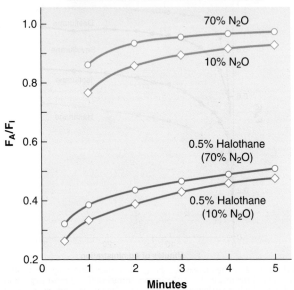

FIGURE 17-3. The concentration effect is demonstrated in the top half of the graph in which 70% nitrous oxide produces a more rapid increase in the alveolar anesthetic concentration (F_A)/inspired anesthetic concentration (F_I) ratio of nitrous oxide than does administration of 10% nitrous oxide. The second gas effect is demonstrated in the lower graphs in which the F_A/F_I ratio for halothane increases more rapidly when administered with 70% nitrous oxide than with 10% nitrous oxide.

G. **Second Gas Effect**
   1. A special case of the concentration effect is administration of two gases simultaneously (nitrous oxide and a potent volatile anesthetic) in which the high volume uptake of nitrous oxide increases the F_A (concentrates) of the volatile anesthetic.

H. **Ventilation Effects**
   1. Inhaled anesthetics with a low blood solubility have a rapid rate of increase in the F_A/F_I with induction of anesthesia such that there is little room to improve this rate of increase by increasing or decreasing ventilation (Fig. 17-3).
   2. To the extent that inhaled anesthetics depress ventilation with an increasing F_I, alveolar ventilation

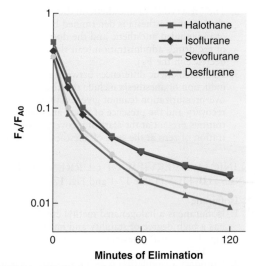

FIGURE 17-4. Elimination of anesthetic gases is defined as the ratio of end-tidal anesthetic concentration (F_A) to the last F_A during administration and immediately before beginning elimination (F_{AO}). During the 120-minute period after ending anesthetic delivery, the elimination of sevoflurane and desflurane is 2 to 2.5 times faster than the elimination of isoflurane or halothane.

decreases, as does the rate of increase of F_A/F_I (negative feedback that results in apnea and may prevent an overdose).

I. **Perfusion Effects**
1. As with ventilation, cardiac output does not greatly affect the rate of increase of the F_A/F_I for poorly soluble anesthetics.
2. Cardiovascular depression caused by a high F_I results in depression of anesthetic uptake from the lungs and increases the rate of increase of F_A/F_I (positive feedback that may result in profound cardiovascular depression).

J. **Exhalation and Recovery**
1. Recovery from anesthesia, similar to induction of anesthesia, depends on the drug's solubility (primary determinant of the rate of decrease in F_A), ventilation, and cardiac output (Fig. 17-4).

2. The "reservoir" of anesthetic in the body at the conclusion of anesthesia is determined by the solubility of the inhaled anesthetic and the dose and duration of the drug's administration (can slow the rate of decrease in the F_A).

3. Pharmacokinetic differences between recovery and induction of anesthesia include the absence of overpressurization (cannot give less than zero) during recovery and the presence of tissue anesthetic concentrations present at the start of recovery (tissue concentration of zero at the start of anesthesia induction).

II. CLINICAL OVERVIEW OF CURRENT INHALED ANESTHETICS (Table 17-1 and Fig. 17-1)

A. Isoflurane

1. Isoflurane is a halogenated methyl ethyl ether that has a high degree of stability and has become the "gold standard" anesthetic since its introduction in the 1970s.

2. Coronary vasodilation is a characteristic of isoflurane, and in patients with coronary artery disease, there has been concern that coronary steal could occur (rare occurrence).

B. Desflurane

1. Desflurane is a completely fluorinated methyl ethyl ether that differs from isoflurane only by replacement of a chlorine with a fluorine atom.

2. Compared with isoflurane, fluorination of desflurane results in low tissue and blood solubility (similar to nitrous oxide), greater stability (near-absent metabolism to trifluoroacetate), loss of potency, and a high vapor pressure (decreased intermolecular attraction). A heated and pressurized vaporizer requiring electrical power is necessary to deliver desflurane.

3. Disadvantages of desflurane include its pungency (it cannot be administered by face mask to an awake patient), transient sympathetic nervous system stimulation when F_I is abruptly increased, and degradation to carbon monoxide when exposed to dry carbon dioxide absorbents (more so than isoflurane).

C. Sevoflurane

1. Sevoflurane is completely fluorinated methyl isopropyl ether with a vapor pressure similar to that of isoflurane. It can be used in a conventional vaporizer.

2. Compared with isoflurane, sevoflurane is less soluble in blood and tissues (it resembles desflurane), is less potent, and lacks coronary artery vasodilating properties.

3. Sevoflurane has minimal odor and pungency (it is useful for mask induction of anesthesia) and is a potent bronchodilator.

4. Similar to enflurane, the metabolism of sevoflurane results in fluoride, but unlike enflurane, this has not been associated with renal concentrating defects.

5. Unlike other volatile anesthetics, sevoflurane is not metabolized to trifluoroacetate but rather to hexafluoroisopropanol, which does not stimulate formation of antibodies and immune-mediated hepatitis.

6. Sevoflurane does not decompose to carbon monoxide or to dry carbon dioxide absorbents but rather is degraded to a vinyl halide (compound A), which is a dose-dependent nephrotoxin in rats. Renal injury has not been shown to occur in patients, even when fresh gas flows are 1 L/min or less.

D. **Xenon**

1. This inert gas has many characteristics of an "ideal" inhaled anesthetic (blood gas partition coefficient of 0.14, provides some analgesia, nonpungent, does not produce myocardial depression).

2. The principal disadvantages of xenon are its expense (difficult to obtain) and high minimum alveolar concentration (MAC) (71%).

E. **Nitrous Oxide**

1. Nitrous oxide is a sweet-smelling, nonflammable gas of low potency and limited blood and tissue solubility that is most often administered as an adjuvant in combination with other volatile anesthetics or opioids.

2. Controversy surrounding the use of nitrous oxide is related to its unclear role in postoperative nausea and vomiting, potential toxicity related to inactivation of vitamin B_{12}, effects on embryonic development, and adverse effects related to its absorption into air-filled cavities and bubbles. (Compliant spaces such as a pneumothorax expand, and noncompliant spaces such as the middle ear experience increased pressure.)

    a. Inhalation of 75% nitrous oxide may expand a pneumothorax to double its size in 10 minutes.

    b. Accumulation of nitrous oxide in the middle ear may diminish hearing after surgery.

III. NEUROPHARMACOLOGY OF INHALED ANESTHETICS

A. Minimum Alveolar Concentration

1. MAC is the F_A of an anesthetic at 1 atm and 37°C that prevents movement in response to a surgical stimulus in 50% of patients (analogous to an ED50 for injected drugs; Table 17-1). Clinical experience is that 1.2 to 1.3 MAC consistently prevents patient movement during surgical stimulation. Although these MAC levels do not absolutely ensure the defining criteria for brain anesthesia (i.e., the absence of self-awareness and recall), it is unlikely for a patient to be aware of or to recall the surgical incision at these anesthetic concentrations unless other conditions exist so that MAC is increased (Table 17-4). Self-awareness and recall are prevented by 0.4 to 0.5 MAC.

2. Standard MAC values are roughly additive (0.5 MAC of a volatile anesthetic and 0.5 MAC of nitrous oxide is equivalent to 1 MAC of the volatile anesthetic).

3. A variety of factors may increase or decrease MAC (Table 17-4).

B. Other Alterations in Neurophysiology.
The currently used volatile anesthetics have qualitatively similar effects on cerebral metabolic rate, the electroencephalogram (EEG), cerebral blood flow (CBF), and flow–metabolism coupling. There are differences in effects on intracerebral pressure, cerebrospinal fluid (CSF) production and resorption, CO_2 reactivity, CBF autoregulation, and cerebral protection. Nitrous oxide departs from the more potent agents in several respects.

1. **Cerebral Metabolic Rate and Electroencephalogram.** All of the potent agents depress cerebral metabolic rate (CMR) to varying degrees in a nonlinear fashion. As soon as spontaneous cortical neuronal activity is absent (isoelectric EEG), no further decreases in CMR are generated.

    a. Desflurane and sevoflurane decrease CMR similar to isoflurane.

TABLE 17-4

FACTORS THAT INFLUENCE (INCREASE OR DECREASE) MINIMUM ALVEOLAR CONCENTRATION

Increase

Increased central neurotransmitter levels (monoamine oxidase inhibitors, acute dextroamphetamine administration, cocaine, ephedrine, levodopa)

Hyperthermia

Chronic ethanol abuse

Hypernatremia

Decrease

Increasing age

Metabolic acidosis

Hypoxia (PaO_2 38 mm Hg)

Induced hypotension (MAP <50 mm Hg)

Decreased central neurotransmitter levels (alpha-methyldopa, reserpine)

α_{-2} Agonists

Hypothermia

Hyponatremia

Lithium

Hypo-osmolality

Pregnancy

Acute ethanol administration

Ketamine

Lidocaine

Opioids

Opioid agonist–antagonist analgesics

Barbiturates

Diazepam

Hydroxyzine

Delta-9-Tetrahydrocannabinol

Verapamil

Anemia (<4.3 mL oxygen/dL blood)

      b. Conflicting data are available concerning whether sevoflurane has proconvulsant effects. (This questions the appropriateness of administering it to patients with epilepsy.)

  2. Cerebral Blood Flow, Flow–Metabolism Coupling, and Autoregulation. All of the potent agents increase CBF in a dose-dependent manner (Fig. 17-5). The dose-dependent increase in CBF caused by volatile anesthetics occurs despite concomitant decreases in cerebral metabolic rate (uncoupling).

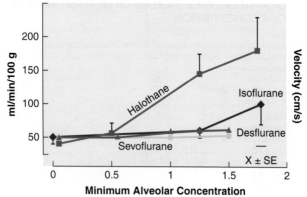

FIGURE 17-5. Cerebral blood flow measured in the presence of normocapnia and in the absence of surgical stimulation in volunteers. At light levels of anesthesia, halothane (but not isoflurane, sevoflurane, or desflurane) increases cerebral blood flow. Isoflurane increases cerebral blood flow at 1.6 minimum alveolar concentration (MAC).

3. **Intracerebral pressure (ICP)** parallels CBF, and mild increases in ICP accompany isoflurane, sevoflurane, and desflurane concentrations above 1 MAC.
4. **Cerebrospinal Fluid Production and Resorption.** Anesthetic effects on ICP via changes in CSF dynamics are less important than anesthetic effects on CBF.
5. **Cerebral Blood Flow Response to Hyper- and Hypocarbia.** Significant hypercapnia is associated with dramatic increases in CBF with or without the administration of volatile anesthetics.
6. **Cerebral Protection.** Cerebral hypoperfusion secondary to hypotension may be associated with better tissue oxygenation than during hypotension by other means. Human neuroprotection outcome studies for sevoflurane and desflurane have not been published.
7. **Processed Electroencephalograms and Neuromonitoring.** All volatile anesthetics produce dose-dependent effects on the EEG, sensory evoked potentials, and motor evoked potentials. Visual evoked potentials are more sensitive to the effects of volatile anesthetics than are somatosensory evoked potentials.

C. **Nitrous Oxide.** The effects of nitrous oxide on cerebral physiology are not clear (these effects vary widely with species). However, nitrous oxide appears to have an antineuroprotective effect.

IV. THE CIRCULATORY SYSTEM

A. **Hemodynamics**
   1. Volatile anesthetics produced dose-dependent and similar decreases in systemic blood pressure (Fig. 17-6). The primary mechanism to decrease blood pressure with increasing dose is related to their potent effects to lower regional and systemic vascular resistance (Fig. 17-7).
   2. In volunteers, sevoflurane to about 1 MAC results in minimal changes in heart rate; isoflurane and desflurane are associated with an increase of 5% to 10% from baseline 10 to 15 (Fig. 17-6).
      a. Rapid increases in the delivered concentration of desflurane (and to a lesser extent, isoflurane) may transiently increase heart rate and systemic blood pressure.
      b. Administration of an opioid or clonidine blunts the heart rate responses evoked by volatile anesthetics, including responses associated with abrupt increases in the delivered concentration of volatile drug.
B. **Myocardial Contractility.** Human studies with isoflurane, sevoflurane, and desflurane have not demonstrated significant changes in echocardiographic-determined indices of myocardial function.
C. **Other Circulatory Effects**
   1. Nitrous oxide is associated with increased sympathetic nervous system activity when administered alone or in combination with other volatile anesthetics.
   2. Isoflurane, sevoflurane, and desflurane do not predispose patients to ventricular arrhythmias or sensitize the heart to the arrhythmogenic effects of epinephrine.
D. **Coronary steal** has not been confirmed to occur with isoflurane, desflurane, or sevoflurane concentrations up to 1.5 MAC.
E. **Myocardial ischemia and cardiac outcome** seem more related to events that alter myocardial oxygen delivery

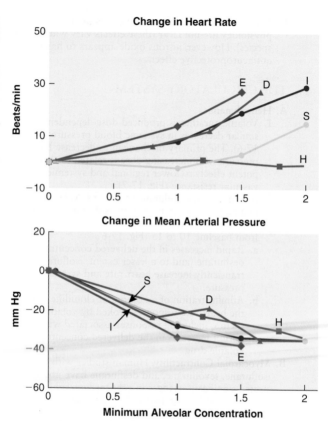

FIGURE 17-6. Heart rate and systemic blood pressure changes (from awake baseline) in volunteers receiving general anesthesia with a volatile anesthetic. Halothane and sevoflurane produced little change in heart rate at less than 1.5 minimum alveolar concentration. All anesthetics caused similar decreases in blood pressure. MAP = mean arterial pressure.

and demand rather than the specific anesthetic drug selected.

F. **Cardioprotection from Volatile Anesthetics**
   1. Volatile anesthetics mimic ischemia preconditioning and initiate a cascade of intracellular events resulting in myocardial protection against ischemia and reper-

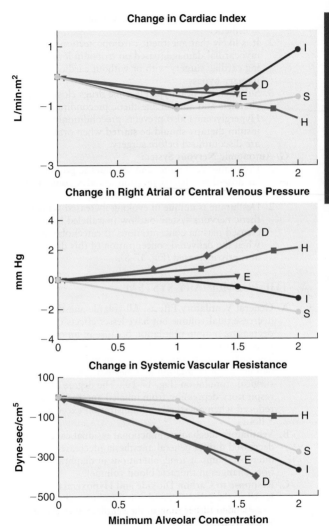

FIGURE 17-7. Cardiac index, systemic vascular resistance, and central venous pressure (CVP) changes from awake baseline in volunteers receiving general anesthesia with a volatile anesthetic. Whereas increases in CVP in the presence of halothane may reflect myocardial depression, increases in the presence of desflurane are more likely caused by venoconstriction.

fusion injury that last beyond elimination of the anesthetic.

2. It is likely that anesthetic cardioprotection lessens myocardial damage (based on troponin levels) during cardiac surgery with or without cardiopulmonary bypass.

3. Sulfonylurea oral hyperglycemic drugs close K_{ATP} channels and abolish anesthetic preconditioning. Hyperglycemia also prevents preconditioning, so insulin therapy should be started when oral agents are discontinued before surgery.

G. **Autonomic Nervous System**
1. Isoflurane, desflurane, and sevoflurane produce similar dose-dependent depression of reflex control of sympathetic nervous system outflow.
2. Desflurane is unique in evoking increased sympathetic nervous system outflow (paralleled by increased plasma concentrations of catecholamine) when the delivered concentration of this drug is abruptly increased (Fig. 17-8).

V. THE PULMONARY SYSTEM

A. **General Ventilatory Effects.** All volatile anesthetics decrease tidal volume but have lesser effects on decreasing minute ventilation because of an offsetting response to increase breathing frequency (Fig. 17-9). The increase in resting $PaCO_2$ as an index of depression of ventilation is somewhat offset by surgical stimulation (Fig. 17-10). The degree of respiratory depression from inhaled anesthetics is reduced when anesthesia administration exceeds 5 hours.

B. **Ventilatory mechanics.** Functional residual capacity is decreased during general anesthesia (decreased intercostal muscle tone, alterations in diaphragm position, changes in thoracic blood volume).

C. **Response to Carbon Dioxide and Hypoxemia**
1. All of the inhaled anesthetics produce a dose-dependent depression in the ventilatory response to hypercarbia (Fig. 17-11).
2. Even subanesthetic concentrations of volatile anesthetics (0.1 MAC) produce depression of chemoreceptors responsible for the ventilatory response to hypoxia.

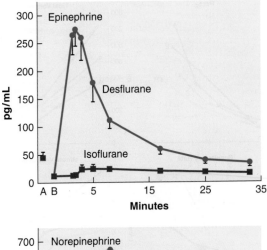

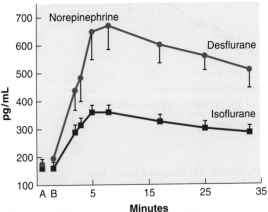

FIGURE 17-8. Stress hormone responses to a rapid increase in anesthetic concentration from 4% to 12% inspired. Data are mean ± SE. A = awake; B = value after 32 minutes of 0.55 minimum alveolar concentration (MAC). *Time* represents minutes after initiation of increased anesthetic concentration.

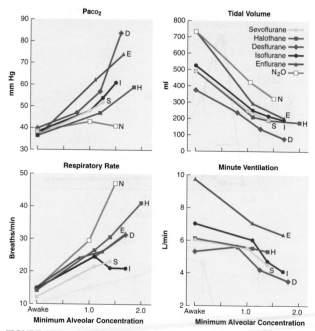

FIGURE 17-9. Comparison of mean changes in resting $PaCO_2$, tidal volume, respiratory rate, and minute ventilation in patients receiving an inhaled anesthetic.

D. **Bronchiolar Smooth Muscle Tone**
   1. Bronchoconstriction during anesthesia is most likely caused by mechanical stimulation of the airway in the presence of minimal concentrations of inhaled anesthetics. This response is enhanced in patients with reactive airway disease.
   2. Volatile anesthetics relax airway smooth muscle by directly depressing smooth muscle contractility and indirectly by inhibiting the reflex neural pathways. Airway resistance increases more with desflurane than sevoflurane (Fig. 17-12).
E. **Pulmonary Vascular Resistance**
   1. The pulmonary vasodilator action of volatile anesthetics is minimal. The effect of nitrous oxide on

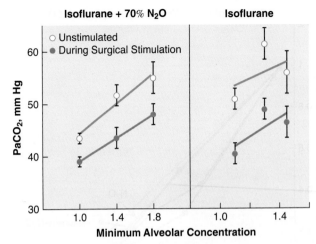

FIGURE 17-10.   The effect of surgical stimulation on the ventilatory depression produced by isoflurane with or without nitrous oxide.

ANESTHETIC AGENTS

pulmonary vascular resistance may be exaggerated in patients with resting pulmonary hypertension.

2. All inhaled anesthetics inhibit hypoxic pulmonary vasoconstriction in animals. Nevertheless, in patients undergoing one-lung ventilation during thoracic surgery, minimal effects on PaO_2 and intrapulmonary shunt fraction occur regardless of the volatile anesthetic being administered (Fig. 17-13).

VI. HEPATIC EFFECTS

A. Postoperative liver dysfunction has been associated to varying degrees with all of the volatile anesthetics in common use. Anesthetics may cause hepatitis that is mild and does not require a previous exposure. Another mechanism requires repeat exposure and probably represents an immune reaction to oxidatively derived metabolites of anesthetics.

B. Ether-based anesthetics (isoflurane, desflurane, sevoflurane) maintain or increase hepatic artery blood flow while decreasing or not changing portal vein blood flow (Fig. 17-14).

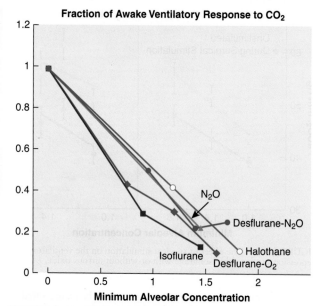

FIGURE 17-11. All inhaled anesthetics produce similar dose-dependent decreases in the ventilatory response to carbon dioxide.

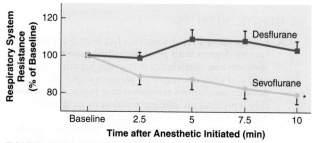

FIGURE 17-12. Changes in airway resistance before (baseline) and after tracheal intubation were significantly different in the presence of sevoflurane compared with desflurane.

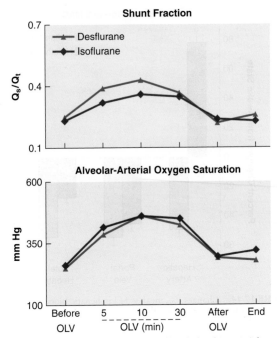

FIGURE 17-13. Shunt fraction (*top panel*) and alveolar–arterial oxygen gradient (*bottom panel*) before, during, and after one-lung ventilation (OLV) in patients anesthetized with desflurane or isoflurane.

VII. NEUROMUSCULAR SYSTEM AND MALIGNANT HYPERTHERMIA

A. Volatile anesthetics (not nitrous oxide) directly relax skeletal muscle (most prominent >1 MAC) and potentiate the action of neuromuscular blocking drugs. (The infusion rate of rocuronium required to maintain neuromuscular blockade is 30% to 40% less with isoflurane, desflurane, and sevoflurane than with propofol.)

B. Although the mechanism of this potentiation is not entirely clear, it appears to be largely caused by a postsynaptic effect at the nicotinic acetylcholine receptors located at the neuromuscular junction. (Volatile anesthetics act synergistically with neuromuscular blocking drugs to enhance their action.)

ANESTHETIC AGENTS

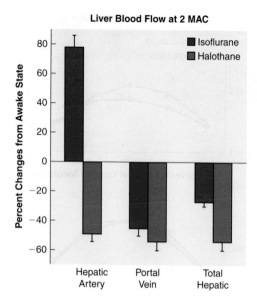

FIGURE 17-14.   Changes (%, mean ≠ SE) in hepatic blood flow during administration of isoflurane or halothane.

  C. All volatile anesthetics serve as triggers for malignant hyperthermia (halothane greatest and desflurane less), but nitrous oxide is only a weak trigger.

VIII. GENETIC EFFECTS, OBSTETRIC USE, AND EFFECTS ON FETAL DEVELOPMENT

  A. The Ames test, which identifies chemicals that act as mutagens and carcinogens, is negative for isoflurane, desflurane, sevoflurane, and nitrous oxide.

  B. Volatile anesthetics can be teratogenic in animals but none of them has been shown to be teratogenic in humans.

  C. Nitrous oxide decreases the activity of vitamin B_{12}-dependent enzymes (methionine synthetase, thymidylate synthetase) by irreversible oxidation of the cobalt atom of vitamin B_{12} by nitrous oxide.

   1. Administration of 70% nitrous oxide results in 50% inactivation of methionine synthetase in 46 minutes.

2. There is concern these changes might have an effect on a rapidly developing embryo or fetus because methionine synthetase and thymidylate synthetase are involved in the formation of myelin and DNA, respectively.

3. A sensory neuropathy that is often combined with signs of posterior lateral spinal cord degenerations has been described in humans who chronically inhaled nitrous oxide for recreational use.

D. Uterine smooth muscle tone is diminished by volatile anesthetics in similar fashion (dose dependent) to the effects of volatile anesthetics on vascular smooth muscle.

1. Uterine relaxation can be troubling at concentrations of volatile anesthetics above 1 MAC and may delay the onset time of newborn respiration. Consequently, for an urgent cesarean section, a common technique is general anesthesia with low concentrations of the volatile anesthetic (0.5–0.75 MAC) combined with nitrous oxide.

2. Uterine relaxation may be desirable when it is necessary to remove a retained placenta.

E. No causal relationship has been shown between exposure to waste anesthetic gases, regardless of the presence or absence of scavenging systems, and adverse health effects. Despite the unproven influence of trace concentrations of volatile anesthetics on fetal development and spontaneous abortions, the use of scavengering systems is common. The National Institute for Occupational Safety and Health recommends exposure levels of 25 parts per million for nitrous oxide and 2 parts per million for halogenated anesthetics.

IX. **ANESTHETIC DEGRADATION BY CARBON DIOXIDE ABSORBERS**

A. **Compound A**

1. Sevoflurane undergoes base catalyzed degradation in carbon dioxide absorbents to form a vinyl ether designated as compound A (Fig. 17-15). The production of compound A is enhanced in low-flow and closed-circuit breathing systems and by warm or very dry carbon dioxide absorbents.

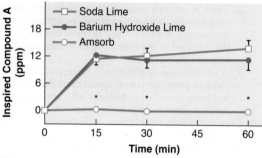

FIGURE 17-15.   Compound A levels produced from three carbon dioxide absorbents during 1 minimum alveolar concentration (MAC) sevoflurane anesthesia delivered at a fresh gas flow of 1 L/min (mean ≠ SE). *$P < 0.05$ versus soda lime and barium hydroxide lime.

    2. Species differences are present in the threshold for compound A–induced nephrotoxicity. (The β-lyase–dependent metabolism pathway for compound A breakdown to cysteine-S conjugates is less in humans than rats.) There is a high probability that renal injury in patients receiving sevoflurane does not occur regardless of the fresh gas flow rate.

B. Carbon Monoxide and Heat

    1. Carbon dioxide absorbents degrade sevoflurane, desflurane, isoflurane, and isoflurane to carbon monoxide (patients at risk for carbon monoxide intoxication) when carbon dioxide absorbent has become desiccated (water content <5%).

        a. The degradation is the result of an exothermic reaction of the anesthetics with the absorbent.

        b. Instances of carbon monoxide poisoning have occurred when the carbon dioxide absorbent has been presumably desiccated because an anesthetic machine has been left on with a high fresh gas flow passing through the carbon dioxide absorbent over an extended period.

    2. Although desflurane produces the most carbon monoxide with anhydrous carbon dioxide absorbents the reaction with sevoflurane produces the most heat. This is an exothermic reaction with the potential for fires and patient injuries.

3. Although sevoflurane is not flammable at less than 11%, formaldehyde, methanol, and formate may result from degradation at high temperatures and when combined with oxygen may be flammable.

C. **Generic Sevoflurane Formulations.** Although the generic formulations of sevoflurane are chemically equivalent, the water content of the formulations differs, resulting in different resistance to degradation to hydrogen fluoride when exposed to Lewis acids (metal halides and metal oxides that are present in modern vaporizers).

X. ANESTHETIC METABOLISM

A. **Fluoride-Induced Nephrotoxicity**
  1. The safety of sevoflurane with regard to fluoride concentrations may be caused by a rapid decline in plasma fluoride concentrations because of less availability of the anesthetic for metabolism from a faster washout compared with enflurane.
  2. Furthermore, a minimal amount of renal defluorination may contribute to the relative absence of renal concentrating defects.

XI. CLINICAL UTILITY OF VOLATILE ANESTHETICS

A. **For Induction of Anesthesia.** There is renewed interest in mask induction of anesthesia (especially pediatric patients) using sevoflurane (which is poorly soluble and nonpungent).

B. **For Maintenance of Anesthesia.** Because of their ease of administration and ability to adjust (titrate) the dose, volatile anesthetics remain the most popular drugs for maintenance of anesthesia.

XII. PHARMACOECONOMICS AND VALUE-BASED DECISIONS

A. In the current environment of cost containment, clinicians are constantly pressured to use less expensive anesthetic agents, including antiemetics, neuromuscular blocking drugs, and volatile anesthetics.

B. Factors involved in value-based decisions include drug efficacy (all volatile anesthetics are similar in efficacy) and side effects (hepatic toxicity and cardiac sensitization cause by halothane offset its low cost).

1. The need for rescue medications to treat nausea and vomiting after volatile anesthesia should be weighed in any cost analysis.

2. Reducing the fresh gas flow of sevoflurane and desflurane can decrease by half the cost per MAC hour of these more expensive anesthetics without compromising their speed and effectiveness.

CHAPTER 18 ■ INTRAVENOUS ANESTHETICS

Despite thiopental's proven clinical usefulness, it has been supplanted by a variety of drugs (midazolam, ketamine, etomidate, propofol) from different groups (Fig. 18-1) (White PF, Eng MR: Intravenous anesthetics. In *Clinical Anesthesia*. Edited by Barash PG, Cullen BF, Stoelting RK, Cahalan MK, Stock MC. Philadelphia: Lippincott Williams & Wilkins, 2009, pp 444–464). These newer compounds combine many of the characteristics of the ideal intravenous (IV) anesthetics but fail in aspects where the other drugs succeed (Table 18-1). Because the desired pharmacologic properties are not equally important in every clinical situation, the anesthesiologist must make the choice that best fits the needs of the individual patient and the operative procedure.

I. GENERAL PHARMACOLOGY OF INTRAVENOUS ANESTHETICS

A. Mechanism of Action

1. A widely accepted theory is that IV hypnotics (benzodiazepines, barbiturates, propofol, etomidate, ketamine) exert their primary effects through an interaction with the inhibitory neurotransmitter γ-aminobutyric acid (GABA) (Fig. 18-2).

2. Activation of the GABA–receptor complex increases transmembrane chloride conductance, resulting in hyperpolarization and functional inhibition of the postsynaptic neuron.

3. Benzodiazepines increase the efficiency of the coupling between GABA and its receptor (ceiling effect).

4. Barbiturates and propofol appear to decrease the dissociation of GABA from its receptor.

5. Ketamine's central nervous system (CNS) effects appear to be primarily related to its antagonistic activity at the N-methyl-D-aspartate (NMDA)

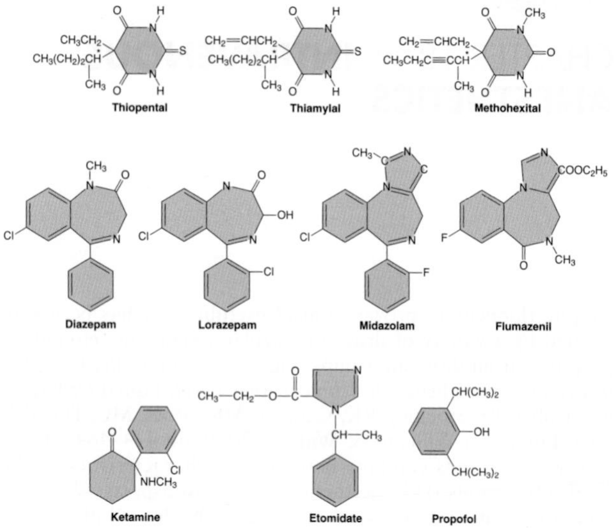

FIGURE 18-1. Chemical structures of nonopioid intravenous anesthetics.

receptor. In addition, ketamine inhibits neuronal sodium channels (modest local anesthetic activity) and calcium channels (cerebral vasodilation).

6. Dexmedetomidine is a centrally active α-2 adrenergic agonist that produces potent sedative and analgesic-

TABLE 18-1

DESIRABLE CHARACTERISTICS OF AN INTRAVENOUS ANESTHETIC

Stable in solution
Absence of pain on injection (venoirritation) or tissue damage from extravasation
Low potential to release histamine
Rapid onset
Prompt metabolism to inactive metabolites
Efficient clearance and redistribution mechanisms
Benign cardiovascular and ventilatory effects
Decrease in cerebral blood flow and metabolism
Prompt and complete return of consciousness
Absence of adverse postoperative effects (e.g., nausea, vomiting, delirium, headache)

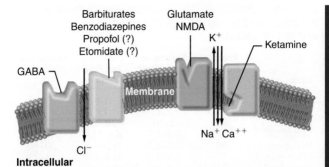

FIGURE 18-2. A model depicting the postsynaptic receptor sites for the inhibitory neurotransmitter γ-aminobutyric acid (GABA) and the excitatory neurotransmitter glutamate in the central nervous system. When GABA occupies the receptor, it allows inward flux of chloride ions, resulting in hyperpolarization of the cell membrane and subsequent resistance of the neurons to stimulation by excitatory neurotransmitters. Barbiturates, benzodiazepines, and possibly propofol and etomidate decrease neuronal excitability by enhancing the effect of GABA at this receptor complex. When glutamate occupies the binding site of *N*-methyl-D-aspartate (NMDA) subtype of the glutamate receptor, the channel opens and allows sodium, potassium, and calcium ions to enter or leave the cell. Flux of these ions leads to depolarization of the postsynaptic neuron and initiation of an action potential. Ketamine blocks these open channels, inhibiting the excitatory response to glutamate.

sparing properties and reduces sympathetic outflow from the CNS.

B. **Pharmacokinetics and Metabolism**
   1. The rapid onset of the CNS effect of most IV anesthetics can be explained by their high lipid solubility and relatively high cerebral blood flow (CBF).
   2. The pharmacokinetics of IV hypnotics are characterized by rapid distribution and subsequent redistribution into several hypothetical compartments, followed by elimination (Table 18-2).
      a. The primary mechanism for terminating the CNS effects of drugs used for the IV induction of anesthesia is redistribution from a central highly perfused compartment (the brain) to larger and well-perfused peripheral compartments (muscle, fat).

TABLE 18-2				
PHARMACOKINETIC VALUES FOR INTRAVENOUS ANESTHETIC DRUGS				
Drug	Protein Binding (%)	Volume at Steady State (L/kg)	Clearance (mL/kg/min)	Elimination Half-Time (hr)
Thiopental	85	2.5	3.4	11
Methohexital	85	2.2	11	4
Propofol	98	2–10	20–30	14–23
Midazolam	94	1.1–1.7	6.4–11.0	1.7–2.6
Diazepam	98	0.7–1.7	0.2–0.5	20–50
Lorazepam	98	0.8–1.3	0.8–1.8	11–22
Etomidate	75	2.5–4.5	18–25	2.9–5.3
Ketamine	12	2.5–3.5	12–17	2–4

b. Most IV anesthetic agents are eliminated via hepatic metabolism (some metabolites are active) followed by renal excretion of more water-soluble metabolites.

c. For most drugs, the hepatic enzyme systems are not saturated at clinically relevant drug concentrations, and the rate of drug elimination decreases as an exponential function of the drug's plasma concentration (first-order kinetics).

d. High steady-state plasma concentrations are achieved with prolonged infusions, hepatic enzyme systems can become saturated, and the elimination rate becomes independent of the drug concentration (zero-order kinetics).

e. **Perfusion-limited clearance** describes hepatic clearance of drugs (etomidate, propofol, ketamine, methohexital, midazolam) in which extraction largely depends on delivery to the liver. (Hepatic blood flow decreases with upper abdominal surgery and increasing age.)

3. **The elimination half-time** (T1/2β) is the time required for the plasma concentration to decrease 50%.

a. Wide variations in T1/2β reflect differences in volume of distribution (Vd), clearance, or both.

b. Careful titration of an anesthetic drug to achieve the desired clinical effect is necessary to avoid

TABLE 18-3

FACTORS THAT CONTRIBUTE TO INTERPATIENT VARIABILITY
IN PHARMACOKINETICS

Degree of protein binding
Efficiency of renal and hepatic clearance mechanisms
Aging (lean body mass decreases)
Pre-existing diseases (hepatic, renal, cardiac)
Drug interactions
Body temperature

   drug accumulation and the resultant prolonged
   CNS effects after the infusion has been
   discontinued.
   4. **Context-sensitive half-time is the time** necessary for
   the plasma concentration to decrease 50% in relation
   to the duration of the infusion. (This is important for
   determining recovery after varying length infusions of
   sedative-hypnotic drugs.)
   5. Many factors contribute to interpatient variability in
   the pharmacokinetics of IV sedative-hypnotic drugs
   (Table 18-3).
C. **Pharmacodynamic Effects**
   1. The principal pharmacologic effect of IV anesthetics is
   to produce dose-dependent CNS depression (dose-
   response curves) manifesting as sedation and hypnosis
   (Fig. 18-3).
   2. When steady-state plasma concentrations are
   achieved, it can be presumed that the plasma concentration is in equilibrium with the effect-site (receptor)
   concentration.
      a. **Efficacy** of an IV anesthetic relates to the maxi-
      mum effect that can be achieved with respect to
      some measure of CNS function (e.g., benzodi-
      azepines are less efficacious than barbiturates in
      depressing electrical activity in the brain).
      b. **Potency** relates to the quantity of drug necessary to
      obtain the maximum CNS effect.
   3. Most sedative-hypnotic drugs (except for ketamine)
   cause a proportional reduction in cerebral metabolism
   ($CMRO_2$) and CBF, resulting in a decrease in
   intracranial pressure (ICP).

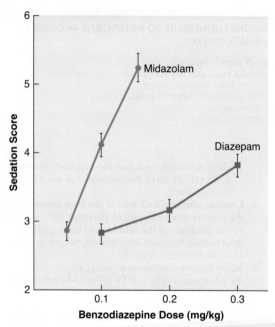

FIGURE 18-3. Dose–response relationships for sedation with midazolam and diazepam. The level of sedation was rated as 2 (awake and alert) to 6 (asleep).

    a. On the electroencephalogram (EEG), it is likely that whereas sedative doses produce activation of high-frequency activity, anesthetic doses produce a burst-suppression pattern.

    b. Most sedative-hypnotic drugs can cause occasional EEG seizure-like activity despite also acting as anticonvulsants. One should differentiate between the epileptogenic activity (methohexital) and myoclonic-like phenomena (etomidate). Myoclonic activity is considered to be the result of an imbalance between excitatory and inhibitory subcortical centers owing to unequal degrees of suppression of these centers by the hypnotic drug.

TABLE 18-4

FACTORS THAT CONTRIBUTE TO HEMODYNAMIC EFFECT OF
INTRAVENOUS INDUCTION

Drugs
Blood volume
Sympathetic nervous system tone
Speed of injection
Cardiovascular drugs
Preanesthetic medication
Direct effects on cardiac contractility or peripheral vasculature

4. Most sedative-hypnotics (exception is ketamine) lower intraocular pressure in parallel with effects on ICP and blood pressure.

5. With the exception of ketamine (and to a lesser extent, etomidate), IV anesthetics produce dose-dependent depression of ventilation (transient apnea followed by decreased tidal volume).

6. Many different factors contribute to the hemodynamic changes associated with IV induction of anesthesia (Table 18-4)

7. The effects of IV anesthetics on neuroendocrine function are also influenced by surgical stimuli (release of vasopressin and catecholamines, decreased glucose tolerance).

8. Most IV sedative-hypnotic drugs lack intrinsic analgesic activity (except ketamine, which has pronounced analgesic-like activity).

D. **Hypersensitivity (Allergic) Reactions**

1. Allergic reactions to IV anesthetics or their solubilizing agents, although rare, can be life threatening.

2. With the exception of etomidate, all IV induction drugs have been alleged to cause some histamine release.

3. Although propofol does not normally trigger histamine release, life-threatening allergic reactions have been reported, especially in patients with a history of allergy to other drugs (most often muscle relaxants).

4. Barbiturates may precipitate episodes of acute intermittent porphyria in vulnerable patients. (The

benzodiazepines, ketamine, etomidate, and propofol are reported to be safe.)

II. COMPARATIVE PHYSIOCHEMICAL AND CLINICAL PHARMACOLOGIC PROPERTIES

A. Barbiturates

1. Thiopental and thiamylal are thiobarbiturates with similar potency (adult induction dose, 3–5 mg/kg IV) and pharmacologic profile. Methohexital is an oxybarbiturate with a greater potency (adult induction dose, 1.5 mg/kg IV) than the thiobarbiturates and is associated with a high incidence of myoclonic-like muscle tremors and other signs of excitatory activity (e.g., hiccoughing).

   a. These drugs are provided as racemic mixtures that are alkaline (thiopental 2.5% has a pH >9) and precipitate when added to acidic solutions (Ringer's lactate).

   b. Geriatric patients require a 30% to 40% reduction in the usual adult dose because of a decrease of the volume of the central compartment and slowed redistribution of thiopental from the vessel-rich tissues to lean muscle.

   c. Thiopental is seldom used to maintain anesthesia because of its long context-sensitive half-time and prolonged recovery period.

   d. Accidental intra-arterial injection of barbiturates may result in formation of crystals in arterioles and capillaries, causing intense vasoconstriction, thrombosis, and even tissue necrosis. (This is treated with intra-arterial administration of papaverine and lidocaine, brachial plexus block, and heparin.)

2. Methohexital is metabolized in the liver to inactive metabolites more rapidly than thiopental.

3. Barbiturates produce a maximum decrease in $CMRO_2$ (55%) when the EEG becomes isoelectric (associated with a decrease in CBF and ICP).

   a. An isoelectric EEG can be maintained with a thiopental infusion rate of 4 to 6 mg/kg/hr IV.

   b. Although barbiturate therapy is widely used to control ICP after brain injury, the results of outcome studies are no better than with other aggressive forms of cerebral antihypertensive therapy.

    c. Barbiturates have no place in the therapy after resuscitation of a cardiac arrest patient.

    d. Barbiturates may improve the brain's tolerance to incomplete ischemia and may be used for cerebro-protection during carotid endarterectomy, profound controlled hypotension, or cardiopulmonary bypass. Moderate degrees of hypothermia (33°C to 34°C) may provide superior neuroprotection without prolonging the recovery phase.

    e. Barbiturates possess potent anticonvulsant activity. Methohexital produces epileptogenic effects in patients with psychomotor epilepsy.

4. Barbiturates cause dose-dependent depression of ventilation. Bronchospasm and laryngospasm are usually the result of airway manipulation in the presence of inadequate anesthesia.

5. Cardiovascular effects of barbiturates include decreases in blood pressure decreased venous return because of peripheral pooling and direct myocardial depression and a compensatory increase in heart rate.

6. Hypotension is exaggerated in the presence of hypovolemia.

B. Propofol

1. As an alkylphenol compound, this drug is virtually insoluble in water, requiring its preparation in an egg-lecithin emulsion as a 1% (10 mg/mL) solution.

    a. An alternative propofol formulation containing sodium metabisulfite (rather than disodium edetate) as an antimicrobial is associated with less pain on injection. The concern regarding use of this formulation in sulphite-allergic patients does not seem to be a clinically important problem.

    b. Ampofol is a lower-lipid formulation of propofol, and the increased free fraction of propofol leads to increased pain with injection into small veins.

    c. Aquavan is a water-soluble prodrug that is rapidly metabolized in the circulation to release propofol. Its onset is slower, but recovery is similar to propofol. Injection site discomfort does not occur, but a transient burning sensation in the perineum may occur after IV injection.

2. Propofol is rapidly cleared from the central compartment by hepatic metabolism and the context-sensitive half-time for continuous IV infusions (≤8 hours) is less than 40 minutes. Emergence and

awakening are prompt and complete even after prolonged infusions.

   a. Hepatic metabolism is prompt to inactive water-
   soluble metabolites that are eliminated by the
   kidneys.

   b. The clearance rate (1.5–2.2 L/min) exceeds hepatic
   blood flow, suggesting that an extrahepatic route
   of elimination (i.e., through the lungs) also contributes to its clearance (this is important during
   the anhepatic phase of liver transplantation).

3. The induction dose in adults is 1.5 to 2.5 mg/kg IV,
   and the recommended IV infusion rate is 100 to 200
   μg/kg/min for hypnosis and 25 to 75 μg/kg/min for
   sedation.

   a. Pain on injection occurs in a high proportion of
   patients when the drug is injected into small hand
   veins; this can be minimized by injection into
   larger veins or by prior administration of 1%
   lidocaine.

   b. Propofol may produce a subjective feeling of well-
   being and euphoria and may have abuse potential
   as a result of these effects.

4. Propofol decreases $CMRO_2$, CBF, and ICP, but the
   associated decrease in systemic blood pressure may
   also significantly decrease cerebral perfusion
   pressure.

   a. Cortical EEG changes produced by propofol
   resemble those of thiopental.

   b. A neuroprotective effect may reflect antioxidant
   properties.

   c. Induction of anesthesia with propofol is occasionally accompanied by excitatory motor activity
   (nonepileptic myoclonia).

   d. This drug is an anticonvulsant. The duration of
   seizure activity after electroconvulsive therapy is
   shorter with propofol than methohexital and is
   effective in terminating status epilepticus.

5. Propofol produces dose-dependent depression of ventilation. Apnea occurs in 25% to 35% of patients
   after induction of anesthesia.

   a. Bronchodilatation may occur in patients with
   chronic obstructive pulmonary disease.

   b. Hypoxic pulmonary vasoconstriction is not inhibited by propofol.

6. Propofol produces greater cardiovascular depressant effects than thiopental, reflecting decreased systemic vascular resistance (arterial and venous dilation) and direct myocardial depressant effects.

7. Propofol appears to possess antiemetic properties that contribute to a low incidence of emetic sequelae after propofol anesthesia. Subanesthetic doses (10–20 mg) may be used to treat nausea and emesis in the early postoperative period. Postulated antiemetic mechanisms include an antidopaminergic activity and a depressant effect on the chemoreceptor trigger zone and vagal nuclei.

8. Propofol decreases the pruritus associated with neuraxial opioids.

9. Propofol does not trigger malignant hyperthermia and may be considered the induction drug of choice in patients who are susceptible to malignant hyperthermia.

C. Benzodiazepines

1. The benzodiazepines of primary interest to anesthesiologists are diazepam, lorazepam, and midazolam and the antagonist flumazenil.

   a. These drugs are primarily used as preoperative medication and adjuvant drugs because of their anxiolytic, sedative, and amnestic properties.

   b. Diazepam and lorazepam are insoluble in water, and their formulation contains propylene glycol, a tissue irritant that causes pain on injection and venous irritation.

   c. Midazolam is a water-soluble benzodiazepine that produces minimal irritation after IV or intramuscular (IM) injection. When exposed to physiologic pH, an intramolecular rearrangement occurs that changes the physiocochemical properties of midazolam such that it becomes more lipid soluble.

2. Benzodiazepines undergo hepatic metabolism via oxidation and glucuronide conjugation. Oxidation reactions are susceptible to hepatic dysfunction and coadministration of other drugs such as H2-receptor antagonists.

   a. The hepatic clearance rate of midazolam is five times greater than that of lorazepam and 10 times greater than that of diazepam.

  b. Diazepam is metabolized to active metabolites, which may prolong its residual sedative effects.

  c. Lorazepam is directly conjugated to glucuronic acid to form pharmacologically inactive metabolites. The primary metabolite of midazolam (1-hydroxy-methylmidazolam) has some CNS depressant activity.

  d. The context-sensitive half-times for diazepam and lorazepam are very long, so only midazolam should be used for continuous infusion.

3. Benzodiazepines decrease $CMRO_2$ and CBF analogous to the barbiturates and propofol, but these drugs have not been shown to possess neuroprotective activity in humans.

  a. In contrast to other compounds, midazolam is unable to produce an isoelectric EEG.

  b. Similar to the other sedative-hypnotic drugs, the benzodiazepines are potent anticonvulsants that are commonly used to treat status epilepticus.

4. Benzodiazepines produce dose-dependent depression of ventilation that is enhanced in patients with chronic respiratory disease, and synergistic depressant effects occur when benzodiazepines are coadministered with opioids.

5. Both midazolam and diazepam produce decreases in systemic vascular resistance and systemic blood pressure (accentuated with hypovolemia) when large doses are administered for induction of anesthesia, but a ceiling effect appears to exist above which little further change in arterial pressure occurs.

6. Short-acting IV sedatives are characterized by water-soluble benzodiazepines with full agonist activity and a higher plasma clearance rate compared with midazolam.

7. In contrast to all other sedative-hypnotic drugs, there is a specific antagonist for benzodiazepines. (Flumazenil has a high affinity for CNS benzodiazepine receptors but possesses minimal intrinsic activity.)

  a. Flumazenil acts as a competitive antagonist in the presence of benzodiazepine agonist compounds.

  b. Recurrence of the CNS effects of benzodiazepines may occur after a single dose of flumazenil (which is rapidly metabolized in the liver with an elimination half-time of about 1 hour) because of residual effects of the more slowly eliminated agonist.

c. In general, 45 to 90 minutes of antagonism can be expected after IV administration of 1 to 3 mg of flumazenil. (Sustained effects require repeated doses or continuous infusion.)

D. **Etomidate**

1. Etomidate is a carboxylated imidazole (only the dextro isomer possesses anesthetic activity) that is structurally unrelated to any other IV anesthetic. but similar to midazolam (which also contains an imidazole nucleus), etomidate undergoes an intramolecular rearrangement at physiologic pH, resulting in a closed ring structure with enhanced lipid solubility.

   a. This drug is formulated with propylene glycol, contributing to a high incidence of pain on injection and occasional venoirritation.

   b. The standard induction dose of etomidate (0.2–0.4 mg/kg IV) produces a rapid onset of anesthesia (myoclonic movements are common because of an alteration in the balance of inhibitory and excitatory influence on the thalamocortical tract), and emergence is prompt. (Extensive ester hydrolysis in the liver, forming inactive water-soluble metabolites.)

   c. The frequency of myoclonic-like activity can be attenuated by prior administration of opioid analgesics, benzodiazepines, or remifentanil or administration of small sedative doses of etomidate (0.03–0.05 mg/kg) before induction of anesthesia.

2. Analogous to the barbiturates, etomidate decreases $CMRO_2$, CBF, and ICP, but the hemodynamic stability associated with etomidate maintains adequate cerebral perfusion pressure.

   a. An inhibitory effect on adrenocortical synthetic function (a single dose inhibits 11-β-hydroxylase for 5 to 8 hours) limits its clinical usefulness for long-term treatment of increased ICP.

   b. Although an anticonvulsant effective in terminating status epilepticus, etomidate is also capable of evoking EEG evidence of seizure activity in attempts to identify seizure foci.

   c. Etomidate produces a significant increase in the amplitude of somatosensory evoked potentials and can be used to facilitate the interpretation of somatosensory evoked potentials when the signal quality is poor.

3. Etomidate causes minimal depression of ventilation and cardiovascular function (it may be recommended for induction of anesthesia in poor-risk patients with cardiopulmonary disease) and does not release histamine (it is an acceptable drug choice for use in patients with reactive airway disease).

4. Etomidate is associated with a high incidence of nausea and vomiting, especially if it is combined with an opioid.

5. Etomidate may inhibit platelet function and prolong bleeding time.

E. **Ketamine**

1. Ketamine is an acrylcyclohexilamine that is structurally related to phencyclidine.

    a. The commercially available preparation is a racemic mixture, although the S+ isomer possesses more potent anesthetic and analgesic properties, reflecting its fourfold greater affinity at the binding sites on the NMDA receptor. Hepatic biotransformation of the S+ isomer is more rapid, contributing to a faster return of cognitive function. Both isomers possess similar cardiovascular-stimulating properties, and the incidence of dreaming is similar with the S+ isomer and the racemic mixture.

    b. Ketamine produces dose-dependent CNS depression, leading to a so-called "dissociative anesthetic state" characterized by profound analgesia and amnesia. Low-dose ketamine (75–200 µg/kg/min IV) produces opioid-sparing effects when administered as an adjuvant during general anesthesia.

    c. Induction of anesthesia can be accomplished with 1 to 2 mg/kg IV (4–8 mg/kg IM), producing an effect that lasts for 10 to 20 minutes, although recovery to full orientation may require an additional 60 to 90 minutes.

    d. Subanesthetic doses of ketamine (0.1–0.5 mg/kg IV) produce analgesic effects. A low-dose infusion of ketamine (4 µg/kg/min IV) is equivalent to morphine (2 mg/hr IV) for production of postoperative analgesia.

2. Ketamine is extensively metabolized in the liver to norketamine, which is one third to one fifth as potent as the parent compound.

3. Psychomimetic reactions during the recovery period from ketamine anesthesia are less likely in patients also treated with benzodiazepines, barbiturates, or propofol.
4. Ketamine increases $CMRO_2$, CBF, and ICP (which is minimized by hyperventilation of the lungs and pretreatment with benzodiazepines).
5. Ketamine can activate epileptogenic foci in patients with known seizure disorders but otherwise appears to possess anticonvulsant activity.
6. Ketamine is often recommended for induction of anesthesia in patients with asthma because of its ability to produce bronchodilation.
   a. Depression of ventilation is minimal in clinically relevant doses.
   b. Increased oral secretions may contribute to the development of laryngospasm.
7. Ketamine has prominent cardiovascular stimulating effects (increased blood pressure, heart rate, pulmonary artery pressure) most likely because of direct stimulation of the sympathetic nervous system. This is possibly undesirable in patients with coronary artery disease.
   a. Ketamine has intrinsic myocardial depressant properties, which may only become apparent in seriously ill patients with depleted catecholamines.
   b. Ketamine can reduce the magnitude of redistribution hypothermia owing to its peripheral arteriolar vasoconstriction.
8. The renewed interest in ketamine is related to the use of smaller doses (100–250 $\mu g/kg$) as an adjuvant during anesthesia.
   a. The anesthetic (sedative) and opioid analgesic-sparing effects of ketamine may reduce ventilatory depression during monitored anesthesia care.
   b. The availability of the stereosimer of ketamine has increased the non-anesthetic adjunctive use of ketamine. The anesthetic and analgesic potency of $S(+)$ ketamine is three times greater than $R(-)$ ketamine and twice that of the racemic mixture.

F. **Dexmedetomidine**
   1. Dexmedetomidine is a highly selective $\alpha\text{-}_2$ agonist that produces sedation and analgesia with less depression of ventilation than other commonly used drugs. The drug is approved for sedation of mechanically

ventilated patients in the intensive care unit (ICU) but is also being used during diagnostic and therapeutic procedures (regional and local anesthesia) outside the ICU ("off-label use").

2. When used for premedication, dexmedetomidine is comparable to midazolam, but the incidence of intraoperative hypotension and bradycardia is increased.

3. The acute hemodynamic response to laryngoscopy and intubation is blunted by dexmedetomidine.

III. CLINICAL USES OF INTRAVENOUS ANESTHETICS

A. Use of Intravenous Anesthetics as Induction Agents (Table 18-5)

1. Propofol has become the IV drug of choice for outpatients undergoing ambulatory surgery.

2. Clinical use of midazolam (often combined with other injected drugs), etomidate (cardiac stability), and ketamine (hypovolemic patients) is restricted to specific situations in which their unique pharmacologic profiles offer advantages over other available IV anesthetics.

B. Use of Intravenous Drugs for Maintenance of Anesthesia

1. The availability of IV drugs with more rapid onset and shorter recovery profiles, as well as easier-to-use infusion delivery systems, has facilitated the maintenance of anesthesia with continuous infusion of IV drugs (total IV anesthetic techniques [TIVA]), producing an anesthetic state that compares favorably with the volatile anesthetics.

2. The optimal IV dose range is influenced by many factors (Table 18-6).

3. Clinical signs of depth of anesthesia, such as skeletal muscle tone, ventilation, blood pressure, and heart rate, may be obscured by adjuvant drugs.
   a. Analysis of the spontaneous EEG (bispectral index [BIS], patient state index [PSI], response entropy [RE]) may provide useful information regarding anesthetic (hypnotic) depth.
   b. The BIS can improve titration of both IV and inhaled anesthetics, thus facilitating the recovery process.

4. When using constant-rate IV infusions, 4.0 to 5.5 times may be required to achieve a steady-state

TABLE 18-5

INDUCTION CHARACTERISTICS AND DOSAGE REQUIREMENTS FOR INTRAVENOUS ANESTHETIC DRUGS

Drug	Induction Dose (mg/kg)	Onset (sec)	Duration (min)	Excitatory Activity	Pain on Injection	Heart Rate	Blood Pressure
Thiopental	3–6	<30	5–10	+	0/+	+	–
Methohexital	1–3	<30	5–10	++	+	++	–
Propofol	1.5–2.5	15–45	5–10	+	++	0/–	–
Midazolam	0.2–0.4	30–90	10–30	0	0	0	0/–
Diazepam	0.3–0.6	45–90	15–30	0	+++	0	0/–
Lorazepam	0.03–0.06	60–120	60–120	0	++	0	0/–
Etomidate	0.2–0.3	15–45	3–12	+++	+++	0	0
Ketamine	1–2	45–60	10–20	+	0	++	++

0 = no change; + = increase; – = decrease.

265

TABLE 18-6

FACTORS THAT INFLUENCE INTRAVENOUS DRUG DOSE
REQUIREMENTS

Concomitant use of adjunctive drugs
Type of operation (superficial, intra-abdominal)
Patient age
Pre-existing diseases (hepatic, renal, cardiac)
Intraoperative interventions (laryngoscopy, skin incision)

anesthetic concentration (offset with an initial loading
[primary] dose) (Fig. 18-4).
  a. Rapid, short-acting, sedative-hypnotics and opioids
     are better suited for continuous administration
     techniques because they can be more precisely
     titrated to meet the unique and changing needs of
     the individual patient.
  b. Context-sensitive half-time is more appropriate in
     choosing drugs for continuous IV administration
     (Fig. 18-5).
  c. None of the currently available IV drugs can pro-
     vide for a complete anesthetic state without pro-
     ducing prolonged recovery times and undesirable
     side effects; therefore, combinations of drugs must

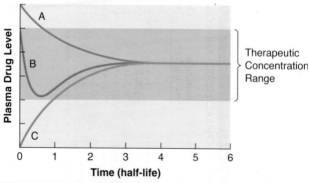

FIGURE 18-4. Simulated drug level curves when a constant infusion is
administered after a full dose (*curve A*), a smaller loading dose (*curve B*),
and no loading dose (*curve C*).

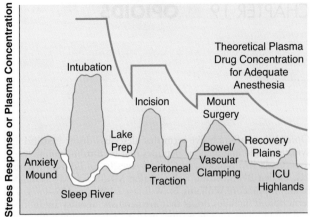

FIGURE 18-5. Context-sensitive half-time values as a function of infusion duration for intravenous anesthetics. The context-sensitive half-times for thiopental and diazepam are significantly longer compared with etomidate, propofol, and midazolam with an increasing infusion duration.

> be administered to achieve hypnosis, amnesia, analgesia, and hemodynamic stability.
>
> C. **Use of Intravenous Anesthetics for Sedation.** The use of sedative-hypnotic drugs as part of a monitored anesthesia care technique in combination with local anesthetics and to provide sedation for the management of patients in the ICU is becoming increasingly popular.

CHAPTER 19 ■ OPIOIDS

Opioid is an all-inclusive term that describes drugs (natural and synthetic) and endogenous peptides that bind to morphine receptors (Coda BA: Opioids. In *Clinical Anesthesia*. Edited by Barash PG, Cullen BF, Stoelting RK, Cahalan MK, Stock MC. Philadelphia: Lippincott Williams & Wilkins, 2009, pp 465–497). The term *opioid* includes drugs that are agonists, agonist-antagonists, and antagonists. *Opiate* is often used interchangeably with *opioid* but historically designates only drugs derived from opium (morphine, codeine). *Narcotic* is a nonspecific designation applicable to any drug that produces sleep.

I. ENDOGENOUS OPIOIDS AND OPIOID RECEPTORS (Table 19-1)

A. All of the endogenous opioids are derived from prohormones, and each of these precursors is encoded by a separate gene. Synthesis of endorphins is from a prohormone principally located in the anterior pituitary. Endogenous opioids bind to a number of opioid receptors to produce their effects.

   1. The expression of endogenous opioids and opioid receptors is not a static phenomenon.

   2. Acute inflammation up-regulates the expression of peripheral μ and ∂-opioid receptors. Chronic inflammation is associated with a down-regulation of μ-opioid receptors.

B. All opioid receptors appear to be coupled to G proteins, which regulate the activity of adenylate cyclase and subsequent ion channel conduction characteristics.

TABLE 19-1

CLASSIFICATION OF OPIOID RECEPTORS AND ACTIONS

Receptor	Analgesia	Respiratory	Gastrointestinal	Endocrine	Other
μ	Peripheral		Slowed gastric emptying Antidiarrheal	Pruritus	Skeletal muscle rigidity Possibly urinary retention Biliary spasm
μ_1	Supraspinal			Prolactin turnover	Acetylcholine release
μ_2	Spinal Supraspinal	Depression	Slowed gastric emptying		Cardiovascular effects
μ_3					Antiinflammatory
K	Peripheral			Decreased ADH release	Sedation
K_1	Spinal				
K_2	?				Antipruretic
K_3	Supraspinal				
∂	Peripheral	Possibly depression	Slowed gastric emptying Antidiarrheal	Possibly growth hormone release	Possibly urinary retention
∂_1	Spinal Supraspinal				Dopamine turnover
∂_2	Supraspinal				
Unknown receptor and subtype					Miosis Nausea Vomiting

ADH = antidiuretic hormone.

269

II. PHARMACOKINETICS AND PHARMACODYNAMICS

A. **Physicochemical properties** of opioids influence both pharmacokinetics and pharmacodynamics (Table 19-2).

1. To reach its sites of action (receptors on neuronal cell membranes in the central nervous system [CNS]), an opioid must cross the blood–brain barrier.

   a. The ability of opioids to cross the blood–brain barrier depends on properties such as molecular size, ionization, lipid solubility, and protein binding.

   b. The degree of ionization depends on the pKa of the opioid and the pH of the tissue (nonionized drugs are 1000 to 10,000 times more lipid soluble than the ionized form).

2. The major plasma proteins to which opioids bind are albumin and *alpha*$_1$-acid glycoprotein.

B. **Biotransformation** and **excretion** are the principal mechanisms for elimination of opioids.

1. Opioids are metabolized in the liver (conjugation, oxidative and reductive reactions) or hydrolyzed in the plasma (unique for remifentanil).

2. With the exception of the N-dealkylated metabolite of meperidine and the 6- and possibly 3-glucuronides of morphine, opioid metabolites are generally inactive.

3. Opioid metabolites, and to a lesser extent, parent compounds are excreted by the kidneys. The biliary system and gastrointestinal (GI) tract are less important routes of opioid excretion.

III. MORPHINE mimics the effects of endogenous opioids by acting as an agonist at μ_1- and μ_2-opioid receptors throughout the body and is considered the agonist with which other μ agonists are compared (Tables 19-3 and 19-4).

A. **Analgesia**

1. Morphine analgesia results from complex interactions at a number of discrete sites in the brain, spinal cord, and under certain conditions, peripheral tissues, and involves both μ_1- and μ_2-opioid effects.

TABLE 19-2

PHYSICOCHEMICAL CHARACTERISTICS AND PHARMACOKINETICS OF COMMONLY USED OPIOID AGONISTS

Parameter	Morphine	Meperidine	Fentanyl	Sufentanil	Alfentanil	Remifentanil
pKa	7.9	8.5	8.4	8.0	6.5	7.3
Nonionized (pH, 7.4) (%)	23	7	8.5	20	89	58
Protein binding (%)	35	70	84	93	92	66–93
Clearance (mL/min)	1050	1020	1530	900	238	3000
Volume of distribution (steady state, L)	224	305	334	123	27	25–30
Elimination half-time (hr)	1.7–3.3	3–5	3.1–6.6	2.2–4.6	1.4–1.5	0.17–0.33

TABLE 19-3

RELATIVE POTENCIES AND PLASMA CONCENTRATIONS FOR VARIOUS OPIOID EFFECTS

Effect	Morphine	Meperidine	Fentanyl	Sufentanil	Alfentanil	Remifentanil
Relative potencies	1	0.1	100	500–1000	10–20	
Analgesic dose (mg)	10	100	0.1	0.01–0.02	0.5–1.5	
Minimum effective analgesic concentration (ng/mL)	10–15	200	0.6	0.03	15	
Moderate to strong analgesia (ng/mL)	20–50	400–600	1.5–5.0	0.05–0.1	40–80	
Decrease MAC 50% (ng/mL)	NA	>500	0.5–2	0.145	200	1.3
Surgical analgesia with 70% nitrous oxide (ng/mL)	NA	NA	15–25	NA	300–500	4.0–7.5
Depression of ventilation threshold (ng/mL)	25	200	1	0.02–0.04	50–100	
Ventilatory response to carbon dioxide decreased 50% (ng/mL)	50	NA	1.5–3.0	0.04	120–350	0.9–1.2
Apnea (ng/mL)	NA	NA	7–22	NA	300–600	
Unconsciousness (not reliably achieved with opioids alone) (ng/mL)		Seizures	15–20	NA	500–1500	

MAC = minimum alveolar concentration; NA = not available.

TABLE 19-4

EFFECTS OF OPIOID AGONISTS*

Central Nervous System (Brain and Spinal Cord)
Analgesia
Sedation
Euphoria
Depression of ventilation (increased $PaCO_2$ [decreased ventilatory response to CO_2 because of brain stem depression] and decreased breathing rate and minute ventilation)
Nausea and vomiting (stimulation of the chemoreceptor trigger zone, especially in ambulatory patients; high doses of opioids depress the vomiting center and may overcome the chemoreceptor trigger zone stimulating effect)
Pruritus
Miosis (diagnostic of opioid administration)
Depressed cough reflex
Skeletal muscle rigidity
Myoclonus (may be confused with seizures)

Gastrointestinal Tract
Slowed gastric emptying
Increased tone of the common bile duct and sphincter of Oddi (reversed by nitroglycerin [as is angina] or naloxone [not angina]; can prevent visualization of contrast material in the duodenum, resulting in the erroneous conclusion that the common bile duct is blocked by a stone)

Genitourinary Tract
Urinary retention

Endocrine System
Antidiuretic hormone release

Autonomic Nervous System
Arterial and venous vasodilation (orthostatic hypotension)
Bradycardia (sympatholytic and parasympathomimetic mechanisms)

Histamine Release (morphine and meperidine are probably not mediated by opioid receptors)

*Similar for all opioid agonists, but the magnitude of effect of equianalgesic doses may differ.

2. Supraspinal opioid analgesia originates in the periaqueductal gray matter, the locus ceruleus, and nuclei within the medulla and primarily involves μ_1-opioid receptors.
3. At the spinal cord level, morphine acts presynaptically on primary afferent nociceptors to decrease

the release of substance P. Morphine also hyperpolarizes interneurons in the substantia gelatinosa of the dorsal spinal cord to decrease afferent transmission of nociceptive impulses. Spinal morphine analgesia is mediated by μ_2-opioid receptors.

4. Peripheral analgesia produced by morphine is most likely attributable to activation of opioid receptors on primary afferent neurons, which occurs only when inflammation is present.

5. The minimum effective analgesic concentration of morphine for postoperative pain relief is 10 to 15 ng/mL. (This is more likely to be maintained by patient-controlled analgesia than by intermittent intravenous [IV] or intramuscular [IM] injections; Table 19-3).

B. **Effect on Minimum Alveolar Concentration of Volatile Anesthetics**

1. The μ agonists are used extensively in conjunction with nitrous oxide with or without a volatile anesthetic to produce "balanced anesthesia."

2. Morphine (1 mg/kg IV) administered with 60% inhaled nitrous oxide blocks the adrenergic response to surgical skin incision in 50% of patients (MAC-BAR).

3. Neuraxial morphine may also decrease minimum alveolar concentration (MAC).

C. **Other Central Nervous System Effects.** Morphine can produce sedation as well as cognitive and fine motor impairment, even at plasma concentrations commonly achieved during management of moderate to severe pain.

D. **Respiratory Depression**

1. Morphine and other μ agonists produce dose-dependent ventilatory depression primarily by decreasing the response of the medullary respiratory center to carbon dioxide.

2. Frequent periods of oxygen desaturation associated with obstructive apnea, paradoxical breathing, and slow respiratory rate may occur in patients who are sleeping and who receive morphine infusions for postoperative analgesia. Sleep apnea increases the risk of morphine-induced respiratory depression.

E. **Cardiovascular Effects**

1. In doses typically used for pain management or as part of balanced anesthesia, morphine has little

effect on blood pressure or heart rate and cardiac rhythm in supine normovolemic patients.

2. Large doses may produce peripheral vasodilation (central sympatholytic activity), especially in patients with high sympathetic nervous system tone (congestive heart failure, severe trauma). Hypotension may reflect sympatholysis and histamine release.

3. Morphine does not depress myocardial contractility but does produce bradycardia probably by both sympatholytic and parasympathomimetic mechanisms.

   a. In clinical anesthesia practice, opioids are often used for cardiac surgery to prevent tachycardia and decrease myocardial oxygen demand.

   b. Morphine (40 mg) suppresses several components of the inflammatory response to cardiopulmonary bypass.

4. Morphine does not directly affect cerebral circulation as long as drug-induced depression of ventilation with retention of carbon dioxide (would produce cerebral vasodilation) is prevented by mechanical support of breathing.

F. **Disposition Kinetics.** After IM administration of morphine, peak plasma concentration is seen at 20 minutes.

G. **Active Metabolites**

1. Morphine's major metabolic pathway is conjugation in the liver to morphine-3-glucuronide (M3G) and morphine-6-glucuronide (M6G). The importance of extrahepatic sites of glucuronidation (kidneys, lungs, GI tract) in humans is unknown.

2. M6G possesses significant μ-receptor affinity and potent antinociceptive activity.

3. Sensitivity of renal failure patients to morphine may reflect the dependence of M6G on renal excretion.

H. **Dosage and Administration of Morphine**

1. Morphine crosses the blood–brain barrier relatively slowly because of its hydrophilicity.

2. Because of its delayed onset of action, morphine can be more difficult to titrate as an anesthetic supplement than the more rapidly acting opioids.

IV. MEPERIDINE

A. **Analgesia and Effect on Minimum Alveolar Concentration of Volatile Anesthetics**

1. Meperidine's analgesic potency is about one tenth that of morphine's and is most likely mediated by μ-opioid receptor activation.
2. Unlike morphine, meperidine's plasma concentrations correlate with its analgesic effects (Table 19-3).
3. Meperidine is unique among the opioids in also possessing a **weak local anesthetic** properly, which is useful for neuraxial administration.

B. **Side effects** resemble those of morphine (Table 19-4).
   1. High doses of meperidine are associated with CNS excitement (seizures) and decreased myocardial contractility (hypotension).
   2. The increase in common bile duct pressure occurs to a lesser extent than with equianalgesic doses of morphine and fentanyl.

C. **Shivering.** Meperidine (25–50 mg IV) is effective in decreasing postoperative shivering; equianalgesic doses of morphine and fentanyl are not effective. The observation that drugs other than opioids (e.g., clonidine, serotonic antagonists, propofol, physostigmine) reduce postoperative shivering suggest that a nonopioid mechanism may be involved.

D. **Disposition Kinetics** (Table 19-2)
   1. After IV administration, meperidine plasma concentrations decrease rapidly.
   2. Meperidine is metabolized mainly in the liver by N-demethylation to form normeperidine, the principal metabolite, and by hydrolysis to form meperidinic acid.

E. **Active Metabolites.** Normeperidine has pharmacologic activity and can produce signs of CNS excitation (daily doses >1000 mg increase the risk of seizures).

F. **Dosage and Administration of Meperidine** (Table 19-3)

V. **METHADONE** is a synthetic μ-opioid receptor agonist that possesses a long elimination half-time. The drug is most often used for long-term pain management (10 mg is similar to morphine) and in treatment of abstinence syndrome.

A. **Side effects** are similar in magnitude and frequency to those of morphine.

B. **Disposition Kinetics.** Methadone is well absorbed after oral administration and reaches peak plasma concentration at 4 hours after oral administration.

C. **Dosage and Administration of Methadone.** Patients with significant pain have no depression of respiration or level of consciousness.

VI. FENTANYL and its related μ-opioid receptor analogs sufentanil and alfentanil are the most frequently used opioids in clinical practice. The clinical potency of fentanyl is 50 to 100 times that of morphine, and there is a direct relationship between plasma concentrations and analgesia (Table 19-3).

A. **Use in Anesthesia**
1. Plasma fentanyl concentrations decrease rapidly after a single IV injection, so the magnitude of MAC reduction varies depending on the time after fentanyl administration. (Computer-assisted continuous infusion provides a constant plasma concentration and associated decrease in anesthetic requirements.)
2. Combining opioids with propofol rather than an inhaled anesthetic can produce general anesthesia (total IV anesthesia). Plasma concentrations of fentanyl and propofol that prevent responses to skin incision in 50% of patients have been determined.
3. Fentanyl has been used as the sole drug for anesthesia (50–150 μg/kg IV or a stable plasma concentration in the range of 20–30 ng/mL) because hemodynamic stability is desirable for patients with heart disease.
   a. When administered rapidly intravenously, high doses of opioids can produce skeletal muscle rigidity.
   b. Combining opioids with other depressant drugs (nitrous oxide, benzodiazepines) changes the stable hemodynamic profile of the opioid alone, and hypotension can occur.

B. **Other Central Nervous System Effects**
1. The effect of fentanyl on intracranial pressure (ICP) is inconsistent with some reports showing an increase and others no change.
2. Fentanyl has been associated with seizure-like movements (most likely myoclonus), but seizure activity is not present on the electroencephalogram.
3. Fentanyl-induced pruritus often presents as facial itching but can be generalized (similar with sufentanil and alfentanil).

C. **Respiratory Depression**
   1. Peak depression of ventilation occurs in about 5 minutes and parallels the plasma concentration and intensity of analgesia (Table 19-3).
   2. The magnitude of respiratory depression can be greatly increased when fentanyl is administered with another sedative drug such as a benzodiazepine.

D. **Airway Reflexes**
   1. Similar to the volatile anesthetics, opioids depress airway reflexes elicited in response to laryngeal stimulation (placement of a laryngeal mask airway).
   2. Cough is the laryngeal reflex that is most vulnerable to depression by fentanyl.

E. **Cardiovascular and Endocrine Effects**
   1. In clinical practice, high-dose fentanyl administration is associated with remarkable hemodynamic stability. (Combination with other anesthetic drugs may result in cardiovascular depression.)
   2. Hypertension in response to median sternotomy is the most common hemodynamic disturbance during high-dose fentanyl anesthesia.
   3. Unlike morphine and meperidine, which induce hypotension, at least partly by histamine release, high-dose fentanyl is not associated with significant histamine release.

F. **Smooth Muscle and Gastrointestinal Effects.** Similar to morphine and meperidine, fentanyl increases common bile duct pressure. Fentanyl can cause nausea and vomiting, especially in ambulatory patients, and can delay gastric emptying.

G. **Disposition Kinetics** (Table 19-2)
   1. Fentanyl's high lipid solubility allows it to cross biologic membranes rapidly (rapid onset) followed by redistribution to inactive tissue sites such as skeletal muscle and fat (short duration). High doses or prolonged administration of fentanyl can saturate redistribution sites, converting this drug to a long-acting opioid.
   2. Clearance of fentanyl is primarily by hepatic metabolism (N-dealkylation to norfentanyl and hydroxylation of both the parent compound and norfentanyl).
   3. A patient with respiratory acidosis will have a higher proportion of unbound (active) fentanyl.

H. **Dosage and Administration of Fentanyl** (Table 19-3)
   1. Fentanyl can be used as a sedative/analgesic premedication when given a short time before induction of

anesthesia (25–50 μg IV or transmucosal delivery system for pediatric and adult patients). Respiratory depression can occur, emphasizing the need to monitor patients treated with these doses of fentanyl.

2. Fentanyl is commonly used as an adjunct to induction drugs to blunt the hemodynamic response to laryngoscopy and tracheal intubation. Because fentanyl's peak effect lags behind the peak plasma concentration by 3 to 5 minutes, fentanyl should be administered about 3 minutes before initiating laryngoscopy.

3. Perhaps the most common use of fentanyl and its derivatives is as an analgesic component of balanced general anesthesia (0.5–2.5 μg/kg IV as dictated by the intensity of the surgical stimulus or 2–10 μg/kg/hr as a continuous infusion).

4. High-dose fentanyl (50–150 μg/kg IV) may be used as the sole anesthetic for cardiac surgery. (It may not provide total amnesia in healthy patients.)

5. Fentanyl has been used as an analgesic in the management of acute and chronic pain. Both transdermal and transmucosal fentanyl delivery systems are effective for relief of cancer pain.

VII. **SUFENTANIL** is a highly selective and potent (10 to 15 times that of fentanyl) μ-opioid receptor agonist that equilibrates rapidly between the blood and the brain.

A. **Use in Anesthesia**
   1. Sufentanil, similar to other opioids, produces a dose-dependent decrease in the MAC of volatile anesthetics.
   2. In clinical practice, sufentanil is used as a component of balanced anesthesia and in high doses (10–30 μg/kg IV) for cardiac surgery. (Similar to fentanyl, sufentanil does not completely block the hemodynamic response to noxious stimuli.)

B. **Other central nervous system effects** resemble those of fentanyl.

C. **Respiratory depression** resembles other μ-opioid receptor agonists and can be especially marked in the presence of inhaled anesthetics.

D. **Disposition Kinetics** (Table 19-2)
   1. Sufentanil is highly lipid soluble and has pharmacokinetic properties that resemble fentanyl. Because of

its higher degree of ionization at physiologic pH and higher degree of plasma protein binding, its volume of distribution is somewhat smaller and its elimination half-time shorter than those of fentanyl. Obesity may increase the volume of distribution and prolong the elimination half-time of sufentanil.

2. Clearance of sufentanil (similar to fentanyl) is rapid, primarily by hepatic metabolism (N-dealkylation and O-demethylation).

E. **Dosage and Administration of Sufentanil** (Table 19-3)
   1. Sufentanil (similar to fentanyl) is most often used as a component of balanced anesthesia or in high doses for cardiac surgery (≤ 50 µg/kg IV).
   2. Doses in the range of 0.3 to 1.0 µg/kg IV given 1 to 3 minutes before laryngoscopy can be expected to blunt hemodynamic responses to tracheal intubation.
   3. For maintenance of balanced anesthesia, sufentanil can be administered in intermittent doses (0.1–0.5 µg/kg IV) or as a continuous infusion (0.3–1.0 µg/kg/hr IV).

VIII. **ALFENTANIL** is a µ-opioid receptor agonist with a potency approximately 10 times that of morphine and one fourth to one tenth that of fentanyl. In contrast to fentanyl and sufentanil, the duration of even very large doses of alfentanil is brief, necessitating its administration by continuous infusion if a sustained effect is desired.

A. **Nausea and Vomiting.** Clinical comparisons between alfentanil and sufentanil or fentanyl and nitrous oxide reveal a similar incidence of nausea and vomiting.

B. **Disposition Kinetics** (Table 19-2)
   1. Alfentanil pharmacokinetics differ from fentanyl and sufentanil with respect to pK (alfentanil 6.8 and all other opioids above 7.4). This results in 90% of unbound plasma alfentanil being unionized at a plasma pH of 7.4. This property, together with moderate lipid solubility, enables alfentanil to rapidly cross the blood–brain barrier (with a blood–brain equilibration half-time of 1.1 minutes versus >6 minutes for fentanyl and sufentanil) and accounts for its rapid onset of action.

2. Alfentanil has a smaller volume of distribution than fentanyl, which is a result of its lower lipid solubility and high protein binding (about 92%, mostly to α_1-acid glycoprotein).

3. Plasma alfentanil concentrations decrease rapidly (90% of an administered dose has left the plasma by 30 minutes) because of rapid distribution to tissues. After a single IV dose, redistribution is the most important mechanism for recovery, but after a very large dose, repeated small doses, or a continuous infusion, elimination are a more important determinant of the duration of alfentanil's effects.

4. Clearance of fentanyl is only half that of fentanyl, but because its volume of distribution is four times smaller than fentanyl's, more alfentanil is available to the liver for metabolism (cirrhosis slows elimination of alfentanil). Alfentanil undergoes *N*-dealkylation and *O*-demethylation in the liver to form inactive metabolites.

C. **Dosage and Administration of Alfentanil** (Table 19-3)

1. Because of its rapid onset of action, alfentanil has been used for the induction of anesthesia (120 μg/kg IV produces unconsciousness in 2.0 to 2.5 minutes but may also be associated with skeletal muscle rigidity).

2. With 2.5 mg/kg of propofol, an alfentanil dose of 10 μg/kg appears optimal for laryngeal mask insertion but is accompanied by apnea for about 2 minutes.

IX. **REMIFENTANIL** is an ultra short-acting μ-receptor opioid agonist that is unique among the opioids in that it contains a methyl ester side chain that is susceptible to hydrolysis by blood and tissue esterases. (It is ultrashort acting because of metabolism rather than redistribution.)

A. **Analgesia** produced by remifentanil 1.5 μg/kg IV and alfentanil 32 μg/kg IV is similar in magnitude and duration (about 10 minutes).

B. **Use in Anesthesia**

1. The rapid onset and brief duration of action of remifentanil suggest that this opioid may be suitable for induction of anesthesia, yet a high incidence of skeletal muscle rigidity and purposeless movements have been described.

ANESTHETIC AGENTS

        a. At doses above 1 µg/kg IV, brief increases in blood pressure and heart rate occur, but histamine release does not occur.

        b. Pediatric patients require twice as much remifentanil as adults (0.15 µg/kg/min vs. 0.08 µg/kg/min) when it is used with propofol for total IV anesthesia.

  2. Recovery from remifentanil is rapid with return of spontaneous ventilation in 2 to 5 minutes, but the disadvantage is that patients may require analgesics soon after remifentanil is discontinued.

  3. The rapid onset and brief duration of remifentanil make this opioid suitable for combination with other injected drugs (propofol) to provide total IV anesthesia.

  4. Remifentanil produces dose-dependent nausea and vomiting similar to those of other short-acting μ-opioid agonists.

  5. Remifentanil is frequently administered with propofol to provide total IV anesthesia. Fixed infusion rates or computer-controlled systems, or target-controlled infusions, that provide target plasma concentrations may be used.

  6. As with other opioids, higher rates of respiratory depression occur when propofol is combined with remifentanil.

C. Disposition Kinetics (Table 19-2)

  1. The key structural feature of remifentanil is the ester side chain that is susceptible to hydrolysis by blood and tissue esterases, resulting in rapid metabolism (elimination half-time, 10–20 minutes).

  2. Because the short duration of action is attributable to metabolism rather than redistribution, remifentanil should be less likely to accumulate with repeated dosing or prolonged infusion.

  3. Pharmacokinetic parameters of remifentanil are unchanged by hepatic or renal disease. Nevertheless, patients with hepatic disease appear to be more sensitive to remifentanil-induced respiratory depression.

  4. Advanced age is associated with a decrease in clearance and volume of distribution of remifentanil as well as an increase in potency.

D. Dosage and Administration of Remifentanil. Because of its short duration of action, remifentanil is best administered as a continuous IV infusion in combination with another anesthetic drug to produce general anesthesia.

1. **Induction Dosage, Intubation, and LMA Placement.** The most common remifentanil-based regimen for anesthetic induction and laryngoscopy consists of remifentanil 0.5 to 1.0 µg/kg IV administered over 60 seconds plus propofol 1 to 2 mg/kg IV followed by remifentanil infusion of 0.25 to 0.5 µg/kg/min IV (with or without midazolam premedication).

2. **Maintenance of General Anesthesia**
   a. In combination with 70% nitrous oxide, remifentanil 0.6 µg/kg/min IV is generally adequate. (There is a wide range of infusion rates.)
   b. A disadvantage of remifentanil related to its short duration of action is that patients may experience substantial pain on emergence from anesthesia.

3. **Monitored Anesthesia Care**
   a. Remifentanil can be used as an adjunct for sedation or analgesia during regional anesthesia (0.5–1.0 µg/kg/min IV), for block placement (retrobulbar block preceded by remifentanil 1.0 µg/kg IV 90 seconds before the block), and as part of monitored anesthetic care (colonoscopy).
   b. The dose requirement for remifentanil for sedation and analgesia is decreased when the opioid is combined with midazolam (as much as 50%) or propofol.
   c. The risk of excessive depression of ventilation or development of chest rigidity after a bolus dose of remifentanil can be minimized by injecting the dose over 30 seconds.

X. **PARTIAL AGONISTS AND MIXED AGONIST–ANTAGONISTS** (Table 19-5). The partial agonist and mixed agonist–antagonist opioids are synthetic or semisynthetic compounds that are structurally related to morphine. These drugs are characterized by binding activity at multiple opioid receptors and differential effects (agonist, partial agonist, antagonist) at each receptor type. The major clinical use of these drugs is the provision of postoperative analgesia, but they have also been used for intraoperative sedation, as adjuncts

RECEPTOR EFFECTS AND RELATIVE POTENCIES OF OPIOID
AGONISTS–ANTAGONISTS

Drug	μ Receptor	K Receptor	Relative Potency*	Analgesic Dose (mg)
Nalbuphine	Partial agonist	Partial agonist	11	10
Butorphanol	Partial agonist	Partial agonist	15	2–3
Buprenorphine	Partial agonist	Possibly an antagonist	30	0.3

*Morphine's relative potency is 1.

during general anesthesia, and to antagonize some of the effects of μ receptor agonists.

A. **Nalbuphine**
1. The modest ability of this drug to decrease MAC (8% vs 65% for morphine) suggests that nalbuphine may not be a useful adjunct for general anesthesia.
2. Analgesia (mediated by K and μ receptors) and associated depression of ventilation (mediated by μ receptors) produced by nalbuphine have a ceiling effect. Nalbuphine has been used to antagonize the ventilatory depressant effects of μ agonists while still providing analgesia by K receptor stimulation.

B. **Butorphanol**
1. This drug has partial agonist activity at μ and K opioid receptors (similar to nalbuphine). Compared with nalbuphine and similar drugs, butorphanol has a pronounced sedative effect, which is probably mediated by K receptors.
2. Increases in intrabiliary pressure do not occur, and this drug may be effective in treatment of postoperative shivering.
3. Butorphanol is indicated for sedation as well as treatment of moderate to severe postoperative pain.

C. **Buprenorphine**
1. Buprenorphine is a highly lipid-soluble thebaine derivative that is 25 to 50 times more potent than morphine. Slow dissociation from μ receptors can lead to prolonged effects that are not easily antagonized by naloxone.

2. Unlike nalbuphine and butorphanol, buprenorphine does not seem to possess agonist activity at *K* receptors. (It may act as an antagonist at these receptors.)

XI. OPIOID ANTAGONISTS (NALOXONE AND NALTREXONE)

A. **Naloxone** is a pure antagonist at μ, *K,* and ∂-opioid receptors.
   1. In clinical practice, naloxone is administered to antagonize opioid-induced respiratory depression and sedation.
   2. Because opioid antagonists reverse all opioid effects, including analgesia, naloxone should be carefully titrated (20–40 μg IV produces peak effects in 1 to 2 minutes) to avoid producing sudden, severe pain in postoperative patients.
      a. Sudden, complete antagonism of opioid effects can cause hypertension, tachycardia, ventricular cardiac dysrhythmias, and pulmonary edema.
      b. Pulmonary edema can occur in the absence of heart disease and is thought to reflect centrally mediated catecholamine release causing acute pulmonary hypertension.
      c. Naloxone precipitates opioid withdrawal symptoms in opioid-dependent individuals.
   3. Because naloxone has a short duration of action (1 to 4 hours), depression of ventilation may recur if large systemic doses of opioids or long-acting opioid agonists or neuraxial opioids have been administered. When prolonged depression of ventilation is anticipated, an initial loading dose of naloxone followed by a continuous IV infusion (3–10 μg/kg/hr) can be used.
B. **Naltrexone** is a long-acting oral antagonist of opioid effects.

XII. USE OF OPIOIDS IN CLINICAL ANESTHESIA (Tables 19-6 and 19-7)

A. Opioids are used alone or in combination with other drugs, such as sedatives or anticholinergics, as pharmacologic preoperative medication.
B. Intraoperatively, opioids are administered as components of balanced anesthesia or alone in high doses.

TABLE 19-6

CLINICAL USES OF OPIOIDS

Premedication
Induction of anesthesia (sole drug or adjuvant)
Blunt hemodynamic responses to noxious stimulation (alfentanil has the most rapid blood–brain equilibration time)
Intraoperative analgesia
Postoperative pain relief (patient-controlled analgesia, neuraxial, parenteral)
Adjuvant to facilitate mechanical ventilation and tolerance to tracheal tube

1. Fentanyl and its derivatives sufentanil and alfentanil are the opioids most often used as supplements to general anesthesia. (They are more easily titrated than morphine because of their rapid onsets of action.)

TABLE 19-7

DOSAGE FOR OPIOID AGONISTS IN ELECTIVE SURGERY IN ADULTS

Anesthetic Phase	Fentanyl	Sufentanil	Alfentanil	Remifentanil
Premedication (μg)	25–50	2–5	250–500	
Induction				
With hypnotic (μg/kg)	1.5–5.0	0.1–1.0	10–50	0.5–1.0 or 0.25–0.5 μg/kg/min
With 60–70% N20 (μg/kg)	8–23	1.3–2.8		
High-dose opioid (μg/kg)	50	10–30	120	2.5 or 2 μg/kg/min
Maintenance				
Balanced anesthesia				
Intermittent bolus(μg)	25–100	5–20	250–500	
Infusion (μg/kg/min)	0.033	0.005–0.015	0.5–1.5	0.25–0.5
High dose opioid (μg/kg/min)	0.5		2.5–10	1.0–3.0
Transition to PACU (μg/kg/min)				0.05–0.15
Monitored Anesthesia Care				
Intermittent bolus (μg/kg)	12.5–50	2.5–10		12.5–25
Infusion (μg/kg/min)				0.01–0.02

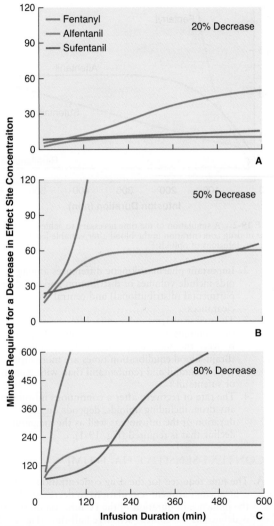

FIGURE 19-1. Overlay of the fentanyl, alfentanil, and sufentanil recovery curves describing the time required for decreases of 20% (**A**), 50% (**B**), and 80% (**C**) from the maintained intraoperative effect site concentration after termination of the infusion.

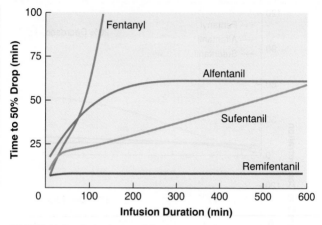

FIGURE 19-2. A simulation of the time necessary to achieve a 50% decrease in drug concentration in the blood after variable-length intravenous infusions of opioids.

2. Important pharmacokinetic differences among opioids include volumes of distribution and intercompartmental (distributional) and central (elimination) clearances.
3. The major pharmacodynamic differences among these opioids are potency and equilibration time between the plasma and the site of drug effect. (Brain–blood equilibration times are more rapid with alfentanil and remifentanil than with fentanyl or sufentanil.)
4. The rate of recovery after a continuous infusion of any drug, including opioids, depends on the duration of the infusion as well as the magnitude of decline that is required (Fig. 19-1).

XIII. CONTEXT-SENSITIVE HALF-TIME

A. The time required for the drug concentration in the central compartment (circulation) to decrease 50% and the influence of duration of the IV infusion on this time is defined as the context-sensitive half-time (Fig. 19-2).
B. Context-sensitive half-time curves are theoretical predictions based on computer models. It is not known if a decrement of 50% provides the most clinically useful description of the rate of offset of opioid effects.

CHAPTER 20 ■ NEUROMUSCULAR BLOCKING AGENTS

The introduction of muscle relaxants (neuromuscular blocking drugs [NMBDs]) into clinical practice more than 60 years ago was an important milestone in the history of anesthesia (Donati F, Bevan DR: Neuromuscular blocking agents. In *Clinical Anesthesia*. Edited by Barash PG, Cullen BF, Stoelting RK, Cahalan MK, Stock MC. Philadelphia: Lippincott Williams & Wilkins, 2009, pp 498–530). In addition to providing immobility and better surgical conditions, NMBDs improve intubating conditions. As important as it is to provide adequate anesthesia while a patient is totally or partially paralyzed, it is also essential to make sure that the effects of NMBDs have worn off or are reversed before the patient regains consciousness. With the introduction of shorter acting NMBDs, it was thought that reversal of blockade could be omitted. However, residual paralysis is still a problem, and the threshold for complete neuromuscular recovery is now considered to be a train-of-four (TOF) of 0.9 rather than 0.7.

I. PHYSIOLOGY AND PHARMACOLOGY

A. **Structure.** The cell bodies of motor neurons supplying skeletal muscle lie in the spinal cord. Information is carried by an elongated axon that ends in a specialized structure, the neuromuscular junction (NMJ), that is designed for the production and release of acetylcholine (Ach) (Fig. 20-1). The endplate is a specialized portion of the membrane of the muscle fiber where nicotinic Ach receptors are concentrated.

B. **Nerve Stimulation.** Under resting conditions, the electrical potential of the inside of a nerve cell is negative with respect to the outside (typically −90 mV).

C. **Release of Ach** into the synaptic cleft occurs when an action potential arrives at the nerve terminal.

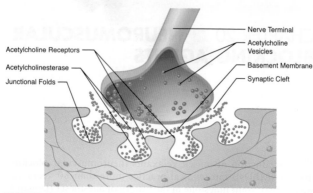

FIGURE 20-1. Diagram of the neuromuscular junction.

D. Postsynaptic Events
1. Activation of the postsynaptic nicotinic receptor requires simultaneous occupation of the receptor's two α subunits by ACh. Skeletal muscle contraction occurs when ACh-induced changes in the muscle cell's transmembrane permeability result in inward movement of sodium sufficient to decrease intracellular negativity (depolarization) and cause an action potential.
2. Propagation of the action potential initiates release of calcium from the sarcoplasmic reticulum, where activation of myosin adenosine triphosphate leads to excitation–contraction coupling of the myofilaments.
3. ACh is hydrolyzed (within milliseconds to prevent prolonged depolarization) by acetylcholinesterase (true cholinesterase) to choline, which is reused for synthesis of new ACh, and acetate.

E. Presynaptic Events
1. The release of ACh normally decreases during high-frequency stimulation under physiologic conditions because the pool of readily releasable ACh becomes depleted faster than it can be replenished. In the presence of muscle relaxants, this decreased release of ACh produces a progressive decrease in skeletal muscle response (fade) with each stimulus.
2. Fade is an important property of nondepolarizing neuromuscular blockade and is useful for monitoring purposes.

TABLE 20-1

DEFINITION OF NEUROMUSCULAR BLOCKING DRUGS ACCORDING TO THE ONSET AND DURATION OF BLOCK AT THE ADDUCTOR POLLICIS

Onset to Maximum Block	
Ultra rapid (<1 min)	Succinylcholine
Rapid (1–2 min)	Rocuronium
Intermediate (2–4 min)	Atracurium
	Vecuronium
	Pancuronium
Long (>4 min)	Cisatracurium
	Doxacurium
Duration to 25% Recovery of T1	
Ultra short (<8 min)	Succinylcholine
Intermediate (20–50 min)	Atracurium
	Cisatracurium
	Rocuronium
	Vecuronium
Long (>50 min)	Doxacurium
	Pancuronium

II. NEUROMUSCULAR BLOCKING AGENTS
(Table 20-1)

A. **Pharmacologic Characteristics of Neuromuscular Blocking Agents.** The effect of NMBDs is measured as the depression of adductor muscle contraction (twitch) after electrical stimulation of the ulnar nerve.

B. **Potency** is determined by constructing the dose–response curves, which describe the relationship between twitch depression and dose.
   1. The ED_{95} is a clinically relevant value that corresponds to 95% block of single twitch (half of patients will reach 95% block, and half will be reach a lower percentage).

C. **Onset time** or time to maximum blockade can be shortened if the dose is increased ($2 \times ED_{95}$).

D. **Duration of action** is the time from injection of the NMBD to return of 25% twitch height (comparisons are usually made at $2 \times ED_{95}$). Categories of NMBDs may be based on their durations of action.

E. **Recovery index** is the time interval between 25% and 75% twitch height (this reflects speed of recovery after return of twitch is manifest). The adductor pollicis is the most commonly monitored muscle for determining the onset and duration of action of NMBDs.

III. DEPOLARIZING BLOCKING DRUGS: SUCCINYLCHOLINE

Succinylcholine (SCh) remains a useful muscle relaxant because of its ultra rapid-onset and short-duration neuromuscular blocking properties, which cannot be duplicated by any of the available nondepolarizing muscle relaxants.

- A. **Neuromuscular Effects.** SCh binds to postsynaptic nicotinic receptors, where it exhibits ACh-like activity. SCh also binds to extrajunctional receptors and presynaptic receptors.
  1. The net effect of SCh-induced depolarization is uncoordinated skeletal muscle activity that manifests clinically as fasciculations.
  2. SCh predictably increases masseter muscle tone (this may be responsible for poor intubating conditions), and masseter muscle spasm may be associated with malignant hyperthermia. It is likely that increased masseter muscle tone is mediated by ACh receptors because it is blocked by nondepolarizing drugs.
  3. Nonparalyzing doses of nondepolarizing drugs (pretreatment) block visible evidence of SCh-induced depolarization, suggesting that presynaptic receptors are principally involved in the production of fasciculations.
  4. The blocking effect of SCh at the NMJ is probably attributable to desensitization (i.e., prolonged exposure to an agonist leads to a state characterized by a lack of responsiveness of the receptors).
- B. **Characteristics of Depolarizing Blockade**
  1. SCh initially produces features characterized as phase I block (Table 20-2).
  2. Phase II block develops after prolonged exposure to SCh or high doses of SCh and has characteristics of a nondepolarizing neuromuscular blockade (Table 20-3). The onset of phase II block coincides with the appearance of tachyphylaxis to the effects of SCh.
- C. **Pharmacology of Succinylcholine**
  1. SCh is rapidly hydrolyzed (the elimination half-time is estimated to be 2–4 minutes) by plasma

TABLE 20-2

CHARACTERISTICS OF PHASE I DEPOLARIZING BLOCKADE

Decreased twitch amplitude
Absence of fade with continuous (tetanic) stimulation
Similar decreases in the amplitude of all twitches in the train-of-four (ratio >0.7)
Absence of posttetanic potentiation
Antagonism by nondepolarizing muscle relaxants
Augmentation by anticholinesterase drugs

cholinesterase (pseudocholinesterase) to choline and succinylmonocholine (which has about 1/20 the neuromuscular blocking properties of the parent drug).

2. The ED_{95} of SCh in the presence of opioid–nitrous oxide anesthesia is 0.30 to 0.35 mg/kg.

3. The onset of neuromuscular blocking effect is usually within 1 minute after high doses of SCh (1–2 mg/kg intravenously [IV]), and the time until full recovery of the electromyographic response is 10 to 12 minutes after a dose of 1 mg/kg IV.

4. A small proportion of patients (1:1500 to 1:3000) have a genetically determined (atypical plasma cholinesterase) inability to metabolize SCh (1–1.5 mg/kg IV lasts for 3–6 hours).

D. **Side Effects** (Table 20-4)

E. **Clinical Uses**

1. The principal indication for SCh is to facilitate tracheal intubation (1 mg/kg IV is the usual dose, which is increased to 1.5–2.0 mg/kg IV if pretreatment is used).

TABLE 20-3

CHARACTERISTICS OF NONDEPOLARIZING NEUROMUSCULAR BLOCKADE

Decreased twitch amplitude
Fade with continuous (tetanic) stimulation
Train-of-four ratio <0.7
Posttetanic potentiation
Absence of fasciculations
Antagonism by anticholinesterase drugs
Augmentation by other nondepolarizing muscle relaxants

TABLE 20-4

SIDE EFFECTS OF SUCCINYLCHOLINE

Bradycardia (especially in children; more likely in adults with second dose)

Allergic reactions

Fasciculations

Muscle pains (relationship to fasciculations not conclusively established)

Increased intragastric pressure (offset by even greater increase in lower esophageal sphincter pressure)

Increased intraocular pressure (caused by the cycloplegic action of succinylcholine and not reliably blunted by pretreatment)

Increased intracranial pressure (small effect and of questionable clinical significance)

Transient increase in plasma potassium concentration (a normal increase of 0.5–1.0 mEq/L is enhanced by denervation injuries, burns, extensive trauma, or unrecognized muscular dystrophy in boys)

Trigger for malignant hyperthermia (masseter muscle spasm may be an early sign)

Prolonged response in the presence of atypical cholinesterase or drug-induced inhibition of plasma cholinesterase activity (neostigmine but not edrophonium)

2. The use of SCh in children is limited largely because of concerns about triggering hyperkalemia in young boys with unrecognized muscular dystrophy and the occasional triggering of malignant hyperthermia in children.

IV. NONDEPOLARIZING DRUGS

Nondepolarizing NMDBs bind to postsynaptic receptors (they must bind to one of the α subunits) in a competitive fashion to produce neuromuscular blockade.

A. **Characteristics of Nondepolarizing Blockade** (Table 20-3)

B. **Pharmacokinetics** (Table 20-5)

1. The pharmacokinetic variables derived from measurements of plasma concentrations of nondepolarizing muscle relaxants depend on the dose administered, the sampling schedule used, and the accuracy of the assay.

TABLE 20-5

TYPICAL PHARMACOKINETIC DATA FOR NONDEPOLARIZING MUSCLE RELAXANTS

	Volume of Distribution (L/kg)	Clearance (mL/kg/min)	Elimination Half-Time (min)
Intermediate-Duration Drugs			
Atracurium	0.14	5.5	20
Cisatracurium	0.12	5	23
Rocuronium	0.3	3	90
Vecuronium	0.4	5	70
Long-Duration Drugs			
Doxacurium	0.2	2.5	95
Pancuronium	0.3	1.8	140

    2. All nondepolarizing muscle relaxants have a volume of distribution that is approximately equal to extracellular fluid volume.

  C. **Onset and Duration of Action** (Table 20-6)

    1. Although peak plasma concentrations of nondepolarizing muscle relaxants occur within 1 to 2 minutes of injection, the onset of maximum blockade is reached only after 2 to 7 minutes, reflecting the time required for drug transfer between plasma and NMJ.

TABLE 20-6

COMPARATIVE PHARMACOLOGY OF NONDEPOLARIZING MUSCLE RELAXANTS

	ED_{95} (mg/kg)	Onset Time (min)	Duration to 25% Recovery (min)	Recovery Index (25%–75% Recovery) (min)
Intermediate-Duration Drugs				
Atracurium	0.2–0.25	3–4	35–45	10–15
Cisatracurium	0.05	5–7	35–45	12–15
Rocuronium	0.3	1.5–3.0	30–40	8–12
Vecuronium	0.05	3–4	35–45	10–15
Long-Duration Drugs				
Doxacurium	0.025	5–10	40–120	30–40
Pancuronium	0.07	2–4	60–120	30–40

AUTONOMIC AND HISTAMINE-RELEASING EFFECTS OF
MUSCLE RELAXANTS

	Nicotinic Receptors at Autonomic Ganglia	Cardiac Muscarinic Receptors	Histamine Release
Succinylcholine	Stimulates	Stimulates	Rare
Atracurium	No effect	No effect	Minimal
Cisatracurium	No effect	No effect	0
Rocuronium	No effect	No effect	0
Vecuronium	No effect	No effect	0
Doxacurium	No effect	No effect	0
Pancuronium	No effect	No effect	0

2. The duration of action of nondepolarizing drugs is determined by the time required for drug concentration at site of action to decrease below a certain level, usually corresponding to 25% first-twitch blockade
   D. **Individual Nondepolarizing Relaxants** (Tables 20-5 to 20-8)

MECHANISMS FOR CLEARANCE OF NONDEPOLARIZING
MUSCLE RELAXANTS

	Renal Excretion (% Unchanged)	Biliary Excretion (% Unchanged)	Hepatic Degradation (% Unchanged)	Hydrolysis in Plasma
Atracurium	Insignificant	Insignificant	?	Spontaneous and enzymatic
Cisatracurium	Insignificant	Insignificant	?	Spontaneous
Rocuronium	10–25	50–70	10–20	0
Vecuronium	15–25	40–75	20–30	0
Doxacurium	70	30	?	0
Pancuronium	80	5–10	10–40	0

1. **Atracurium** is an intermediate-acting benzylisoquinolinium-type nondepolarizing NMDB.
   a. **Metabolism** is by ester hydrolysis (which accounts for an estimated two thirds of the drug's metabolism) and Hofmann elimination (nonenzymatic degradation at body temperature and pH). A metabolite of atracurium, laudanosine is a cerebral stimulant, but it is unlikely that this is clinically significant with the usual clinical doses of atracurium administered.
   b. **Hypotension and tachycardia** may accompany high doses of atracurium ($>2 \times ED_{95}$), reflecting dose-related histamine release (attenuated by injection of the muscle relaxant over 1–3 minutes).
   c. **Dose requirements** are similar in all age groups, presumably reflecting the absence of atracurium's dependence on renal or hepatic clearance mechanisms. The dose of atracurium, as for all nondepolarizing drugs, should be decreased on a milligram per kilogram basis to reflect lean body mass.
2. **Cisatracurium** is an intermediate-acting benzylisoquinolinium-type NMDB.
   a. As one of the 10 isomers of atracurium, this drug resembles atracurium in onset, duration of action, rate of recovery, and clearance mechanisms (Hofmann elimination rendering both drugs independent of hepatic and renal function). Cisatracurium does not undergo significant hydrolysis by nonspecific plasma esterases.
   b. The metabolites of cisatracurium include laudanosine (peak plasma concentrations are about fivefold less than present with atracurium) and monoquaternary acrylate. These metabolites are not active at the NMJ.
   c. In contrast to atracurium, cisatracurium is more potent (ED_{95}, 0.05 mg/kg), is devoid of histamine-releasing properties even at high doses ($8 \times ED_{95}$), and lacks cardiovascular effects.
   d. Neuromuscular block is easily maintained at a stable level by continuous infusion of cisatracurium at a constant rate and does not diminish over time. The rate of recovery is independent of the dose of cisatracurium or the duration of administration, presumably reflecting independence

　　　of its clearance mechanisms from hepatic and
　　　renal function.
　　e. Recovery from drug-induced neuromuscular
　　　blockade can be facilitated by administration of
　　　an anticholinesterase drug.
3. **Doxacurium** is a long-acting nondepolarizing
　　NMBD that is devoid of histamine-releasing and
　　cardiovascular side effects.
4. **Gantacurium** is a nondepolarizing NMBD whose
　　main degradation pathway involves cysteine in the
　　plasma and is independent of plasma
　　cholinesterase. The ED_{95} is approximately 0.19
　　mg/kg. Cardiovascular effects at doses exceeding
　　$3 \times ED_{95}$ are most likely related to histamine
　　release. At doses required for tracheal intubation
　　(0.4 to 0.6 mg/kg), onset at the adductor pollicis is
　　1.5 minutes, and duration to 25% first-twitch
　　recovery is 8 to 10 minutes.
5. **Pancuronium** is a long-acting nondepolarizing
　　NMBD with a steroid structure but lacking any
　　endocrine effects.
　　a. The drug is metabolized to a 3-OH compound
　　　that has one half the neuromuscular blocking
　　　activity of the parent compound.
　　b. Pancuronium is associated with modest (usually
　　　<15%) increases in heart rate, blood pressure,
　　　and cardiac output.
　　c. Pancuronium does not release histamine.
　　d. The use of pancuronium to provide muscle relax-
　　　ation may offer some advantage over the use of
　　　cardiovascularly neutral muscle relaxants in
　　　patients anesthetized with high doses of
　　　opioids.
　　e. Compared with newer and more expensive short-
　　　and intermediate-acting nondepolarizing NMDBs,
　　　pancuronium's continued popularity is because of
　　　its cost. Generic pancuronium is the least expen-
　　　sive muscle relaxant to provide neuromuscular
　　　blockade for long surgeries (>2 hours), but its
　　　routine use in these situations may result in an
　　　increased incidence of postoperative skeletal
　　　muscle weakness.
　　f. Pancuronium neuromuscular blockade is more
　　　difficult to reverse than blockade of the interme-
　　　diate-acting nondepolarizing NMDBs.

6. **Rocuronium** is an aminosteroid NMBD that has a more rapid onset (intubating conditions 60 seconds after administration of 1 mg/kg IV resemble conditions after administration of SCh 1 mg/kg IV) but similar duration of action and pharmacokinetic characteristics as vecuronium.

   a. As for other short- and intermediate-acting NMBDs, the onset of action of rocuronium is more rapid at the diaphragm and laryngeal muscle than at the adductor pollicis, and about twice as much drug is required to produce the same degree of paralysis.

   b. Hemodynamic changes or release of histamine does not occur after administration of even high doses ($4 \times ED_{95}$) of rocuronium.

7. **Vecuronium** is an intermediate-acting aminosteroid NMBD that is devoid of histamine-releasing and cardiovascular side effects.

   a. Vecuronium is a monoquaternary ammonium compound produced by demethylation of the pancuronium molecule. This demethylation decreases the ACh-like characteristics of the molecule and increases its lipophilicity, which encourages hepatic uptake.

   b. Vecuronium undergoes spontaneous deacetylation. The most potent of the resulting metabolites, 3-OH vecuronium, has about 60% of the activity of vecuronium, is excreted by the kidneys, and may contribute to prolonged paralysis. (It is incriminated in prolonged weakness after chronic use to maintain patients on mechanical ventilation.)

   c. Vecuronium is less potent and has a shorter duration of action in men than women, probably as a result of a decrease in the volume of distribution, which results in increased plasma concentrations in women.

   d. Accidental mixing of vecuronium and thiopental in the IV tubing may form a precipitate of barbituric acid and obstruct the IV cannula.

   e. The cardiovascular neutrality and intermediated duration of action make vecuronium a suitable drug for use in patients with ischemic heart disease and those undergoing short ambulatory surgery.

TABLE 20-9

DRUG INTERACTIONS INVOLVING MUSCLE RELAXANTS

Volatile anesthetics (dose-dependent potentiation of all muscle relaxants; impact on initial dose of muscle relaxant may be greater with sevoflurane or desflurane, reflecting rapid equilibration of these poorly soluble drugs)

Local anesthetics (potentiate effects of all muscle relaxants)

Nondepolarizing muscle relaxants (depending on the combination, produce synergistic or additive effects; clinical significance is doubtful)

Nondepolarizing–depolarizing muscle relaxants (response depends on the sequence; administering a nondepolarizer before SCh interferes with SCh blockade, and administering a nondepolarizer after SCh is potentiated)

Antibiotics (aminoglycosides and polymyxins are most likely to potentiate muscle relaxants)

Anticonvulsants (resistance to nondepolarizing muscle relaxants)

SCh = succinylcholine.

V. DRUG INTERACTIONS (Table 20-9)

VI. ALTERED RESPONSES TO NEUROMUSCULAR BLOCKING AGENTS (Table 20-10)

VII. MONITORING NEUROMUSCULAR BLOCKADE

TABLE 20-10

ALTERED RESPONSES TO NEUROMUSCULAR BLOCKING AGENTS

Myopathy (enthusiasm for liberal use of neuromuscular blockings agents has waned because of myopathy)

Myasthenia gravis (usually resistant to SCh and highly sensitive to nondepolarizing muscle relaxants)

Myotonia (sustained contracture in response to SCh; normal response to nondepolarizing muscle relaxants)

Muscular dystrophy (SCh is contraindicated)

Neurologic diseases (isolated reports of hyperkalemia in response to SCh)

Hemiplegia or paraplegia (hyperkalemia in response to SCh; resistant to nondepolarizing muscle relaxants)

Burn injury (hyperkalemia in response to SCh; resistant to the effects of nondepolarizing muscle relaxants)

SCh = succinylcholine.

TABLE 20-11

ASSESSMENT OF THE ADEQUACY OF ANTAGONISM OF
NEUROMUSCULAR BLOCKADE

Responses to electrical stimulation of a peripheral nerve
  (ulnar, facial)
Head lift for 5 seconds
Tongue protrusion
Tongue depressor
Hand grip strength
Maximum negative inspiratory pressure (>-25 cm H_2O)

A. **Why Monitor?** The margin of safety is narrow because
   blockade occurs over a narrow range of receptor occu-
   pancy. Furthermore, there is considerable interindividual variability in response to the same dose of NMDB.
   To test the function of the NMJ, a peripheral nerve
   (ulnar nerve or the facial nerve) is electrically
   stimulated with a peripheral nerve stimulator, and
   the response of the skeletal muscle is assessed.
B. **Stimulator Characteristics.** The response of the nerve to
   electrical stimulation depends on three factors: the current applied, the duration of the current, and the position of the electrodes.
C. **Monitoring Modalities** (Table 20-11)
D. **Recording the Response**
   1. **Visual and tactile evaluation** is the easiest and least
      expensive way to assess the response to electrical
      stimulation applied to a peripheral nerve. The disad-
      vantage of this technique is the subjective nature of
      its interpretation.
   2. **Measurement of force** using a force transducer pro-
      vides accurate assessment of the response elicited by
      electrical stimulation of a peripheral nerve.
   3. **Electromyography** measures the electrical rather
      than mechanical response of the skeletal muscle.
E. **Choice of Muscle**
   1. The **adductor pollicis** supplied by the ulnar nerve is
      the most common skeletal muscle monitored
      clinically. This muscle is relatively sensitive to
      nondepolarizing muscle relaxants, and during
      recovery, it is blocked more than some respiratory
      muscles such as the diaphragm and laryngeal
      adductors.

2. There seem to be important differences in the responses of muscles innervated by the facial nerve (stimulated 2–3 cm posterior to the lateral border of the orbit) around the eye.
   a. The response of the orbicularis oculi over the eyelid is similar to that of the adductor pollicis.
   b. The response the eyebrow (corrugator supercilii) parallels the response of the laryngeal adductors (onset is more rapid and recovery is sooner than at the adductor pollicis). This response is useful for predicting intubating conditions.

F. **Clinical Application**
   1. **Monitoring Onset.** After induction of anesthesia, the intensity of neuromuscular blockade must be assessed to determine the time for tracheal intubation (maximum relaxation of laryngeal and respiratory muscles). Single-twitch stimulation is often used to monitor the onset of neuromuscular blockade.
   2. **Surgical relaxation** is usually adequate when fewer than two or three visible twitches of the TOF are observed in response to stimulation of the adductor pollicis muscle.
   3. **Monitoring recovery** is useful in determining whether spontaneous recovery has progressed to a degree that allows reversal drugs to be given (preferably 4 twitches visible) and to assess the effect of these drugs (supplement with other clinical observations) (Table 20-11).
      a. Traditionally, a TOF of 0.7 has been considered to be the threshold below which residual weakness of the respiratory muscles could be present. Evidence suggests, however, that significant weakness and impairment of swallowing may be present at a TOF ratio of 0.9.
      b. A sustained head lift test may not guarantee full skeletal muscle recovery.
      c. The upper airway muscles used to retain a tongue depressor between the teeth are very sensitive to residual effects of muscle relaxants.
   4. **Factors Affecting the Monitoring of Neuromuscular Blockade**
      a. If the monitored hand is cold, the degree of paralysis will appear to be increased.
      b. If the monitored limb is characterized by nerve damage (from stroke, spinal cord transection,

peripheral nerve trauma), there is inherent resistance to the effect of muscle relaxants, and the degree of skeletal muscle paralysis will be underestimated.

VIII. ANTAGONISM OF NEUROMUSCULAR BLOCKADE

In most circumstances, all efforts should be made to ensure that the patient leaves the operating room with unimpaired muscle strength (respiratory and upper airway muscles functioning normally to permit breathing, coughing, swallowing, and maintaining a patent airway). Strategies to achieve this goal include titrating the NMBDs so that no residual effect is manifest at the end of surgery, administering a reversal drug, and selective binding of NMBDs with a cyclodextrin molecule to restore neuromuscular function.

A. **Assessment of Neuromuscular Blockade.** Spontaneous breathing (adequate to prevent hypercapnia if a patent airway is maintained) can resume even if relatively deep degrees of paralysis are present because of the relative diaphragm-sparing effect of NMBDs. Swallowing is impaired, and laryngeal aspiration may occur in the presence of vecuronium when the TOF ratio is 0.9 or below.

1. **Residual paralysis** (neuromuscular blockade) is frequent in patients in the recovery room after surgery. The most important reason for the high incidence of residual paralysis seems to be omission of reversal.

2. **Clinical Importance.** Residual paralysis in the recovery room is associated with significant morbidity.

B. **Reversal Agents.** The pharmacologic principle involved is inhibition of Ach breakdown to increase its concentration of Ach at the NMJ, thus tilting the competition for receptors in favor of the neurotransmitter.

1. **Mechanism of Action of Anticholinesterases**

   a. Inhibition of acetylcholinesterase by anticholinesterase drugs (neostigmine, pyridostigmine, edrophonium) results in an increase in the amount of ACh that reaches the receptor.

   b. Anticholinesterase drugs may also have presynaptic effects.

2. **Neostigmine Block.** Large doses of anticholinesterases, especially if given in the absence of neuromuscular block, may produce evidence of neuromuscular

TABLE 20-12

PHARMACOKINETICS OF ANTICHOLINESTERASE DRUGS

	Patient Status	Volume of Distribution (L/kg)	Clearance (mL/kg/min)	Elimination Half-Time (min)
Neostigmine	Normal	0.7	9.2	177
	Renal failure	1.6	7.8	181
Edrophonium	Normal	1.1	9.6	110
	Renal failure	0.7	2.7	206
Pyridostigmine	Normal	1.1	8.6	112
	Renal failure	1.0	2.1	379

dysfunction. Although there are no clinical reports of postoperative weakness attributed to reversal agents, it seems prudent to reduce the dose of anticholinesterase agent if recovery from neuromuscular block is almost complete.

3. **Potency** ratios are difficult to determine because the slopes of the edrophonium and neostigmine dose–response curves are not parallel.

4. The **pharmacokinetics** of anticholinesterase drugs reflect the dependence of these drugs on renal clearance (Table 20-12).

5. **Pharmacodynamics.** The onset of action of edrophonium to peak effect (1–2 minutes) is much more rapid than the onsets of action of neostigmine (7–11 minutes) and pyridostigmine (15–20 minutes).

   a. Recovery of neuromuscular activity reflects spontaneous recovery plus augmented (accelerated) recovery induced by the anticholinesterase drug.

   b. **Recurarization** should not be expected as long as the duration of the anticholinesterase drug exceeds that of the muscle relaxant.

C. **Factors Affecting Reversal** (Table 20-13)

   1. The dose of anticholinesterase drug selected and the time to effective recovery are directly related to the intensity of blockade at the time of reversal (Table 20-14).

      a. Neostigmine is more effective than edrophonium or pyridostigmine in antagonizing intense neuromuscular blockade.

TABLE 20-13

FACTORS AFFECTING REVERSAL

Block intensity (the time to drug-augmented recovery is directly proportional to the intensity of blockade present at the time of antagonism; see Table 20-15)
Anticholinesterase dose
Muscle relaxant administered
Age
Renal failure
Acid–base balance (impairment of antagonism by acidosis is difficult to document)

      b. Because of the ceiling effect, there is little benefit in administering more than 0.7 mg/kg of neostigmine.
  2. The overall rate of recovery (spontaneous plus drug enhanced) is more rapid from atracurium or vecuronium than from pancuronium. Furthermore, the doses of antagonist drugs required to produce the same degree of antagonism are greater after administration of the long-acting than after the administration of the intermediate- and short-acting muscle relaxants.
  3. Recovery of neuromuscular activity occurs more rapidly with lower doses of anticholinesterase drugs in infants and children than in adults.

TABLE 20-14

RECOMMENDED DOSES OF ANTICHOLINESTERASE DRUGS AND ANTICHOLINERGIC DRUGS BASED ON TRAIN-OF-FOUR STIMULATION

Visible	Fade	Anticholinesterase	Dose (mg/kg IV)	Anticholinergic Dose (μg/kg IV)
<2	++++	Neostigmine	0.07	Glycopyrrolate 7 or atropine 15
3–4	+++	Neostigmine	0.04	Glycopyrrolate 7 or atropine 15
4	++	Edrophonium	0.5	Atropine 7
4	+/−	Edrophonium	0.25	Atropine 7

D. **Anticholinesterases: Other Effects**
  1. **Cardiovascular Effects**
     a. Anticholinesterase drugs evoke profound vagal stimulation that can be prevented by concomitant administration of an anticholinergic drug.
     b. Because of its rapid onset (1 minute), atropine is appropriate for use in combination with edrophonium. Glycopyrrolate (onset 2–3 minutes) may be more suitable for use with neostigmine or pyridostigmine.
     c. Atropine requirements are lower when combined with edrophonium (7–10 μg/kg IV) than with neostigmine (15–20 μg/kg IV).
  2. **Other cholinergic effects of** anticholinesterase drugs include increased salivation, enhanced bowel motility (concern about increase in bowel anastomotic leakage), and an alleged increased incidence of nausea and vomiting after ambulatory surgery.
  3. **Respiratory Effects.** Anticholinesterases may cause an increase in airway resistance, but anticholinergics reduce this effect.
E. Pharmacologically assisted recovery is expected in most cases because it is illusory to aim for complete recovery only by careful titration of NMBDs.
  1. Administration of anticholinesterase agents accelerate recovery, no matter when they are given in the course of recovery. However, there are advantages in giving reversal agents when spontaneous recovery is underway.
  2. If 4 twitches are not visible after TOF stimulation, it is recommended to keep the patient anesthetized and mechanically ventilated until 4 twitches reappear and then administer anticholinesterases.
F. **Sugammadex**
  1. This cyclodextrin leads to restoration of normal neuromuscular function by selectively binding to rocuronium (and to a lesser extent to vecuronium and pancuronium). Because it does not bind to any known receptors, it is devoid of cardiovascular and other side effects.
  2. **Pharmacology.** If sugammadex is given upon return of the second twitch in the TOF, doses of 2 to 4 mg/kg result in return of the TOF ratio to 0.9 in about 2 minutes. The availability of sugammadex may make Sch obsolete for intubation.

3. **Pharmacokinetics.** Sugammadex and sugammadex–rocuronium complexes are excreted unchanged via the kidney.
4. For reversal of rocuronium blockade when spontaneous recovery has already started (2 to 4 twitches present), administration of 2 to 4 mg/kg will produce faster recovery than neostigmine and without cardiovascular side effects. The response of a patient who has received sugammadex who needs reexploration is unknown.

CHAPTER 21 ■ LOCAL ANESTHETICS

Local anesthetics block the conduction of impulses in electrically excitable tissues (Liu SS, Lin Y: Local anesthetics. In *Clinical Anesthesia*. Edited by Barash PG, Cullen BF, Stoelting RK, Cahalan MK, Stock MC. Philadelphia: Lippincott Williams & Wilkins, 2009, pp 531–548). One of the important uses of local anesthetics is to provide anesthesia and analgesia by blocking the transmission of pain sensation along nerve fibers.

I. MECHANISM OF ACTION OF LOCAL ANESTHETICS

A. Anatomy of Nerves

1. Nerves in both the central nervous system (CNS) and peripheral nervous system are differentiated by the presence or absence of a myelin sheath that is interrupted at short intervals by specialized regions called *nodes of Ranvier*.

2. Nerve fibers are commonly classified according to their size, conduction velocity, and function (Table 21-1).

B. Electrophysiology of Neural Conduction and Voltage-Gated Sodium Channels

1. Transmission of electrical impulses along cell membranes is the basis of signal transduction. Energy necessary for the propagation and maintenance of the electric potential is maintained on the cell surface by ionic disequilibria across the permeable cell membrane. The resting membrane potential (about -60 to -70 mV) is predominantly attributable to a difference in the intracellular and extracellular concentrations of potassium and sodium ions.

2. The flow of ions responsible for action potentials is mediated by a variety of channels and pumps, the

TABLE 21-1

CLASSIFICATION OF NERVE FIBERS

Classification	Diameter (μ)	Myelin	Conduction (m/sec)	Location	Function
A-α	6–22	+	30–120	Afferents/efferents for muscles and joints	Motor
A-β					Proprioception
A-γ	3–6	+	15–35	Efferent to muscle spindle	Muscle tone
A-δ	1–4	+	5–25	Afferent sensory nerve	Pain Touch Temperature
A B	<3	+	3–15	Preganglionic sympathetic	Autonomic function
C	0.3–1.3	−	0.7–1.3	Postganglionic sympathetic	Autonomic function
				Afferent sensory nerve	Pain Temperature

most important of which are the voltage-gated sodium channels. (Nine isoforms of voltage-gated sodium channels have been identified.)

C. **Molecular Mechanisms of Local Anesthetics**
   1. It is widely accepted that local anesthetics induce anesthesia and analgesia through direct interactions with the sodium channels (they reversibly bind the intracellular portion of voltage-gated sodium channels).
   2. Application of local anesthetics typically produces a concentration-dependent decrease in the peak sodium current.

D. **Mechanism of Nerve Blockade**
   1. Local anesthetics block peripheral nerves by disrupting the transmission of action potentials along nerve fibers. Only about 1% to 2% of the injected local anesthetics ultimately penetrate into the nerve to

reach the site of action (voltage-gated sodium channels).

2. The degree of nerve blockade depends on the local anesthetic's concentration and volume (needed to suppress the regeneration of nerve impulses over a critical length of nerve fiber).

3. Not all sensory and motor modalities are equally blocked by local anesthetics (sequential disappearance of temperature sensation, proprioception, motor function, sharp pain, and last light touch). This differential blockade had been thought to be simply related to the diameter of the nerve fiber (smaller fibers are inherently more susceptible to drug blockade than large fibers), but this does not appear to be universally true. In this regard, small nerve fibers require a shorter length (<1 cm) exposed to local anesthetic for block to occur than do large fibers.

II. PHARMACOLOGY AND PHARMACODYNAMICS

A. Chemical Properties and Relationship to Activity and Potency

1. Most clinically relevant local anesthetics are made up of a lipid-soluble, aromatic benzene ring connected to an amide group via either an amide or ester moiety.

2. The type of linkage divides the local anesthetics into aminoesters (metabolized in the liver or by plasma cholinesterase) and aminoamides (metabolized in the liver).

3. All clinically used local anesthetics are weak bases that can exist as either the lipid-soluble, neutral form or as the charged, hydrophilic form. The combination of pH and pKa of the local anesthetic determines how much of the compound exists in each form (Table 21-2).

4. A ratio with high concentration of the lipid-soluble form favors entry into cells because the main pathway for entry is by passive absorption of lipid-soluble form through the cell membrane. Clinically, alkalization of the anesthetic solution increases the ratio of the lipid-soluble form to the cationic form, thereby facilitating drug entry.

TABLE 21-2

PHYSIOCHEMICAL PROPERTIES OF CLINICALLY USED
LOCAL ANESTHETICS

Local Anesthetic	pKa	% Ionized (at pH 7.4)	Partition Coefficient (Lipid Solubility)	% Protein Binding
Amides				
Bupivacaine*	8.1	83	3420	95
Etidocaine	7.7	66	7317	94
Lidocaine	7.9	76	366	64
Mepivacaine	7.6	61	130	77
Prilocaine	7.9	76	129	55
Ropivacaine	8.1	83	775	94
Esters				
Chloroprocaine	8.7	95	810	NA
Procaine	8.9	97	100	6
Tetracaine	8.5	93	5822	94

*Levo-bupivacaine is the same as bupivacaine.
NA = not applicable.

ANESTHETIC AGENTS

5. Anesthetic activity and potency are affected by the stereochemistry of local anesthetics.
   a. Ropivacaine and levo-bupivacaine are single enantiomers that were initially developed as less cardiotoxic alternatives to bupivacaine.
   b. The desired improvement in the safety index seems to be present, but it comes at the expense of a slight decrease in potency and shorter duration of action compared with the racemic mixtures.
B. **Additives to Increase Local Anesthetic Activity** (Table 21-3)
   1. **Epinephrine** added to the local anesthetic solution may prolong the local anesthetic block, increase the intensity of the block and decrease systemic absorption of the local anesthetic.
      a. Vasoconstrictive effects produced by epinephrine augment local anesthetics by antagonizing inherent vasodilating effects of local anesthetics, thus decreasing systemic absorption and intraneural clearance, and perhaps by redistribution of intraneural local anesthetic.

TABLE 21-3

EFFECTS OF THE ADDITION OF EPINEPHRINE TO
LOCAL ANESTHETICS

	Increase Duration	Decrease Blood Levels (%)	Dose or Concentration of Epinephrine
Nerve Block			
Bupivacaine	Inconsistent	10–20	1:200,000
Lidocaine	Yes	20–30	1:200,000
Mepivacaine	Yes	20–30	1:200,000
Ropivacaine	Doubtful	0	1:200,000
Epidural			
Bupivacaine	Inconsistent	10–20	1:300,000–1:200,000
Levo-bupivacaine	Inconsistent	10	1:200,000–1:400,000
Chloroprocaine	Yes		1:200,000
Lidocaine	Yes	20–30	1:600,000–1:200,000
Mepivacaine	Yes	20–30	1:200,000
Ropivacaine	Doubtful		1:200,000
Spinal			
Bupivacaine	Inconsistent		0.2 mg
Lidocaine	Yes		0.2 mg
Tetracaine	Yes		0.2 mg

    b. Analgesic effects of epinephrine via interaction with α_2-adrenergic receptors in the spinal cord and brain may play a role in the effects of epinephrine added to the local anesthetic solution.

    c. The effectiveness of epinephrine depends on the local anesthetic administered, the type of regional block performed, and the amount of epinephrine added to the local anesthetic solution.

  2. Opioids added to the local anesthetic solution placed into the epidural or subarachnoid space result in synergistic analgesia and anesthesia without increasing the risk of toxicity.

  3. α_2-Adrenergic agonists such as clonidine produce synergistic analgesia via supraspinal and spinal adrenergic receptors. Clonidine also has direct inhibitory effects on peripheral nerve conduction (A and C nerve fibers).

III. **PHARMACOKINETICS OF LOCAL
ANESTHETICS** (Tables 21-4 and 21-5). Plasma
concentration of local anesthetics is a function of the dose
administered and the rates of systemic absorption, tissue
distribution, and drug elimination.

TABLE 21-4

TYPICAL PEAK PLASMA CONCENTRATIONS (C_{max}) AFTER
REGIONAL ANESTHETICS

Local Anesthetic or Technique	Dose (mg)	Peak Plasma Concentration ($\mu g/mL$)	Time to Peak Plasma Concentration ($\mu g/mL$)	Toxic Plasma Concentration ($\mu g/mL$)
Bupivacaine				
Brachial plexus	150	1.0	20	3
Celiac plexus	100	1.5	17	
Epidural	150	1.26	20	
Intercostal	140	0.90	30	
Lumbar sympathetic	52.5	0.49	24	
Sciatic/ Femoral	400	1.89	15	
Levo-bupivacaine				
Epidural	75	0.36	50	4
Brachial plexus	250	1.2	55	
Lidocaine				
Brachial plexus	400	4.0	25	5
Epidural	400	4.27	20	
Intercostal	400	6.8	15	
Mepivacaine				
Brachial plexus	500	3.68	24	5
Epidural	500	4.95	16	
Intercostal	500	8.06	9	
Sciatic/ Femoral	500	3.59	31	
Ropivacaine				
Brachial plexus	190	1.3	53	4
Epidural	150	1.07	40	
Intercostal	140	1.10	21	

TABLE 21-5

PHARMACOKINETIC PARAMETERS OF LOCAL ANESTHETICS

Local Anesthetic	Volume of Distribution at Steady State (VDss) (L/kg)	Clearance (L/kg/hr)	Elimination Half-Time (hr)
Bupivacaine	1.02	0.41	3.5
Levo-bupivacaine	0.78	0.32	2.6
Chloroprocaine	0.50	2.96	0.11
Etidocaine	1.9	1.05	2.6
Lidocaine	1.3	0.85	1.6
Mepivacaine	1.2	0.67	1.9
Prilocaine	2.73	2.03	1.6
Procaine	0.93	5.62	0.14
Ropivacaine	0.84	0.63	1.9

A. **Systemic Absorption** (Table 21-6)
   1. Decreasing systemic absorption of local anesthetics increases their safety margin in clinical uses. The rate and extent of systemic absorption depends on the site of injection, the dose, the drug's intrinsic pharmacokinetic properties, and the addition of a vasoactive agent.
B. **Distribution**
   1. Regional distribution of local anesthetics after systemic absorption depends on organ blood flow, the partition coefficient of the local anesthetic between compartments, and protein binding.
   2. Organs that are well perfused, such as the heart and brain, have higher drug concentrations.

TABLE 21-6

DETERMINANTS OF THE RATE AND EXTENT OF SYSTEMIC ABSORPTION OF LOCAL ANESTHETICS

Site of injection (intercostal > caudal > brachial plexus > sciatic or femoral)
Dose
Physiochemical properties (lipid solubility, protein binding)
Addition of epinephrine

C. Elimination
   1. Clearance of aminoester local anesthetics primarily depends on clearance by plasma cholinesterase.
   2. Aminoamides are transformed by hepatic carboxylesterases and cytochrome P450 enzyme.
D. Clinical Pharmacokinetics
   1. The primary benefit of knowledge of the systemic pharmacokinetics of local anesthetics is the ability to predict C_{max} (maximum plasma concentration) after the drugs are administered, thus reducing the likelihood of administration of toxic doses.
   2. Pharmacokinetics are difficult to predict in any given circumstance because both physical and pathophysiologic characteristics affect individual pharmacokinetics.

ANESTHETIC AGENTS

IV. CLINICAL USE OF LOCAL ANESTHETICS
(Tables 21-7 and 21-8)

V. TOXICITY OF LOCAL ANESTHETICS

A. Central Nervous System Toxicity
   1. Local anesthetics readily cross the blood–brain barrier, and generalized CNS toxicity may occur from systemic absorption or direct vascular injection.
   2. Development of CNS toxicity is more likely with certain local anesthetics (Table 21-9), and the signs of generalized CNS toxicity from local anesthetics are dose dependent (Table 21-10).
   3. Factors that increase CNS toxicity include decreased protein binding, acidosis, vasoconstriction, and hyperdynamic circulation caused by epinephrine being added to the local anesthetic solution.
   4. Factors that decrease CNS toxicity include drugs (barbiturates, benzodiazepines) and decreased systemic absorption caused by epinephrine being added to the local anesthetic solution.

TABLE 21-7

CLINICAL USE OF LOCAL ANESTHETICS

Regional anesthesia and analgesia
Intravenous regional anesthesia
Peripheral nerve blocks (single injection or continuous infusion)
Topical (airway, eye, skin)
Blunt responses to tracheal intubation

TABLE 21-8

CLINICAL PROFILE OF LOCAL ANESTHETICS

Local Anesthetic	Concentration (%)	Clinical Use	Onset	Duration (hr)	Recommended Maximum Single Dose (mg)
Amides					
Bupivacaine (levo-bupivacaine)	0.25	Infiltration	Fast	2–8	175/225 + epinephrine
	0.25–0.5	Peripheral nerve block	Slow	4–12	175/225 + epinephrine
	0.5–0.75	Epidural anesthesia	Moderate	2–5	175/225 + epinephrine
Lidocaine	0.5–1	Infiltration	Fast	2–8	300/500 + epinephrine
	0.25–0.5	Intravenous regional	Fast	0.5–1.0	300
	1.0–1.5	Peripheral nerve block	Fast	1–3	300/500 + epinephrine
	1.5–2.0	Epidural anesthesia	Fast	1–2	300/500 + epinephrine
	1.5–2.0	Topical	Fast	0.5–1.0	100
	4	Topical	Fast	0.5–1.0	300
Mepivacaine	0.5–1.0	Infiltration	Fast	1–4	400/500 + epinephrine
	1.0–1.5	Peripheral nerve block	Fast	2–4	400/500 + epinephrine
	1.5–2.0	Epidural anesthesia	Fast	1–3	400/500 + epinephrine
	2–4	Spinal anesthesia	Fast	1–2	100
Prilocaine	0.5–1.0	Infiltration	Fast	1–2	600
	0.25–0.5	Intravenous regional	Fast	0.5–1.0	600
	1.5–2.0	Peripheral nerve block	Fast	1.5–3.0	600
	2–3	Epidural	Fast	1–3	600

Ropivacaine	0.2–0.5	Infiltration	Fast	2–6	200
	0.5–1.0	Peripheral nerve block	Slow	5–8	250
	0.5–1.0	Epidural anesthesia	Moderate	2–6	200
Mixture					
Lidocaine + prilocaine	2.5/2.5	Skin topical	Slow	3–5	20 g
Esters					
Benzocaine	≤20%	Skin topical	Fast	0.5–1.0	200
Chloroprocaine	1	Infiltration	Fast	0.5–1.0	800/1000 + epinephrine
	2	Peripheral nerve block	Fast	0.5–1.0	800/1000 + epinephrine
	2–3	Epidural anesthesia	Fast	0.5–1.0	800/1000 + epinephrine
Cocaine	4–10	Topical	Fast	0.5–1.0	150
Procaine	10	Spinal anesthesia	Fast	0.5–1.0	1000
Tetracaine	2	Topical	Fast	0.5–1.0	20
	0.5	Spinal anesthesia	Fast	0.5–1.0	20

TABLE 21-9

CENTRAL NERVOUS SYSTEM AND CARDIOVASCULAR
SYSTEM TOXICITY

Local Anesthetic	Relative Potency for CNS Toxicity	Ratio of Dose Needed for CVS:CNS Toxicity
Bupivacaine	4.0	2.0
Levo-bupivacaine	2.9	2.0
Chloroprocaine	0.3	3.7
Etidocaine	2.0	4.4
Lidocaine	1.0	7.1
Mepivicaine	1.4	7.1
Prilocaine	1.2	3.1
Procaine	0.3	3.7
Ropivacaine	2.9	2
Tetracaine	2.0	

CNS = central nervous system; CVS = cardiovascular system.

5. The incidence of CNS toxicity with epidural injection of local anesthetics is estimated to be three in 10,000; for peripheral nerve blocks, the incidence is one in 10,000.

B. **Cardiovascular Toxicity of Local Anesthetics**
   1. In general, much greater doses of local anesthetics are required to produce cardiovascular toxicity than CNS toxicity (Table 21-10).
      a. Use of single-optical isomer (S/L) preparations of ropivacaine and levo-bupivacaine may improve the safety profile for long-lasting regional anesthesia.

TABLE 21-10

DOSE-DEPENDENT SYSTEMIC EFFECTS OF LIDOCAINE

Plasma Concentration (μg/mL)	Effect
1–5	Analgesia
5–10	Light-headedness
	Tinnitus
	Numbness of tongue
10–15	Seizures
	Unconsciousness
15–25	Coma
	Respiratory arrest
>25	Cardiovascular depression

      b. Reduced potential for cardiotoxicity is likely because of reduced affinity for brain and myocardial tissue from their single isomer preparation.

      c. In addition to the stereoselectivity, the larger butyl side chain in bupivacaine may also have more of a cardiodepressant effect as opposed to the propyl side chain of ropivacaine.

  2. Cardiovascular toxicity (hypotension, bradycardia, arterial hypoxemia) produced by less lipid-soluble and potent local anesthetics such as lidocaine is different from that produced by more potent and lipid-soluble anesthetics such as bupivacaine (sudden cardiovascular collapse because of ventricular cardiac dysrhythmias that are resistant to resuscitation).

  3. All local anesthetics block the cardiac conduction system via a dose-dependent block of sodium channels.

  4. Compared with lidocaine cardiotoxicity, bupivacaine cardiotoxicity is enhanced by bupivacaine's stronger binding affinity to resting and inactivated sodium channels.

  5. Local anesthetics bind to sodium channels during systole and dissociate during diastole.

      a. Bupivacaine dissociates more slowly from sodium channels during cardiac diastole than lidocaine.

      b. Bupivacaine dissociates so slowly that the duration of diastole at heart rates between 60 and 180 bpm does not allow enough time for complete recovery of sodium channels, so bupivacaine conduction block increases.

      c. Lidocaine fully dissociates from sodium channels during diastole, and little accumulation of conduction block occurs.

  6. Bupivacaine may inhibit cyclic adenosine monophosphate (cAMP) production, suggesting that large doses of epinephrine (resuscitative effects modulated by cAMP) may be needed during resuscitations from bupivacaine overdose.

C. Treatment of Systemic Toxicity From Local Anesthetics (Table 21-11)

  1. The best method for avoiding systemic toxicity from local anesthetics is through prevention, including using frequent syringe aspirations, a small local anesthetic test dose (3 mL), and slow injection or fractionation of the dose of local anesthetic.

TABLE 21-11

TREATMENT OF SYSTEMIC TOXICITY FROM LOCAL ANESTHETICS

Stop injection of local anesthetic
Administer supplemental oxygen
Support ventilation
Insert tracheal intubation and control ventilation if necessary
Suppress seizure activity (thiopental, midazolam, propofol)
Treat ventricular dysrhythmias (electrical cardioversion,
   epinephrine, vasopressin, amiodarone; 20% lipid solutions
   should be considered to remove bupivacaine from its sites of
   action)

2. Treatment of systemic toxicity is primarily supportive.
3. A promising treatment for cardiac toxicity from bupivacaine is intravenous administration of lipid to theoretically remove the local anesthetic from sites of
   action.

D. **Neural Toxicity of Local Anesthetics**
   1. Although all clinically used local anesthetics can cause
      concentration-dependent nerve fiber damage in
      peripheral nerves when used in high concentrations, it
      is believed that clinically used concentrations are safe
      for peripheral nerves.
   2. Compared with peripheral nerves, the spinal cord and
      nerve roots are more prone to injury.
      a. Lidocaine and tetracaine may be especially neuro-
         toxic in a concentration-dependent fashion, and
         this neurotoxicity may theoretically occur with
         clinically used concentrations.
      b. Despite laboratory findings that all local anesthet-
         ics may cause neurotoxicity, spinal administration
         of local anesthetics in patients has not manifested a
         neurotoxic potential.

E. **Transient Neurologic Symptoms After Spinal Anesthesia**
   1. Transient neurologic symptoms (TNS; pain or sensory
      abnormalities in the lower back and extremities) may
      occur after administration of all local anesthetics used
      for spinal anesthesia (Table 21-12).
   2. Increased risk of TNS is associated with lidocaine, the
      lithotomy position, and ambulatory anesthesia but
      not the baricity of the solution or the dose of local
      anesthetic.

TABLE 21-12

INCIDENCE OF TRANSIENT NEUROLOGIC SYMPTOMS AFTER SPINAL ANESTHESIA

Local Anesthetic	Concentration (%)	Type of Surgery	Approximate Incidence of Transient Neurologic Symptoms (%)
Lidocaine	2–5	Lithotomy position	30–36
	2–5	Knee arthroscopy	18–22
	0.5	Knee arthroscopy	17
	2–5	Mixed supine position	4–8
Mepivacaine	1.5–4.0	Mixed	23
Bupivacaine	0.5–0.75	Mixed	1
Levo-bupivacaine	0.5	Mixed	1
Prilocaine	2–5	Mixed	1
Ropivacaine	0.5–0.75	Mixed	1

3. The potential neurologic cause of this syndrome coupled with the known concentration-dependent toxicity of lidocaine has led to concerns over a neurotoxic cause for TNS from spinal lidocaine (Table 21-13).
4. Preservative-free 2-chloroprocaine provides an anesthetic profile similar to lidocaine's without TNS.

F. **Myotoxicity of Local Anesthetics.** Local anesthetics have the potential for myotoxicity in clinically applicable concentrations (dysregulation of intracellular calcium concentrations).

TABLE 21-13

POSSIBLE CAUSES OF TRANSIENT NEUROLOGIC SYMPTOMS

Concentration-dependent neurotoxicity
Patient positioning
Early ambulation
Needle trauma
Neural ischemia
Pooling secondary to maldistribution

G. **Allergic Reactions to Local Anesthetics**
   1. True allergic reactions to local anesthetics, especially aminoamides, are rare.
   2. Increased allergenic potential with ester local anesthetics may be caused by metabolism to para-aminobenzoic acid, which is a known antigen.
   3. Preservatives such as methylparaben and metabisulfite can also provoke an allergic response.

CHAPTER 22 ■ **DRUG INTERACTIONS**

Modern drug regimens often involve use of multiple drugs in combination, which introduces the risk of drug interactions (Rosow C, Levine WC: Drug interactions. In *Clinical Anesthesia*. Edited by Barash PG, Cullen BF, Stoelting RK, Cahalan MK, Stock MC. Philadelphia: Lippincott Williams & Wilkins, 2009, pp 549–566).

I. PROBLEMS CREATED BY DRUG–DRUG INTERACTIONS

A. The probability of a drug–drug interaction increases with the number of drugs administered.

B. Drug interactions are uncommon even though many patients take multiple drugs (antihypertensives, antidepressants, gastrointestinal drugs) before surgery and then receive five to 10 drugs during anesthesia. (Many reactions are not significant. Drugs have a large safety margin, and many interactions are not recognized.)

C. **Why Combine Drugs?** The goal of combining drugs is to decrease toxicity while maintaining efficacy (hypertension, chemotherapy, prophylaxis against grand mal seizures).

II. PHARMACEUTICAL INTERACTIONS

A. A chemical or physical interaction may occur between drugs before they are administered to form a precipitate (e.g., thiopental or ketamine injected with succinylcholine; epinephrine injected with sodium bicarbonate as during cardiopulmonary resuscitation).

B. A chemical or physical interaction may occur between drugs before they are administered to form a toxic compound (e.g., desflurane or isoflurane in contact with dry soda lime forms carbon monoxide; nitric oxide in contact with oxygen forms nitrogen dioxide).

III. PHARMACOKINETIC INTERACTIONS

A. A pharmacokinetic interaction occurs when one drug alters the absorption, metabolism, or elimination of another drug.

B. **Absorption** may be altered because of direct chemical or physical interaction between drugs in the body (e.g., orally administered tetracycline is inactivated by chelation with antacids; opioids slow gastric emptying) or changes in regional blood flow (e.g., local administration of epinephrine slows absorption of local anesthetics; congestive heart failure or shock may alter the onset and intensity of drug effect by decreasing tissue perfusion).

C. **Distribution**-related drug interactions occur when distribution of a second drug is altered by hemodynamics (drug-induced changes in cardiac output), drug ionization ("ion trapping"), or binding to plasma and tissue proteins (α_1-acid glycoprotein concentrations increase postoperatively; after myocardial infarction or trauma, albumin concentrations may be decreased by hepatic cirrhosis).

   1. A drug that is highly bound to plasma protein effectively exists in a depot (similar to a drug given by intramuscular administration).

   2. Altered protein binding or displacement from protein binding sites has been dogma for many years, but the true clinical relevance of this type of interaction is not clear.

D. **Metabolism**

   1. Drugs administered to inhibit acetylcholinesterase (as for reversal on nondepolarizing neuromuscular blocking drugs) also inhibit pseudocholinesterase and prolong the duration of action of succinylcholine.

E. **Monoamine Oxidase Interactions**

   1. Inhibition of monoamine oxidase (MAO), which is present in tissues throughout the body, by MAO inhibitors may produce interactions with drugs that affect sympathetic neurotransmission (e.g., ephedrine produces an exaggerated response as more presynaptic transmitter is available for release; "wine and cheese" interaction caused by the tyramine content of foods) or interactions that involve central nervous system depressants (e.g., hyperpyrexia and

hypertension that may progress to seizures and coma in patients receiving meperidine).
  2. Current clinical opinion favors continuing MAO inhibitor therapy up to the time of surgery.
  3. Patients taking MAO inhibitors have the potential for perioperative hemodynamic instability, yet beta-blockers, direct vasodilators, and direct-acting vasopressors appear to be safe and effective treatments in most circumstances.
F. **Hepatic Biotransformation**
  1. Many anesthetic drugs undergo oxidative metabolism by one of the isoforms of cytochrome P450 found in liver microsomes.
    a. P450 isoforms have low substrate specificity such that drugs of diverse structures (general anesthetics, opioids, barbiturates, benzodiazepines) can be biotransformed by a single group of enzymes.
    b. Inhibitors or inducers or these enzymes may also affect the clearance of broad groups of drugs (Table 22-1).

TABLE 22-1

CLASSIFICATION OF PHARMACODYNAMIC DRUG INTERACTIONS

Additive Interactions (most likely to occur when drugs with identical mechanisms of action are combined)
Administration of two aminosteroid nondepolarizing muscle relaxants
Administration of nitrous oxide with a volatile anesthetic

Antagonistic Drug Interactions
Deliberate
  Administration of neostigmine, naloxone, flumazenil
Unintended
  Succinylcholine and a nondepolarizing muscle relaxant
  Epidural opioid administered after establishing a block with chloroprocaine

Synergistic Drug Interactions (most likely to occur when drugs of different classes or mechanisms are administered to produce the same effect)
Potentiation of opioids by NSAIDs
Potentiation of nondepolarizing muscle relaxants by volatile anesthetics
Potentiation between hypnotics that have related mechanisms of action (act on γ-aminobutyric acid, a chloride ionophore)

NSAID = nonsteroidal antiinflammatory drug.

2. Removal of a drug from the blood by hepatic biotransformation (hepatic clearance) is dependent on hepatic blood flow and intrinsic clearance (the maximal ability of the liver to metabolize that drug or extraction ratio).

   a. For drugs with a high extraction ratio (lidocaine, morphine, propranolol), hepatic blood flow is the rate-limiting factor in overall hepatic clearance. Decreases in hepatic blood flow (anesthesia, congestive heart failure) result in increased plasma concentrations.

   b. For drugs with a low extraction ratio (diazepam, alfentanil), hepatic enzyme activity is the rate-limiting factor.

3. The most common reason for increased intrinsic clearance is enzyme induction of cytochrome P450 enzymes (microsomal or CYP enzymes). The most important subfamily appears to be CYP3A, which is found in greatest abundance in human liver and is responsible for the metabolism of a large number of drugs.

4. Drugs may also inhibit the hepatic biotransformation of other drugs by competing for the same P450 enzymes (e.g., protease inhibitors may inhibit the metabolism of midazolam and fentanyl by inhibiting CYP3A4).

G. **Drug elimination** may result in pharmacokinetic drug interactions via alterations in renal or pulmonary clearance.

IV. PHARMACODYNAMIC INTERACTIONS

A. A pharmacodynamic interaction occurs when one drug alters the sensitivity of a target receptor or tissue to the effects of a second drug. Pharmacokinetic interaction

---

TABLE 22-2

DRUGS THAT INDUCE OR INHIBIT HEPATIC DRUG METABOLISM

Inhibitors	Inducers
Phenobarbital	Cimetidine
Phenytoin	Ketoconazole
Rifampicin	Erythromycin
Carbamazepine	Disulfiram
Ethanol	Ritonavir

is a change in the amount of active drug reaching
receptor sites.

B. The dose–response curve or concentration–response curve
for one drug is shifted by another drug (Table 22-2).

V. PHARMACODYNAMIC INTERACTIONS AFFECTING HEMODYNAMICS

A. Prior recommendations that cardiovascular stimulant
or depressant drugs should be discontinued before

TABLE 22-3

EFFECTS OF ANTIHYPERTENSIVE DRUGS DURING ANESTHESIA

Class	Drugs	Effects
α-Blockers	Phenoxybenzamine Phentolamine Prazosin	Hypotension or vasodilation Reflex tachycardia
Beta-blockers	Propranolol Metoprolol Atenolol	Hypotension Decreased myocardial contractility Bradycardia, heart block
Mixed α/beta blocker	Labetalol	Hypotension or vasodilation, bradycardia, heart block
Calcium channel blockers	Verapamil Diltiazem Nifedipine Nicardipine	Hypotension or vasodilation Decreased myocardial contractility Bradycardia Heart block
Direct vasodilators	Nitroglycerin Isosorbide Hydralazine	Hypotension or vasodilation Reflex tachycardia
Angiotensin-converting enzyme inhibitors	Captopril Enalapril Lisinopril	Hypotension or vasodilation Hyperkalemia
Angiotensin II blockers	Losartan Valsartan Thiazides Furosemide Bumetanide	Hypotension or vasodilation Hyperkalemia Hypovolemia Hypokalemia Possible vasodilation

TABLE 22-4

DRUG INTERACTIONS BETWEEN COMBINATIONS OF CENTRAL NERVOUS SYSTEM DEPRESSANTS

Opioid–Hypnotic
Fentanyl decreases dose requirements for thiopental (more rapid awakening after short surgical procedures).
Opioids potentiate propofol.
Infusions of remifentanil or alfentanil decrease the needed infusion rate of propofol.

Opioid–Benzodiazepine
Alfentanil (weak hypnotic but highly selective depressant of central nervous system [sedation]) decreases the hypnotic (sleep) dose of midazolam.

Benzodiazepine–Hypnotic
Midazolam potentates the hypnotic effects of propofol.

Volatile Anesthetic–Opioid
Opioids produce dose-dependent decreases in MAC.

α_2-Agonist Interactions
Clonidine and dexmedetomidine potentiate opioid analgesia and decrease MAC (may reflect depression of the locus ceruleus, which is the main adrenergic nucleus in the brain as well as being important for sleep, memory, and analgesia).

MAC = minimum alveolar concentration.

surgery because they interfere with protective responses to the trauma of anesthesia and surgery are no longer advocated.

1. Patients with hypertension who remain well controlled are less likely to have wide swings in systemic blood pressure during surgery.
2. Abrupt discontinuation of vasoactive medications may actually increase cardiovascular instability (rebound hypertension, cardiac dysrhythmias).

B. The majority of cardiovascular drug interactions are extensions of the known pharmacology of the drugs (Table 22-3).

1. There is currently no consensus on the preoperative management of patients taking angiotensin-converting enzyme inhibitors.

a. Continuation through the perioperative period may be associated with an increased incidence of hypotension during induction of general anesthesia.

TABLE 22-5

EVIDENCE FOR HERBAL TOXICITY

Herb	Common Use	Claimed Toxicity	Supporting Evidence
Ephedra	Weight loss Antitussive Bacteriostatic	Cardiac dysrhythmias Enhanced sympathomimetic effects Stroke Hypertension	Oral ephedra is known to cause adverse CNS and cardiac events
Echinacea	Common cold prevention Urinary tract infections Bronchitis	Hepatotoxicity Decrease corticosteroid effect	No evidence Laboratory evidence of macrophage activation
Garlic	Lipid lowering	Potentiates warfarin	No evidence of interaction with warfarin Decreased platelet aggregation *in vitro*
Ginger	Hypertension Antiplatelet Antioxidant Nausea Antispasmodic	Inhibits thromboxane synthetase	*In vitro* evidence of thromboxane synthetase inhibition Inhibits platelet function when dose exceeds 5 g
Ginkgo Goldenseal	Circulatory stimulant Diuretic Antiinflammatory Laxative Hemostatic	Inhibits platelet activating factor Oxytocic Paralysis in overdose Edema Hypertension	Reports of increased bleeding No evidence

(continued)

329

TABLE 22-5

EVIDENCE FOR HERBAL TOXICITY *(Continued)*

Herb	Common Use	Claimed Toxicity	Supporting Evidence
Kava	Anxiolytic	Hepatotoxicity Potentiates barbiturates and benzodiazepines	Reports of hepatotoxicity Clinical studies demonstrating sedation and anxiolysis
Licorice	Gastric or duodenal ulcer Gastritis Bronchitis	Hypokalemia Hypertension Edema	Hypokalemia with abuse
St John's Wort	Depression	Decreased digoxin level Enzyme induction Prolonged anesthesia	Supportive clinical data Supportive clinical data Reports of prolonged emergence
Valerian	Sedative Anxiolytic	Potentiates barbiturates	Small clinical trial shows decreased sleep latency
Vitamin E	Anti-aging Prevents stroke Prevents pulmonary emboli Prevents atherosclerosis Promotes wound healing	Hypertension Bleeding	No evidence Decreased platelet aggregation *in vitro*

CNS = central nervous system.

  b. Withholding these drugs for 24 hours may decrease hypotension but may also make blood pressure extremely labile during surgery.

  c. Chronic blockade of the angiotensin system reduces the vasoconstrictor response to norepinephrine. (This may explain why drug-induced hypotension is resistant to sympathetic drugs.)

C. Patients with **acute cocaine intoxication** may present with hypertension, tachycardia, and myocardial ischemia (resembles pheochromocytoma). Administration of a beta-blocker alone may allow unopposed α-adrenergic stimulation and large increases in systemic vascular resistance.

VI. PHARMACODYNAMIC INTERACTIONS AFFECTING ANALGESIA OR HYPNOSIS (Table 22-4)

VII. HERBAL PREPARATIONS AND DRUG INTERACTIONS (Table 22-5)

CHAPTER 23 ■ **PREOPERATIVE PATIENT ASSESSMENT AND MANAGEMENT**

The goals of preoperative evaluation are to reduce patient risk and the morbidity of surgery, as well as to promote efficiency and reduce costs (Hata TM, Moyers JR: Preoperative patient assessment and management. In *Clinical Anesthesia*. Edited by Barash PG, Cullen BF, Stoelting RK, Cahalan MK, Stock MC. Philadelphia: Lippincott Williams & Wilkins, 2009, pp 567–597).

I. INTRODUCTION

A. The Joint Commission requires that all patients receive a preoperative anesthetic evaluation.

B. The American Society of Anesthesiologists (ASA) approved its Basic Standards for Preanesthetic Care, which outlines the minimum requirements for a preoperative evaluation.

C. Conducting a preoperative evaluation is based on the premise that it will modify patient care and improve outcome.

  1. Based on the history and physical examination, the appropriate laboratory tests and preoperative consultations should be obtained.

  2. Guided by the history and physical examination, the anesthesiologist should choose the appropriate anesthetic and care plan.

II. CHANGING CONCEPTS IN PREOPERATIVE EVALUATION

A. The first time the anesthesiologist performing the anesthetic sees the patient may be just before anesthesia and surgery. (The patient has been seen previously by others in a preoperative evaluation clinic.)

B. Information technology using preoperative question-naires and computer-driven programs has helped anesthesiologists preview upcoming patients that will be anesthetized.

III. APPROACH TO THE HEALTHY PATIENT

A. The preoperative evaluation form is the basis for formulating the best anesthetic plan tailored to the patient. It should aid the anesthesiologist in identifying potential complications, as well as serve as a medico-legal document. The information obtained must be complete, concise, and legible.

B. The approach to the patient should always begin with a thorough history and physical examination (may be sufficient without additional routine laboratory tests).

1. The indication for the surgical procedure may also have implications on other aspects of perioperative management.

   a. Small bowel obstruction has implications regard-ing the risk of aspiration and the need for a rapid sequence induction.

   b. The extent of a lung resection dictates the need for further pulmonary testing and perioperative monitoring.

   c. Patients undergoing carotid endarterectomy may require a more extensive neurologic examination as well as testing to rule out coronary artery disease (CAD).

2. The ability to review previous anesthetic records is helpful in detecting the presence of a difficult airway, a history of malignant hyperthermia, and the individual's response to surgical stress and specific anesthetics.

3. The patient should be questioned regarding any pre-vious difficulty with anesthesia and other family members having difficulty with anesthesia. (History relating an "allergy" to anesthesia should make one suspicious of malignant hyperthermia.)

4. The history should include a complete list of medica-tions, including over-the-counter and herbal products, to define a preoperative medication regimen, anticipate potential drug interactions, and provide clues to underlying disease.

TABLE 23-1

COMPONENTS OF THE AIRWAY PHYSICAL EXAMINATION

Airway Examination Component	Findings Suggestive of Difficult Intubation
Length of upper incisors	Long compared with rest of dentition
Relation of maxillary and mandibular incisors during normal jaw closure	Prominent overbite
Relation of maxillary and mandibular incisors during voluntary protrusion of mandible	Patient cannot bring mandibular incisors anterior to maxillary incisors
Interincisor distance	<3 cm
Visibility of uvula	Not visible when the tongue is protruded with the patient in the sitting position
Shape of palate	Highly arched or very narrow
Compliance of mandibular space	Stiff, indurated, occupied by a mass, or nonresilient
Thyromental distance	<3 finger breadths
Length of neck	Short neck
Thickness of neck	Thick neck
Range of motion of head and neck	Patient cannot touch the tip of the chin to the chest or is unable to extend the neck

C. Systems Approach
   1. Airway
      a. Evaluation of the airway involves determination of the thyromental distance; the ability to flex the base of the neck and extend the head; and examination of the oral cavity, including dentition (Table 23-1).
      b. The Mallampati classification has become the standard for assessing the relationship of the tongue size relative to the oral cavity, although by itself the Mallampati classification has a low positive predictive value in identifying patients who are difficult to intubate (Table 23-2).
      c. In appropriate patients, the presence of pain or symptoms of cervical cord compression on movement should be assessed. In other instances, radiographic examination may be required.

TABLE 23-2

AIRWAY CLASSIFICATION SYSTEM

Class	Direct Visualization (Patient Seated)	Laryngoscopic View
I	Soft palate, fauces, uvula, pillars	Entire glottic opening
II	Soft palate, fauces, uvula	Posterior commissure
III	Soft palate, uvular base	Tip of epiglottis
IV	Hard palate only	No glottal structures

2. **Pulmonary** (Table 23-3)
3. **Cardiovascular System** (Table 23-4)
4. **Neurologic System.** The patient's ability to answer health history questions practically ensures a normal mental status (exclude the presence of increased intracranial pressure, cerebrovascular disease, seizure history, pre-existing neuromuscular disease, or nerve injuries).
5. **Endocrine System.** The patient should be screened for endocrine diseases (diabetes mellitus, adrenal cortical suppression) that may affect the perioperative course.

TABLE 23-3

SCREENING EVALUATION FOR THE PULMONARY SYSTEM

History
Tobacco use
Shortness of breath
Cough
Wheezing
Stridor
Snoring or sleep apnea
Recent history of an upper respiratory tract infection

Physical Examination
Respiratory rate
Chest excursion
Use of accessory muscles
Nail color
Ability to walk and carry on a conversation without dyspnea
Auscultation to detect decreased breath sounds, wheezing, stridor, and rales

EVALUATION

TABLE 23-4

SCREENING EVALUATION FOR THE CARDIOVASCULAR SYSTEM

Uncontrolled hypertension
Unstable cardiac disease
Myocardial ischemia (unstable angina)
Congestive heart failure
Valvular heart disease (aortic stenosis, mitral valve prolapse)
Cardiac dysrhythmias
Auscultation of the heart (murmur radiating to the carotid
  arteries)
Bruits over the carotid arteries
Peripheral pulses

IV. EVALUATION OF THE PATIENT WITH KNOWN SYSTEMIC DISEASE

A. Cardiovascular Disease

1. The goals are to define risk; determine which patients will benefit from further testing; devise an appropriate anesthetic plan; and identify patients who will benefit from perioperative beta-blockade, intervention therapy, or even surgery (Table 23-5).

TABLE 23-5

AMERICAN SOCIETY OF ANESTHESIOLOGISTS PHYSICAL
STATUS CLASSIFICATION

ASA Class	Disease State
1	No organic, physiologic, biochemical, or psychiatric disturbance
2	Mild to moderate systemic disturbance that may not be related to the reason for surgery
3	Severe systemic disturbance that may or may not be related to the reason for surgery
4	Severe systemic disturbance that is life threatening with or without surgery
5	Moribund patient who has little chance of survival but is submitted to surgery as a last resort (resuscitative effort)

ASA = American Society of Anesthesiologists.
E = emergency operation.

2. Independent predictors of complications in the Goldman risk index include high-risk type of surgery, history of ischemic heart disease, history of congestive heart failure, history of cerebrovascular disease, preoperative treatment with insulin, and preoperative serum creatinine above 2.0 mg/dL.
3. The presence of unstable angina has been associated with a high perioperative risk of myocardial infarction (MI).
4. The presence of active congestive heart failure before surgery is associated with an increased incidence of perioperative cardiac morbidity.
5. The importance of the intervening time interval between an acute MI and elective surgery (traditionally 6 months or longer) may no longer be valid in the current era of interventional therapy (Table 23-6).

TABLE 23-6

CLINICAL PREDICTORS OF INCREASED PERIOPERATIVE CARDIOVASCULAR RISK (MYOCARDIAL INFARCTION, CONGESTIVE HEART FAILURE)

Major
Unstable coronary syndromes
Recent myocardial infarction
Unstable or severe angina
Decompensated congestive heart failure
Significant arrhythmias
High-grade atrioventricular block
Symptomatic ventricular arrhythmias
Supraventricular arrhythmias with uncontrolled ventricular rate
Severe valvular disease

Intermediate
Mild angina pectoris
Prior myocardial infarction by history or pathologic Q waves
Compensated or prior congestive heart failure
Diabetes mellitus
Renal Insufficiency

Minor
Advanced age
Abnormal electrocardiogram (left ventricular hypertrophy, left bundle branch block, ST-T abnormalities)
Rhythm other than sinus (atrial fibrillation)
Low functional capacity (inability to climb one flight of stairs with a bag of groceries)
History of stroke
Uncontrolled systemic hypertension

EVALUATION

B. **Patients with Coronary Artery Disease**
1. For patients without overt symptoms or history, the probability of CAD varies with the type and number of atherosclerotic risk factors present (peripheral arterial disease, diabetes mellitus [autonomic neuropathy the best predictor of silent CAD], hypertension [left ventricular hypertrophy], atherosclerosis associated with tobacco use, hypercholesterolemia).
   a. Although there has been a suggestion in the literature that surgery should be delayed if the diastolic pressure is 110 mm Hg or above, the study often quoted as the basis for this determination demonstrated no major morbidity in that small group of patients.
   b. Other authors state that there is little association between blood pressures of less than 180 mm Hg systolic or 110 mm Hg diastolic and postoperative outcomes (such patients are prone to perioperative myocardial ischemia, ventricular dysrhythmias, and lability in blood pressure).
C. **Importance of Surgical Procedure** (Table 23-7)

TABLE 23-7

CARDIAC RISK STRATIFICATION FOR NONCARDIAC
SURGICAL PROCEDURES

High (reported cardiac risk often >5%)
Emergent major operations, particularly in elderly patients
Aortic and other major vascular
Peripheral vascular
Anticipated prolonged surgical procedures associated with large
  fluid shifts or blood loss

Intermediate (reported cardiac risk generally <5%)
Carotid endarterectomy
Head and neck
Intraperitoneal and intrathoracic
Orthopedic
Prostate

Low (reported cardiac risk generally <1%)
Endoscopic procedures
Superficial procedure
Cataract
Breast

1. The surgical procedure influences the scope of pre-operative evaluation required by determining the potential range of physiologic flux during the perioperative period.
   a. Peripheral procedures performed as ambulatory surgery are associated with an extremely low incidence of morbidity and mortality.
   b. High-risk procedures include major vascular, abdominal, thoracic, and orthopedic surgery.
D. **Importance of Exercise Tolerance**
   1. Exercise tolerance is one of the most important determinants of perioperative risk and the need for further testing and invasive monitoring.
   2. An excellent exercise tolerance, even in patients with stable angina, suggests that the myocardium can be stressed without failing.
      a. If a patient can walk a mile without becoming short of breath, the probability of extensive CAD is small.
      b. If patients experience dyspnea associated with chest pain during minimal exertion, the probability of extensive CAD is high, which has been associated with greater perioperative risk.
   3. There is good evidence to suggest that minimal additional testing is necessary if the patient has good exercise tolerance.

V. **INDICATIONS FOR FURTHER CARDIAC TESTING** (Fig. 23-1).

No preoperative cardiovascular testing should be performed if the results will not change the perioperative management.

A. **Cardiovascular Tests**
   1. **Electrocardiography**
      a. Abnormal Q waves in high-risk patients are highly suggestive of a past MI. (It is estimated that approximately 30% of MIs occur without symptoms and can only be detected on routine electrocardiograms [ECGs].)
      b. The presence of Q waves on a preoperative ECG in a high-risk patient, regardless of symptoms, should alert the anesthesiologist to an increased perioperative risk and the possibility of active ischemia.

EVALUATION

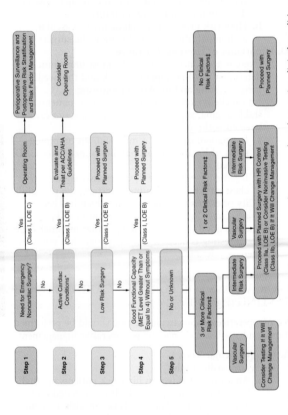

FIGURE 23-1. Cardiac evaluation and care algorithm for noncardiac surgery based on active clinical conditions, known cardio-vascular disease, or cardiac risk factors for patients 50 years of age or greater. (Reused with permission from ACC/AHA 2007 Guidelines on Perioperative Cardiovascular Evaluation and Care for Noncardiac Surgery. Circulation 2007;116:e418–e500.)

    c. It has not been established that information obtained from the preoperative ECG affects clinical care.

    d. Although controversy exists, current recommendations for a resting 12-lead preoperative ECG include patients with at least one clinical risk factor who are undergoing a vascular surgical procedure and for patients with known CAD, peripheral vascular disease, or cerebrovascular disease who are undergoing intermediate-risk surgical procedures.

2. **Noninvasive Cardiovascular Testing**

    a. The exercise ECG represents the most cost effective and least invasive method of detecting ischemia.

    b. Pharmacologic stress thallium imaging is useful in patients who are unable to exercise.

    c. In patients who cannot exercise, dopamine can be used to increase myocardial oxygen demand by increasing heart rate and blood pressure.

    d. The ambulatory ECG (Holter monitoring) provides a means of continuously monitoring the ECG for significant ST-segment changes before surgery.

    e. Stress echocardiography may be of value in evaluating patients with suspected CAD.

    f. Dobutamine echocardiography has been found to have among the best predictive values.

    g. Current recommendations are that patients with active cardiac conditions (unstable angina, congestive heart failure, arrhythmias, valve disease) should undergo noninvasive testing before noncardiac surgery.

3. **Assessment of Ventricular and Valvular Function**

    a. Both echocardiography and radionuclide angiography may assess cardiac ejection fraction at rest and under stress, but echocardiography is less invasive and is also able to assess regional wall motion abnormalities, wall thickness, valvular function, and valve area.

    b. Conflicting results exist regarding the predictive value of ejection fraction determinations.

    c. It is reasonable for those with dyspnea of unknown origin and for those with current or prior heart failure with worsening dyspnea to

EVALUATION

> have preoperative evaluation of left ventricular function.
>
> d. Aortic stenosis has been associated with a poor prognosis in noncardiac surgical patients, and knowledge of valvular lesions may modify perioperative hemodynamic therapy.

4. **Coronary angiography** is the best method of defining coronary artery anatomy. (Narrowing of the left main coronary artery may be associated with a greater perioperative risk.)

B. **Perioperative Coronary Interventions**

1. The long-term survival of some patients scheduled for high-risk surgery may be enhanced by revascularization (transluminal coronary angioplasty, coronary stent placement).

2. Early surgery after coronary stent placement has been associated with adverse cardiac events. Antiplatelet therapy (aspirin, clopidogrel) requires perioperative management to balance the risk of bleeding versus stent thrombosis. The risk of regional versus general anesthesia is a consideration in the presence of antiplatelet therapy.

VI. PULMONARY DISEASE

A. **Introduction**

1. The site and type of surgery (thoracic and upper abdominal surgery) are the strongest predictors of pulmonary complications.

2. Diaphragmatic dysfunction occurs despite adequate analgesia and is theorized to be caused by phrenic nerve inhibition.

3. Duration of anesthesia is a well-established risk factor for postoperative pulmonary complications, with morbidity rates increasing after 2 to 3 hours.

B. **Patient-Related Factors**

1. Preoperative evaluation of patients with pre-existing pulmonary disease should include assessment of the type and severity of disease, as well as its reversibility.

2. Inquiries should be made regarding exercise intolerance, chronic cough, and unexplained dyspnea.

3. On physical examination, findings of wheezing, rhonchi, decreased breath sounds, dullness to percussion, and a prolonged expiratory phase are important.

4. **Tobacco** is an important risk factor but usually cannot be influenced. Cessation of smoking for 2 days may decrease carboxyhemoglobin levels, abolish nicotine's effects, and improve mucous clearance, but smoking cessation for at least 8 weeks is necessary to reduce the rate of postoperative pulmonary complications.

5. **Asthma**
   a. Frequent use of bronchodilators, hospitalizations for asthma, and the requirement for systemic steroids are all indicators of the severity of the disease.
   b. After an episode of asthma, airway hyperreactivity may persist for several weeks.
   c. The possibility of adrenal insufficiency is another concern in patients who have received more than a "burst and taper" of steroids in the previous 6 months.

6. **Obstructive sleep apnea (OSA)** (periodic obstruction of the upper airway during sleep leading to episodic oxygen saturation and hypercarbia, chronic sleep deprivation, and daytime somnolence) is estimated to be present (often undiagnosed) in 9% of females and 24% of males (Table 23-8). Preoperative identification of these patients may lead to a formal sleep study to identify the severity of symptoms and the need for preoperative initiation of continuous positive airway pressure (CPAP). A general consensus exists that preoperative institution of CPAP reduces perioperative risk.
   a. Patients with OSA are exquisitely sensitive to the respiratory depressant effects of inhaled anesthetics, sedatives, and opioids.
   b. The ASA has published practice guidelines for the perioperative management of patients with OSA.

EVALUATION

TABLE 23-8

FACTORS COMMONLY ASSOCIATED WITH AN INCREASED RISK OF OBSTRUCTIVE SLEEP APNEA

Body mass index >35 kg/m^2
Increased neck circumference
Severe tonsillar hypertrophy
Anatomic abnormalities of the upper airway

TABLE 23-9

QUESTIONS TO ASK DURING THE PREOPERATIVE EVALUATION
REGARDING THE PRESENCE OF SYMPTOMS AND SIGNS OF
OBSTRUCTIVE SLEEP APNEA

Does the patient snore loudly?
Are there observed pauses in breathing during sleep?
Are there frequent arousals during sleep or awakening with a
  choking sensation?
Is daytime somnolence present?
Do the child's parents notice restless sleep or difficulty breathing?
Is the child aggressive or have trouble concentrating?

During the preoperative evaluation, specific questions may be asked to determine the patient's likelihood of having OSA (Table 23-9).

c. Preoperative communication between the surgeon and anesthesia professional is important for planning the management of a patient with OSA (Table 23-10).

d. Postoperative hospitalization is recommended for OSA patients with other coexisting diseases. When procedures are performed on an outpatient basis, postoperative monitoring (pulse oximetry) should be continued to ensure that the patient is able to maintain room air saturation without obstruction when left undisturbed.

TABLE 23-10

MANAGEMENT DECISIONS IN COORDINATION WITH THE
SURGEON FOR PATIENTS WITH OBSTRUCTIVE SLEEP APNEA

Determine if noninvasive approaches for performing the surgery
  would reduce the need for postoperative opioids.
Discuss if it is feasible to perform the surgery under neuraxial,
  regional, or local anesthesia to decrease the amount of
  anesthesia or opioids needed.
Determine if NSAIDs are acceptable for postoperative analgesia.
Discuss whether outpatient surgery is a safe option.
Determine if the patient will be able to use CPAP postoperatively.
Determine if postoperative admission to an ICU is needed for a
  patient who is a first-time user of CPAP.

CPAP = continuous positive airway pressure; ICU = intensive care unit;
NSAID = nonsteroidal antiinflammatory drug.

VII. ENDOCRINE DISEASE

A. **Diabetes mellitus** is the most common endocrinopathy (0.4% of the US population has type 1, and 8% to 10% of the US population has type 2). This incidence increases increasing with the greater incidence of obesity. Critical illness–induced hyperglycemia (blood glucose >200 mg/dL) in the absence of known diabetes occurs frequently, especially in elderly individuals.

1. Individuals with diabetes have an increased risk of developing CAD (silent angina caused by diabetic neuropathy), perioperative MI, hypertension, and congestive heart failure.

   a. Peripheral neuropathies (documented preoperatively) and vascular disease make patients with diabetes at risk for positioning injuries.

   b. Autonomic neuropathy is common and may contribute to hemodynamic instability and pulmonary aspiration from gastroparesis.

   c. Stiff joint syndrome caused by glycosylation of proteins may contribute to limited motion of the temporomandibular joint and cervical vertebra, leading to difficult airway management (this should be evaluated preoperatively).

2. Patients with type 1 diabetes must receive exogenous insulin to avoid development of ketoacidosis.

3. Elective surgery should be delayed if there is evidence of suboptimal blood glucose control (hemoglobin A1c >6% to 8%, abnormal electrolytes, ketonuria).

4. Administration of perioperative beta-blockers (no evidence of drug-induced glucose intolerance or masking of hypoglycemic symptoms) should be considered in diabetic patients with CAD to help limit perioperative myocardial ischemia.

5. **Preoperative Glucose Management.** Evidence is lacking to be able to set standards for the perioperative management of diabetic patients, but at a minimum, an attempt should be made to control the glucose level within a range of 100 to 200 mg/dL (some argue for a top limit of 150 mg/dL) (Table 23-11).

B. **Adrenal Disorders.** There is consensus that for patients taking corticosteroids for long periods that perioperative steroid supplementation is indicated to cover the stresses of anesthesia and surgery.

TABLE 23-11

RECOMMENDATIONS FOR PERIOPERATIVE GLUCOSE MANAGEMENT IN DIABETIC PATIENTS

Schedule as the first case of the day to avoid prolonged fasting.

Hold oral hypoglycemic drugs on the day of surgery to avoid reactive hypoglycemia (the exception is metformin, which should be held for 24 hours).

Continue usual insulin regimen through the evening before surgery.

Advise the patients to take a glucose tablet or clear juice if hypoglycemia occurs before arrival at the hospital.

Schedule the patient to arrive NPO in early morning and check blood glucose, electrolytes, and ketones.

For type 1 diabetics, administer half the usual morning does of intermediate- or long-acting insulin after arrival for surgery (hold the usual dose of rapid or short-acting insulin).

Continue use of insulin pumps for brief surgeries or convert the pump to an IV insulin infusion for moderate or major surgeries.

Use the patient's own sliding scale to administer short-acting insulin subcutaneously to maintain the blood glucose concentration 100 to 200 mg/dL before surgery.

Measure blood glucose concentrations every 1 to 2 hours during surgery.

Prevent postoperative nausea and vomiting and encourage early resumption of diet and return to the previous insulin regimen.

IV = intravenous; NPO = nil per os.

VIII. OTHER ORGAN SYSTEMS

A. Renal disease has important implications for fluid and electrolyte management, as well as metabolism of drugs.

B. Liver disease is associated with altered protein binding and volume of distribution of drugs, as well as coagulation abnormalities (this may influence the choice of regional anesthesia).

C. Musculoskeletal disorders have been associated with an increased risk of malignant hyperthermia.

D. Osteoarthritis may result in difficulty exposing the glottic opening for tracheal intubation or difficulty in positioning the patient for regional anesthesia.

IX. PERIOPERATIVE LABORATORY TESTING

A. **The Value of Preoperative Testing: Normal Values**
   1. The vast majority of tests only increase or decrease the probability of disease.

2. To determine the clinical relevance, a test must be interpreted within the context of the clinical situation. (There is a high incidence of false-positive test results when tests are performed in normal patients.)

B. **Risks and Costs versus Benefits**
   1. The use of medical testing is associated with significant cost, both in real dollars and in potential harm to the patient.
   2. Even if testing better defines a disease state, the risks of any intervention based on the results may outweigh the benefit.

C. **Recommended Laboratory Testing** (Table 23-12)
   1. **Complete Blood Count and Hemoglobin Concentration.**
      a. The current recommendations of the National Blood Resource Education Committee is that a hemoglobin of 7 g/dL is acceptable in patients without systemic disease.
      b. In patients with systemic disease, signs of inadequate systemic oxygen delivery (tachycardia, tachypnea) are an indication for transfusion.
   2. **Electrolytes**
      a. The only consensus is the lack of routine testing in asymptomatic adults, although creatinine and glucose testing have been recommended in older patients.
      b. In patients with systemic diseases and those taking medications that affect the kidneys, blood urea nitrogen and creatinine testing are indicated.
   3. **Coagulation Studies**
      a. Patients with abnormal laboratory study results but without clinical abnormalities rarely have perioperative problems.
      b. A prothrombin and partial thromboplastin time analysis are indicated in the presence of previous bleeding disorders (after injuries; after tooth extraction or surgical procedures; and in patients with known or suspected liver disease, malabsorption or malnutrition, and taking certain medications such as antibiotics or chemotherapeutic agents).
   4. **Pregnancy Testing.** Regarding the need to routinely test women without a pregnancy history, current practice varies dramatically among centers and anesthesiologists and may be a function of the population served.

EVALUATION

TABLE 23-12

RECOMMENDED LABORATORY TESTING

Blood Count
Neonates
Physiologic age ≥75 yr
Class C procedure
Malignancy
Renal disease
Tobacco use
Anticoagulant use or bleeding
  disorder

Electrolytes
Renal disease
Diabetes
Diuretic, digoxin, or steroid
  use
CNS disease
Endocrine disorders

Blood Glucose
Physiologic age ≥75 yr
Diabetes
Steroid use
CNS disease

Electrocardiography
Physiologic age ≥75 yr
Class C procedure
Cardiovascular disease
Pulmonary disease
Radiation Therapy
Diabetes
Digoxin use
CNS disease

Coagulation Studies
Chemotherapy
Hepatic disease

Bleeding disorder
Anticoagulants

BUN and Creatinine
Physiologic age ≥75 yr
Class C procedure
Cardiovascular disease
Renal disease
Diabetes
Direct or digoxin use
CNS disease

Liver Function Tests
Hepatic disease
Hepatitis exposure
Malnutrition

Chest Radiography
Recent upper respiratory
  infection
Physiologic age ≥75 yr
Cardiovascular disease
Pulmonary disease
Malignancy
Radiation therapy
Tobacco ≥20 pack years

Pregnancy Test
Possible pregnancy

Albumin
Physiologic age ≥75 yr
Class C procedure
Malnutrition

CNS = central nervous system; BUN = blood urea nitrogen.

5. **Chest Radiography**
    a. Preoperative chest radiography may identify
       abnormalities that may lead to delay or cancella-
       tion of the planned surgical procedure or modifi-
       cation of perioperative care.

b. Routine testing in a population without risk factors can lead to more harm than benefit.

c. Preoperative chest radiography is indicated in patients with a history or clinical evidence of active pulmonary disease and may be indicated routinely only in patients with advanced age.

6. **Pulmonary function tests** can be divided into spirometry and an arterial blood gas (ABG) analysis.

a. With the advent of pulse oximetry, the use of preoperative ABG sampling has become less important.

b. A normal serum bicarbonate level virtually excludes the diagnosis of CO_2 retention.

X. PREOPERATIVE MEDICATION consists of psychological and pharmacologic preparation of patients before surgery. Ideally, all patients should enter the preoperative period free from apprehension, sedated but easily arousable, and fully cooperative.

A. **Psychological preparation** is provided by the preoperative visit and interview with the patient and family members serving as a nonpharmacologic antidote to apprehension (Table 23-13).

B. **Pharmacologic Preparation**

1. Drugs selected for preoperative medication are administered orally with up to 150 mL of water 1 to 2 hours before the anticipated induction of anesthesia. Drugs may be administered intramuscularly (IM)

EVALUATION

TABLE 23-13

AREAS TO BE DISCUSSED DURING A PREOPERATIVE INTERVIEW

Review the medical history with patient, including coexisting diseases, chronic drug therapy, and prior anesthetic experience.
Describe the anesthetic techniques available and their associated risks.
Review the planned preoperative medication and the time of the scheduled surgery.
Describe what to expect on arrival in the operating room.
Describe the anticipated duration of surgery and expected time to return to the room.
Describe methods available to manage postoperative pain, including patient-controlled analgesia and neuraxial opioids.

TABLE 23-14

GOALS FOR PREOPERATIVE MEDICATION

Relief of anxiety
Sedation
Amnesia
Analgesia
Drying of airway secretions
Prevention of autonomic reflex responses
Reduction of gastric fluid volume and increased pH
Antiemetic effects
Reduction of anesthetic requirements
Facilitation of smooth induction of anesthesia
Prophylaxis against allergic reactions

if the oral route of administration is not judged to be effective or possible. Alternatively, drugs may be administered intravenously (IV) in the immediate preoperative period.

2. **Various Goals for Pharmacologic Premedication** (Table 23-14)
3. **Determinant of Drug Choice and Dose** (Table 23-15)
4. Several classes of drugs are available to facilitate achievement of the desired individual goals for pharmacologic premedication (Table 23-16).
5. There is no best drug or drug combination for preoperative medication.
    a. The choice may be influenced by tradition and the anesthesiologist's previous experience.
    b. Timing of drug delivery is as important as drug selection.

TABLE 23-15

DETERMINANT OF DRUG CHOICE AND DOSE

Patient age and weight
ASA physical status classification
Level of anxiety
Tolerance for depressant drugs
Prior adverse experiences with premedication
Drug allergies
Elective versus emergency surgery
Inpatient versus outpatient

ASA = American Society of Anesthesiologists.

TABLE 23-16

DRUGS USED FOR PHARMACOLOGIC PREMEDICATION

Drug	Route of Administration	Adult Dose (mg)
Lorazepam	PO, IV	0.5–4.0
Midazolam	PO (children)	0.5 mg/kg
	IV	1.0–2.5
Fentanyl	IV	25–100 µg
Morphine	IV	1.0–2.5
Meperidine	IV	10–25
Cimetidine	PO, IV	150–300
Ranitidine	PO	50–200
Metoclopramide	IV	5–10
Atropine	IV	0.3–0.4
Glycopyrrolate	IV	0.1–0.2
Scopolamine	IV	0.1–0.4

IV = intravenous; PO = per os.

6. Ideally, the specific drugs selected are based on the goals of premedication balanced against the potential undesirable effects these drugs may produce. It is important to recognize that some patients (e.g., elderly patients and those with decreased level of consciousness, intracranial hypertension, severe pulmonary disease, or profound hypovolemia) may not need or should not receive depressant drugs for preoperative medication.

7. **Benzodiazepines** act on specific brain receptors (γ-aminobutyric acid) to produce selective antianxiety effects at doses that do not produce excessive sedation, depression of ventilation, or adverse cardiac effects.

   a. **Lorazepam** produces intense amnesia, but sedation and prolonged duration of action detract from its use for short surgical procedures and in outpatients. Peak effects after oral administration may not occur for 2 to 4 hours.

   b. **Midazolam** has replaced diazepam in its use for preoperative medication and conscious sedation. An oral form of midazolam is particularly useful for preoperative medication in children. The incidence of side effects after administration of midazolam is low, although depression of ventilation and sedation may be greater than expected, especially in elderly patients and when the drug is combined with other central nervous system depressants. The onset after IV administration of midazolam is in 1 to 2 minutes, and recovery occurs rapidly, reflecting this drug's poor lipid solubility and rapid distribution to peripheral receptors compared with diazepam. Furthermore, the metabolites of midazolam are not likely to be pharmacologically active. For all these reasons, midazolam should usually be administered within 1 hour of induction of anesthesia.

8. **Opioids** are used for preoperative medication when there is a need to provide analgesia, such as before institution of a regional anesthetic or when patients have pain owing to their surgical disease. Anesthesiologists often use a combination of an opioid, benzodiazepine, and scopolamine for preoperative medication in patients who are likely to be unusually apprehensive, as before cardiac surgery or cancer surgery. Administration of opioids has the potential to produce multiple side effects, which may be exaggerated when other depressant drugs are also included in the preoperative medication (Table 23-17).

   a. **Morphine** produces peak effects within 45 to 90 minutes after IM injection. Inclusion of morphine in the preoperative medication decreases the likelihood that undesirable increases in heart rate will accompany surgical stimulation.

   b. **Meperidine** is often administered in combination with promethazine. Peak effects after IM injection of meperidine may be unpredictable.

TABLE 23-17

SIDE EFFECTS OF OPIOIDS AS USED FOR PHARMACOLOGIC PREMEDICATION

Depression of ventilation
Nausea and vomiting
Synergistic effects, especially when administered with
  benzodiazepines
Orthostatic hypotension
Delayed gastric emptying
Pruritus
Choledochoduodenal sphincter spasm

TABLE 23-18

SUMMARY OF FASTING RECOMMENDATIONS TO REDUCE THE
RISK OF PULMONARY ASPIRATION*

Ingested Material	Minimum Fasting Period (Applied to All Ages) (hours)
Clear liquids (water, fruit juice without pulp, carbonated beverages, clear tea, black coffee)	2
Breast milk	4
Infant formula	6
Non-human milk	6
Light meal (toast and clear liquids)	6

*These recommendations apply only to healthy patients who are undergoing
elective procedures and are not intended for women in labor. Following these
guidelines does not guarantee complete gastric emptying.

  c. **Fentanyl** (which is 75 to 125 times more potent
     than morphine as an analgesic) may be administered IV to provide a rapid onset of preoperative
     analgesia.
C. **Gastric Fluid pH and Volume**
  1. Despite the predictable presence of acidic fluid in the
     stomach at the time of induction of anesthesia, clinically significant pulmonary aspiration of gastric fluid
     is rare in healthy patients undergoing elective
     surgery. The ASA has adopted guidelines for preoperative fasting (Table 23-18).
    a. Maintenance of a patent airway is more important than routine pharmacologic prophylaxis in
       otherwise healthy patients undergoing elective
       surgery.
    b. Ingestion of clear fluids in the 2 hours preceding
       the induction of anesthesia does not increase gastric fluid volume. Patients who are permitted to
       ingest clear fluids before surgery are more comfortable than those who have fasted. Under no
       circumstances are solid foods permitted in the
       period preceding induction of anesthesia for elective surgery.
  2. **Drugs Used to Decrease Gastric Fluid Volume and
     Increase Gastric Fluid pH** (Table 23-19)
D. **Antiemetics** may be administered in the preoperative
   or intraoperative period as prophylaxis against

TABLE 23-19

DRUGS USED TO DECREASE GASTRIC FLUID VOLUME AND INCREASE GASTRIC FLUID pH

Anticholinergics (do not reliably increase gastric fluid pH at clinical doses and may relax the lower esophageal sphincter, making gastroesophageal reflux more likely)

H_2-receptor antagonists (not 100% effective in increasing gastric fluid pH)

    Cimetidine (inhibits mixed-function oxidase enzyme systems and decreases hepatic blood flow, which may prolong the elimination half-time of some drugs)

    Ranitidine (more potent and longer lasting than cimetidine)

    Famotidine (has the longest duration of action of all H_2-receptor antagonists)

Antacids (nonparticulate antacids are recommended to decrease the risk of pulmonary reaction if the antacid is inhaled; in contrast to H_2-receptor antagonists, there is no lag time before gastric fluid pH is increased)

Omeprazole (increases gastric fluid pH by blocking secretion of hydrogen ions by parietal cells)

Gastrokinetic agents

    Metoclopramide (onset in 30–60 minutes after oral administration and 3–5 minutes after IV administration; gastric emptying effects may be offset by opioids, anticholinergics, or antacids)

IV = intravenous.

postoperative nausea and vomiting, especially in patients considered to be at increased risk for this complication (history of vomiting, obesity, ophthalmologic or gynecologic surgery) (Table 23-20).

E. **Anticholinergics**

1. Routine inclusion of anticholinergics as part of the pharmacologic premedication is not mandatory but

TABLE 23-20

ANTIEMETICS USED TO PREVENT OR TREAT POSTOPERATIVE NAUSEA AND VOMITING

Droperidol (sedation and dysphoria may be side effects; inexpensive; its use is limited by rare risk of prolongation of the QTc interval)

Possibly metoclopramide

Transdermal scopolamine patch (should be applied several hours before induction of anesthesia)

Ondansetron or granisetron

TABLE 23-21

COMPARATIVE EFFECTS OF ANTICHOLINERGICS*

	Atropine	Scopolamine	Glycopyrrolate
Antisialagogue effect	+	+++	++
Sedative and amnesic effects	+	+++	0
Central nervous system toxicity	+	++	0
Relaxation of gastroesophageal sphincter	++	++	++
Mydriasis and cycloplegia	+	++	0
Increased heart rate	+++	+	++

*Intravenous administration.
0 = none; + = mild; ++ = moderate; +++ = marked.

should be individualized based on the patient's needs and the pharmacology of the anticholinergic (Table 23-21).

   2. **Indications for Anticholinergics** (Table 23-22)

   3. **Side Effects of Anticholinergic Drugs** (Table 23-23)

F. **Adrenergic Agonists**

   1. Clonidine (5 mg/kg orally as preoperative medication) produces sedation, decreases the anesthetic requirements for inhaled and injected drugs, and attenuates the sympathetic nervous system response (hypertension, tachycardia, catecholamine release) to tracheal intubation.

   2. Dexmedetomidine is a more selective α-adrenergic agonist than clonidine that has also been used for preoperative medication.

TABLE 23-22

INDICATIONS FOR ANTICHOLINERGICS

Antisialagogue effect (not necessary when regional anesthesia planned)

Sedation and amnesia (doses should be decreased in elderly patients; scopolamine is the most effective)

Vagolytic action (IM administration is not as effective as IV injection just before the anticipated vagal stimulus)

IM = intramuscular; IV = intravenous.

TABLE 23-23

SIDE EFFECTS OF ANTICHOLINERGIC DRUGS

Central nervous system toxicity (restlessness and confusion, especially in elderly patients; this is unlikely with glycopyrrolate because it minimally crosses the blood–brain barrier)
Relaxation of the lower esophageal sphincter (may not be clinically significant)
Mydriasis and cycloplegia (miotic eye drops should be continued in patients with glaucoma)
Increased physiologic dead space
Drying of airway secretions
Interference with sweating (an important consideration in febrile patients, especially children)
Increased heart rate (unlikely after IM administration)

IM = intramuscular.

3. Side effects (hypotension, bradycardia, dry mouth) limit the usefulness of these drugs for preoperative medication.
G. **Other Drugs Given with Preoperative Medication** (Table 23-24)
H. **Differences in Preoperative Medication Between Pediatric and Adult Patients**
1. Children differ from adults regarding preoperative medication in terms of psychological preparation,

TABLE 23-24

OTHER DRUGS GIVEN WITH PREOPERATIVE MEDICATION

Beta-blockers (patients with known or suspected CAD may be protected; the goal is to achieve a heart rate of 50–70 bpm and systolic blood pressure <110 mm Hg)
Statins (may protect patients with CAD; they should be continued in the perioperative period if the patient is being treated preoperatively)
Antibiotics (these should be administered 1 hour before incision [2 hours for vancomycin]; if a tourniquet is used, they should be administered before cuff inflation; they may potentiate neuromuscular blocking drugs)
Steroids (history of hypoadrenocorticism or treatment of nonadrenal diseases)
Insulin

CAD = coronary artery disease.

greater use of oral medications, and more frequent use of anticholinergics to reduce vagal activity.

2. **Psychological Factors in Pediatric Patients**
   a. Age is probably the most important factor in the success of a preoperative visit and interview.
   b. Children who do not ask questions or appear disinterested during the preoperative interview may be masking a high level of anxiety.
   c. Some children wish to take an active part in the induction of anesthesia. In this regard, it may be helpful to have the parents accompany these children to the operating room.

3. **Differences in Pharmacologic Preparation**
   a. Use of pharmacologic premedication in children older than age 6 months is controversial and has not been proven to decrease unwanted psychological outcomes. More important in avoiding long-lasting psychological problems is a pleasant induction of anesthesia.
   b. Oral administration (often midazolam in a flavored liquid) is preferred to IM injections in children.
   c. Some anesthesiologists prefer to administer atropine IM or IV just before the induction of anesthesia to protect against vagal reflexes in response to airway manipulations.

EVALUATION

CHAPTER 24 ■ MALIGNANT HYPERTHERMIA AND OTHER INHERITED DISORDERS

Malignant hyperthermia (MH) or malignant hyperpyrexia is perhaps the most significant inherited disorder triggered by exposure to anesthetic drugs (Rosenberg H, Brandom BWD, Sambuughin S: Malignant hyperthermia and other inherited disorders. In *Clinical Anesthesia*. Edited by Barash PG, Cullen BF, Stoelting RK, Cahalan MK, Stock MC. Philadelphia: Lippincott Williams & Wilkins, 2009, pp 598–621).

I. MALIGNANT HYPERTHERMIA

A. **Historical Aspects.** MH was first formally described in 1960, and a clinically useful test for MH with limited sensitivity was introduced in 2003. Some deaths formerly attributed to MH were actually the result of destruction of muscle cells that occurred during anesthesia with volatile anesthetics and succinylcholine (Sch) in patients with unrecognized dystrophinopathies (Duchenne and Becker muscular dystrophy).

B. **Clinical Presentation**
   1. MH is a hypermetabolic disorder of skeletal muscle that may or may not have a heritable component.
   2. An important pathophysiologic process in this disorder is intracellular hypercalcemia, which activates metabolic pathways, resulting in adenosine triphosphate depletion, acidosis, membrane destruction, and cell death.

C. **Classic Malignant Hyperthermia**
   1. The first manifestations of this syndrome most often occur in the operating room but may also occur within the first few hours of recovery from anesthesia (Table 24-1).
   2. Sch may accelerate the onset of MH (entire course over 5–10 minutes) in some patients; in others, a

TABLE 24-1

MANIFESTATIONS OF MALIGNANT HYPERTHERMIA

Hypercarbia (reflects hypermetabolism and is responsible for
  many of the signs of sympathetic nervous system stimulation;
  this may be masked by hyperventilation of the patient's lungs)
Tachycardia
Tachypnea
Temperature increase (1°–2°C increase every 5 minutes)
Hypertension
Cardiac dysrhythmias
Acidosis
Arterial hypoxemia
Hyperkalemia
Skeletal muscle activity
Myoglobinuria

volatile anesthetic plus Sch is necessary to trigger the
response. Some susceptible patients may develop MH
despite multiple prior uneventful exposures to triggering drugs.

3. Even with successful treatment, patients with MH are
   at risk for myoglobinuric renal failure and disseminated intravascular coagulation. Creatine kinase
   (CK) levels may exceed 20,000 U in the first 12 to
   24 hours. Increased CK may not be present if the
   syndrome is detected promptly and treatment
   instituted. Recrudescence of the syndrome may
   occur in the first 24 to 36 hours.

D. **Masseter Muscle Rigidity** (Table 24-2)
   1. Rigidity of the jaw muscles after administration of
      Sch is referred to as masseter muscle rigidity (MMR)
      or masseter spasm. Although MMR probably occurs
      in patients of all ages, it is more common in children
      and young adults. Repeat doses of Sch or nondepolar-
      izing relaxants do not relieve MMR (peripheral nerve
      stimulator reveals flaccid paralysis).

TABLE 24-2

EVENTS THAT MIMIC MASSETER SPASM

Inadequate dose of succinylcholine
Inadequate time for onset of action of succinylcholine
Temporomandibular joint dysfunction
Myotonic syndrome

EVALUATION

TABLE 24-3

RECOMMENDATIONS FOR MANAGEMENT OF MASSETER MUSCLE RIGIDITY

Discontinue the anesthetic and postpone surgery or continue with a nontriggering anesthetic using end-tidal CO_2 monitoring with the availability of dantrolene.

Give dantrolene if generalized rigidity and signs of hypermetabolism.

After event, admit the patient for 12 to 24 hours and monitor for myoglobinuria. Consider administration of dantrolene 1 to 2 mg/kg.

Inform the patient's family of the event and its potential implication.

Monitor CK levels at 6, 12, and 24 hours.

If CK is above 20,000 IU and a concomitant myopathy is not present, the diagnosis of MH is likely.

If contracture test results are normal, it is not recommended that family members be tested, but succinylcholine should be avoided.

CK = creatine kinase.

2. If the anesthetic is continued with a triggering agent, the initial signs of MH most commonly appear in 20 minutes or more. Conversely, if the anesthetic is discontinued, the patient appears to recover uneventfully.

3. **Recommendations for Management of MMR** (Table 24-3)

E. **Variations in Presentation of Malignant Hyperthermia** (Table 24-4)

TABLE 24-4

VARIATIONS IN THE PRESENTATION OF MALIGNANT HYPERTHERMIA

Multiple prior uneventful anesthetics

Present several hours postoperatively

Rigidity may not be present

Temperature increase may be unimpressive

Postoperative myoglobinuria may be the only sign (succinylcholine-induced rhabdomyolysis should be ruled out in patients with skeletal muscle disorders and patients taking cholesterol inhibitors)

F. **Myodystrophies Exacerbated by Anesthesia**
   1. **Duchene muscular dystrophy** occurs in one in 3000 males. Boys are usually asymptomatic until the age of 4 or 5 years, but elevated CK is present from birth. Hyperkalemia and cardiac arrest may occur after the administration of Sch. Because of potentially fatal hyperkalemia in patients with undiagnosed myopathy, Sch should not be used routinely in children and young adolescents (patients with airway emergencies and full stomachs are exceptions).
   2. **Congenital myopathies** (central core disease) is often characterized by weakness of the spine and pelvis and may include foot deformities. There is a risk of MH in these patients.
   3. **Myotonias and periodic paralyses** are caused by point mutations in an ion channel. Muscle contractures occur in response to the administration of Sch.
G. **Syndromes with a Clinical Resemblance to Malignant Hyperthermia** (Table 24-5)
H. **Malignant Hyperthermia Outside the Operating Room.** Exercise-induced rhabdomyolysis may occur in patients with myopathies with or without exposure to myotoxic drugs (cholesterol-lowering drugs).
I. **Neuroleptic Malignant Syndrome and Other Drug-Induced Hyperthermic Reactions**
   1. Neuroleptic malignant syndrome may mimic MH (dantrolene may be effective). Unlike MH, this syndrome is associated with prolonged drug therapy with psychoactive drugs (phenothiazines or haloperidol) or sudden withdrawal of drugs used to treat Parkinson's disease. Bromocriptine (a dopamine agonist) is useful in treatment, suggesting that this syndrome may reflect depletion of central nervous system dopamine stores by psychoactive drugs.

EVALUATION

TABLE 24-5

SYNDROMES WITH A CLINICAL RESEMBLANCE TO MALIGNANT HYPERTHERMIA

Pheochromocytoma
Thyrotoxicosis
Sepsis
Hypoxic encephalopathy
Mitochondrial myopathies (avoid succinylcholine)

TABLE 24-6

DRUGS THAT MAY OR MAY NOT TRIGGER
MALIGNANT HYPERTHERMIA

Unsafe Drugs	
Succinylcholine	Volatile anesthetics

Safe Drugs	
Antibiotics	Antihistamines
Antipyretics	Vasoactive drugs
Barbiturates	Benzodiazepines
Droperidol	Ketamine (inherent circulatory effects may mimic malignant hyperthermia)
Propofol	Nitrous oxide
Local anesthetics	Propranolol
Opioids	Nondepolarizing neuromuscular blocking drugs

    a. From an anesthesiologist's point of view, it is best to treat patients with neuroleptic malignant syndrome as though they are susceptible to MH.

    b. The recommendation is to conduct electroconvulsive therapy without the use of Sch or other triggering drugs.

  2. Similar signs have been observed in some patients taking serotonin uptake inhibitors.

J. Drugs That Trigger Malignant Hyperthermia (Table 24-6)

K. Incidence and Epidemiology

  1. A better understanding of the prevalence of MH is being provided by use of molecular genetics for the diagnosis of MH susceptibility.

  2. Although the incidence of reported cases of MH has increased, the mortality rate from MH has declined (<5%), reflecting both a greater awareness of the syndrome and earlier diagnosis followed by better treatment.

L. Diagnostic Tests for Malignant Hyperthermia

  1. Halothane–Caffeine Contracture Test

    a. Although several tests have been described, this test remains the standard (100% sensitivity).

    b. Skeletal muscle biopsy specimens (usually vastus lateralis) are bathed in a solution containing 1.5% to 3% halothane plus caffeine or either drug alone. A response indicative of MH susceptibility is based on a previously established contracture threshold.

2. **Other Agents Used in Contracture Tests**
   a. **Ryanodine.** This test was based on the premise that a defect in the ryanodine receptor (calcium release channel of skeletal muscle) was the only cause of MH that would afford maximum specificity (premise no longer valid).
   b. **4-Chloro-m-cresol** is a potent activator of ryanodine receptor-mediated calcium release. Contractures occur in 100% of skeletal muscles from patients who are MH susceptible.
3. **Pitfalls of the Contracture Test**
   a. Because of the variation in the presentation of MH, it may not be possible to achieve agreement on the status of a patient based on clinical history.
   b. MH trigger agents should be avoided if a patient has a positive contracture test result.
4. **Tests with More Limited Usefulness in Malignant Hyperthermia Diagnosis**
   a. Use of resting CK levels for screening for MH is neither sensitive nor specific, but a relationship exists between postoperative CK levels associated with MMR and the probability of a positive contracture test result.
   b. Elevated CK levels may be useful in identifying family members to be referred for contracture testing and in identifying MH in children who are too young to undergo contracture testing.
5. **Clinical Diagnosis of Malignant Hyperthermia: The Grading Scale** (Table 24-7).
6. **Molecular Genetic Testing for Malignant Hyperthermia Susceptibility**
   a. Multiple mutations on the *RYR1* gene and mutations in other genes have been shown to be causal for MH.
   b. Ultimately, genetic testing is likely to replace more invasive diagnostic tests.
   c. The presence of a ryanodine mutation predicts MH susceptibility.
M. **Treatment of Malignant Hyperthermia.** MH is a treatable disorder that should have a mortality near zero when recognized early and treated promptly. All institutions in which anesthetic drugs are administered (hospitals, ambulatory surgery facilities, doctors' offices) should have **dantrolene** available (36 ampoules [720 mg])

EVALUATION

TABLE 24-7

CRITERIA USED IN THE MALIGNANT HYPERTHERMIA CLINICAL
GRADING SCALE*

Process 1: Muscle Rigidity	
Generalized rigidity	15
Masseter rigidity	15
Process II: Myonecrosis	
Elevated CK >20,000 (after succinylcholine administration)	15
Elevated CK >10,000 (without succinylcholine)	15
Cola-colored urine	10
Myoglobin in urine >60 μg/mL	5
Serum potassium >6 mEq/L	3
Process III: Respiratory Acidosis	
End-tidal CO_2 >55 mm Hg with controlled ventilation	15
$PaCO_2$ >60 mm Hg with controlled ventilation	15
End-tidal CO_2 >60 mm Hg with spontaneous ventilation	15
Inappropriate hypercarbia	15
Inappropriate tachypnea	10
Process IV: Temperature Increase	
Rapid increase in temperature	15
Inappropriate temperature (>38°C) in perioperative period	10
Process V: Cardiac Involvement	
Inappropriate tachycardia	3
Ventricular tachycardia or fibrillation	3

*A total of 50 points (termed "D6") is almost certainly a case of MH.
A total of 35 to 49 points (termed "D5") is very likely a case of MH.
CK = creatine kinase.

and an established management plan in place (see inside
back cover for a malignant hyperthermia protocol).
1. **Acute Episode** (Table 24-8)
2. **Management After an Acute Episode** (Table 24-9)
3. **Dantrolene**
   a. This drug acts in skeletal muscle cells to decrease
   intracellular levels of calcium, most likely by
   decreasing sarcoplasmic reticulum release or
   inhibiting excitation–contracture coupling at the
   transverse tubular level.
   b. **Therapeutic levels** of dantrolene (2.5 mg/mL) usually persist for 4 to 6 hours after an intravenous
   (IV) dose of 2.5 mg/kg. (This is a reason to supplement every 4 hours.)

TABLE 24-8

MANAGEMENT OF THE ACUTE EPISODE OF
MALIGNANT HYPERTHERMIA

Discontinue inhaled anesthetics and succinylcholine.

Hyperventilate the lungs with oxygen at 10 L/min (this hastens purging of residual anesthetic gases).

Use an Ambu bag and E cylinder (do not spend time replacing anesthesia machine).

Administer dantrolene (2.5 mg/kg IV) with repeated doses (2–3 mg/kg is often sufficient but may require >10 mg/kg) based on $PaCO_2$, heart rate, and body temperature.

Place a bladder catheter (each 20 mg of dantrolene contains 300 mg of mannitol).

Treat persistent acidosis with sodium bicarbonate (1–2 mEq/kg IV).

Control body temperature (gastric lavage, external ice packs until the patient's temperature is 38°C).

Monitor with capnography (best clinical measurement to guide therapy) and arterial blood gases.

Be prepared to treat hyperkalemia (glucose, insulin, hyperventilation, calcium) and cardiac dysrhythmias (avoid verapamil; lidocaine is acceptable).

Obtain baseline laboratory tests (creatinine, coagulation studies, CK [increases may not occur for 6 to 12 hours], liver function tests, myoglobin levels).

CK = creatine kinase.

EVALUATION

      c. **Prophylaxis** for MH should be carried out with IV or oral dantrolene (5 mg/kg).

    4. **Management of Patients Susceptible to Malignant Hyperthermia** (Table 24-10)

      a. There have been no deaths from MH in previously diagnosed MH-susceptible patients when the

TABLE 24-9

MANAGEMENT OF MALIGNANT HYPERTHERMIA AFTER AN
ACUTE EPISODE

Continue dantrolene (1–2 mg/kg IV) every 6 hours for at least 24 to 36 hours.

Anticipate complications.

  Recrudescence

  Disseminated intravascular coagulation

  Myoglobinuric renal failure (alkalinize urine if acidic and administer mannitol to facilitate excretion of myoglobin)

  Skeletal muscle weakness

  Electrolyte abnormalities

TABLE 24-10

MANAGEMENT OF MALIGNANT HYPERTHERMIA-SUSCEPTIBLE PATIENTS

Administer the standard preoperative medication.

Administer dantrolene (2.5 mg/kg IV) 15–30 minutes before induction of anesthesia.

Clean the anesthesia machine (disposable circuit, new soda lime, drain vaporizers, oxygen flow 10 L/min for 10 minutes or longer to flush the system).

Modern anesthesia workstations are larger than traditional anesthesia machines (it may require more than 10 minutes to purge inhalational agents).

Capnography (increased end-tidal CO_2 concentration is the earliest sign of malignant hyperthermia).

Monitor body temperature.

Use nontriggering drugs and techniques (regional if possible).

Closely observe the patient after surgery (routine administration of dantrolene is not indicated in the absence of signs of malignant hyperthermia).

Rehydration (decreases chance that fever caused by dehydration will occur).

anesthesiologist was prospectively aware of the problem. This information is useful to allay the patient's preoperative anxiety.

   b. Dantrolene need not be repeated after the anesthetic is terminated if there were no signs of MH during surgery.

   c. In MH-susceptible parturients, an acceptable approach to management of routine labor is epidural analgesia without dantrolene pretreatment and close monitoring of vital signs. If general anesthesia is necessary for delivery, an acceptable approach is to administer dantrolene IV and use nontriggering drugs. No adverse fetal effects of dantrolene have been observed.

II. DISORDERS OF PLASMA CHOLINESTERASE

A. Succinylcholine-Related Apnea

1. Hydrolysis of Sch by plasma cholinesterase is slowed to absent in patients with inherited alterations on the gene locus responsible for production of this enzyme by the liver (Table 24-11).

TABLE 24-11

GENOTYPES FOR PLASMA CHOLINESTERASE ENZYME

Genotype	Dibucaine Number	Fluoride Number	Cholinesterase Activity	Response to Succinylcholine	Incidence
EuEu	78–86	55–65	Normal	Normal	96%
EaEa	18–26	16–32	Decreased	Greatly prolonged	1 in 2000
EuEa	51–70	38–55	Intermediate	Slightly prolonged	1in 25
EuEf	74–80	47–48	Intermediate	Slightly prolonged	1 in 200
EfEa	49–59	25–33	Intermediate	Greatly prolonged	1 in 20,000
EfEs	63	26	Decreased	Moderately prolonged	1 in 150,000

      a. When there is a question about the rate of hydrolysis of Sch, the plasma cholinesterase activity as well as dibucaine and fluoride numbers should be measured.

      b. Patients who are homozygous for atypical cholinesterase enzyme should wear Medic-Alert bracelets indicating that Sch will result in prolonged apnea (often longer than 2 hours).

  2. Depression of plasma cholinesterase activity in the absence of atypical genotypes can be seen after administration of anticholinesterase drugs or plasmapheresis and in the presence of advanced liver disease (Table 24-12). This usually results in only moderate prolongation of Sch-induced skeletal muscle paralysis (rarely longer than 30 minutes).

  3. **Treatment of Succinylcholine Apnea**

      a. The safest course of treatment after a patient fails to breathe spontaneously within 10 to 15 minutes after Sch administration is to continue mechanical ventilation of the patient's lungs until adequate skeletal muscle strength has returned.

      b. The use of anticholinesterase drugs in treating patients with Sch apnea is controversial.

B. **Plasma Cholinesterase Abnormalities and the Metabolism of Local Anesthetics**

  1. Ester local anesthetics are metabolized by plasma cholinesterase.

  2. Despite the theoretical argument that the action of these drugs might be prolonged, there is evidence that the response of homozygous atypical patients is usually normal.

III. PORPHYRIAS

A. These inherited defects of heme synthesis can mimic surgical diseases and may be provoked by administration of certain drugs (Table 24-13).

B. **Management of Patients with Porphyria**

  1. Triggering drugs (barbiturates, perhaps benzodiazepines and ketamine) should be avoided. Nontriggering drugs include propofol, nitrous oxide, volatile anesthetics, opioids, and muscle relaxants. Regional anesthesia may be avoided to prevent confusion if neurologic changes occur postoperatively.

TABLE 24-12

CAUSES OF CHANGES IN CHOLINESTERASE ACTIVITY

Inherited
Cholinesterase variants (silent gene, C5 variant)

Physiologic
Decreases in last trimester of pregnancy
Decreases in newborn

Acquired Decreases
Liver disease
Cancer
Debilitating diseases
Collagen diseases
Uremia
Malnutrition
Myxedema

Acquired Increases
Obesity
Alcoholism
Thyrotoxicosis
Nephrosis
Psoriasis
Electroshock therapy

Drug-Related Decreases
Echothiophate iodide
Anticholinesterases
Chlorpromazine
Cyclophosphamide
Monoamine oxidase inhibitors
Pancuronium
Contraceptives
Organophosphate insecticides
Hexafluorenium

Other Causes of Decreased Activity
Plasmapheresis
Extracorporeal circulation
Tetanus
Radiation therapy
Burns

EVALUATION

TABLE 24-13

MANIFESTATIONS OF PORPHYRIA

Abdominal pain
Fever
Vomiting
Confusion
Tachycardia
Seizures
Hypertension
Somnolence
Neuropathy

   2. Glucose infusions are important in prevention (starvation can induce an attack) and treatment of porphyria.

IV. GLYCOGEN STORAGE DISEASES

   A. These inherited diseases are characterized by dysfunction of one of the many enzymes involved in glucose metabolism.
   B. Associated problems that may influence anesthetic management include hypoglycemia, acidosis, and cardiac and hepatic dysfunction.

V. OSTEOGENESIS IMPERFECTA occurs in

approximately one in 50,000 births. Minor trauma can lead to fractures, and airway management may be difficult because of cervical spine involvement. Inhalation anesthetics have been administered to many of these patients without complications of MH.

CHAPTER 25 ■ **RARE AND COEXISTING DISEASES**

A variety of rare disorders may influence the selection and conduct of anesthesia (Table 25-1) (Dierdorf SF, Walton JS: Anesthesia for patients with rare coexisting diseases. In *Clinical Anesthesia*. Edited by Barash PG, Cullen BF, Stoelting RK, Cahalan MK, Stock MC. Philadelphia: Lippincott Williams & Wilkins, 2009, pp 622–643). Anesthesiologists must periodically update their diagnostic skills and clinical knowledge to recognize when additional evaluation or treatment may be required and how these diseases influence the management of anesthesia.

I. MUSCULOSKELETAL DISEASES are characterized by a progressive loss of skeletal muscle function. (Cardiac and smooth muscle are also affected.)

A. **Duchenne's muscular dystrophy** is caused by a lack of production of dystrophin, a major component of the skeleton of the muscle membrane characterized by painless degeneration and atrophy of skeletal muscle.
   1. The genetic defect is sex linked (manifests only in males), and symptoms manifest between 2 and 5 years of age (creatine kinase may be increased before symptoms appear). Death is usually secondary to congestive heart failure or pneumonia.
   2. Axial skeletal muscle imbalance produces **kyphoscoliosis,** which often requires surgical correction.
   3. Involvement of cardiac muscle is reflected by a progressive loss of the R-wave amplitude on the lateral precordial leads of the electrocardiogram (ECG). Routine echocardiography can provide important information about cardiac function. Progressive loss of myocardial tissue results in cardiomyopathy, ventricular dysrhythmias, and mitral regurgitation.

TABLE 25-1

COEXISTING DISEASES THAT INFLUENCE
ANESTHESIA MANAGEMENT

Musculoskeletal	**Anemias**
Muscular dystrophy	Nutritional deficiency
Myotonic dystrophy	Hemolytic
Myasthenia gravis	Hemoglobinopathies
Myasthenic syndrome	Thalassemias
Familial periodic paralysis	
Guillain-Barré syndrome	**Collagen Vascular**
	Rheumatoid arthritis
Central Nervous System	Systemic lupus erythematosus
Multiple sclerosis	Scleroderma
Epilepsy	Polymyositis
Parkinson's disease	
Alzheimer's disease	**Skin**
Amyotrophic lateral sclerosis	Epidermolysis bullosa
Creutzfeldt-Jakob disease	Pemphigus

4. Treatment of cardiac dysfunction includes angiotensin-converting enzyme inhibitors, beta-adrenergic blockers, and dysrhythmia surveillance.

5. Degeneration of respiratory muscles (reflected by spirometry) results in an ineffective cough with retention of secretions and pneumonia.

6. **Management of Anesthesia.** Significant complications from anesthesia in patients with muscular dystrophy are secondary to the effects of anesthetic drugs on myocardial and skeletal muscle.

   a. Reports of cardiac arrest associated with rhabdomyolysis and hyperkalemia have occurred with volatile anesthetics alone or in combination with succinylcholine (Sch).

   b. Susceptibility to malignant hyperthermia is unpredictable.

   c. It may be prudent to use intravenous anesthetics and avoid volatile anesthetics and Sch for patients with muscular dystrophy.

   d. Degeneration of gastrointestinal smooth muscle with hypomotility of the intestinal tract and delayed gastric emptying in conjunction with impaired swallowing mechanisms may increase the risk of perioperative aspiration.

B. **THE MYOTONIAS** are characterized by delayed relaxation of skeletal muscle after voluntary contraction owing to dysfunction of ion channels in the muscle membrane.

1. Clinical features include diabetes mellitus, thyroid dysfunction, adrenal insufficiency, and cardiac abnormalities (conduction delays, heart block [sudden death], tachydysrhythmias, cardiomyopathy).

2. Pulmonary function studies demonstrate a restrictive lung disease pattern, mild arterial hypoxemia, and diminished ventilatory responses to hypoxia and hypercapnia.

3. Pregnancy may produce an exacerbation of myotonic dystrophy, and congestive heart failure is more likely to occur during pregnancy.

4. **Management of Anesthesia**

   a. Sch produces myotonia and should not be administered to these patients. The response of these patients to nondepolarizing muscle relaxants may be enhanced. Reversal with neostigmine may provoke myotonia. The response to the peripheral nerve stimulator must be carefully interpreted because muscle stimulation may produce myotonia (misinterpreted as sustained tetanus when significant neuromuscular block still exists).

   b. Patients with myotonia are very sensitive to the ventilatory depressant effects of opioids, barbiturates, benzodiazepines, and volatile anesthetics.

   c. No specific anesthetic technique has been shown to be superior for patients with myotonic dystrophy. Propofol infusions may be acceptable. Inhaled anesthetics may be used, but close monitoring of cardiac rhythm and cardiovascular function is indicated.

C. **Familial Periodic Paralysis.** The familial periodic paralyses are a subgroup of diseases referred to as skeletal muscle channelopathies. The common mechanism for these diseases appears to be a persistent sodium inward current depolarization causing muscle membrane inexcitability and subsequent muscle weakness (Table 25-2).

   1. **Hyperkalemic periodic paralysis** is characterized by episodes of myotonia and muscle weakness that may last for hours after exposure to a trigger (Table 25-2).

   2. **Hypokalemic periodic paralysis** is caused by a defect in the calcium ion channel (Table 25-2).

TABLE 25-2
CLINICAL FEATURES OF FAMILIAL PERIODIC PARALYSIS

Hyperkalemic
Sodium channel defect
Potassium level normal or >5.5 mEq/L during symptoms
Rest after exercise
Potassium infusions
Metabolic acidosis
Hypothermia
Skeletal muscle weakness may be localized to the tongue and
  eyelids

Hypokalemic
Calcium channel defect
Potassium level <3 mEq/L during symptoms
Large glucose meals
Strenuous exercise
Glucose-insulin infusions
Stress
Hypothermia
Chronic myopathy with aging

3. **Management of Anesthesia**
   a. The primary goal of the perioperative management of patients with both forms of periodic paralysis is the maintenance of normal potassium levels and avoidance of events that precipitate muscle weakness (alkalosis owing to hyperventilation, carbohydrate loads, hypothermia).
   b. Short-acting muscle relaxants are preferred, and the response should be monitored with a peripheral nerve stimulator. Sch should be avoided because it may enhance potassium release from skeletal muscle cells.
   c. The ECG should be monitored for evidence of hypokalemia and associated cardiac dysrhythmias (serum potassium concentration should be measured during prolonged operations).
   d. Avoidance of carbohydrate loads, hypothermia, and excessive hyperventilation is prudent.

D. **Myasthenia gravis** is an autoimmune disease with antibodies directed against the nicotinic acetylcholine receptor or other muscle membrane proteins (Table 25-3). The majority of patients have abnormalities of the thymus (thymoma, thymic hyperplasia, thymic atrophy).

TABLE 25-3

SUMMARY OF THE DIFFERENT PRESENTATIONS OF MYASTHENIA GRAVIS

	Etiology	Onset (y)	Gender	Thymus	Course
Neonatal myasthenia	Passage of antibodies from myasthenic mother across the placenta	Neonatal	Both genders	Normal	Transient
Congenital myasthenia	Congenital endplate pathology; genetic autosomal recessive pattern of inheritance	0–2	Male > female	Normal	Nonfluctuating, compatible with long survival
Juvenile myasthenia	Autoimmune disorder	2–20	Female > male (4:1)	Hyperplasia	Slowly progressive, tendency to relapse and remission
Adult myasthenia	Autoimmune disorder	20–40	Female > male	Hyperplasia	Maximum severity within 3 to 5 years
Elderly myasthenia	Autoimmune disorder	>40	Male > female	Thymoma (benign or locally invasive)	Rapid progress, higher mortality

1. The clinical hallmark of myasthenia gravis is skeletal muscle weakness (increased by repetitive muscle use) with periods of exacerbation and remission.
   a. Neonatal myasthenia begins 12 to 48 hours after birth and reflects transplacental passage of anti-acetylcholine antibodies.
   b. Focal myocarditis and atrioventricular heart block may be present.
2. **Treatment** includes administration of anticholinesterase drugs, thymectomy, corticosteroids, and immunosuppressants. Whereas underdosage with anticholinesterase drugs results in skeletal muscle weakness, overdosage leads to a "cholinergic crisis." The role of thymectomy for the treatment of myasthenia is not clearly established.
3. **Management of Anesthesia**
   a. The primary concern is the potential interaction between the disease, treatment of the disease, and neuromuscular blocking drugs. Patients with uncontrolled or poorly controlled myasthenia are exquisitely sensitive to even small (defasciculating) doses of nondepolarizing muscle relaxants.
   b. The variability in response to different muscle relaxants warrants careful monitoring with a peripheral nerve stimulator and its correlation with clinical signs of recovery from neuromuscular blockade. Short- or intermediate-acting non-depolarizing muscle relaxants are usually recommended.

E. **Myasthenic Syndrome (Lambert-Eaton Syndrome)**
   1. The myasthenic syndrome is a disorder of neuromuscular transmission associated with carcinomas, particularly small cell carcinoma of the lung (this should be suspected in patients undergoing diagnostic procedures, such as diagnostic bronchoscopy, mediastinoscopy, or exploratory thoracotomy for possible cancer) (Table 25-4).
   2. **Management of Anesthesia**
      a. Patients with myasthenic syndrome are sensitive to the effects of both depolarizing and nondepolarizing muscle relaxants.
      b. Administration of 3,4-diaminopyridine should be continued until the time of surgery.

F. **Guillain-Barré syndrome (polyradiculoneuritis)** is the acute form of a group of disorders classified as

TABLE 25-4

COMPARISON OF MYASTHENIA GRAVIS AND
MYASTHENIC SYNDROME

	Myasthenia Gravis	Myasthenic Syndrome
Manifestations	Extraocular, bulbar, and facial muscle weakness	Proximal limb weakness (legs > arms)
	Fatigue with exercise	Exercise improves strength
	Muscle pain is uncommon	Muscle pain is common
	Normal reflexes	Absent or decreased reflexes
Gender	Female > male	Male > female
Coexisting pathology	Thymoma	Cancer (especially small cell carcinoma of the lung)
Response to muscle relaxants	Resistant to succinylcholine	Sensitive to succinylcholine and nondepolarizing muscle relaxants
	Sensitive to nondepolarizing muscle relaxants	
Response to anticholinesterases	Poor response to anticholinesterases	Poor response to anticholinesterases

inflammatory polyneuropathies (autoimmune disease caused by a bacterial or viral infection that triggers an immune response, producing antibodies that damage the myelin sheath and cause axonal degeneration).

1. This syndrome is characterized by the acute or subacute onset of skeletal muscle weakness or paralysis of the legs, which spreads cephalad and may result in difficulty swallowing and impaired ventilation from paralysis of the intercostal muscles.

   a. The most serious immediate problem is hypoventilation. (Vital capacity should be monitored frequently. If it decreases below 15 to 20 mL/kg, mechanical ventilation of the lungs is indicated.)

   b. Although 85% of patients with this syndrome achieve a good recovery, chronic recurrent neuropathy develops in 3% to 5% of patients.

   c. **Autonomic nervous system** dysfunction may be associated with wide fluctuations in blood pressure (physical stimulation may precipitate hypertension),

tachycardia, cardiac dysrhythmias, and cardiac arrest.
2. **Management of Anesthesia**
   a. Compensatory cardiovascular responses may be absent (autonomic nervous system dysfunction), resulting in significant hypotension secondary to postural changes, blood loss, or positive airway pressure. Conversely, stimuli such as laryngoscopy and tracheal intubation may produce hypertension and tachycardia.
   b. Sch is not recommended because drug-induced potassium release may result in hyperkalemia and cardiac arrest. The response to nondepolarizing muscle relaxants ranges from sensitivity to resistance.
   c. It is likely that mechanical ventilation is required during the immediate postoperative period.

III. CENTRAL NERVOUS SYSTEM DISEASES

A. **Multiple sclerosis** is characterized by multiple sites of demyelination in the brain and spinal cord, leading to visual disturbances, limb weakness, and paresthesias.
   1. Therapy for multiple sclerosis is directed at modulating the immunologic and inflammatory responses that damage the central nervous system (CNS) (corticosteroids, interferon, glatiramer, mitoxantrone [maybe cardiotoxic]).
   2. **Management of Anesthesia.** The effect of anesthesia and surgery on the course of multiple sclerosis is controversial.
      a. Regional and general anesthesia have been reported to exacerbate or have no effect on multiple sclerosis. Factors other than anesthesia, such as infection, emotional stress, and hyperpyrexia, may contribute to an increased risk of perioperative exacerbation.
      b. A neurologic examination before anesthesia and surgery is helpful to document coexisting neurologic deficits.
      c. Patients being treated with corticosteroids may require perioperative supplementation, and immunosuppressants may produce cardiotoxicity and subclinical cardiac dysfunction.
      d. Autonomic dysfunction caused by multiple sclerosis may produce exaggerated hypotensive effects in response to volatile anesthetics.

TABLE 25-5

THE MOST FREQUENTLY ENCOUNTERED TYPES OF SEIZURES

Grand Mal Seizure
All respiratory activity is arrested, leading to arterial hypoxemia
Diazepam and thiopental are effective for acute generalized
 seizures

Focal Cortical Seizure
May be motor or sensory
Usually no loss of consciousness

Absence Seizure (Petit Mal)
Brief (30 seconds) loss of awareness
Most common in children and young adults

Akinetic Seizure
Sudden, brief loss of consciousness
Usually occur in children; a fall may result in head injury

Status Epilepticus
Defined as two consecutive tonic-clonic seizures without regaining
 consciousness or seizure activity that is unabated for 30 minutes
 or more
Ventilation is impaired
Diazepam and lorazepam are drugs of choice (thiopental effective,
 but its effect is brief)

EVALUATION

    e. Respiratory muscle weakness and dysfunction may
       increase the likelihood of the need for postopera-
       tive mechanical ventilation.
  B. **Epilepsy** (Table 25-5)
    1. The sudden onset of seizures in a young to middle-
      aged adult should arouse the suspicion of focal brain
      disease (tumor); onset after 60 years of age is usually
      secondary to cerebrovascular disease.
    2. The availability of new antiseizure drugs has
      increased the therapeutic options for patients with
      epilepsy (Table 25-6).
    3. **Management of Anesthesia**
      a. Antiseizure medications should be maintained
        throughout the perioperative period.
      b. An anesthetic technique should be used that mini-
        mizes the risk of seizure activity. Although most
        inhaled anesthetics, including nitrous oxide, have
        been reported to produce seizure activity, such
        activity during the administration of isoflurane and

TABLE 25-6

ANTICONVULSANT DRUGS

Drug	Seizure Type	Therapeutic Blood Level (μg/mL)	Side Effects
Phenobarbital	Generalized	15–35	Sedation
			Increased drug metabolism
Valproate	Generalized Absence	50–100	Pancreatitis
			Hepatic dysfunction
			Thrombocytopenia
Felbamate	Generalized Partial		Insomnia
			Ataxia
			Nausea
Phenytoin	Generalized Partial	10–20	Gingival hyperplasia
			Dermatitis
			Resistance to nondepolarizing muscle relaxants
Fosphenytoin	Generalized Partial		Paresthesias
			Hypotension
Carbamazepine	Generalized Partial	6–12	Cardiotoxicity
			Hepatitis
			Resistance to nondepolarizing muscle relaxants
Lamotrigine	Generalized Partial	2–16	Rash
			Stevens-Johnson syndrome
Topiramate	Generalized Partial	4–10	Severe metabolic acidosis
			Hyperthermia
Gabapentin	Generalized Partial	4–16	Fatigue
			Somnolence
Primidone	Generalized Partial	6–12	Nausea
			Ataxia
Clonazepam	Absence	0.01–0.07	Ataxia
Ethosuximide	Absence	40–100	Leukopenia
Levetiracetam	Generalized	5–45	Erythema multiforme
	Partial		Dizziness
			Headache
Oxycarbazepine	Partial	10–35	Hyponatremia
			Diplopia
			Somnolence
Tiagabine	Partial		Tremor
			Depression
Zonisamide	Generalized	10–40	Anorexia
			Decreased cognition

TABLE 25-7
CLINICAL FEATURES OF PARKINSON'S DISEASE

Increases in spontaneous movements
Cogwheel rigidity of the extremities (shuffling gait, stooped posture)
Facial immobility
Rhythmic tremor at rest
Seborrhea
Sialorrhea
Orthostatic hypotension
Bladder dysfunction
Diaphragmatic spasm
Oculogyric crises
Mental depression

desflurane is extremely rare. (Sevoflurane may be eliptogenic, but the clinical significance is uncertain.) Ketamine may produce seizure activity in patients with known seizure disorders. Reported seizure activity after administration of opioids may reflect myoclonic activity.

C. **Parkinson's disease** is a degenerative disease of the CNS caused by the loss of dopaminergic fibers in the basal ganglia of the brain (occurs in 1% of population older than age 60 years)

1. Typical clinical features are secondary to depletion of dopamine from the basal ganglia (Table 25-7).

2. Treatment protocols involve combinations of drugs designed to increase dopamine levels in the brain while blunting the peripheral effects of dopamine. The therapeutic regimen for patients with Parkinson's disease is complex and requires a skilled neurologist to individualize therapy.

   a. The combination of levodopa and carbidopa (which blocks peripheral conversion of levodopa to dopamine) is the most frequent treatment.

   b. Side effects of levodopa include depletion of myocardial norepinephrine stores, peripheral vasoconstriction, hypovolemia, and orthostatic hypotension.

   c. Use of surgical pallidotomy (local anesthesia) and implantation of deep brain stimulators may be a good option for selected patients.

EVALUATION

3. **Management of Anesthesia**
    a. Drugs that may antagonize the effects of dopamine in the CNS (droperidol, metoclopramide, and possibly alfentanil) should be avoided.
    b. Levodopa has a brief half-time, and interruption of therapy for more than 6 to 12 hours may result in skeletal muscle rigidity that interferes with ventilation.
    c. Success with the use of selegiline for the treatment of parkinsonism increases the likelihood of having to anesthetize a patient who is receiving a monoamine oxidase B inhibitor. (Meperidine should be avoided in these patients.)
    d. **Autonomic dysfunction** is common and manifests as esophageal dysfunction (risk of aspiration) and orthostatic hypotension (exaggerated decreases in blood pressure in response to volatile anesthetics).
    e. Postoperatively, these patients may develop mental confusion.
D. **Alzheimer's disease** is the major cause of dementia in the United States.
    1. The incidence of Alzheimer's disease is 1% in 60 year olds and 30% in 85 year olds.
    2. Administration of cholinesterase inhibitors is considered the standard of care for patients with early Alzheimer's disease.
    3. **Management of anesthesia** is guided by the patient's general physiologic condition, the degree of neurologic impairment, and the potential for interaction between anesthetics and medications the patient is receiving.
        a. Sedative drugs for preoperative medication may result in further mental confusion.
        b. Anesthetics (propofol, desflurane, sevoflurane) known to result in prompt postoperative recovery may be advantageous by permitting a more rapid return to the patient's preoperative state. Although isoflurane may increase amyloid beta protein generation and aggregation in isolated human neurons, the clinical significance is unknown.
        c. If an anticholinergic drug is required, glycopyrrolate, which does not easily cross the blood–brain barrier, is preferable to scopolamine or atropine, which cross blood–brain barrier and may exacerbate dementia.

TABLE 25-8

TYPES OF ANEMIA

Nutritional
Iron deficiency
Vitamin B_{12} deficiency
Folic acid deficiency
Chronic illness

Hemolytic
Spherocytosis
Glucose-6-phosphate dehydrogenase deficiency
Immune-mediated
Drug-induced ABO incompatibility

Genetic
Hemoglobin S (sickle cell)
Thalassemia major (Cooley's anemia)
Thalassemia intermedia
Thalassemia minor

> **d.** Patients receiving cholinesterase inhibitors may have a prolonged response to Sch.

IV. **ANEMIAS** (Table 25-8)

A. In an otherwise healthy person, symptoms do not develop from anemia until the hemoglobin level decreases below 7 g/dL. (Physiologic compensation includes increased blood volume and cardiac output and decreased blood viscosity.) There is no universally accepted hemoglobin level that mandates blood transfusion. The patient's physiologic status and coexisting diseases must be factored into this highly subjective decision.

B. **Nutritional Deficiency Anemias**
1. **Iron deficiency anemia** may be an absolute deficiency caused by decreased oral intake of iron or a relative deficiency of iron caused by a rapid turnover of red blood cells (chronic blood loss, hemolysis). Severe iron deficiency produces microcytic anemia and may result in thrombocytopenia and neurologic abnormalities.
2. **Vitamin B_{12} deficiency** results in megaloblastic anemia and nervous system dysfunction (peripheral neuropathy secondary to degeneration of the lateral and

EVALUATION

posterior columns of the spinal cord manifesting as symmetric paresthesias with loss of proprioception and vibratory sensation, especially in the lower extremities). Prolonged exposure to nitrous oxide (inactivates the vitamin B_{12} component of methionine synthetase) results in megaloblastic anemia and neurologic changes similar to those that occur in pernicious anemia.

3. **Folic acid deficiency** (because of alcoholism, pregnancy, malabsorption [phenytoin, methotrexate]) results in megaloblastic anemia, but peripheral neuropathy is not as common as with vitamin B_{12} deficiency.

C. **Hemolytic anemias** reflect premature destruction (before 120 days) of red blood cells.

D. **Glucose-6-phosphate dehydrogenase (G6PD) deficiency** is the most common enzymopathy in humans. It affects 400 million people worldwide and may confer malarial resistance.

1. A deficiency of G6PD results in decreased levels of glutathione when erythrocytes are exposed to oxidants. This increases the rigidity of the red blood cell membrane (hemolysis) and accelerates clearance of erythrocytes from the circulation.

2. A number of drugs may enhance the destruction of erythrocytes in patients with G6PD deficiency (Table 25-9). Characteristically, the hemolytic episode begins 2 to 5 days after drug administration.

3. Patients with G6PD deficiency are unable to reduce methemoglobin produced by sodium nitrate, so sodium nitroprusside should not be administered in these patients.

TABLE 25-9

DRUGS THAT PRODUCE HEMOLYSIS IN PATIENTS WITH GLUCOSE-6-PHOSPHATE DEHYDROGENASE DEFICIENCY

Phenacetin	Chloramphenicol
Nalidixic acid	Quinidine
Aspirin (high doses)	Sulfacetamide
Isoniazid	Doxorubicin
Penicillin	Sulfanilamide
Primaquine	Methylene blue
Streptomycin	Sulfapyridine
Quinine	Nitrofurantoin

4. Anesthetic drugs have not been implicated as hemolytic agents, but early postoperative evidence of hemolysis might suggest G6PD.

E. **Hemoglobinopathies** are diseases caused by genetic errors in hemoglobin synthesis and production. (These diseases convey survival protection in malaria-endemic areas.)

1. **Sickle cell disease (SCD)** results from mutation of chromosome 11, which causes substitution of valine for glutamic acid. Whereas persons heterozygous for the sickle cell gene (HbSA) are usually asymptomatic, homozygous individuals (HbSS) have SCD.

2. **Clinical Manifestations** (Table 25-10). Acute chest syndrome (dyspnea, wheezing, chest pain, hypoxemia, pulmonary infiltrates) represents the single greatest threat to patients with SCD.

3. **Treatment** of SCD is supportive and directed at early treatment of complications.

4. **Management of Anesthesia.** Preparation of patients with SCD for surgery should be done in close collaboration with the SCD specialty service that provides the patient's routine care. Prevention of conditions that favor sickling is the basis of perioperative management.

   a. Supplemental oxygen is recommended during and after regional and general anesthesia.

   b. Circulatory stasis can be prevented with hydration and anticipation of intraoperative blood loss in order to avoid acute hypovolemia.

   c. Normothermia is desirable because hyperthermia increases the rate of gel formation, and hypothermia produces vasoconstriction that impairs organ blood flow.

   d. The use of a tourniquet or preoperative transfusion is controversial.

   e. Hemoglobin and hematocrit should be measured preoperatively and adequate oxygen-carrying capacity maintained by transfusion to keep the hematocrit near 30%.

   f. Drugs commonly used for anesthesia do not have significant effects on the sickling process, assuming arterial hypoxemia, vascular stasis, and reduced cardiac output are avoided. Regional anesthesia has been successfully used for surgery, labor and delivery, and pain management.

EVALUATION

TABLE 25-10

CLINICAL MANIFESTATIONS OF SICKLE CELL DISEASE

System	Clinical Manifestations
Hematologic	Hemolytic anemia (hemoglobin 7–8 g/dL)
	Aplastic anemia
	Leukocytosis
Spleen	Infarction
	Hyposplenism
	Splenic sequestration
Central nervous system	Stroke
	Hemorrhage
	Aneurysms
	Meningitis
Musculoskeletal	Painful episodes
	Bone marrow hyperplasia
	Avascular necrosis
	Osteomyelitis
	Bone infarcts
	Skeletal deformity
	Growth retardation
	Cutaneous ulceration
Cardiac	Cardiomegaly
	Pulmonary hypertension
	Cor pulmonale
	Diastolic dysfunction
	Cardiomyopathy
Renal	Papillary necrosis
	Glomerular sclerosis
	Renal failure
Pulmonary	Acute chest syndrome
	Hypoxemia
	Pulmonary infarction
	Fibrosis
	Asthma
	Thromboembolism
	Pneumonia
Genitourinary	Priapism
	Infection
Hepatobiliary	Jaundice
	Hepatitis
	Cirrhosis
	Cholelithiasis
	Cholestasis
Eye	Retinopathy
	Hemorrhage
	Visual loss
Immune system	Immunosuppression
	Leukocytosis
Psychosocial	Depression
	Anxiety
	Substance abuse
	Opioid dependence

TABLE 25-11

TYPES OF COLLAGEN VASCULAR DISEASES

Rheumatoid Arthritis

Lupus
Systemic lupus erythematosus
Drug-induced lupus
Discoid lupus

Scleroderma
Progressive systemic sclerosis
CREST syndrome (Raynaud's phenomenon, esophageal
  dysfunction, sclerodactyly, telangiectasis)
Focal scleroderma

Polymyositis
Dermatomyositis

Overlap Syndromes

V. COLLAGEN VASCULAR DISEASES (Table 25-11)

A. **Rheumatoid arthritis** is a chronic inflammatory disease
   characterized by symmetric and significant polyarthropa-
   thy (hands and wrists first, cervical spine as reflected by
   magnetic resonance imaging) and systemic involvement
   (Table 25-12).
   1. The goals of therapy are induction of a remission,
      improved function, and maintenance of a remission.
      Drugs used for treatment include nonsteroidal antiin-
      flammatory drugs, corticosteroids, and disease-modi-
      fying antirheumatic drugs. (Methotrexate may the
      first-line treatment for patients with early rheumatoid
      arthritis.)
   2. **Management of Anesthesia**
      a. The joint effects of rheumatoid arthritis (temporo-
         mandibular joints, cervical spine, cricoarytenoid
         joints) can render direct laryngoscopy and tracheal
         intubation difficult.
      b. **Atlantoaxial instability** is relatively common, and
         flexion of the neck may compress the spinal cord.
      c. The need for postoperative ventilatory support
         should be anticipated if severe restrictive pul-
         monary disease is present.
      d. Restriction of joint mobility necessitates careful
         positioning to minimize the risk of neurovascular
         compression.

EVALUATION

TABLE 25-12

EXTRA-ARTICULAR MANIFESTATIONS OF RHEUMATOID ARTHRITIS

Skin Raynaud's phenomenon Digital necrosis	**Peripheral Nervous System** Compression syndromes Mononeuritis
Eyes Scleritis Corneal ulceration	**Central Nervous System** Dural nodules Necrotizing vasculitis
Lungs Pleural effusion Pulmonary fibrosis	**Liver** Hepatitis
Heart Pericarditis Cardiac tamponade Coronary arteritis Aortic insufficiency	**Blood** Anemia Leukopenia
Kidneys Interstitial fibrosis Glomerulonephritis Amyloid deposition	

B. **Systemic lupus erythematosus** (SLE) is an autoimmune disease with diverse clinical (polyarthritis, dermatitis, renal failure, pericarditis, pulmonary hypertension) and immunologic manifestations.
   1. Drug-induced SLE (phenytoin, hydralazine, isoniazid) is usually mild and resolves within 4 weeks of discontinuation of the drug.
   2. **Management of anesthesia** is influenced by disease-induced organ dysfunction and drugs used in treatment.
      a. Renal dysfunction is common and necessitates preoperative evaluation.
      b. Laryngeal involvement may manifest postoperatively as laryngeal edema or stridor.
      c. Supplemental steroids may be necessary in patients being treated with corticosteroids.
C. **Scleroderma** is an autoimmune collagen vascular disease that affects the skin (thickened and swollen), joints, and visceral organs (pulmonary interstitial fibrosis and impaired diffusing capacity, pericardial effusion, renal dysfunction, decreased gastrointestinal motility).
   1. Raynaud's phenomenon occurs in 95% of patients with scleroderma.

2. **Management of anesthesia** is influenced by the degree of organ dysfunction.

   a. The risk for aspiration pneumonitis during induction of anesthesia may be increased because of the high incidence of gastroesophageal reflux.

   b. Tracheal intubation may be difficult because fibrotic and taut skin can hinder active and passive opening of the mouth and severely restrict mobility of the temporomandibular joint.

   c. Chronic arterial hypoxemia may reflect restrictive lung disease and impaired oxygen diffusion.

   d. Venous access may be difficult.

   e. Skeletal muscle involvement may increase the sensitivity to muscle relaxants.

D. **Polymyositis and dermatomyositis (inflammatory myopathies)** are characterized by severe muscle weakness and noninfectious inflammation. Patients with dermatomyositis manifest a characteristic erythematous rash over the face, neck, and upper chest.

   1. Pulmonary diseases (interstitial pneumonitis, alveolitis, bronchopneumonia) are often present.

   2. Aspiration pneumonitis (dysphagia and gastroesophageal reflux) is a common complication.

   3. The most effective treatment is with corticosteroids.

   4. **Management of Anesthesia**

      a. Tracheal intubation may be difficult in patients with restricted joint mobility.

      b. Despite the theoretical potential for Sch to produce hyperkalemia in these patients, there is no evidence that this occurs.

      c. It should be anticipated that considerable individual variation will occur in response to nondepolarizing muscle relaxants.

VI. SKIN DISORDERS

A. **Epidermolysis bullosa** is characterized by abnormal collagen that is insufficient for anchoring skin layers to each other. (Laryngeal involvement is rare.)

   1. Pressure applied perpendicular to the skin is less likely to produce separation of skin layers (intradermal fluid accumulation and bullae formation) than are lateral shearing forces.

   2. **Management of anesthesia** is based on avoidance of trauma to the skin and mucous membranes from

EVALUATION

adhesive tape, blood pressure cuffs, tourniquets, and adhesive electrodes.
   a. Lubrication of the face mask is useful for decreasing trauma to the face.
   b. Use of upper airway instruments and passage of an esophageal stethoscope should be avoided. The safety of tracheal intubation has been established for patients with the dystrophic form of this disease.
   c. Ketamine is useful anesthesia for superficial surgical procedures.
B. **Pemphigus** is an autoimmune vesiculobullous disease that involves the skin and mucous membranes. Oral lesions are common, and corticosteroids are effective in therapy.

CHAPTER 26 ■ THE ANESTHESIA WORKSTATION AND DELIVERY SYSTEMS

Modern anesthesia machines are properly referred to as anesthesia workstations (Riutort KT, Brockwell RC, et al: The anesthesia workstation and delivery systems In *Clinical Anesthesia*. Edited by Barash PG, Cullen BF, Stoelting RK, Cahalan MK, Stock MC. Philadelphia: Lippincott Williams & Wilkins, 2009, pp 644–694).The anesthesia workstation is a system for administering anesthetics to patients. The workstation consists of the anesthesia gas supply device, the anesthesia ventilator, monitoring devices, and protection devices (designed to prevent hazardous output caused by incorrect delivery or barotrauma).

I. ANESTHESIA WORKSTATION STANDARDS AND PRE-USE PROCEDURES Workstations may have computer-assisted self-tests that automatically perform all or part of the pre-use machine checkout procedure. Ultimately, performing adequate pre-use testing of the anesthesia workstation is the responsibility of the individual.

II. STANADARDS FOR ANESTHESIA MACHINES AND WORKSTATIONS These standards provide guidelines to manufacturers regarding minimum performance, design characteristics, and safety requirements for anesthesia machines. To comply with the American Society for Testing and Materials Standards, newly manufactured workstations must have monitors to measure specific parameters and possess a prioritized alarm system (Table 26-1).

III. FAILURE OF ANESTHESIA EQUIPMENT The most common malfunction of the medical-gas delivery system is related to the breathing circuit. Pulse oximetry is the principal monitor for alerting the anesthesia professional to an equipment problem.

AMERICAN SOCIETY FOR TESTING AND MATERIALS STANDARDS
FOR MANUFACTURED WORKSTATIONS

Parameters Monitored
Continuous breathing system pressure
Exhaled CO_2 concentration
Anesthetic vapor concentration
Inspired O_2 concentration
O_2 supply pressure
Arterial hemoglobin oxygen saturation
Arterial blood pressure
Continuous electrocardiogram

Prioritized Alarm Systems
High, medium, and low categories
Alarms automatically or manually enabled

IV. SAFETY FEATURES OF NEWER ANESTHESIA WORKSTATIONS (Table 26-2)

V. CHECKOUT OF THE ANESTHESIA WORKSTATION
A complete anesthesia apparatus checkout procedure must be performed each day before the first use of the anesthesia workstation. (A "machine checklist" is most applicable to older anesthesia machines.) Newer workstations may perform an automated checkout. The three most important preoperative checks are O_2 analyzer calibration, the low-pressure circuit leak test, and the circle system test (Table 26-3).

VI. ANESTHESIA WORKSTATION PNEUMATICS

A. **The Anatomy of an Anesthesia Workstation** (Fig. 26-1)
   1. Gases such as O_2, nitrous oxide (N_2O), and air are usually supplied from a central pipeline with cylinders on the machine as a backup. The pipeline source is usually at 50 psig (pounds per square inch gauge). A full O_2 cylinder contains only gas, and the tank pressure decreases linearly from a maximum of about 2200 psig as it is consumed. N_2O is compressed to a liquid in tanks and maintains a pressure of 745 psig until all the liquid is dissipated.

TABLE 26-2

COMPARISON OF ANESTHESIA WORKSTATION FUNCTIONS

Anesthesia Workstation Function	Draeger Fabius GS 1.3	GE Aisys
Increase in FGF increases Vt	No	No
Pre-use system leakage is measured	Yes	Yes
Proximal leak compression	No	Yes
Leakage measurement during operation	No	Yes
Hose compliance compensation	Yes	Yes
System compliance compensation	Yes	Yes
Reported exhaled Vt is adjusted for hose compliance	Yes	Yes
Fresh gas flow is distal to:	Absorber	Absorber
Fresh gas inflow is proximal to:	Decoupling valve	Inspiratory valve
At low FGF, what gas fills the reservoir bag?	Scrubbed	Exhaled
Mechanism of VCV	Displacement	Metered, calculated
Limiting of pressure control ventilation	Flow/pressure	Flow/pressure limited
FiO₂ compensated for volatile agent	No	Yes
Synchronized intermittent mechanical ventilation	No	Yes
Manufacturer specified minimum Vt	20	20
FGF control	Needle valve	Digital control
FGF measurement	Electronic	Electronic
Backup flow tube	Yes	Yes (fail-safe mode)
Integrated capnography	No	Yes
Integrated anesthetic gas monitoring	No	Yes
Effect of lost oxygen pressure on FGR	Air available	Air available
Sample gas returned to circuit	No	No
Mechanical airway pressure gauge	Yes	No
Absorber removable during VCV	Yes	Yes (optional)

EVALUATION

(*continued*)

TABLE 26-2

COMPARISON OF ANESTHESIA WORKSTATION
FUNCTIONS (*Continued*)

Anesthesia Workstation Function	Draeger Fabius GS 1.3	GE Aisys
Room air entrained during a circuit leak	Yes	No
Room air entrained with inadequate FGF	Yes	No
Effect of oxygen flush during VCV inspiration	None	Greater Vt, end at pressure release
Failsafe integrate with the ratio controller	Yes, pneumatic	Yes, electronic
Method to find a low pressure/vaporizer leak	Automatic, vaporizer open	Automatic
Ventilator drive gas scavenging	NA	Yes

FGF = fresh gas flow; NA = not applicable; VCV = volume control
ventilation; Vt = tidal volume.

2. **Oxygen failure cut-off** ("**fail safe**") **valves** are located
   downstream from the N_2O supply source and serve as
   an interface between the O_2 and N_2O supply sources.
   This value shuts off or proportionally decreases the
   supply of N_2O if the O_2 of supply decreases.
3. **Regulators** downstream from the O_2 supply source
   adjust the pressure to about 14 psig before entering
   the flow meter assembly.

TABLE 26-3

PREOPERATIVE ANESTHESIA WORKSTATION CHECKLIST

Oxygen analyzer calibration (evaluates the integrity of low-
pressure circuit; this is the only machine monitor that detects
problems downstream from the flow control valves)
Low-pressure circuit leak test (checks the integrity of the anesthesia
machine from flow control valves to the common outlet; leaks in
the low-pressure circuit may cause hypoxia and awareness)
Circle system tests (evaluate the integrity of the system from the
common gas outlet to the Y-piece)
  Leak test (close the pop-off valve, occlude the Y-piece, and
  pressurize the circuit to 30 cm H_2O using the oxygen flush
  valve)
  Flow test (confirms the integrity of the unidirectional valves; it is
  performed by disconnecting the Y-piece and breathing
  individually through each corrugated tube)

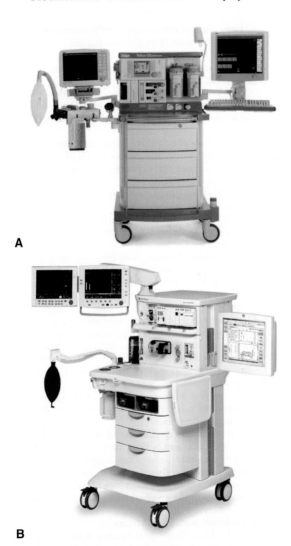

A

B

FIGURE 26-1. Draeger Medical Fabius GS anesthesia workstation (**A**) and GE Healthcare Aisys anesthesia workstation (**B**).

4. **Flow control valves** separate the intermediate-pressure circuit from the low-pressure circuit (the part of the machine that is downstream from the flow control valves). The operator regulates flow entering the low-pressure circuit by adjusting the flow control valves. After leaving the flow tubes, the mixture of gases travels through a common manifold and may be directed to a calibrated vaporizer.

5. A one-way check valve located between the vaporizer and common gas outlet prevents backflow into the vaporizer during positive pressure ventilation.

6. The O_2 flush connection joins the mixed-gas pipeline between the one-way check valve and the machine outlet. When the O_2 flush valve is activated, the pipeline O_2 pressure is reflected in the common gas outlet.

B. **Pipeline Supply Source.** Most hospitals have a central piping system to deliver medical gases such as O_2, N_2O, and air to the operating room at appropriate pressures for the anesthesia workstation to function properly.

C. **Flow meter assemblies** precisely measure gas flow to the common gas outlet. Depending on the setting of the flow control valve, gases flow through variable orifice, tapered tubes at a rate indicated by the position of a float indicator in relation to a calibrated scale.

1. At low flow rates, the viscosity of the gas is dominant in determining flow; density is dominant at high flow rates.

2. Safety features include use of standardized colors for each gas, an O_2 flow meter dial that is distinct from the others, and positioning of the O_2 flow meter immediately proximal to the common gas outlet to minimize the chance of delivery of hypoxic mixtures in the event of leaks in the flow meter assembly.

3. **Problems with Flow Meters**

   a. **Leaks** are hazardous because flow meters are located downstream from all machine safety devices except the O_2 analyzer. The use of electronic flow meters and the removal of conventional glass flow tubes helps eliminate this potential source of leak and risk for delivery of hypoxic gas mixtures (minimized if the O_2 flow meter is located downstream from all other flow meters).

    b. Inaccuracy of flow measurement may occur (dirt or static electricity may cause a float to stick)

    c. With an **ambiguous scale,** the operator reads the float position beside an adjacent but erroneous scale (this is minimized by etching the scale into the tube).

D. Dilution of Inspired Oxygen Concentration by Volatile Inhaled Anesthetic. When added to the inhaled gases downstream from flow meters and proportioning system, concentrations of less potent volatile anesthetics (maximum desflurane dial setting, 18%) may result in a gas–vapor mixture that contains an inspired O_2 concentration below 21%.

VII. WEB-BASED ANESTHESIA SOFTWARE SIMULATION: THE VIRTUAL ANESTHESIA MACHINE (Fig. 26-2)

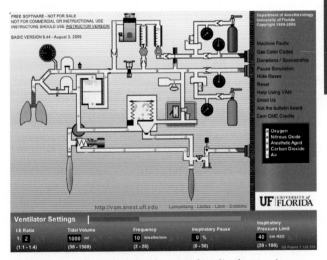

FIGURE 26-2. The Virtual Anesthesia Machine Simulator, an interactive model of an anesthesia machine.

TABLE 26-4

VAPORIZER MODELS AND CHARACTERISTICS

Type of Vaporizer	Tec 4, Tec 5, SevoTec, Vapor 19.n, Vapor 2000, Aladin	Tec 6 (Desflurane) D-Vapor (Desflurane)	MAQUET 950 Series Injection Vaporizer
Carrier gas flow	Variable bypass	Dual circuit	Concentration-calibrated injector
Vaporization method	Flow-over	Gas/vapor blender	None (injected)
Temperature compensation	Automatic	Thermostatically controlled at 39°C	None needed*
Calibration	Agent specific	Agent specific	Agent specific
Position	Out of circuit	Out of circuit	Out of circuit
Fill capacity	Tec 4: 125 mL Tec 5: 300 mL Vapor 19.n: 200 mL (dry wick) Aladin: 250 mL	Tec 6: 425 mL d-Vapor: 300 mL	125 mL (105 mL between minimum and maximum fill levels)

*A 10°C increase in temperature will result in a 10% increase in output concentration.

VIII. VAPORIZERS (Table 26-4)

A. Variable Bypass Vaporizers

1. The Datex-Ohmeda Tec 4, 5, and 7 and the North American Draeger Vapor 19n and 20n are classified as variable bypass (method for regulating output concentration), flow-over, temperature-compensated, agent-specific (keyed filling devices), out-of-breathing circuit vaporizers.

2. **Basic Operating Principles**

   a. As gas flow enters the vaporizer's inlet, the setting of the concentration dial determines the ratio of flow that goes through the bypass chamber and through the vaporizing chamber. The gas diverted to the vaporizing chamber flows over the liquid anesthetic and becomes saturated with vapor.

   b. The amount of gas diverted into the vaporizing chamber is primarily a function of the anesthetic

TABLE 26-5

SAFETY FEATURES OF VARIABLE BYPASS VAPORIZERS

Agent specific (keyed filling devices)
Filler port placed at a maximum safe liquid level (prevents overfilling)
Secured to vaporizer manifold (prevents tipping and spillage of liquid anesthetic into the bypass chamber and delivery of an overdose)
Interlock system (prevents simultaneous delivery of more than one volatile anesthetic)

vapor pressure. A temperature-compensating device helps maintain a constant vaporizer output over a wide range of temperatures.

3. **Safety Features** (Table 26-5)
4. **Hazards** (Table 26-6)

B. **The Datex-Ohmeda Tec 6 vaporizer for desflurane** is an electrically heated, pressurized device specifically designed to deliver desflurane.
   1. Desflurane boils at 22.8°C, and its vapor pressure is three to four times that of other contemporary inhaled anesthetics.
   2. Desflurane's high volatility and moderate potency preclude its use with contemporary variable bypass vaporizers.
   3. **Factors that Influence Vaporizer Output**
      a. **Varied altitudes** influence the output of this vaporizer that is unlike contemporary variable

TABLE 26-6

HAZARDS ASSOCIATED WITH VARIABLE BYPASS VAPORIZERS

Misfilling
Contamination of volatile agent added to vaporizer
Tipping (unlikely if properly mounted on manifold)
Overfilling
Underfilling
Simultaneous inhaled anesthetic administration (unlikely with newer machines)
Leaks (loose filler cap the most common cause; risk of patient awareness)
Internal ferrous components, a risk in the MRI suite

MRI = magnetic resonance imaging.

bypass vaporizers, which deliver a constant partial pressure of anesthetic. At a given concentration dial setting, the Tec 6 provides a lower partial pressure of the anesthetic as altitude increases. For example, at 2000-m elevation, the concentration dial setting of the Tec 6 must be increased from 10% to 12.5% to deliver the same partial pressure as at sea level.

b. **Carrier Gas Composition.** The vaporizer output approximates the dial setting when O_2 is the carrier gas. At low flow rates using N_2O as the carrier gas (decreased viscosity compared with O_2), the vaporizer output is approximately 20% less than with the dial setting.

4. **Safety Features.** The agent-specific filler cap of the desflurane bottle prevents its use with traditional vaporizers.

C. **The Datex-Ohmeda Aladin Cassette vaporizer** is a unique, single, electronically controlled vaporizer designed to deliver five different volatile drugs (halothane, isoflurane, enflurane, desflurane, sevoflurane).

D. **The MAQUET 950 series injector vaporizer** is designed to be used with the MAQUET Servo Ventilator.

IX. ANESTHETIA BREATHING CIRCUITS

A. An anesthetic circuit is interposed between the anesthesia machine, the common gas outlet, and the patient. The function of the circuit is to deliver anesthetic gases and O_2 to the patient and to remove exhaled carbon dioxide (CO_2).

B. **Mapleson Systems**

1. In 1954, Mapleson described and analyzed five different semiclosed anesthetic systems (Mapleson Systems A–E) in which the amount of CO_2 rebreathing associated with each system is multifactorial (Table 26-7 and Fig. 26-3).

2. The **Bain circuit** is a modification of the Mapleson D circuit, in which fresh gas flow is delivered at the end nearest the patient through a small inner tube located within the larger corrugated tubing (Fig. 26-2).

TABLE 26-7

VARIABLES THAT DETERMINE THE AMOUNT OF CARBON DIOXIDE REBREATHING ASSOCIATED WITH MAPLESON SYSTEMS

Fresh gas inflow rate
Minute ventilation
Mode of ventilation (spontaneous or controlled)
Tidal volume
Breathing rate
Inspiratory/expiratory ratio
Duration of expiratory pause
Peak inspiratory flow rate
Volume of reservoir tube
Volume of breathing bag
Ventilation by mask or tracheal tube
CO_2 sampling site

    3. The advantages of all these systems are that they are lightweight and convenient. The main disadvantage is that high fresh gas flows are required.

  C. Circle Breathing Systems

    1. Technological changes in the traditional circle breathing system include application of single-circuit piston-type ventilators and use of new spirometry devices that are located at the Y-connector instead of at the traditional location on the expiratory circuit limb.

    2. **The Traditional Circle Breathing System.** The circle system (fresh gas inflow, inspiratory and expiratory unidirectional valves, inspiratory and expiratory corrugated tubing, Y-piece connector, overflow or pop-off valve, reservoir bag, and a canister containing a CO_2 absorbent) is the most popular breathing system in the United States (Table 26-8 and Fig. 26-4).

      a. The unidirectional valves are placed so that gases flow in only one direction and through the CO_2 absorber (Fig. 26-4).

      b. If the valves are functioning properly, the only dead space in the system is between the Y-piece and the patient.

    3. A **closed system** exists when the fresh gas flow equals that being consumed by the patient (about 300 mL/min of O_2 plus uptake of anesthetic gases)

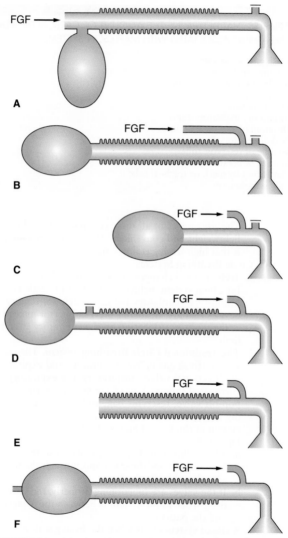

FIGURE 26-3. Schematic diagram of the Mapleson systems and the Bain system. FGF = fresh gas flow.

TABLE 26-8

CHARACTERISTICS OF A CIRCLE SYSTEM

Advantages	Disadvantages
Conservation of gases	Complex design
Conservation of moisture	Tubing disconnection or misconnection
Conservation of heat	Leaks
Minimal operating room pollution	CO_2 absorbent exhaustion
	Failure of unidirectional valves (rebreathing, circuit occlusion)
	Obstructed bacterial filter in expiratory limb
	Poor portability

and the overflow (pop-off) valve is closed. If high fresh gas flows are used, the system is semi-closed or semi-open.

D. Carbon Dioxide Absorbents
 1. Undesirable chemical reactions between desiccated Baralyme (no longer commercially available in the

EVALUATION

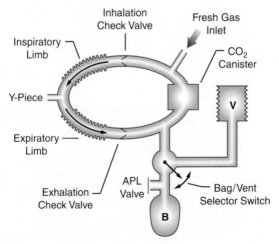

FIGURE 26-4. Components of the circle system. APL = adjustable pressure-limiting valve or "pop-off" valve.

TABLE 26-9

CHEMICAL REACTIONS OF CARBON DIOXIDE WITH SODA LIME

$$CO_2 + H_2O \rightarrow H_2CO_3$$
$$H_2CO_3 + 2NaOH(KOH) \rightarrow Na_2CO_3(K_2CO_3) + 2H_2O + heat$$
$$Na_2CO_3(K_2CO_3) + Ca(OH)_2 \rightarrow CaCO_3 + 2NaOH(KOH)$$

United States) include exothermic reactions with sevoflurane (fires in the breathing system) and production of carbon monoxide (desflurane) and compound A (sevoflurane).

2. **Chemistry of Absorbents**
   a. Available formulations of CO_2 absorbents are soda lime and calcium hydroxide lime (Amsorb).
   b. Advantages of calcium hydroxide are the lack of strong bases (sodium and potassium hydroxide) and the absence of undesirable chemical reactions and formation of heat, compound A, and carbon monoxide.
   c. Absorption of CO_2 is accomplished in a circle system by a chemical reaction that results in water and heat as byproducts (Table 26-9).

3. **Absorptive Capacity.** The maximum amount of CO_2 that can be absorbed by soda lime is 26 L of CO_2 per 100 g of absorbent. The absorptive capacity of calcium hydroxide is lower (10.2 L of CO_2 per 100 g of absorbent).

4. **Indicators**
   a. Ethyl violet is the pH indicator added to soda lime that changes from colorless to violet in color when the pH of the absorbent decreases as a result of CO_2 absorption.
   b. Prolonged exposure of ethyl violet to fluorescent lights can produce photodeactivation of the dye (the absorbent appears white even though it may have a reduced pH and its absorptive capacity has been exhausted).
   c. Clinical signs that the CO_2 absorbent is exhausted may occur even in the absence of color changes (Table 26-10).

TABLE 26-10

CLINICAL SIGNS THAT THE CARBON DIOXIDE ABSORBENT
IS EXHAUSTED

Increased spontaneous respiratory rate (assuming that no muscle
relaxant has been used)
Initial increase in hemodynamics (blood pressure, heart rate)
followed by a decrease
Increased sympathetic nervous system activity (skin flushing,
sweating, tachyarrhythmia, hypermetabolic state [malignant
hyperthermia should be ruled out])
Respiratory acidosis (arterial blood gases)
Increased surgical bleeding (hypertension, coagulopathy)

X. INTERACTIONS OF INHALED ANESTHETICS
   WITH ABSORBENTS (Table 26-11)

The likelihood of adverse chemical reactions between CO_2
absorbents and volatile anesthetics is minimized by avoiding the
use of desiccated CO_2 absorbents.

XI. ANESTHESIA VENTILATORS

   A. **Classification**
      1. Ventilators can be classified according to their power
         source (electricity or compressed gas), drive mecha-
         nism (pneumatically driven), and cycling mechanism
         (time cycled, pressure cycled).
      2. **Bellows Classification**
         a. The direction of the bellows movement during
            the expiratory phase determines the bellows clas-
            sification.

TABLE 26-11

INTERACTIONS OF INHALED ANESTHETICS WITH CARBON
DIOXIDE ABSORBENTS

Sevoflurane and formation of compound A
Formation of carbon monoxide (increased carboxyhemoglobin;
formation is greatest with desflurane and least with sevoflurane)
Fires in the breathing circuit (desiccated Baralyme and
sevoflurane)*

*Baralyme is no longer commercially available in the United States.

EVALUATION

TABLE 26-12
HAZARDS ASSOCIATED WITH VENTILATORS
Accidental disconnection Delivery of excessive pressure Leaks in bellows Erroneous connection of tubing to anesthetic circuit Failure of the ventilator relief valve Failure of the driving mechanism

      b. Ascending (standing) bellows ascend during the expiratory phase, and descending (hanging) bellows descend during the expiratory phase.

      c. Ascending bellows will not fill if a total disconnection occurs, and a descending bellows ventilator will continue its up and down movement despite a patient disconnection (driving gas pushes bellows up during the inspiratory phase).

      d. An essential safety feature of any anesthesia workstation that uses a descending bellows is an integrated CO_2 apnea alarm that cannot be disabled while the ventilator is in use.

  B. Problems and Hazards (Table 26-12)

XII. ANESTHESIA WORKSTATION VARIATIONS

  A. The Datex-Ohmeda S/5 ADU and Aisys eliminates gas flow tubes and conventional anesthesia vaporizes in exchange for a computer screen with digital fresh gas flow scales and a built-in Aladin Cassette vaporizer system.

    1. Entry of the fresh gas inflow on the patient side of the inspiratory valve is more efficient in delivering fresh gas flow to the patient and preferentially eliminating exhaled gases.

    2. This arrangement is also less likely to result in desiccation of the CO_2 absorbent.

  B. The Draeger Medical Narkomed 6000 Series, Fabius GS, and Appolo Workstations are characterized by the absence of flow tubes and glowing electronic fresh gas flow indicators.

    1. Fresh gas decoupling decreases the risk of barotrauma (fresh gas coming into the system from the patient is isolated while the ventilator exhaust valve is closed) and volutrauma.

TABLE 26-13

HAZARDS INTRODUCED BY SCAVENGING SYSTEMS

Transmission of excessive positive pressure to the breathing
system (obstruction of scavenging pathways)
Application of excessive negative pressure to the breathing system
(obstructing the relief valve or port)
Loss of means of monitoring (conceals odor of excessive
anesthetic concentration)

2. A disadvantage of the anesthesia circle systems that
use fresh gas decoupling is the possibility of entrain-
ing room air into the patient gas circuit. High-priority
audible and visual alarms are needed to notify the
user that fresh gas flow is inadequate and room air
is being entrained.

XIII. SCAVENGING SYSTEMS

A. Scavenging systems are designed to collect and subsequently vent gases from operating rooms.
B. These systems minimize operating room pollution but
increase the complexity of the anesthesia system (Table
26-13).
C. The two major causes of waste gas contamination in
the operating room are incorrect anesthetic technique
(failure to discontinue gas delivery from the anesthesia
machine at the conclusion of anesthesia, poorly fitting
face mask, flushing the breathing circuit) and
equipment failure (leaks).

EVALUATION

CHAPTER 27 ■ STANDARD MONITORING TECHNIQUES

Monitoring represents the process by which anesthesiologists recognize and evaluate potential physiologic problems by identifying prognostic trends in patients in a timely manner (Greenberg SB, Murphy GS, Vender JS: Standard monitoring techniques. In *Clinical Anesthesia*. Edited by Barash PG, Cullen BF, Stoelting RK, Cahalan MK, Stock MC. Philadelphia: Lippincott Williams & Wilkins, 2009, pp 695–714). Effective monitoring decreases the potential for poor outcomes that may occur after anesthesia by identifying derangements before they result in serious or irreversible injury. Monitoring devices increase the specificity and precision of clinical judgments. Standards for Basic Anesthesia Monitoring have been adopted by the American Society of Anesthesiologists (ASA).

I. INSPIRATORY AND EXPIRED GAS MONITORING

The concentration of oxygen in the anesthetic circuit must be measured. Manufacturers of gas machines place oxygen (O_2) sensors on the inspired limb of the anesthesia circuit to ensure that hypoxic gas mixtures are not delivered to patients. Monitoring inspired O_2 concentration does not guarantee the adequacy of arterial oxygenation.

II. MONITORING OF EXPIRED GASES

A. Carbon Dioxide

1. Monitoring of expiratory CO_2 (end-tidal CO_2 or $P_{ET}CO_2$) has evolved as an important physiologic and safety procedure for **identifying placement** of the endotracheal tube (this does not confirm placement above the carina) and for **assessing variables** such as

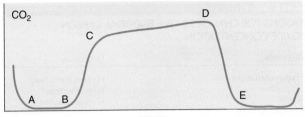

TIME

FIGURE 27-1. The capnogram is divided into four distinct phases. The first phase (A–B) represents the initial stage of expiration (gas from anatomic dead space) and is usually devoid of CO_2. At point B, CO_2-containing gas is present at the sampling site, and a sharp upstroke (B–C) is seen in the capnogram. Phase C–D represents the ventilation-weighted average concentration of CO_2 in alveolar gas. Point D is the highest value and is designated as the end-tidal CO_2 concentration. At point D, the patient begins to inspire CO_2-free gas, and there is a steep downstroke (D–E) back to baseline. Normally, unless rebreathing of CO_2 occurs, the baseline approaches zero.

ventilation ($PaCO_2$), rebreathing, cardiac output, distribution of blood flow, and metabolic activity.

2. **Capnometry** is the measurement and numeric representation of the CO_2 concentration (in millimeters of mercury [mm Hg]).

   a. A **capnogram** is a continuous concentration–time display of the CO_2 concentration (divided into four distinct phases) sampled at the patient's airway during ventilation (Fig. 27-1).

   b. **Capnography** is the continuous monitoring of the patient's capnogram.

3. The end-tidal CO_2 concentration provides a clinical estimate of the $PaCO_2$, assuming ventilation and perfusion in the lungs are appropriately matched (normal gradient, 5–10 mm Hg) and no sampling errors occur during measurement. (Sidestream analyzers may dilute a patient's tidal breath with fresh gas, especially when tidal volume is small, as in young patients. Loose connections and system leaks also dilute end-tidal CO_2.)

   a. **Dead space** (ventilation without perfusion) and a resulting increase in the difference between the $PaCO_2$ and the end-tidal CO_2 (dead space gases containing little or no CO_2 greatly dilute the end-tidal CO_2 concentration) may reflect

TABLE 27-1

REASONS FOR CHANGES IN THE END-TIDAL CARBON
DIOXIDE CONCENTRATION

Increases	Decreases
Hypoventilation	Hyperventilation
Hyperthermia	Hypothermia
Sepsis	Hypoperfusion
Malignant hyperthermia	Pulmonary embolism
Rebreathing	Slowed metabolism
Increased skeletal muscle activity	

     hypoperfusion states, chronic obstructive pulmonary
disease, and embolic phenomena (thrombus, air).
   b. Shunt (perfusion without ventilation) causes minimal changes in the gradient between $PaCO_2$ and end-tidal CO_2.
4. Capnography has decreased the potential for unrecognized accidental esophageal intubation.
   a. Because the esophageal or gastric gas concentration is primarily composed of inspired gas, it should contain exceedingly small amounts of CO_2. After an accidental esophageal intubation, the first one or two "breaths" may contain some CO_2, but the concentration should approach zero after four or five "breaths."
   b. A continuous stable CO_2 waveform ensures the presence of alveolar ventilation (tube in the trachea) but does not necessarily indicate that the endotracheal tube is properly positioned above the carina.
5. Common causes of gradual increases or decreases in end-tidal CO_2 reflect changes in CO_2 production or changes in CO_2 elimination (Table 27-1).

TABLE 27-2

EXPLANATIONS FOR ABRUPT DECREASES IN THE END-TIDAL
CARBON DIOXIDE CONCENTRATION

Malposition of the tracheal tube into the pharynx or esophagus
Disruption of airway integrity (disconnection or obstruction)
Disruption of the sampling line
Pulmonary embolism
Low cardiac output
Cardiac arrest

TABLE 27-3

INFORMATION DERIVED FROM THE CAPNOGRAM WAVEFORM

Slow Rate of Rise of Upstroke
Chronic obstructive pulmonary disease
Acute airway obstruction

Normally Shaped but Increased End-Tidal CO_2 Concentration
Alveolar hypoventilation
Increased CO_2 production

Transient Increases in End-Tidal CO_2 Concentration
Tourniquet release or aortic unclamping
Administration of bicarbonate
Insufflation of CO_2 during laparoscopy

Failure of the Baseline to Return to Zero
Rebreathing

6. A sudden decrease in end-tidal CO_2 to near zero requires a rapid assessment of possible causes (Table 27-2).
7. The adequacy of cardiopulmonary resuscitation can be assessed by capnography, as reflected by a reappearance or an increase in end-tidal CO_2 with restoration of pulmonary blood flow.
8. The size and shape of the capnogram waveform may be informative (Table 27-3).
   B. **Multiple Expired Gas Analysis.** Many critical events may be detected by analysis of respiratory and anesthetic gases (Table 27-4). Nitrogen (N_2) monitoring provides quantification of washout during preoxygenation. A sudden increase in the N_2 concentration in the exhaled gas indicates either introduction of air from leaks in the anesthesia delivery system or venous air embolism.

III. ARTERIAL OXYGENATION MONITORING

A. **Pulse Oximetry**
   1. Measurement of the peripheral O_2 saturation of hemoglobin (SpO_2) on a continual basis is the **standard of care for measuring oxygenation** during anesthesia and in the postanesthesia care unit.

MANAGEMENT

TABLE 27-4

GAS ANALYSIS AND THE DETECTION OF CRITICAL EVENTS

Event	Monitored Gas
Error in gas delivery system	Oxygen
	Carbon dioxide
	Nitrogen
	Inhaled anesthetic
Anesthesia machine malfunction	Oxygen
	Carbon dioxide
	Nitrogen
	Inhaled anesthetic
Disconnection	Carbon dioxide
	Oxygen
	Inhaled anesthetic
Vaporizer malfunction or contamination	Volatile anesthetic
Anesthesia circuit leaks	Nitrogen
	Carbon dioxide
Tracheal tube cuff leaks	Nitrogen
	Carbon dioxide
Poor mask fit	Nitrogen
	Carbon dioxide
Air embolism	Nitrogen
	Carbon dioxide
Hypoventilation	Carbon dioxide
Airway obstruction	Carbon dioxide
Malignant hyperthermia	Carbon dioxide
Circuit hypoxia	Oxygen

2. Overwhelming evidence supports the capability of pulse oximetry for detecting desaturation before it is clinically apparent.
3. No definitive data demonstrate a decrease in morbidity and mortality associated with the use of pulse oximetry.
4. The absence of a pulsatile waveform limits the ability of a pulse oximeter to calculate the SpO_2.
5. A relationship exists between hemoglobin saturation and O_2 tension (in mm Hg) as depicted by the oxyhemoglobin dissociation curve (Fig. 27-2).
6. The SpO_2 measured by pulse oximetry is not the same as the arterial O_2 saturation (SaO_2) measured by a laboratory co-oximeter. In clinical circumstances when other hemoglobin moieties (methemoglobin, carboxyhemoglobin) are present in low

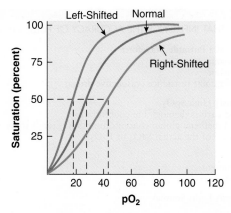

FIGURE 27-2. The relationship between arterial hemoglobin saturation with oxygen (%) and PO_2 is represented by the sigmoid-shaped oxyhemoglobin dissociation curve.

concentrations, the SpO_2 value is higher than the SaO_2 reported by the blood gas laboratory.

7. Many factors may influence the accuracy or ability of a pulse oximeter to calculate SpO_2 (Table 27-5).

IV. **BLOOD PRESSURE MONITORING** Intraoperative measurements and recordings of arterial blood pressure (at least every 5 minutes) are important indicators of the adequacy of circulation.

A. **Indirect Measurement of Arterial Blood Pressure**
   1. The simplest method of blood pressure determination estimates systolic blood pressure by palpating the return of the arterial pulse or Doppler sounds while an occluding cuff is deflated.
   2. **Auscultation** of Korotkoff sounds (which result from turbulent flow within an artery in response to the mechanical deformation from the blood pressure cuff) is a common method of blood pressure measurement.
      a. Systolic blood pressure is considered to be equivalent to the appearance of the first Korotkoff sound, and disappearance of the sounds or a muffled tone is considered to be equivalent to the diastolic

MANAGEMENT

TABLE 27-5
FACTORS THAT INFLUENCE THE ACCURACY OF PULSE OXIMETRY

Absence of a Pulsatile Waveform
Hypothermia
Hypotension
Altered vascular resistance (vasoactive drugs)

Factitiously High SpO_2
Increased carboxyhemoglobin concentration
Increased methemoglobin concentration (SpO_2 tends to be 85% regardless of the actual SaO_2 or PaO_2)

Motion
Awake patient
Shivering

Extraneous Light Sources

Factitiously Low SpO_2
Methylene blue
Fingernail polish

PaO_2 = arterial oxygen partial pressure; SaO_2 = arterial oxygen saturation; SpO_2 = peripheral oxygen saturation of hemoglobin.

blood pressure. Mean arterial pressure (MAP) is calculated as the diastolic blood pressure plus one third of the pulse pressure (systolic blood pressure minus diastolic blood pressure).
 b. The detection of sound changes is subjective, requires pulsatile flow (unreliable during low flow), and is prone to mechanical errors (Table 27-6).

TABLE 27-6
MECHANICAL ERRORS ASSOCIATED WITH AUSCULTATORY MEASUREMENT OF BLOOD PRESSURE

Falsely High Estimates of Blood Pressure
The cuff is too small (bladder width should approximate 40% of the circumference of the extremity)
The cuff is applied too loosely
Uneven compression of the underlying artery
The extremity is below heart level

Falsely Low Estimates of Blood Pressure
The cuff is too large
Cuff deflation is at a rate more rapid than 3 mm Hg per second
The extremity is above heart level

TABLE 27-7

PROBLEMS ASSOCIATED WITH NONINVASIVE AUTOMATIC CYCLED CUFF-BASED BLOOD PRESSURE MONITORING SYSTEMS

Edema of the extremity

Petechiae formation

Ulnar neuropathy (an encircling cuff should be applied proximal to the ulnar groove)

Interference with timing of intravenous drug administration when the access site is located in the same extremity as the monitoring system

Hydrostatic effect (this should be corrected by adding or subtracting 0.7 mm Hg for every centimeter the cuff is above or below the level of the heart)

   3. **Automated oscillometry** has replaced auscultatory and palpatory techniques for routine intraoperative blood pressure monitoring.
      a. Oscillometry accurately measures systolic blood pressure, diastolic blood pressure, and MAP (discrepancy with centrally placed arterial line <5 mm Hg).
      b. A variety of cuff sizes makes it possible to use oscillometry in patients of all ages.
   B. **Problems with Noninvasive Blood Pressure Monitoring.** Complications may accompany repeated inflations of automatically cycled blood pressure cuffs placed on the upper extremity (Table 27-7).
   C. **Invasive Measurement of Vascular (Arterial Blood) Pressure**
      1. Indwelling arterial cannulation not only offers anesthesiologists the opportunity to monitor beat-to-beat changes in arterial blood pressure but also provides vascular access for arterial blood sampling.
      2. Intra-arterial measurement of blood pressure is subject to many sources of error based on the physical properties of fluid motion and the performance of the catheter–transducer–amplification system used to sense, process, and display the pressure pulse wave. Ideally, the catheter and tubing are stiff, the volume of fluid in the connecting tubing is small, the number of stopcocks is limited, and the connecting tubing length is not excessive.

MANAGEMENT

3. Because many therapeutic decisions are based on changes in arterial blood pressure, it is imperative that anesthesiologists understand the physical limitations imposed by fluid-filled pressure transducer systems.

   a. In clinical practice, underdamped catheter–transducer systems tend to overestimate systolic blood pressure by 15 to 30 mm Hg and to amplify artifact ("catheter whip").

   b. Air bubbles cause overdamping and underestimation of systolic blood pressure.

   c. MAP is accurately measured even in the presence of overdamping or underdamping.

   d. In clinical practice, it is sufficient to calibrate the transducer to atmospheric pressure, usually with the transducer located at the level of the right atrium.

D. **Arterial Cannulation**

   1. The radial artery remains the most popular site for cannulation because of its accessibility and the presence of a collateral blood supply (Fig. 27-3).

   2. The prognostic value of the Allen test in assessing the adequacy of the ulnar collateral circulation has not been confirmed.

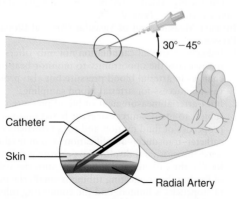

FIGURE 27-3.   Technique for radial artery cannulation.

E. **Complications of Invasive Arterial Monitoring** (Table 27-8)

1. Traumatic cannulation has been associated with median nerve dysfunction, hematoma formation, and thrombosis.

2. Abnormal radial artery blood flow after the removal of an arterial catheter (a nontapered 20- to 22-gauge Teflon catheter is recommended) occurs frequently (presumably because of radial artery thrombosis), with normalization of blood flow usually occurring in 3 to 7 days.

3. Direct arterial pressure monitoring requires constant vigilance and correlation of the measured blood pressure with other clinical parameters before therapeutic interventions are initiated.

TABLE 27-8

CANNULATION SITES FOR DIRECT ARTERIAL BLOOD PRESSURE MONITORING

Site	Clinical Points
Radial artery	Preferred cannulation site Ischemia most likely reflects arterial thrombosis Aneurysm formation Arteriovenous fistula formation Infection Fluid overload in neonates from continuous flush techniques (3–6 mL/hr)
Ulnar artery	Complications similar to those of radial artery Principal source of blood flow to the hand
Brachial artery	Insertion site medial to biceps tendon Median nerve damage
Axillary artery	Insertion site at junction of pectoralis major and deltoid muscles
Femoral artery	Easy access in low-flow states Potential for local and retroperitoneal hemorrhage Catheter with increased length preferred
Dorsalis pedis artery	Collateral circulation via posterior tibial artery Higher systolic blood pressure

MANAGEMENT

    a. Sudden increases or decreases in blood pressure may represent a hydrostatic error when the position of the transducer is not adjusted after changes in the position of the operating room table.

    b. A sudden decrease in blood pressure may be caused by a damped tracing from a partially occluded or kinked arterial catheter.

    c. Before initiating therapy based on a change in blood pressure, the calibration of the transducer system and the patency of the arterial cannula should be verified.

V. CENTRAL VENOUS AND PULMONARY ARTERY MONITORING

The **right internal jugular vein** is the most common site for cannulation (Table 27-9 and Figs. 27-4 to 27-6). Ultrasound-guided placement of the right internal jugular vein venous catheter may decrease complications and improve first attempt success rates.

A. Central Venous Pressure Monitoring

1. Central venous pressure is essentially equivalent to right atrial pressure, and the normal waveform consists of three peaks (a, c, and v waves) and two descents (x, y) (Table 27-10 and Fig. 27-7).

2. The possibility of venous air embolism is decreased by positioning the patient in a head-down position during placement or removal of the central venous catheter.

3. Central venous catheter placement is an important source of nosocomial infection and sepsis, emphasizing the importance of sterile technique during catheter placement and of the application of appropriate dressings (Table 27-11).

B. Pulmonary Artery Monitoring

1. **Indications** for placement of a pulmonary artery catheter are broadly defined. (Intracardiac pressures, thermodilution cardiac output, and mixed venous O_2 saturations should be measured, and derived hemodynamic indices should be calculated.) The measured and derived information is used to help define the clinical problem, monitor the progression of hemodynamic dysfunction, and guide the response to therapy.

TABLE 27-9

CENTRAL VENOUS PRESSURE CANNULATION SITES

Site	Advantages	Disadvantages
Right internal jugular vein	Accessible from head of operating room table Predictable anatomy High success rate in both adults and children Good landmarks	Carotid artery puncture Trauma to the brachial plexus Pneumothorax
Left internal jugular vein	Same as for right internal jugular vein	Damage to thoracic duct Difficulty in maneuvering the catheter through the jugular–subclavian junction Carotid artery puncture and embolization of the left dominant cerebral hemisphere
External jugular vein	Superficial location Safety	Lower success rate Kinks at the subclavian vein
Subclavian vein	Accessible Good landmarks	Pneumothorax Hemothorax Chylothorax Pleural effusion
Antecubital vein	Few complications	Lowest success rate Thrombosis Thrombophlebitis
Femoral vein	High success rate Thrombophlebitis	Catheter sepsis

    a. Pulmonary artery catheter monitoring may decrease perioperative complications if its use is tailored to the clinical condition of the patient as it changes with time.

    b. The ASA has developed Practice Guidelines for Pulmonary Artery Catheterization.

  2. Correct placement of a pulmonary artery catheter is most often guided by observing changes in vascular waveforms (Fig. 27-8).

MANAGEMENT

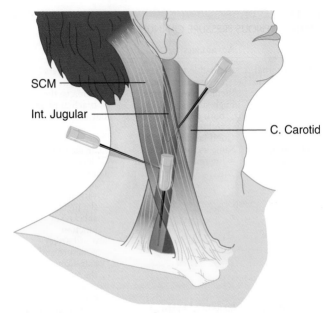

FIGURE 27-4. Three anatomic approaches for placement of a catheter in the internal jugular vein. The patient is placed head down with the head turned away from the intended venipuncture site. A 22-gauge locator needle may be inserted initially to identify the vein and thus minimize the likelihood of accidental carotid artery puncture when the larger needle is placed. Return of desaturated blood or transduction of the catheter (venous pressure) confirms entry into the internal jugular vein. SCM = sternocleidomastoid.

    3. Pulmonary capillary wedge pressure is used to indirectly assess left ventricular end-diastolic volume by reflecting changes in left ventricular end-diastolic pressure. Right-sided filling pressures often are poor indicators of left ventricular filling, either as absolute numbers or in terms of direction of change in response to therapy.

  C. **Factors Affecting the Accuracy of Pulmonary Artery Catheter Data** (Table 27-12)

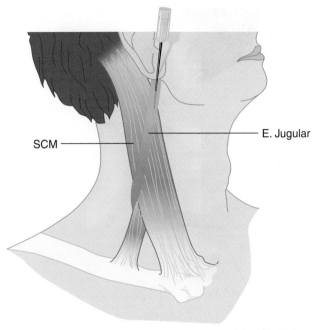

FIGURE 27-5. Placement of a catheter in the external jugular vein. SCM = sternocleidomastoid.

D. **Complications of Pulmonary Artery Catheter Monitoring** (Tables 27-13 and 27-14)
E. **Mixed Venous Oximetry**
   1. Advances in fiberoptic technology have led to the development of pulmonary artery catheters that can continuously measure **mixed venous** O_2 saturation (SvO_2).
   2. SvO_2 varies directly with cardiac output, hemoglobin concentration, and SaO_2 and inversely with minute O_2 consumption.
      a. When all other variables are constant, SvO_2 reflects corresponding changes in cardiac output.
      b. The normal SvO_2 is 75%, and anaerobic metabolism occurs when SvO_2 is below 30%.

MANAGEMENT

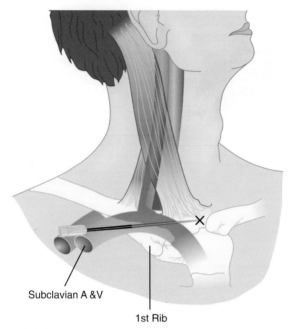

FIGURE 27-6.   Placement of a catheter (infraclavicular approach) in the subclavian vein. The patient is placed head down with the head turned away from the intended venipuncture site. Placing a roll between the scapulas opens the space between the clavicle and first rib. The needle is inserted 1 cm below the midpoint of the clavicle and advanced toward the anesthesiologist's finger in the suprasternal notch, keeping close to the posterior surface of the clavicle. Return of desaturated blood or transduction of the catheter (venous pressure) confirms entry into the subclavian vein.

F. **Central Venous Oxygen and Its Relation to Mixed Venous Oxygen**
  1. Central venous O_2 ($ScvO_2$) represents O_2 extraction from the upper body and brain but may serve as a surrogate measure of SvO_2.
  2. $ScvO_2$ may not reflect SvO_2 in the presence of septic shock.

TABLE 27-10

DIAGNOSTIC VALUE OF CENTRAL VENOUS PRESSURE WAVEFORMS

Waveform	Associated Conditions
Large a waves	Tricuspid stenosis
	Pulmonic stenosis
	Pulmonary hypertension
	Decreased right ventricular compliance
Large v waves	Tricuspid regurgitation
	Right ventricular papillary muscle ischemia or right ventricular failure
	Constrictive pericarditis
	Cardiac tamponade

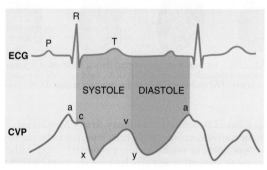

FIGURE 27-7. Central venous pressure (CVP) waveforms in relation to electrical events on the electrocardiogram (ECG).

TABLE 27-11

COMPLICATIONS COMMON TO ALL CENTRAL VENOUS PRESSURE CATHETER PLACEMENT TECHNIQUES

Accidental arterial puncture (hematoma, false aneurysm, arteriovenous fistula)
Poor positioning of the catheter during placement (vascular or cardiac chamber perforation, cardiac dysrhythmias)
Injury to surrounding structures
Clot and fibrinous sleeve formation
Thrombosis of the vein (embolus)
Catheter-related sepsis (see guidelines for prevention of catheter-related infections developed by the Centers for Disease Control and Prevention)
Bleeding

MANAGEMENT

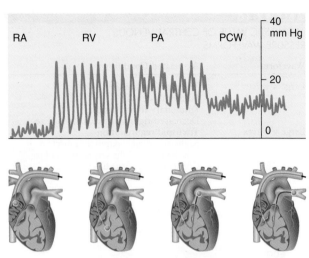

FIGURE 27-8. Pressure tracing observed during flotation of a pulmonary artery catheter through the right atrium (RA), right ventricle (RV), and pulmonary artery (PA) and into a pulmonary capillary wedge (PCW) position.

G. **Clinical Benefits of Pulmonary Artery Monitoring.** Perioperative outcomes have been reported to be improved, worsened, or unchanged by pulmonary artery catheter usage. Several recent articles have illustrated insufficient

TABLE 27-12

FACTORS AFFECTING THE ACCURACY OF PULMONARY ARTERY CATHETER DATA

Pulmonary vascular resistance (any disease- or drug-induced increase alters the relationship between pulmonary capillary wedge pressure and pulmonary artery end-diastolic pressure)

Alveolar–pulmonary artery pressure relationships (flow-directed pulmonary artery catheters usually advance to gravity-dependent areas of highest pulmonary blood flow; the location of the catheter should be confirmed with lateral chest radiography)

Intracardiac factors (mitral stenosis interferes with validity of left atrial pressure as a reflection of left ventricular end-diastolic pressure; decreased left ventricular compliance interferes with the validity of pulmonary capillary wedge pressure as a reflection of left ventricular end-diastolic pressure)

TABLE 27-13

COMPLICATIONS OF PULMONARY ARTERY CATHETER PASSAGE

Cardiac dysrhythmias (this is the most common complication; it is usually transient)
Catheter knotting, kinking, or coiling
Cardiac valve damage
Heart block
Perforation of the pulmonary artery, right atrium, or right ventricle
Trauma to the right ventricular endocardium

evidence for an outcome benefit from the use of a pulmonary artery catheter.

VI. TEMPERATURE MONITORING

A. The potential for accidental heat loss or the risk of triggering malignant hyperthermia requires the continued observation of temperature changes.
B. **Perioperative hypothermia** commonly results from anesthetic-induced inhibition of thermoregulation as well as a cold ambient environment in the operating room and heat loss owing to surgical exposure of tissues.
   1. Anesthetized patients often behave like poikilotherms until the core temperature approaches a new set point for thermoregulation.
   2. Patients at greatest risk for perioperative hypothermia include elderly patients, burn patients, neonates, and patients with spinal cord injuries.

TABLE 27-14

COMPLICATIONS OF PULMONARY ARTERY CATHETER PRESENCE

Thrombosis
Pulmonary infarction
Pulmonary artery rupture
Thrombocytopenia
Sepsis or infection
Cardiac valve damage
Endocarditis
Thromboembolism
Balloon rupture
Cardiac dysrhythmias
Trauma to the right ventricular endocardium

MANAGEMENT

C. **Perioperative hyperthermia** occurs rarely, and potential explanations other than malignant hyperthermia include exposure to endogenous pyrogens, increases in metabolic rate secondary to thyrotoxicosis or pheochromocytoma, and anticholinergic blockade of sweating.

D. Central temperature is customarily measured using temperature probes placed in the nasopharynx, esophagus, blood (pulmonary artery catheter), bladder, or rectum.

1. During routine noncardiac surgery, temperature differences between these sites are small.

2. During and after cardiopulmonary bypass or deliberate hypothermia, gradients between these sites are predictable.

   a. During cooling in anesthetized patients, changes in rectal temperature often lag behind changes in central (core) temperature.

   b. During rewarming, probe locations residing in regions of high blood flow often reflect blood temperature rather than central temperature, emphasizing that the adequacy of rewarming is best judged by measuring temperature at more than one location.

CHAPTER 28 ■
ECHOCARDIOGRAPHY

With its ability to provide comprehensive evaluation of myocardial, valvular, and hemodynamic performance, echocardiography is the first imaging technique to enter the mainstream of intraoperative patient monitoring (Table 28-1). (Perrino AC, Popescu WM, Skubas NJ: Perioperative echocardiography. In *Clinical Anesthesia*. Edited by Barash PG, Cullen BF, Stoelting RK, Cahalan MK, Stock MC. Philadelphia: Lippincott Williams & Wilkins, 2009, pp 715–750). In conjunction with the National Board of Echocardiography, the American Society of Anesthesiologists is establishing a second certification pathway in basic perioperative echocardiography.

I. **PRINCIPLES AND TECHNOLOGY OF ECHOCARDIOGRAPHY** Echocardiography generates dynamic images of the heart from the reflections of sound waves.
   A. **Physics of Sound.** In clinical echocardiography, a mechanical vibrator, known as the *transducer*, is placed in contact with the esophagus (transesophageal echocardiography [TEE]), the skin (transthoracic echocardiography), or the heart (epicardial echocardiography) to create tissue vibrations.
   B. **Properties of Sound Transmission in Tissue.** Echocardiographic imaging relies on the transmission and subsequent reflection of ultrasound energy back to the transducer.
   C. **Instrumentation**
      1. **Transducers.** Ultrasound transducers use piezoelectric crystals to create a brief pulse of ultrasound.
      2. **Beam Shape.** The ultrasound transducer emits a three-dimensional ultrasound beam similar to a movie

427

TABLE 28-1

APPLICATION OF INTRAOPERATIVE ECHOCARDIOGRAPHY

Guide placement of intracardiac and intravascular catheters and devices
Assessment of the severity of valve pathology
Immediate evaluation of a surgical intervention
Rapid diagnosis of acute hemodynamic instability
Directing appropriate therapies

projection. (The beam is narrow in the near field and then diverges into the far field zone.)

3. **Resolution.** Three parameters are evaluated when assessing the resolution of an ultrasound system: the resolution of objects lying along the axis of the ultrasound beam (*axial resolution*), the resolution of objects horizontal to the beam's orientation (*lateral resolution*), and the resolution of objects lying vertical to the beam's orientation (*elevational resolution*).

D. **Signal Processing.** To convert echoes into images, the returning ultrasound pulses are received, electronically processed, and displayed.

E. **Image Display.** Ultrasonic imaging is based on the amplitude and time delay of the reflected signals.

1. With B-mode echocardiography, the amplitude of the returning echoes from a single pulse determines the display brightness of the representative pixels.

2. Motion-mode (M-mode) echocardiography provides a one-dimensional, single-beam view through the heart but updates the B-mode images at a very high rate, providing dynamic real-time imaging. M-mode echocardiography remains the best technique for examining the timing of cardiac events.

3. Two-dimensional (2-D) echocardiography is a modification of B-mode echocardiography and is the mainstay of the echocardiographic examination.

F. **Spatial versus Dynamic Image Quality.** These selections determine whether sector size, spatial resolution, or dynamic motion is best displayed. A common approach is to focus each part of the examination on a given structure of interest and select the imaging plane that best delineates the structure in the near field. In situations in which the maximal frame rate is desired, M-mode echocardiography is chosen.

II. TWO-DIMENSIONAL AND THREE DIMENSIONAL TRANSESOPHAGEAL ECHOCARDIOGRAPHY

is the favored approach to intraoperative echocardiography. In the operating room, TEE is useful because the probe does not interfere with the operative field and can be left in situ, providing continuous, real-time hemodynamic information used to diagnose and manage critical cardiac events. TEE is also useful in situations in which the transthoracic examination is limited by various factors (e.g., obesity, emphysema, surgical dressings, prosthetic valves) and for examining cardiac structures that are not well visualized with TEE (e.g., left atrial appendage). However, the diagnostic capability of TEE depends on image acquisition and interpretation.

A. **Probe Insertion.** The TEE probe is inserted in the anesthetized patient in a manner similar to insertion of an orogastric tube. For improved image quality, the stomach is emptied of gastric contents and air before probe insertion. The TEE probe is advanced beyond the larynx and the cricopharyngeal muscle (around 25 to 30 cm from the teeth) until a loss of resistance is appreciated. At this point, the TEE probe lies in the upper esophagus, and the first cardiovascular images are seen.

B. **TEE Safety.** When performed by qualified operators, TEE has a low incidence of complications. Various studies have suggested an association between swallowing dysfunction after cardiac surgery and the use of intraoperative TEE. (Postoperative swallowing dysfunction is associated with pulmonary complications.)

C. **Contraindication to TEE Probe Placement** (Table 28-2). To maintain the safety profile of TEE, each patient should be evaluated before the procedure for signs, symptoms, and history of esophageal pathology. The most feared complication of TEE is esophageal or gastric perforation.

D. **Probe Manipulation.** Image acquisition is dependent on precise manipulation of the TEE probe. By advancing the shaft of the probe, the probe position can be moved from the upper esophagus to the midesophagus and into the stomach. The shaft can also be manually rotated to the left or right. By using the large knob on the probe handle, the head of the probe can be anteflexed (turning the knob clockwise) and retroflexed (turning the knob counterclockwise). The smaller knob, located on top of

MANAGEMENT

TABLE 28-2

CONTRAINDICATIONS TO TRANSESOPHAGEAL
ECHOCARDIOGRAPHY PROBE PLACEMENT

Esophageal strictures, rings, or webs
Esophageal masses (malignant tumors)
Recent bleeding of esophageal varices
After radiation of the neck
Recent gastric bypass surgery

the large knob, is used to tilt the head of the probe to
the right or left. Using the electronic switch on the probe
handle, the operator can rotate the ultrasound beam
from 0 degrees (transverse plane) to 180 degrees in
1-degree increments.

E. **Orientation.** An understanding of the basic rules of
imaging orientation is essential to echocardiographic
interpretation.

1. The ultrasound beam is always directed perpendicular to the probe face. An easy way to understand
this orientation is to place your right hand in front
of your chest with the palm facing down, the
thumb oriented left, and the fingers oriented anterior right. The scan lines that generate the TEE
image start at your fingers and sweep toward your
thumb.

2. Consequently, the right anatomical structures are displayed on the left side of the monitor (similar to chest
radiography orientation) (Fig. 28-1).

F. **Goals of the Two-Dimensional Examination.** A comprehensive evaluation is preferred with each cardiac chamber and valve imaged in at least two orthogonal planes.
However, in an emergency situation, such examination
may not be possible. In these cases, most echocardiogra-
phers focus the TEE examination to views that are most
likely to provide a diagnosis, including the transgastric
short axis view of the left ventricle (LV) for diagnosing
hypovolemia, coronary ischemia, and acute heart failure
(Table 28-3).

G. **Three-Dimensional Echocardiography.** This technology
is capable of acquiring full volumes of the left ventricle,
visualizing heart valves in three dimensions, and assessing the synchrony of LV contraction.

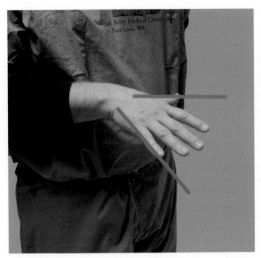

FIGURE 28-1. Orientation of the examiner's hand for an imaging plane of 0 degrees. The imaging plane is projected like a wedge anteriorly through the heart. The image is created by multiple scan lines traveling back and forth from the patient's left (*green line*) to the patient's right (*red line*). The resulting image is displayed on the monitor as a sector with the green edge (*green line*) on the right side of the monitor and the red edge (*red line*) on the left.

III. DOPPLER ECHOCARDIOGRAPHY AND HEMODYNAMICS

A. **Doppler Echocardiography and Hemodynamics.** 2-D echocardiography captures high-fidelity motion images of cardiac structures but not blood flow. Blood flow indices, such as blood velocities, stroke volume, and pressure gradients, are the domain of Doppler echocardiography. The combination of 2-D images and quantitative Doppler measurements create a uniquely powerful diagnostic tool.

1. The motion of an object causes a sound wave to be compressed in the direction of the motion and expanded in the direction opposite to the motion. This alteration in frequency is known as the *Doppler effect.*

2. By monitoring the frequency pattern of reflections of red blood cells, Doppler echocardiography can determine the speed, direction, and timing of blood flow.

MANAGEMENT

TABLE 28-3

MAIN USES OF VARIOUS TRANSESOPHAGEAL
ECHOCARDIOGRAPHY VIEWS

Midesophageal Ascending Aorta Short-Axis View
Evaluate the ascending aorta for dissection flaps.
Evaluate the pulmonary artery (position of catheter, presence
  of thrombus).
Align the Doppler beam parallel to the blood flow in the main
  pulmonary artery.

Midesophageal Aortic Valve Short-Axis View
Evaluate the AV cusps.
Evaluate aortic stenosis and to measure the area of the AV
  orifice (planimetry).
Evaluate aortic insufficiency by applying CFD.
Evaluate the interatrial septum for PFO or ASD.

Midesophageal Aortic Valve Long-Axis View
Evaluate the AV annulus, sinus of Valsalva, sinotubular
  junction, and abdominal aorta dimensions.
Evaluate aortic insufficiency by using CFD.
Evaluate vegetations or masses attached to the AV.
Evaluate left ventricular outflow track pathology.
Evaluate the presence of calcification or dissection flaps in
  the proximal abdominal aorta.

Midesophageal Bicaval View
Evaluate the interatrial septum, including CFD, to detect a
  PFO or ASD.
Determine the passage of air across the interatrial septum.
Guide placement of catheters and cannulas (pulmonary artery
  catheter, pacemaker wires).
Detect the presence of thrombus or tumors.

Midesophageal Right Ventricular Inflow–Outflow View
Evaluate the pulmonic valve by measuring the pulmonary
  annulus (required for Ross procedure) and detect pulmonary
  insufficiency by applying CFD on top of the
  two-dimensional view.
Evaluate the structure and function of the RV and RV
  outflow tract.
Evaluate the tricuspid valve.
Evaluate the location of the pulmonary artery.

Midesophageal Four-Chamber View
Evaluate the size and function of the LA, RA, RV, and LV
  (inferoseptal and anterolateral walls).
Evaluate tricuspid valve and mitral valve structure and function.
  (CFD will detect valvular pathology.)
Evaluate diastolic function.

(continued)

TABLE 28-3

MAIN USES OF VARIOUS TRANSESOPHAGEAL
ECHOCARDIOGRAPHY VIEWS (*Continued*)

Midesophageal Two-Chamber View
Evaluate LV anterior and inferior wall function.
Evaluate the LV apex.
Diagnose apical thrombus.

Midesophageal Long-Axis View
Evaluate LV anteroseptal and posterior wall function.
Evaluate LV outflow tract pathology.
Evaluate the mitral valve.

Transgastric Midpapillary Short-Axis View (considered to be the
most useful view in situations of intraoperative
hemodynamic instability because it allows immediate
diagnosis of hypovolemic state, pump failure, and coronary
ischemia)
Evaluate LV size (enlargement, hypertrophy) and cavity volume.
Evaluate global ventricular systolic function and regional wall
motion.

Transgastric Two-Chamber View
Evaluate function of the LV anterior and inferior walls

Transgastric Long-Axis View
Evaluate the systolic function of the anteroseptal and posterior
LV walls.

Deep Transgastric Long-Axis View
Perform Doppler assessment of the LV outflow tract and aortic
blood velocities.

Aortic Short-Axis and Long-Axis Views
Identify pathology of the descending aorta (atheroma, dissection
flaps, aneurysm).
Assist with placement of guidewires and cannulas (intra-aortic
balloon pump, aortic cannula).

Upper Esophageal Aortic Arch Short-Axis View
Evaluate the presence of pathology in the distal aortic arch.
Perform Doppler assessment of the pulmonary arterial blood
velocities.

ASD = atrial septal defect; AV = aortic valve; CFD = color flow Doppler;
LA = left atrium; LV = left ventricle; PFO = patent foramen ovale; RA = right
atrium; RV = right ventricle.

MANAGEMENT

B. **Doppler Techniques.** Two Doppler techniques, *pulsed-wave* (PW) and *continuous-wave* (CW) Doppler are commonly used to evaluate blood flow.
   1. **PW Doppler** offers the ability to sample blood flow from a particular location. Doppler data are frequently presented as a velocity–time plot known as the *spectral display*.
   2. **CW Doppler** avoids the maximal velocity limitation of PW systems, and blood flows with very high velocities are recorded accurately (determining the high-velocity jet of aortic stenosis).
C. **Color-Flow Doppler** (CFD) provides a dramatic display of both blood flow and cardiac anatomy by combining 2-D echocardiography and PW Doppler methods (Fig. 28-2). Red hues indicate flow toward the transducer, and blue hues indicate flow away from the transducer.
   1. The ability to provide a real-time, integrated display of flow and structural information makes CFD useful for assessing valvular function, aortic dissection, and congenital heart abnormalities.
   2. CFD is susceptible to alias artifacts.

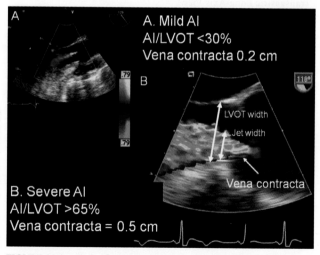

FIGURE 28-2. Color flow Doppler of the aortic valve (AV) in the midesophageal long-axis (ME AV LAX) view. Aortic insufficiency (AI) is graded using the relative ratio of the AI jet thickness to the diameter of left ventricular outflow tract (LVOT).

D. **Hemodynamic Assessment.** The ability of Doppler echocardiography to quantitatively measure blood velocity yields a wealth of information on the hemodynamic state (stroke volume, chamber pressures, valvular disease, pulmonary vascular resistance, systolic and diastolic ventricular function, anatomic defects).

E. **Echocardiographic Evaluation of Systolic Function**
   1. Evaluation of global and regional left ventricular (LV) systolic function is a primary component of every echocardiographic examination (Figs. 28-3 and 28-4). Modalities used are 2-D and M-mode echocardiography, which image the LV walls and cavity, and Doppler echocardiography, which measures the velocity of blood flow and moving tissue.

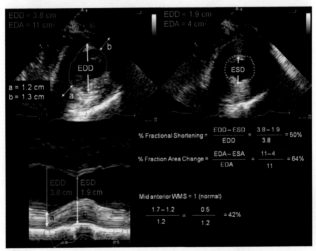

FIGURE 28-3. Two-dimensional evaluation of left ventricular (LV) global and regional function. Regional and global evaluation of the LV using the transgastric short-axis view at the midpapillary level. Measurements are performed at end-diastole (ED) and end-systole (ES). *Top panels:* Measurement of diameters (D), areas (A), and wall thickness. Wall thickness is measured at ED in the anteroseptal and inferolateral wall segments. *Bottom panel:* Diameter and wall thickness measured using M-mode echocardiography with the cursor crossing the middle of inferior (top) and anterior (bottom) segments. The percent change of wall thickness of the midanterior wall segment can be used to grade its regional function. In this example, wall motion score (WMS) is 1 (normal) because the segment thickens more than 30%.

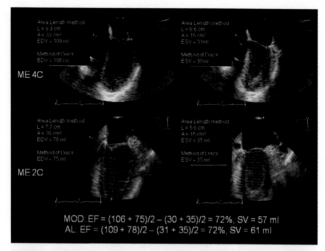

FIGURE 28-4. Quantitation of left ventricular (LV) systolic function. The midesophageal LV (ME) four-chamber (ME 4C) and two-chamber (ME 2C) views are obtained. The images are examined in end-diastole (ED) and end-systole (ES). The LV endocardium is traced. This automatically defines the LV area (A) and long axis (L). The system software will calculate LV volumes using either the method of discs (MOD) or the area-plane method (A-L). EDV = end-diastolic volume; EF = ejection fraction; ESV = end-systolic volume; SV = stroke volume.

2. **Ejection fraction** (EF) is the most frequently used estimate of LV systolic function. EF and stroke volume are affected by factors such as preload, afterload, and heart rate and thus are not always indicators of intrinsic systolic function.

3. **Stroke volume** is calculated as the difference between the end-diastolic volume (EDV) and the end-systolic volume (ESV), and the percentage of EF is calculated as %EF = SV/EDV = (EDV – ESV)/EDV.

4. Normal values for EDV are 67 to 155 mL in men and 56 to 104 mL in women. Normal values for ESV are 22 to 58 mL in men and 19 to 49 mL in women. The normal value for EF (%) is above 55%.

F. **Evaluation of Left Ventricular Diastolic Function**

1. Echocardiographic studies have suggested that patients with diastolic dysfunction presenting for cardiac surgery may be prone to intraoperative hemodynamic instability and worse outcomes.

2. Doppler echocardiography is the preferred technique for assessing diastolic performance and grading the severity of the disease process. Diastolic dysfunction is defined as the inability of the LV to fill at normal left atrium (LA) pressures and is characterized by a decrease in relaxation, LV compliance, or both.

3. Diastolic dysfunction may be present in the absence of clinical symptoms of heart failure. When these symptoms occur in the presence of diastolic dysfunction, the diagnosis of diastolic heart failure is made.

G. **Pericardial Disease: Constrictive Pericarditis and Pericardial Tamponade**

1. Pericardial pathologies, such as constrictive pericarditis or pericardial tamponade, impede diastolic flow (this resembles a diastolic restrictive filling pattern).

2. Pericardial effusions may be global, surrounding the entire heart, or loculated, as seen mostly after cardiac surgery (Fig. 28-5).

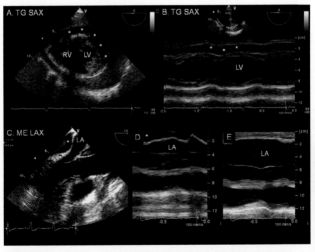

FIGURE 28-5. Echocardiographic findings in pericardial effusion. **A.** Transgastric short-axis (TG SAX) view showing global pericardial effusion (*asterisk*) surrounding both the right ventricle (RV) and left ventricle (LV). **B.** M-mode echocardiography demonstrating separation of the epicardium from the pericardium (*asterisk*) from pericardial effusion. **C.** Regional pericardial effusion (*asterisk*) compressing the left atrium (LA), seen in the midesophageal long-axis (ME LAX) view. **D.** M-mode echocardiography revealing systolic compression of the LA. **E.** After evacuation of the fluid collection, the LA size increases.

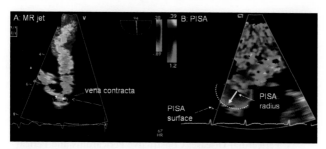

FIGURE 28-6. Doppler evaluation of mitral regurgitation severity. Mitral regurgitation (MR) severity is evaluated using color Doppler. **A.** An MR jet is imaged with color-flow Doppler (midesophageal two-chamber view). The Nyquist limit is moved upward to demonstrate flow acceleration inside the left ventricle (LV) and the neck (vena contracta) of the MR jet. **B.** Zoom of the proximal MR jet allows measurement of the proximal isovelocity surface area (PISA) radius and calculation of the incompetent mitral valve orifice.

IV. EVALUATION OF VALVULAR HEART DISEASE

2-D echocardiography (valve anatomy and function) and Doppler (physiologic consequences and severity of the lesion) are complementary methods in valve assessment (aortic, mitral, pulmonic) (Figs. 28-2, 28-6, and 28-7).

    A. **Diseases of the Aorta.** The evaluation of the aorta is an important part of perioperative TEE. In routine cases such as coronary artery bypass surgery, evaluation of the aorta may reveal previously unknown, significant atheromatous disease of the aorta and alter the surgical plan (off-pump bypass, alternative sites for cannulation).

    B. **Cardiac Masses.** The potential of myxomas to obstruct the inflow or outflow region of a ventricle is demonstrated with Doppler echocardiography.

V. CONGENITAL HEART DISEASE (CHD)

Echocardiography is the primary imaging modality for diagnostic assessment of patients with CHD (atrial septal defect, ventricular septal defect, patent ductus arteriosus, coarctation of the aorta, bicuspid aortic valve, repaired tetralogy of Fallot).

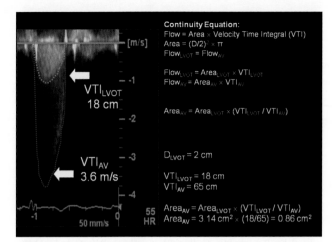

Continuity Equation:

$Flow = Area \times Velocity\ Time\ Integral\ (VTI)$

$Area = (D/2)^2 \times \pi$

$Flow_{LVOT} = Flow_{AV}$

$Flow_{LVOT} = Area_{LVOT} \times VTI_{LVOT}$

$Flow_{AV} = Area_{AV} \times VTI_{AV}$

$Area_{AV} = Area_{LVOT} \times (VTI_{LVOT} / VTI_{AV})$

$D_{LVOT} = 2\ cm$

$VTI_{LVOT} = 18\ cm$

$VTI_{AV} = 65\ cm$

$Area_{AV} = Area_{LVOT} \times (VTI_{LVOT} / VTI_{AV})$

$Area_{AV} = 3.14\ cm^2 \times (18/65) = 0.86\ cm^2$

FIGURE 28-7. Evaluation of aortic stenosis with calculation of aortic valve area using the "double envelope" technique. The cursor of continuous-wave Doppler is placed in the middle of the blood flow traversing the stenosed aortic valve, and two envelopes are identified. The one with the slower velocity is from the left ventricular outflow tract (LVOT), and the one with the fastest is from the aortic valve. The envelopes of the velocities are traced to derive the respective velocity–time integrals (VTIs). The aortic valve area is calculated using the continuity equation. D = diameter.

VI. ECHOCARDIOGAPHY-ASSISTED PROCEDURES

In addition to its role in diagnostics, echocardiography is also used to assist during various procedures such as placement of central venous catheter, intra-aortic balloon pump catheter, coronary sinus cannula, and guidewires for other venous or arterial cannulas.

VII. ECHOCARDIOGRAPHY OUTSIDE THE OPERATING ROOM Echocardiography offers rapid diagnosis by differentiating among the potential complications faced in postoperative care (hypovolemia, aortic dissection, myocardial infarction, endocarditis, pulmonary embolism).

MANAGEMENT

CHAPTER 29 ■ AIRWAY MANAGEMENT

Although the role of the supraglottic airway (SGA) is firmly established in routine anesthetic care as well as airway rescue, the advent of video laryngoscopy promises to remove many of the failings of a technique (translaryngeal tracheal intubation) that has been in use for more than 100 years (Rosenblatt WH, Sukhupragarn WA: Airway management. In *Clinical Anesthesia*. Edited by Barash PG, Cullen BF, Stoelting RK, Cahalan MK, Stock MC. Philadelphia: Lippincott Williams & Wilkins, 2009, pp 751–792). The decrease in claims related to airway events at the induction of anesthesia is not matched with a decrease during emergence and the postoperative period. Management of the airway is paramount to safe perioperative care, and specific steps are necessary to favorably affect outcome (Table 29-1).

I. REVIEW OF AIRWAY ANATOMY

A. The term "airway" refers to the upper airway, consisting of the nasal and oral cavities, pharynx, larynx, trachea, and principal bronchi.

1. The laryngeal skeleton consists of nine cartilages (three paired and three unpaired) that together house the vocal folds that extend in the anterior–posterior plane from the thyroid cartilage to the laryngeal cartilages.

2. The larynx is innervated by two branches of the vagus nerve, superior laryngeal nerve, and recurrent laryngeal nerve.

   a. The recurrent laryngeal nerve supplies all the intrinsic muscles of the larynx with the exception of the cricothyroid muscle.

   b. Vocal cord dysfunction accompanies trauma to these nerves. Unilateral nerve injury is unlikely to impair airway function, but the protective role of

TABLE 29-1

STEPS TO FAVORABLY AFFECT OUTCOME AS RELATED TO
AIRWAY MANAGEMENT

Airway history and physical examination
Consideration of the ease of rapid tracheal intubation (direct or
  indirect laryngoscopy)
Formulation of management plans for use of supraglottic means
  of ventilation
Weighing the risk of aspiration of gastric contents
Estimating the relative risk to the patient of failed airway
  maneuvers

     the larynx in preventing aspiration may be com-
     promised.

3. The cricothyroid membrane covers the cricothyroid
   space (~9 mm).
4. The cricoid cartilage is at the base of the larynx and is
   suspended by the underside of the cricothyroid membrane.
5. The trachea in adults measures about 15 cm and is
   supported circumferentially by 17 to 18 C-shaped cartilages with a posterior membranous aspect overlying
   the esophagus.
   a. The first tracheal ring is anterior to the sixth cervi-
      cal vertebra.
   b. The trachea ends at the fifth thoracic vertebra
      (carina), where it bifurcates into the right and left
      bronchi. The right mainstem bronchus is larger
      than the left and deviates from the plane of the tra-
      chea at a less acute angle. (Aspirated materials as
      well as deeply placed tracheal tubes are more likely
      to enter the right than the left bronchus.)

B. **Patient History and Physical Examination**
   1. Preoperative evaluation of the patient should elicit a
      thorough history of airway-related untoward events
      as well as related airway symptoms (obstructive sleep
      apnea, chipped teeth, dysphagia, stridor, cervical spine
      pain or limited range of motion, temporomandibular
      joint pain or dysfunction).
   2. Physical findings that may indicate subsequent
      difficult airway management include a short, muscu-
      lar neck with full dentition; a receding mandible; pro-
      truding maxillary central incisor teeth; decreased

MANAGEMENT

TABLE 29-2

SENSITIVITY AND SPECIFICITY OF PREOPERATIVE FINDINGS FOR DIFFICULT AIRWAY MANAGEMENT

	Sensitivity (%)	Specificity (%)	Positive Predictive Value*
Mouth opening (<4 cm)	26.3	94.8	25
Thyromental distance (<6 cm)	7	99.2	38.5
Mallampati class III	44.7	89.0	21
Neck movement <80 degrees	10.4	99.4	29.5
Inability to prognath	16.5	95.8	20.6
Body weight >110 kg	11.1	94.6	11.8
History of difficult intubation	4.5	99.9	69.0

*For finding of a grade III or IV view on direct laryngoscopy.

mobility at the temporomandibular joints; a long, high, arched palate; and increased alveolar–mental distance.

3. No common index for difficult airway prediction has proven to be both sensitive and specific (Table 29-2).

a. The Mallampati classification (based on tongue size in the intraoral cavity) is determined with the patient seated, the head in neutral position, the mouth opened as widely as possible, and the tongue protruded. The extent to which the base of the tongue is able to mask the visibility of the pharyngeal structures is the basis of classifying the airway as Mallampati I (uvula is fully visible) to IV (only the hard palate is visible). The practical value of this classification is its ease of application, but this index (like most others) has not proven to be sensitive or specific (there are many false-positive results) in identifying patients who may be difficult to intubate or the ease of using a SGA (laryngeal mask airway [LMA], fiberoptic bronchoscope).

b. The multivariate index (MI) assigns relative weights to each examination finding (thyromental distance, mouth opening, Mallampati score, head and neck movement, ability to prognath). Compared with the Mallampati classification, the MI has an improved positive predictive value and specificity.

II. CLINICAL MANAGEMENT OF THE AIRWAY

A. Preoxygenation

1. This procedure entails the replacement of the lung's nitrogen volume ("denitrogenation") with oxygen to provide a reservoir for diffusion of oxygen into the alveolar capillary bed after the onset of apnea (as associated with direct laryngoscopy for tracheal intubation).

   a. Breathing room air results in desaturation to below 90% after about 2 minutes of apnea.

   b. Breathing oxygen for 5 minutes maintains oxyhemoglobin saturation at 90% for about 6 minutes. As an alternative to breathing oxygen for 5 minutes, the patient may take four vital capacity breaths of oxygen over 30 seconds (or eight vital capacity breaths over 60 seconds).

2. Alveolar carbon dioxide increases during any period of apnea independent of preoxygenation.

B. Support of the Airway with the Induction of Anesthesia

1. With the induction of anesthesia and the onset of apnea, ventilation and oxygenation are supported by the anesthesiologist using traditional methods (face mask, tracheal tube) or a newer SGA device (LMA).

2. **The anesthesia face mask** is the most ubiquitous device used to deliver anesthetic gases and oxygen as well as to ventilate a patient who has been rendered apneic. Appropriate positioning of the patient's head and neck ("sniffing position") is paramount to successful mask ventilation.

   a. After induction of anesthesia, the face mask is held firmly on the patient's face with downward pressure on the mask applied by the anesthesiologist's thumb and first or second fingers with concurrent upward displacement of the mandible with the other fingers (known as a jaw thrust), which raises the soft tissues of the anterior airway off the pharyngeal wall and allows for improved ventilation.

   b. In patients who are obese, edentulous, or have beards, two hands may be required to ensure a tight-fitting face mask (when two hands are required, a second operator is needed).

c. In the presence of normal lung compliance, the lung inflation pressure should not exceed 20 to 25 cm H_2O.

d. If more pressure is required, it may be prudent to consider other devices to aid in the creation of a patent upper airway (oral airway, nasal airway, LMA) to create an artificial passage between the roof of the mouth, tongue, and posterior pharyngeal wall.

e. Oral airways may provoke coughing, vomiting, or laryngospasm when placed into the pharynx of a semiconscious patient.

C. **Supraglottic Airways.** The advent of the LMA and other SGA devices has led some to question the relative safety of tracheal intubation (vocal cord edema, increased airflow resistance). Pharyngeal mucosal changes as a result of SGA use appear to be delayed compared with the effects of tracheal intubation.

1. **The Laryngeal Mask Airway Classic** is composed of a small "mask" designed to sit in the hypopharynx with an aperture overlying the laryngeal inlet. The rim of the mask is composed of an inflatable silicone cuff that fills the hypopharyngeal space, creating a seal that allows positive-pressure ventilation with up to 20 cm H_2O pressure and tidal volumes of 8 mL/kg.

2. **The Laryngeal Mask Airway Flexible** is designed to permit sharing of the airway with the surgical team (designed to be used with a tonsillar mouth gag).

3. **The Laryngeal Mask Airway and Bronchospasm.** As a SGA, the LMA appears to be well suited for patients with a history of bronchospasm (asthma) who are not at risk for reflux and aspiration.

4. **Laryngeal Mask Airway Removal.** The timing of removal of the LMA at the end of surgery is critical. The LMA should be removed when the patient is deeply anesthetized or after protective reflexes have returned and the patient is able to open the mouth on command.

5. **Contraindications to Laryngeal Mask Airway Use** (Table 29-3)

6. **Complications of Laryngeal Mask Airway Use** (Table 29-4)

TABLE 29-3

CONTRAINDICATIONS TO USE OF A LARYNGEAL MASK AIRWAY

Risk of pulmonary aspiration of gastric contents (patient with a "full stomach"
Hiatal hernia with significant gastroesophageal reflux
Morbid obesity
Intestinal obstruction
Delayed gastric emptying
Poor pulmonary compliance
Increased airway resistance
Glottic or subglottic airway obstruction
Limited mouth opening (<1.5 mm)

7. **The Laryngeal Mask Airway Proseal.** This device incorporates a gastric drain and increases the maximum airway seal during positive-pressure ventilation (possible use in obese patients during laparoscopic cholecystectomy) (Table 29-5).
8. **The laryngeal tube** consists of a single-lumen tube and two (distal and proximal) low-pressure cuffs. When inserted correctly, the proximal cuff seals the oral and nasal pharynx, and the distal cuff sits within the upper esophageal sphincter.
9. **The Cobra pharyngeal laryngeal airway** is a disposable supralaryngeal device with a single lumen that terminates in a widened distal end. A fiberscope or tracheal tube may be passed through this device.

TABLE 29-4

COMPLICATIONS WITH USE OF A LARYNGEAL MASK AIRWAY

Gastroesophageal reflux and aspiration
Laryngospasm
Coughing
Bronchospasm
Sore throat (less than with tracheal intubation)
Transient changes in vocal cord function (possibly related to cuff overinflation during prolonged procedures)
Nerve injury (recurrent laryngeal, hypoglossal, or lingual; LMA cuff pressure should not exceed 60 cm H_2O)
Diffusion of nitrous oxide into the cuff, increasing pressure

LMA = laryngeal mask airway.

MANAGEMENT

TABLE 29-5

FEATURES OF THE LARYNGEAL MASK AIRWAY PROSEAL

Feature	Clinical Impact
Gastric drain	Position confirmation
	Active gastric emptying
	Passive gastric emptying
	Protection from gastric content aspiration
Posterior cuff	Increased seal pressure
Bite block	Prevents patient biting obstruction
Wire reinforced airway barrel	Reduced overall size
	Decreased ability to tracheally intubate
Large barrel or bite block configuration	First attempt insertion less successful than
	LMA classic
	Confers rotational stability
	Size choice—size down from LMA classic

LMA = laryngeal mask airway.

D. Tracheal Intubation

1. **Routine Laryngoscopy.** Repeated attempts at tracheal intubation often result in edema and bleeding of the anterior upper airway structures, hindering subsequent attempts at visualization and causing increased airway obstruction (first attempt at laryngoscopy in a best attempt).

2. **Direct Laryngoscopy.** Successful laryngoscopy involves the distortion of the normal anatomic planes of the supralaryngeal airway to produce a line of direct visualization ("sniff position of the patient's head") from the operator's eyes to the larynx (this requires alignment of the oral, pharyngeal, and laryngeal axes) (Fig. 29-1).

   a. Lateral external pressure over the larynx may be applied in an attempt to improve the laryngoscopist's view.

   b. The mouth can be opened by hyperextension of the atlanto-occipital joint using the laryngoscopist's hand placed under the patient's occiput or by application of downward pressure on the patient's chin.

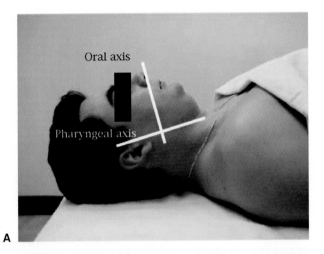

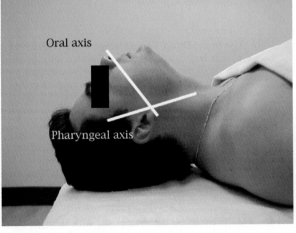

FIGURE 29-1. With the patient in the supine position with no head support, the oral, pharyngeal, and tracheal axes do not overlap (**A**). The "sniff" position maximally overlaps the three axes (**B**).

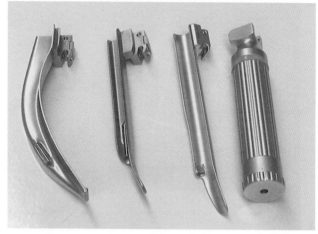

FIGURE 29-2.   Macintosh (curved) and Miller (straight) laryngoscope blades and small and regular-sized handles.

3. **Use of the Direct Laryngoscope Blade** (Fig. 29-2)
   a. The laryngoscope blade is inserted into the right side of the patient's mouth (with care taken not to compress the upper lip against the teeth or to rotate the blade on the upper incisors) and advanced toward the epiglottis as the tongue is displaced to the left.
   b. Whereas the Macintosh blade tip is advanced into the vallecula, the Miller blade is advanced until it is positioned beneath the epiglottis while the laryngoscopist's arm and shoulder lift in an anterior and caudad direction.
   c. The view of the larynx may be complete, partial, or not possible (Fig. 29-3).
   d. The tracheal tube is inserted with the right hand and passed through the vocal folds to a depth of at least 2 cm after the disappearance of the tracheal tube cuff past the vocal folds (represents the midtrachea, which corresponds to the 21- and 23-cm external marking on the tracheal tube at the teeth for the typical adult woman and man, respectively.

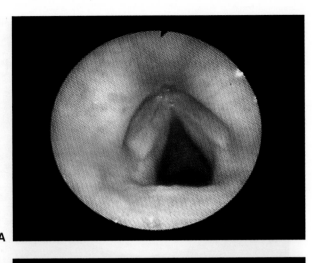

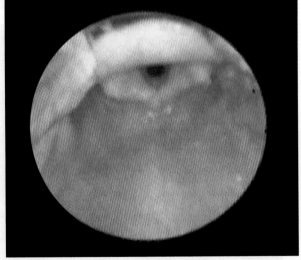

FIGURE 29-3.   The Cormack and Lehane laryngeal view scoring system. **A.** Grade I, visualization of the entire glottic aperture. **B.** Grade II, visualization of only the posterior aspects of the glottic aperture.

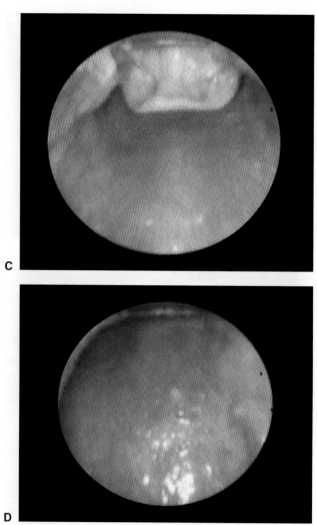

FIGURE 29-3. *Continued.*   C. Grade III visualization of the tip of the epiglottis. D. Grade IV, visualization of no more than the soft palate.

e. The gold standard for confirmation that the tube has been placed in the trachea is sustained detection of exhaled carbon dioxide as measured with capnography.

4. **NPO Status and Rapid Sequence Induction.** In the rapid sequence induction of anesthesia, intravenous administration of an induction drug is followed by a rapidly acting neuromuscular blocking drug. Direct laryngoscopy and tracheal intubation are performed as soon as muscle relaxation is confirmed.

5. **The Intubating Laryngeal Mask Airway (LMA-Fastrach).** Blind fiberoptic-aided, stylet-guided, and laryngoscopy-directed intubation via the LMA can be accomplished in adults and children.
   a. A limiting factor is the size of the tracheal tube that may be passed through the airway.
   b. LMA-Fastrach can accommodate up to an 8-mm cuffed tracheal tube and is indicated for routine elective intubation and for anticipated and unanticipated difficult intubation.

6. **LMA CTrach** is functionally identical to the Intubating LMA-Fastrach with the addition of integrated fiberoptic channels.

E. **Extubation of the trachea** is often performed after the return of consciousness (after the patient can follow simple commands) and spontaneous ventilation (resolution of neuromuscular blockade). A patient who presents with a "difficult airway" at the time of induction of anesthesia must also be considered having "difficult extubation" at the time of extubation.

1. **Laryngospasm** is a possible cause of airway compromise after tracheal extubation. (It is treated with administration of oxygen with continuous positive airway pressure and, if necessary, the use of a small dose of a rapidly acting muscle relaxant.) Negative-pressure pulmonary edema may result from airway obstruction in a patient who develops laryngospasm and who continues to create negative intrathoracic pressure as a result of voluntary respiratory effort.

2. **Approach to Difficult Extubation.** When it is suspected that a patient may have difficulty with oxygenation or ventilation after tracheal extubation, the clinician may choose from a variety of management strategies (standby reintubation equipment, placement of a guide for reintubation or oxygenation).

MANAGEMENT

III. THE DIFFICULT AIRWAY

A. The Difficult Airway Algorithm (Fig. 29-4)

1. A difficult airway is defined as the situation in which a conventionally trained anesthesiologist experiences difficulty with mask ventilation (unassisted anesthesiologist unable to maintain $SpO_2 > 90\%$ using 100% oxygen) or the inability to place a tracheal tube with conventional laryngoscopy (more than three attempts or more than 10 minutes).

2. The incidence of failed tracheal intubation is estimated to be 0.05% to 0.35%, and the incidence of failed intubation plus an inability to achieve mask ventilation is estimated to be 0.01% to 0.03%.

3. Even if the patient's oxygen saturation remains adequate during unsuccessful attempts at tracheal intubation, it is prudent to limit the number of attempts to three because significant soft tissue trauma can result from multiple laryngoscopies. At this stage, the clinician may consider alternatives to direct laryngoscopy and tracheal intubation that include fiberoptic laryngoscopy, use of an LMA, or establishment of a surgical airway. In some instances, it may be best to allow the patient to resume spontaneous ventilation and awaken.

B. Awake Airway Management

1. Awake airway management (LMA, fiberoptic intubation) is indicated if, after a thorough airway examination or a review of previous anesthetics, the ability to safely control ventilation and oxygenation without the risk of pulmonary aspiration is in question.

2. Important to the success of awake intubation techniques is administration of drugs to reduce anxiety and secretions.

3. Local anesthetics (topical lidocaine, benzocaine spray, phenylephrine, oxymetazoline) are a cornerstone of awake airway techniques. Local anesthetic therapy should be directed to the nasal cavity or nasopharynx (cotton-tipped applicators soaked with local anesthetic solution), pharynx, base of the tongue (aerosolized local anesthetic solution or voluntary "swish and swallow," superior laryngeal nerve block), and the larynx or trachea (transtracheal injection of local anesthetic solution).

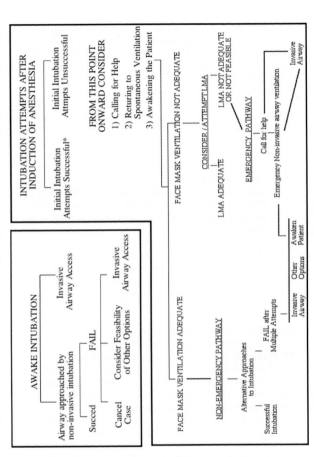

FIGURE 29-4. The American Society of Anesthesiologists' difficult airway algorithm. LMA = laryngeal mask airway.

MANAGEMENT

C. **Use of a Fiberoptic Bronchoscope in Airway Management**
 1. The fiberoptic bronchoscope has proven to be the most versatile tool for anesthesiologists dealing with an awake or unconscious patient who is or appears to be difficult to intubate.
 2. **Use of a Fiberoptic Bronchoscope**
    a. A variety of intubation airways are available and designed to provide a clear visual path from the oral aperture to the pharynx, keep the bronchoscope in the midline, prevent the patient from biting the insertion cord, and provide a clear airway for the spontaneously or mask-ventilated patients.
    b. After successful navigation through the SGA, the endoscopist visualizes the vocal folds. After the larynx is entered, a landmark (the carina) is selected to serve as an identifying landmark as the tracheal tube is advanced.
    c. An estimated 20% to 30% of tracheal tube advancements are accompanied by "hang up."
D. **Video-Macintosh laryngoscope** consists of a conventional-appearing laryngoscope and a fiberoptic cable that enters the handle where the camera elements are housed. The video image is displayed, and the operator or second operator directs the tube into position.
E. **Retrograde wire intubation** is performed with the patient in a sitting position by percutaneous placement of an 18-gauge catheter placed through the cricothyroid membrane. A radiographic guidewire is placed through the catheter until it appears in the mouth, and a 7.0 tracheal tube is place over the guidewire and guided into the trachea.
F. **Use of Esophageal Tracheal Combitube**
 1. The tube is inserted blindly, and the oropharyngeal balloon and distal cuff balloon are inflated.
 2. In the majority of patients, tube placement results in an esophageal position, and ventilation occurs via this lumen's hypopharyngeal perforations.
 3. Advantages include rapid airway control, airway protection from regurgitation, easy use by an inexperienced operator, no need to visualize the glottic opening, and the ability to maintain the neck in a neutral position.
G. **The Laryngeal Mask Airway in the Failed Airway**
 1. It is estimated that one in 10,000 patients cannot be ventilated by mask and cannot be intubated by tradi-

TABLE 29-6

PERCUTANEOUS TRANSTRACHEAL JET VENTILATION

An intravenous catheter (12, 14, or 16 gauge) is attached to a
 syringe ($\geq$5 mL) that is empty or partially filled with saline.
 (Alternatively, a commercially available emergency
 cricothyroidotomy catheter set is used.)
The larynx is stabilized with the anesthesiologist's nondominant
 hand, and the catheter needle is advanced through the caudad
 third of the cricothyroid membrane.
Constant aspiration on the syringe plunger is applied, and free
 aspiration of air confirms entrance into the trachea.
The catheter is advanced into the trachea.
The oxygen source is attached. A fresh gas outlet of anesthesia
 machine is acceptable by placing a cuffed tracheal tube into the
 barrel of a 5- to 10-mL syringe to engage the catheter while the
 15-mm adapter of the tracheal tube is fitted into the fresh gas
 outlet of the anesthesia machine.
Manual closure of the mouth and nose may be needed during
 insufflation but not exhalation.

tional means. It is also estimated that one in 800,000
patients cannot be managed with an LMA.

2. The major disadvantage of the LMA is the lack of
   mechanical protection from regurgitation and
   aspiration.

H. **Minimally Invasive Transtracheal Procedures**

1. **Cricothyrotomy** is the procedure of choice in
   emergency situations.

2. **Percutaneous transtracheal jet ventilation** is a form of
   cricothyrotomy that is an option in the "cannot ventilate, cannot intubate" situation (Table 29-6).

MANAGEMENT

CHAPTER 30 ■ PATIENT POSITIONING AND RELATED INJURIES

Positioning of a patients for a surgical procedure is frequently a compromise between what the anesthetized patient can tolerate (structurally and physiologically) and what the surgical team requires for anatomic access (Warner MA: Patient positioning and related injuries. In *Clinical Anesthesia*. Edited by Barash PG, Cullen BF, Stoelting RK, Cahalan MK, Stock MC. Philadelphia: Lippincott Williams & Wilkins, 2009, pp 793–814).There is a lack of solid scientific information on basic mechanisms of position-related complications. Notations about positions used during anesthesia and surgery, as well as brief comments about special protective measures such as eye care and pressure-point padding, are useful information to include in the anesthesia record.

I. DORSAL DECUBITUS POSITIONS

    A. **Variations of Dorsal Decubitus Positions** (Table 30-1)

    B. **Complications of Dorsal Decubitus Positions** (Table 30-2)

II. BRACHIAL PLEXUS AND UPPER EXTREMITY INJURIES (Table 30-3)

    A. **Ulnar Neuropathy** is characterized by an occurrence predominately in men (70% to 90%), high frequency of contralateral nerve dysfunction (suggesting that many patients have asymptomatic but abnormal ulnar nerves before undergoing anesthesia), and an often delayed appearance of symptoms (48 hours after the surgical procedure).

        1. Elbow flexion (>110 degrees) can cause ulnar nerve damage by compression of the nerve by the aponeurosis of the flexor carpi ulnaris muscle and cubital retinaculum. Conversely, in some patients, the roof of the cubital is poorly formed such that the ulnar nerve

TABLE 30-1

DORSAL DECUBITUS POSITIONS

Supine
Horizontal (the arms are padded and restrained alongside the trunk or abducted on padded arm boards; this does not place the hips and knees in a neutral position, resulting in discomfort for awake patients)
Contoured (the arms are placed as for the horizontal position; the hips and knees are slightly flexed; this is a good position for routine use)
Lateral uterine or abdominal mass displacement (leftward tilt of the table or placement of a wedge under the right hip)

Lithotomy
Standard (the lower extremities are flexed at the hips and knees and simultaneously elevated to expose the perineum; at the end of surgery, both legs are lowered together to minimize torsion stress on the lumbar spine)
Exaggerated (this stresses the lumbar spine and restricts ventilation because of abdominal compression by the thighs)

Head-Down Tilt (this should be avoid in patients with intracranial pathology)
Trendelenburg position (30 to 45 degrees head down; this may require some means of preventing the patient from sliding cephalad; shoulder braces should be avoided if possible; this position should only be used when a unique surgical issue requires it for exposure and only for as long as needed)

subluxes over the medial epicondyle of the humerus during elbow flexion, producing recurrent mechanical trauma.
2. External compression in the absence of elbow flexion may occur within the condylar groove or distal to the

TABLE 30-2

COMPLICATIONS OF DORSAL DECUBITUS POSITIONS

Postural hypotension (this is the most common complication of the head-up position; the legs should be lowered simultaneously from the lithotomy position if the patient has hypovolemia)
Pressure alopecia (padded head supports should be used)
Pressure-point reactions (to the heels, elbows, or sacrum; these should be protected against skin and soft tissue compression and ischemia, but there is no evidence that this is beneficial in reducing peripheral neuropathies in the perioperative period)

MANAGEMENT

TABLE 30-3

BRACHIAL PLEXUS AND UPPER EXTREMITY INJURIES

Brachial plexus neuropathy (most likely if the head is turned away from an excessively abducted arm; it may be associated with first rib fracture during median sternotomy)

Long thoracic nerve dysfunction (winging of the scapula reflecting serratus anterior muscle dysfunction; a viral origin should be considered)

Axillary trauma from the humeral head (abduction of the arm on an arm board to >90 degrees may thrust the head of the humerus into the axillary neurovascular bundle)

Radial nerve compression (a vertical bar of screen forces the nerve against the humerus; wrist drop)

Ulnar nerve compression (trauma occurs as the nerve passes behind the medial epicondyle of the humerus; sensory loss of the fifth finger and lateral border of the fourth finger may occur)

medial epicondyle, where the nerve and its associated artery are relatively superficial.

3. Anatomic differences between men and women may explain the higher incidence of ulnar nerve neuropathy in men (e.g., the tubercle of the coronoid process is approximately 1.5 times larger in men, men have less adipose tissue over the medial aspect of the elbow, and men have thicker flexor cubital retinacula).

4. The time of recognition of digital anesthesia associated with ulnar nerve dysfunction may be important in establishing the origin of the postoperative syndrome.

   a. If ulnar hypesthesia or anesthesia is noted promptly after the end of anesthesia (in the postanesthesia care unit [PACU]), it is likely to be associated with events that occurred during anesthesia and surgery.

   b. If recognition is delayed for many hours, the likelihood of cause shifts to postoperative events despite accepted methods of padding and positioning during the intraoperative period.

   c. Opioids may mask dysesthesias and pain after surgery but not loss of sensation caused by nerve dysfunction. It may be helpful to assess ulnar nerve function and record these observations before discharging patients from the PACU.

TABLE 30-4

OTHER DORSAL DECUBITUS PROBLEMS

Arm complications (abduction of the arm to >90 degrees should be avoided to avoid forcing the head of the humerus into the axillary neurovascular bundle)

Lumbar backache (ligamentous relaxation during anesthesia; the lithotomy position worsens pain from a herniated intervertebral disk)

Perineal crush injury (occurs on the fracture table for repair of a fractured hip when the pelvis is retained in place by a vertical pole at the perineum)

Compartment syndrome (characterized by systemic hypotension and impaired perfusion pressure to the legs that is augmented by elevation of the extremities; decompressive fasciotomies are necessary to relieve increased tissue pressure)

Finger injury (occurs when the digits are caught between the leg and thigh sections of the operating table as the leg section is returned to the horizontal position at the termination of an operation performed in the lithotomy position)

III. **OTHER DORSAL DECUBITUS PROBLEMS** (Table 30-4)

IV. **LATERAL DECUBITUS POSITIONS**

   A. Several positioning concepts should be considered when placing a patient into a lateral decubitus position.
      1. Wrapping the legs and thighs in compressive bandages is commonly used to combat venous pooling.
      2. A small support placed just caudad to the downside axilla (inappropriately called an *axillary roll*) can be used to lift the thorax to relieve pressure on the axillary neurovascular bundle and prevent decreased blood flow to the arm and hand. This chest support has not been shown to protect against ischemia or nerve damage but may decrease shoulder discomfort after surgery.
      3. Any padding support should be observed periodically to ensure that it does not impinge on the neurovascular structures of the axilla.
   B. **Variations of Lateral Decubitus Positions** (Table 30-5)
   C. **Complications of Lateral Decubitus Positions** (Table 30-6)

MANAGEMENT

TABLE 30-5

LATERAL DECUBITUS POSITIONS

Standard (Horizontal) Lateral Position
The downside thigh and knee are flexed, and pillows are placed between the legs and under the head to maintain alignment of the cervical and thoracic spines

Flexed Lateral Positions
Lateral jackknife (the downside iliac crest is over the table hinge to allow stretch of the upside flank; venous pooling occurs in the legs)
Kidney (an elevated table rest under the iliac crest further increases lateral flexion to expose the kidney; venous pooling and ventilation-to-perfusion mismatch may occur)

V. VENTRAL DECUBITUS (PRONE) POSITIONS

A. **Variations of Ventral Decubitus Positions** (Table 30-7)
B. **Complications of Ventral Decubitus Positions** (Table 30-8)
   1. Blindness after nonocular surgery may reflect compromise of oxygen delivery to elements of the visual pathway and include ischemic optic neuropathy, retinal artery occlusion, and cortical blindness.
   2. Positioning appears to be a risk factor for some of these events (spine surgery).
   3. Prolonged spine surgery, intraoperative hypotension, and massive blood loss, which may prevent adequate oxygen delivery to the visual apparatus, have been described in patients experiencing visual loss.

TABLE 30-6

COMPLICATIONS OF LATERAL DECUBITUS POSITIONS

Damage to the eyes or ears (pressure should be avoided)
Neck injury (lateral flexion is a risk, especially in patients with arthritis)
Suprascapular nerve injury (placement of a pad caudad to the dependent axilla prevents circumduction of the nerve; injury manifests as diffuse shoulder pain)
Long thoracic nerve dysfunction may reflect lateral flexion of the neck and stretch of the nerve

TABLE 30-7

VENTRAL DECUBITUS POSITIONS

Full prone (supportive pads should be used under the abdomen)
Prone jackknife
Kneeling

4. The American Society of Anesthesiologists Task Force on Perioperative Blindness has published an advisory based on a review of cases and the literature (Table 30-9).

VI. HEAD-ELEVATED POSITIONS

A. The sitting position permits improved surgical exposure for surgeries involving the posterior fossa and cervical spine.
   1. Mean arterial pressure should be measured at the level of the circle of Willis (with the transducer placed at the level of the external ear canal) because this site provides an accurate reflection of the perfusion pressure to the brain.
   2. Compressive wraps about the legs decrease pooling of blood in the lower extremities.
B. **Complications of Head-Elevated Positions** (Table 30-10)

TABLE 30-8

COMPLICATIONS OF VENTRAL DECUBITUS POSITIONS

Damage to the eyes or ears (pressure should be avoided; the use of protective goggles should be considered)
Blindness
Neck injury (an arthritic neck may be best managed in the sagittal plane; head rotation may decrease carotid and vertebral blood flows)
Brachial plexus injuries
Thoracic outlet syndrome (it may be useful to ask patients before surgery if they are able to sleep with their arms elevated overhead)
Breast injuries
Impaired venous return (supportive pads should be used under the abdomen)

MANAGEMENT

TABLE 30-9

SUMMARY OF PRACTICE ADVISORY FOR PERIOPERATIVE VISUAL LOSS ASSOCIATED WITH SPINE SURGERY

A subset of patients who undergo spine procedures in the supine position under general anesthesia have an increased risk for development of perioperative visual loss. High-risk patients are those who undergo prolonged spine procedures and those who have substantial blood loss.

The anesthesiologist should consider informing high-risk patients that there is a small, unpredictable risk of perioperative visual loss.

Use of deliberate hypotensive techniques during spine surgery has not been shown to be associated with the development of perioperative visual loss.

Colloids should be used along with crystalloids to maintain intravascular volume in patients who have substantial blood loss.

There is no apparent transfusion threshold that would eliminate the risk of perioperative visual loss related to anemia.

High-risk patients should be positioned so that the head is level or higher than the heart when possible. In addition, the head should be maintained in a neutral forward position (without significant neck flexion, extension, lateral flexion, or rotation) when possible.

Consideration should be given to the use of staged spine procedures in high-risk patients.

TABLE 30-10

COMPLICATIONS OF THE SITTING POSITION

Postural hypotension (normal compensatory reflexes are inhibited by anesthesia)

Air embolus (the potential increases with the degree of elevation or the operative site above the heart; air may pass through a probe patent foramen ovale if right atrial pressure exceeds left atrial pressure)

Pneumocephalus

Ocular compression

Edema of the face and tongue

Midcervical tetraplegia

Sciatic nerve injury

TABLE 30-11

SUMMARY OF AMERICAN SOCIETY OF ANESTHESIOLOGISTS'
ADVISORY ON PREVENTION OF PERIPHERAL NEUROPATHIES

Preoperative Assessment
When appropriate, it is helpful to determine if the patient can
comfortably tolerate the position required for the planned
operation.

Upper Extremity Positioning
Arm abduction should be limited to 90 degrees in supine patients.
The arms should be positioned to decrease pressure on the
postcondylar groove of the humerus (tucked at the side in a
neutral forearm position or abducted on arm boards in either a
neutral or supinated forearm position).

Lower Extremity Positioning
Lithotomy positions may stretch the sciatic nerve.
Prolonged pressure on the peroneal nerve at the fibular head
should be avoided.

Protective Padding
Padded arm boards may decrease the risk of upper extremity
neuropathy.
Padding at the elbow and fibular head may decrease the risk of
neuropathies.

Equipment
Properly functioning automatic blood pressure cuffs on the upper
arms do not affect the risk of neuropathies.
Shoulder braces in steep head-down positions may increase the
risk of brachial plexus neuropathies.

Postoperative Assessment
Assessment of extremity nerve function may lead to early
recognition of peripheral neuropathies.

Documentation
Charting specific positioning actions during patient care may
result in improvement in care.

VII. PERIOPERATIVE PERIPHERAL NEUROPATHIES
   A. **Prevention** (Table 30-11)
   B. **Practical Considerations**
      1. **Padding-Exposed Peripheral Nerves**
         a. Many types of padding are available to protect
            exposed peripheral nerves. There are no data to
            suggest that one material is more effective than

MANAGEMENT

another or that any padding is better than no padding.

b. The goal is to position and pad the exposed peripheral nerves to prevent their stretch beyond normally tolerated limits while awake, avoid direct compression of peripheral nerves if possible, and distribute over as large area as possible any compressive forces that must be placed on the peripheral nerve.

2. Prolonged Duration in One Position

a. Prolonged duration in the lithotomy position increases the risk of lower extremity neuropathy.

b. As much as practical, it may be prudent to limit the time spent in a single position. However, intermittent movement of the limbs or head during the intraoperative period may increase the risk of other problems, including moving an extremity into a suboptimal position.

C. Course of Action for the Patient with a Neuropathy

1. Sensory versus Motor Neuropathy

a. Sensory symptoms are usually transient (many resolve in the first 5 days). Typically, the patient is reassured and advised to avoid postures that might compress or stretch the involved nerve. If symptoms persist, a consultation with a neurologist may be indicated.

b. If the neuropathy has a motor component, a neurologist should be consulted promptly because electromyographic studies may be needed to assess the location of any acute lesion and to determine the presence of any chronic abnormalities such as in the contralateral but asymptomatic extremity.

CHAPTER 31 ■ **MONITORED ANESTHESIA CARE**

During monitored anesthesia care, the continuous attention of the anesthesiologist is directed at optimizing patient comfort and safety (Hillier SC, Mazurek MS: Monitored anesthesia care. In *Clinical Anesthesia*. Edited by Barash PG, Cullen BF, Stoelting RK, Cahalan MK, Stock MC. Philadelphia: Lippincott Williams & Wilkins, 2009, pp 815–832).

I. TERMINOLOGY

It is important to distinguish between the terms *monitored anesthesia* care and *sedation/analgesia*. Monitored anesthesia care implies the potential for a deeper level of sedation than that provided by *sedation/analgesia* and is always administered by an anesthesiologist provider. The standards for preoperative evaluation, intraoperative monitoring, and the continuous presence of a member of the anesthesia care team are no different from those for general or regional anesthesia. Conceptually, monitored anesthesia care is attractive because it should invoke less physiologic disturbance and allow a more rapid recovery than general anesthesia.

II. PREOPERATIVE ASSESSMENT

The preoperative assessment of a patient scheduled for surgery under monitored anesthesia care should be as comprehensive as that performed before a general or regional anesthetic is administered. Additional considerations in the preoperative assessment of the patient scheduled to undergo monitored anesthesia care include evaluation of the patient's ability to remain immobile and cooperative. Verbal communication between the anesthesiologist and patient is important in order to evaluate the level of sedation, reassure the patient, and provide a mechanism when the patient is required to cooperate. The presence of a persistent cough may make it difficult for the patient to remain immobile (attempts to attenuate the cough with sedation are not likely to be successful). Additionally, orthopnea may make it impossible for the patient to lie flat.

III. TECHNIQUES OF MONITORED ANESTHESIA CARE

A variety of medications are commonly administered during monitored anesthesia care with the desired endpoints of providing patient comfort, maintaining cardiorespiratory stability, improving operating conditions, and preventing recall of unpleasant perioperative events.

A. Monitored anesthesia care usually involves intravenous (IV) administration of drugs with anxiolytic, hypnotic, analgesic, and amnestic properties either alone or as a supplement to a local or regional anesthetic.

B. The drug(s) selected should allow rapid and complete recovery with a minimal incidence of nausea and vomiting or residual cardiorespiratory depression.

C. A level of sedation that allows verbal communication is optimal for the patient's comfort and safety. If the level of sedation is deepened to the extent that verbal communication is lost, most of the advantages of monitored anesthesia care are also lost, and the risks of the technique approach those of general anesthesia with an unprotected and uncontrolled airway.

D. Increased patient agitation may be a result of pain or anxiety (Table 31-1).

IV. PHARMACOLOGIC BASIS OF MONITORED ANESTHESIA CARE TECHNIQUES: OPTIMIZING DRUG ADMINISTRATION

A. The ability to predict the effects of drugs demands an understanding of their pharmacokinetic and pharmacodynamic properties (context-sensitive half-time, effect site equilibration time, drug interactions).

B. To avoid excessive levels of sedation, drugs should be titrated in increments rather than administered in larger doses according to predetermined notions of efficacy.

C. Continuous infusions (e.g., propofol) are superior to intermittent bolus dosing because they produce less-fluctuation in drug concentration, thus reducing the number of episodes of inadequate or excessive sedation and contributing to a more prompt recovery (Fig. 31-1).

TABLE 31-1

CAUSES OF PATIENT AGITATION DURING MONITORED ANESTHESIA CARE

Pain or anxiety
Life-threatening factors
   Hypoxemia
   Hypoventilation
   Impending local anesthetic toxicity
   Cerebral hypoperfusion
Less ominous but often overlooked factors
   Distended bladder
   Hypothermia or hyperthermia
   Pruritus
   Nausea
   Positional discomfort
   Uncomfortable oxygen masks or nasal cannulas
   Intravenous cannulation site infiltration
   Member of surgical team leaning on the patient
   Prolonged pneumatic tourniquet inflation

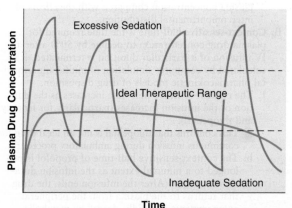

FIGURE 31-1. Schematic depiction of the changes in drug concentration during continuous infusion of the drug (*heavy line* indicates maintenance of a therapeutic concentration) or intermittent bolus injection of the drug (*lighter line* indicates that the drug concentration is often above or below the desired therapeutic concentration).

MANAGEMENT

V. DISTRIBUTION, ELIMINATION, ACCUMULATION, AND DURATION OF ACTION

After administration of IV drugs, the immediate distribution phase causes a rapid decrease in plasma levels as the drug is quickly transported to the vessel-rich group of rapidly equilibrating tissues. Accumulation of drug in poorly perfused tissues during prolonged IV infusion may contribute to delayed recovery when the drug is released back into the central compartment after drug administration is discontinued.

A. **Elimination half-life** is often cited as a determinant of a drug's duration of action, when it is actually often difficult to predict the clinical duration of action from this value.

   1. The elimination half-life represents a single-compartment model in which elimination is the only process that can alter drug concentration.

   2. Most drugs used by anesthesiologists for monitored anesthesia care are lipophilic and much more suited to multicompartmental modeling than single-compartment modeling. In multicompartmental models, the metabolism and excretion of some IV drugs may make only a minor contribution to changes in plasma concentration compared with the effects of intercompartmental distribution.

B. **Context-sensitive half-time** is the time required for the plasma drug concentration to decline by 50% after an IV infusion of a particular duration is terminated. It is calculated by computer simulation of multicompartmental pharmacokinetic models of drug disposition.

   1. The context-sensitive half-time increases as the duration of the infusion increases (particularly for fentanyl and thiopental).

      a. This confirms that thiopental is not an ideal drug for continuous infusion during ambulatory procedures.

      b. The context-sensitive half-time of propofol is prolonged to a minimal extent as the infusion duration increases. (After the infusion ends, the drug that returns to the plasma from the peripheral compartments is rapidly cleared by metabolic processes and is therefore not available to slow the decay in plasma levels.)

   2. The context-sensitive half-times of drugs bear no constant relationship to their elimination half-times.

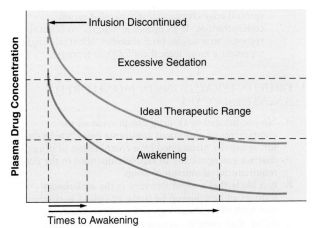

FIGURE 31-2. The time to awakening is determined by the duration of infusion (context-sensitive half-time), the difference in the plasma concentration at the end of the procedure, and the plasma concentration below which awakening will occur.

C. **How Does the Context-Sensitive Half-Time Relate to the Time to Recovery?** The context-sensitive half-time does not directly describe how long it will take for the patient to recover from sedation/analgesia but rather how long it will take for the plasma concentration or drug to decrease by 50%. The time to recovery depends on how far the plasma concentration must decrease to reach levels compatible with awakening (Fig. 31-2).

D. **Effect site equilibration** describes the time from rapid IV administration of a drug until its clinical effect is manifest. (A delay occurs because the blood is not usually the site of action but is merely the route via which the drug reaches its effect site.)

1. Thiopental, propofol, and alfentanil have a short effect site equilibration times compared with midazolam, sufentanil, and fentanyl. This is an important consideration when determining bolus spacing of doses.

2. A distinct time lag between the peak serum fentanyl concentration (which is an important consideration when determining bolus spacing of doses) and the peak electroencephalographic (EEG) slowing can be seen, but after administration of alfentanil, the EEG

spectral edge changes closely parallel serum concentrations. If an opioid is required to blunt the response to a single, brief stimulus, alfentanil might represent a more logical choice than fentanyl.

VI. DRUG INTERACTIONS IN MONITORED ANESTHESIA CARE

A. No one inhaled or IV drug can provide all the components of monitored anesthesia care. Patient comfort is usually maintained by a combination of drugs that act synergistically to enable reductions in the dose requirements of individual drugs.

B. It is likely that a rapid recovery in the ambulatory setting can be achieved by using an opioid in combination with other drugs (especially a benzodiazepine) rather than using an opioid as the sole anesthetic.

1. Opioid and benzodiazepine combinations are frequently used to achieve the components of hypnosis, amnesia, and analgesia.

2. The opioid–benzodiazepine combination displays marked synergism in producing hypnosis. This synergism also extends to unwanted effects of these drugs. (Whereas midazolam alone produces no significant effects on ventilation, the combination with fentanyl produces apnea in many patients.)

3. The advantage of synergy between opioids and benzodiazepines should be carefully weighed against the disadvantages of the potential adverse effect of this drug combination on the cardiovascular system and breathing.

VII. SPECIFIC DRUGS USED DURING MONITORED ANESTHESIA CARE (Table 31-2)

A. **Propofol** has many of the ideal properties of a sedative-hypnotic for use in sedation/analgesia.

1. The context-sensitive half-time of propofol remains short even after prolonged IV infusions (in contrast to midazolam), and the short effect site equilibration time makes propofol an easily titratable drug that has an excellent recovery profile.

2. The prompt recovery combined with a low incidence of nausea and vomiting make propofol well suited to ambulatory sedation/analgesia procedures.

TABLE 31-2

DOSE RANGES FOR DRUGS USED TO PRODUCE
SEDATION/ANALGESIA

Drug	Typical Adult Intravenous Dose (Titrated to Effect in Increments)
Benzodiazepines	
Midazolam	1–2 mg before propofol or remifentanil infusion
Diazepam	2.5–10.0 mg
Opioids	
Alfentanil	5–20 µg/kg bolus 2 minutes before stimulus
Fentanyl	0.5–2 µg/kg bolus 2 minutes before stimulus
Remifentanil	0.1 µg/kg/min infusion 5 minutes before stimulus and then weaned to 0.05 µg/kg/min as tolerated (adjust up or down in increments of 0.025 µg/kg/min; decrease dose accordingly when coadministered with midazolam or propofol)
Propofol	250–500 µg/kg boluses 25–75 µg/kg/min infusion
Ketamine	4–6 mg/kg PO 2–4 mg/kg IM 0.25–1 mg/kg IV
Dexmedetomidine	0.5–1.0 µg/kg over 10–20 minutes followed by 0.2–0.7 µg/kg/hr

IM = intramuscular; IV = intravenous; PO = per os.

    3. Propofol in typical sedation/analgesia doses (25–75 µg/kg/min IV) has minimal analgesic properties and does not reliably produce amnesia.

B. **Benzodiazepines** are commonly used during sedation/analgesia for their anxiolytic, amnestic, and hypnotic properties.

    1. Midazolam has many advantages over diazepam and is the most commonly used benzodiazepine for sedation/analgesia (Table 31-3).

       a. Despite a short elimination half-time, there is often prolonged psychomotor impairment after sedation/analgesia techniques using midazolam as the main component.

MANAGEMENT

TABLE 31-3

COMPARISON OF THE IMPORTANT PROPERTIES OF MIDAZOLAM AND DIAZEPAM

Midazolam	Diazepam
Water soluble (does not require propylene glycol for solubilizing)	Lipid soluble (requires propylene glycol for solubilizing)
Not a veno-irritant (usually painless on injection)	Venoirritant (pain on injection)
Thrombophlebitis is rare	Thrombophlebitis is common
Short elimination half-time (4 hours)	Long elimination half-time (>20 hours)
Clearance is unaffected by H_2 antagonists	Clearance is reduced by H_2 antagonists
Inactive metabolites (1-hydroxy midazolam)	Active metabolites (desmethy-diazepam, oxazepam)
Resedation is unlikely	Resedation is more likely

    b. Midazolam may be better used in a modified role by administering lower doses before the start of a propofol infusion to provide the specific amnestic and anxiolytic component of a balanced sedation technique.

    c. The analgesic component of a balanced sedation technique could be provided by regional/local techniques or opioids. (There is a risk of significant respiratory depression when a benzodiazepine is combined with an opioid.)

    d. The dose of benzodiazepine required to reach a desired clinical endpoint is decreased in elderly patients compared with younger patients (reflecting pharmacodynamic factors) (Fig. 31-3).

  2. Flumazenil Antagonism of Benzodiazepines (Table 31-4). Routine use of flumazenil-antagonized benzodiazepine sedation is not cost effective.

C. Opioids. The analgesic component of "balanced sedation/analgesia" is provided by an opioid, and sedation is provided by drugs (propofol, midazolam) with specific and potent hypnotic and amnestic properties (Tables 31-2 and 31-5).

  1. Remifentanil is a μ opioid agonist with a rapid onset (brain equilibration time, 1.0–1.5 minutes) and offset (ester hydrolysis) that facilitate titration to effect during monitored anesthesia care (MAC).

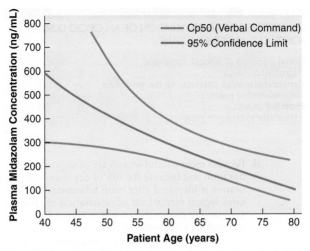

FIGURE 31-3. The plasma concentration of midazolam at which 50% of subjects will fail to respond to verbal command (Cp50) is a function of age.

a. The likelihood of depression of ventilation or chest wall rigidity is decreased by administering remifentanil over 30 to 90 seconds or using a continuous IV infusion technique.

b. A bolus dose (1 μg/kg IV) administered over 30 seconds administered 90 seconds before placement of a retrobulbar block is effective in preventing pain during subsequent placement of the block.

c. Administration of midazolam (2 mg IV) in combination with remifentanil results in decreased dose requirements for the opioid and relieves patient anxiety.

TABLE 31-4

RECOMMENDED REGIMEN FOR USE OF FLUMAZENIL

The initial recommended dose is 0.2 mg IV.
If the desired level of consciousness is not achieved within 45 seconds, repeat 0.2 mg dose IV.
If necessary, repeat 0.2 mg IV every 60 seconds to a maximum of 1.0 mg.
Recognize the potential for resedation.

IV = intravenous.

MANAGEMENT

TABLE 31-5

INDICATIONS FOR ADMINISTRATION OF AN OPIOID DURING MONITORED ANESTHESIA CARE

Initial injection of a local anesthetic
Retrobulbar block
Patient discomfort unrelated to the procedure
Uncomfortable position
Propofol injection
Pneumatic tourniquet pain

       d. Because most painful stimuli are of unpredictable duration and because the risk of depression of ventilation is increased after bolus administration, the most logical method for administration of remifentanil during monitored anesthetic care is by adjustable IV infusion (see Table 31-2).

       e. Discontinuation or accidental interruption of the remifentanil infusion will result in abrupt offset of effect, which may result in patient discomfort, hemodynamic instability, and patient movement.

D. Ketamine is an intense analgesic that is frequently used as a component of pediatric sedation techniques (0.25–0.5 mg/kg IV produces minimal respiratory and cardiovascular depression) (see Table 31-2).

    1. Increased oral secretions make laryngospasm more likely (an antisialagogue should be administered).

    2. Ketamine is frequently combined with a benzodiazepine to reduce the incidence of hallucinations.

    3. Patient movement may make ketamine less than ideal for procedures requiring the patient to remain motionless.

E. Dexmedetomidine stimulates α-2 receptors to produce sedation, analgesia, decreases in sympathetic outflow, and an increase in cardiac vagal activity (bradycardia and hypotension) (see Table 31-2).

    1. Respiratory function is not depressed to the same extent as with other sedatives, and patients sedated with dexmedetomidine are more easily aroused from a given level of sedation. However, airway intervention to relieve obstruction and apnea may be required during dexmedetomidine administration, particularly when used in combination with other respiratory depressants.

TABLE 31-6

COMPARATIVE PROPERTIES OF PROPOFOL
AND DEXMEDETOMIDINE

	Propofol	Dexmedetomidine
Pain upon injection	Yes	Minimal
Analgesic properties with subhypnotic doses	Minimal	Yes
Amnestic properties with subhypnotic doses	Significant	Insignificant
Time of onset with typical administration	Rapid	5–10 minutes
Restrictive regulations on use by non-anesthesiologist providers	Yes	No
Potential for significant bradycardia	Minimal	Significant

2. Episodes of bradycardia and sinus arrest have been associated with dexmedetomidine administration in young healthy volunteers with a high vagal tone, particularly during rapid IV injection.
3. Dexmedetomidine may be used for pediatric magnetic resonance imaging and computed tomography studies.

F. **Amnesia During Sedation with Dexmedetomidine or Propofol** (Table 31-6). All sedative-hypnotics have the potential to impair memory formation. In contrast to propofol and benzodiazepines, it is unlikely that dexmedetomidine has amnestic properties at subhypnotic doses.

VIII. PATIENT-CONTROLLED SEDATION AND ANALGESIA

A. Techniques that allow the patient some direct control of the level of sedation increases patient satisfaction and eliminates the unpredictable variability in dose requirements between patients.

B. A conventional patient-controlled analgesia delivery system that is set to deliver 0.5 mg midazolam and 25 μg fentanyl with a 5-minute lockout interval is useful. Alfentanil as a 5-μg/kg IV bolus with a 3-minute lockout period results in patient acceptability and an outcome comparable to physician-controlled analgesia.

MANAGEMENT

IX. RESPIRATORY FUNCTION AND SEDATIVE-HYPNOTICS

During monitored anesthesia care, there is a risk of depression of ventilation as a result of drug-induced effects (with opioids, there is the potential for hypotension resulting in brainstem hypoperfusion). During sedation, it is likely that protective upper airway reflexes will be attenuated.

A. Sedation and the Upper Airway

1. The coordinated activation of the diaphragm and upper airway muscles (important for maintaining airway patency) is extremely sensitive to sedative-hypnotic drug administration.

2. Elderly patients and those with pre-existing chronic obstructive pulmonary disease often have limited respiratory reserve and are unable to increase their respiratory muscle activity in response to the increased work of breathing induced by sedation; they may become hypercarbic, acidotic, and hypoxemic.

B. Sedation and Protective Airway Reflexes

1. Protective laryngeal and pharyngeal (swallowing) reflexes are depressed by drugs that produce sedation.

   a. Aspiration of gastric contents may occur either in the operating room or during recovery, particularly if oral intake is allowed before the return of adequate upper airway protective reflexes.

   b. Advanced age and debilitation may compromise the protective upper airway reflexes, placing these patients at increased risk for aspiration during sedation.

2. Ideally, patients should be awake enough to recognize the regurgitation of gastric contents and be able to protect their own airways.

C. Sedation and Respiratory Control

1. It is likely that during regional anesthesia, there is a degree of deafferentation that will potentiate the respiratory depressant effects of sedative-hypnotic drugs, especially opioids.

2. When used in combination, opioids and benzodiazepines appear to have the potential to produce marked depressant effects on respiratory responsiveness.

X. SUPPLEMENTAL OXYGEN ADMINISTRATION

A. Arterial hypoxemia as a result of alveolar hypoventilation is a risk after the administration of sedatives, hypnotics, or analgesics.

B. In the absence of significant lung disease, the administration of only modest concentrations of supplemental oxygen is usually effective in restoring oxygenation to an acceptable level.
   1. A patient who is receiving minimal supplemental oxygen may have acceptable oxygenation despite significant alveolar hypoventilation.
   2. Before making the decision to discharge a patient to a less well-monitored environment without supplemental oxygen, it is useful to measure oxygen saturation with a pulse oximeter while the patient is breathing room air.

XI. MONITORING DURING MONITORED ANESTHESIA CARE

A. **American Society of Anesthesiologists (ASA) Standards for Basic Anesthetic Monitoring** are applicable to all levels of anesthesia care, including monitored anesthesia care.
B. **Communication and Observation**
   1. The presence of a vigilant anesthesiologist is the single most important monitor in the operating room.
   2. The effectiveness of this vigilance is enhanced by monitoring techniques and devices (Table 31-7).
   3. It is important that the anesthesiologist continually evaluates the patient's response to verbal stimulation to titrate the level of sedation and to allow the early detection of neurologic or cardiopulmonary dysfunction.
C. **Preparedness to Recognize and Treat Local Anesthetic Toxicity**
   1. Because monitored anesthesia care is often provided in the context of regional or local anesthetic techniques, it is important that the anesthesiologist maintains a high index of suspicion for the risk of local anesthetic toxicity, especially in elderly and debilitated patients.
   2. Even if the anesthesiologist does not perform the block, he or she is in a unique position to advise the surgeon about the most appropriate volume, concentration, and type of local anesthetic drug or technique to be used.
   3. The clinically recognizable toxic effects of local anesthetics on the central nervous system and the

---

TABLE 31-7

MONITORING TECHNIQUES AND DEVICES USED DURING
MONITORED ANESTHESIA CARE

Visual, Tactile, and Auditory Assessment
Rate, depth, and pattern of breathing
Palpation of the arterial pulse
Peripheral perfusion based on temperature of the extremities
    and capillary refill
Diaphoresis
Pallor
Shivering
Cyanosis
Acute changes in neurologic status

Auscultation
Heart and breath sounds (precordial stethoscope)

Pulse Oximetry (an ASA standard)
Capnography (most effective in intubated patients but can be
    adapted [side stream] to MAC)

Electrocardiography

Temperature (forced-air heating is an effective means of
    maintaining normothermia)
Bispectral Index (value <80 minimizes the possibility of recall
    during sedation)

ASA = American Society of Anesthesiologists; MAC = minimum alveolar
concentration.

cardiovascular system are concentration dependent.
Cardiovascular toxicity usually occurs at a higher
plasma concentration than neurotoxicity, but when it
does occur, it is usually more difficult to manage than
neurotoxicity.
   a. At low plasma concentrations, sedation and numb-
       ness of the tongue and circumoral tissues and a
       metallic taste are prominent features of local anes-
       thetic toxicity.
   b. As plasma concentrations increase, restlessness,
       vertigo, tinnitus, and difficulty in focusing may
       occur.
   c. Higher plasma concentrations may result in slurred
       speech and skeletal muscle twitching, which often
       herald the onset of tonic-clonic seizures.

  d. Cardiotoxicity may manifest before neurotoxicity when bupivacaine local anesthetic toxicity occurs.

4. The conduct of monitored anesthesia care may modify the individual's response to the potentially toxic effects of local anesthetic administration and adversely affect the margin of safety of a regional or local anesthetic technique.

  a. Any decrease in cardiac output and hepatic blood flow during sedation may decrease the clearance of local anesthetics that are dependent on metabolism in the liver.

  b. Drug-induced depression of ventilation during sedation leads to acidosis, which increases delivery of local anesthetic to the brain via increases in cerebral blood flow, increases intracellular concentrations of the active non-ionized form of the local anesthetic, and potentiates the cardiovascular toxicity of local anesthetics.

  c. Administration of sedative-hypnotic drugs may interfere with the patient's ability to communicate the symptoms of impending local anesthetic.

  d. The anticonvulsant properties of benzodiazepines and barbiturates may attenuate the seizures associated with local anesthetic toxicity.

XII. SEDATION AND ANALGESIA BY NON-ANESTHESIOLOGISTS

A. The ASA has developed practice guidelines to guide the level of sedation and analgesia that should be provided by non-anesthesiologist providers.

1. Four levels of sedation are defined in the ASA practice guidelines: minimal sedation, moderate sedation, deep sedation, and general anesthesia (Table 31-8).

2. These practice guidelines emphasize that sedation and analgesia represent a continuum of sedation in which patients can easily pass into a level of sedation that is deeper than intended.

3. Certain high-risk patient groups (extremes of age, severe comorbid diseases, morbid obesity, sleep apnea, pregnancy, alcohol abuse) should be evaluated by appropriate physician consultation before administration of sedation and analgesia by non-anesthesiologists.

MANAGEMENT

TABLE 31-8

CONTINUUM OF DEPTH OF SEDATION

	Minimal Sedation	Moderate Sedation	Deep Sedation	General Sedation
Responsiveness	Normal response to verbal stimulation	Purposeful response to verbal or tactile stimulation	Purposeful response after repeated or painful stimulation	Unarousable, even with a painful stimulus
Airway	Unaffected	No intervention is required	Intervention may be required	Intervention is often required
Spontaneous ventilation	Unaffected	Adequate	May be inadequate	Frequently inadequate
Cardiovascular function	Unaffected	Usually maintained	Usually maintained	May be impaired

B. Controversy exists regarding the level of training required for non-anesthesiologists to be credentialed to provide moderate and deep sedation. The ASA recommends that practitioners should complete formal training in the safe administration drugs used to establish a level of moderate sedation and rescue of patients who exhibit adverse physiologic consequences of a deeper-than-intended level of sedation.

CHAPTER 32 ■ **AMBULATORY ANESTHESIA**

Ambulatory surgery is popular both for patients and those who own the facility (Lichtor JL: Anesthesia for ambulatory surgery. In *Clinical Anesthesia*. Edited by Barash PG, Cullen BF, Stoelting RK, Cahalan MK, Stock MC. Philadelphia: Lippincott Williams & Wilkins, 2009, pp 833–846).

I. PLACE, PROCEDURES, AND PATIENT SELECTION

A. Ambulatory surgery occurs in a variety of settings (hospitals, freestanding satellite facilities, physician's offices).

B. The Centers for Medicare and Medicaid Services (CMS) generally pays ambulatory centers 65% of what hospital outpatient surgical facilities receive.

C. Procedures appropriate for ambulatory surgery are those associated with postoperative care that is easily managed at home and with low rates of complications that require intensive physician or nursing management.

D. Scoring systems have been developed to help determine the likelihood of hospital admission after ambulatory surgery (older than 65 years, operating times longer than 120 minutes, regional anesthesia).

1. Many facilities set a 4-hour limit as a criterion for performing a procedure.

2. The need for a transfusion is not a contraindication for ambulatory procedures. Some patients undergoing liposuction as outpatients are given autologous blood.

3. Infants whose postconceptual age is less than 46 weeks or whose age is less than 60 weeks but who also have a history of chronic lung or neurologic disease or have anemia (hemoglobin <6 mmol/L) should be monitored for 12 hours after the procedure because they are at risk of developing apnea even

without a history of apnea. Infants older than 46 weeks and younger than 60 weeks without disease should be monitored for 6 hours after the procedure.

4. Advanced age alone is not a reason to disallow surgery in an ambulatory setting. Age, however, does affect the pharmacokinetics of drugs. Even short-acting drugs such as midazolam and propofol have decreased clearance in older individuals.

5. Hospital admission by itself is not necessarily bad if it results in a better quality of care or uncovers the need for more extensive surgery.

E. Obese patients are not more likely to have adverse outcomes, but they have a higher incidence of obstructive sleep apnea (OSA). The American Society of Anesthesiologists (ASA) has published practice guidelines for the perioperative management of patients with OSA.

F. Patients who undergo ambulatory surgery should have someone to take them home and stay with them afterward to provide care.

1. After the patient has returned home, he or she must be able to tolerate the pain from the procedure, assuming adequate pain therapy is provided.

2. Patients undergoing certain procedures, such as laparoscopic cholecystectomy or transurethral resection of the prostate, should live close to the ambulatory facility because postoperative complications may require their prompt return.

II. PREOPERATIVE EVALUATION AND REDUCTION OF PATIENT ANXIETY

Each outpatient facility should develop its own method of preoperative screening to be conducted before the day of surgery (history, medications, previous anesthetics, transportation and child care needs, dietary restrictions, attire, arrival times, laboratory tests). The preoperative screening is the ideal time for the anesthesiologist to talk with the patient. Automated history taking may also prove beneficial during the screening of a patient.

A. Upper Respiratory Tract Infection

1. Airflow obstruction has been shown to persist for up to 6 weeks after viral respiratory infections in adults. For this reason, surgery should be delayed if an adult presents with an upper respiratory infection (URI) until 6 weeks have elapsed.

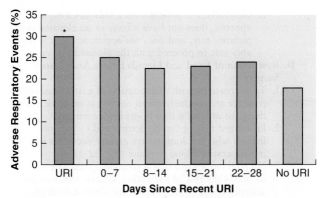

FIGURE 32-1. Adverse respiratory events are similar between children with an upper respiratory infection (URI) and a recent URI, and this similarity persists for at least 4 weeks after the URI. *$P < .05$ versus no URI. (Reprinted with permission from Tait AR, Malviya S, Voepel-Lewis T, et al: Risk factors for perioperative adverse respiratory events in children with upper respiratory tract infections. *Anesthesiology* 95:299, 2001.)

2. In the case of children, whether surgery should be delayed for this length of time is questionable. There seems to be no difference in the incidence of laryngospasm or bronchospasm if the child has had active URIs, a URI within 4 weeks, or no symptoms (Fig. 32-1). Children with active or recent URIs have more episodes of breathholding, incidences of desaturation below 90%, and more respiratory events compared with children without symptoms (Table 32-1).
   a. Although surgery may be canceled because a child is symptomatic, the child may develop another URI when the procedure is rescheduled.

TABLE 32-1

INDEPENDENT RISK FACTORS FOR ADVERSE RESPIRATORY EVENTS IN CHILDREN WITH UPPER RESPIRATORY TRACT INFECTIONS

Use of an endotracheal tube versus laryngeal mask airway
Prematurity
Reactive airway disease
Parenteral smoking
Surgery involving the airway
Presence of copious secretions
Nasal congestion

MANAGEMENT

  b. Generally, if a patient with a URI has a normal appetite, does not have a fever or an elevated respiratory rate, and does not appear toxic, it is probably safe to proceed with the planned procedure.
 B. Restriction of Food and Liquids Before Ambulatory Surgery
  1. To decrease the risk of aspiration of gastric contents, patients are routinely asked not to eat or drink anything for at least 6 to 8 hours before surgery.
  2. Prolonged fasting can be detrimental to patients. Infants who fast longer have greater decreases in intraoperative blood pressure (Fig. 32-2).
  3. No trial has shown that a shortened fluid fast increases the risk of aspiration. Gastric volumes are actually lower when patients are allowed to drink some fluids before surgery.
  4. ASA practice guidelines for preoperative fasting allow a patient to have a light meal up to 6 hours before an elective procedure and support a fasting period for

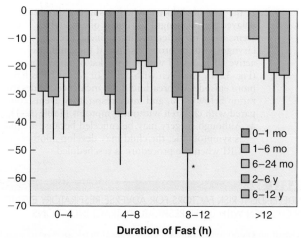

FIGURE 32-2. Blood pressure is lower in children 1 to 6 months of age who fast more than 8 hours compared with those who fast for less than 4 hours. *$P < .05$ versus 0- to 4-hour fasting group. (Reprinted with permission from Friesen RH, Wurl JL, Friesen RM: Duration of preoperative fast correlates with arterial blood pressure response to halothane in infants. *Anesth Analg* 95:1572, 2002.)

clear liquids of 2 hours for all patients (including taking chronic medications). Coffee and tea are considered clear liquids.

  a. Coffee or tea drinkers should follow fasting guidelines but should be encouraged to drink coffee before the procedure because physical signs of caffeine withdrawal (headache) can easily occur.

  b. It is not clear if these fasting guidelines should apply to patients with diabetes or dyspepsia.

C. Anxiety Reduction

  1. Preoperative reassurance from non-anesthesia staff and the use of booklets reduce preoperative anxiety. However, the use of booklets is less effective than a preoperative visit by the anesthesiologist. Audiovisual instructions also reduce preoperative anxiety.

  2. Much of a child's anxiety before surgery concerns separation from the parent or parents. If the parents are calm and can effectively manage the physical transfer to a friendly and playful anesthesiologist or nurse, premedication may not be necessary.

  3. Family-centered care (videotapes, pamphlets, mask practice kits) has become popular and is useful for decreasing children's preoperative anxiety.

III. MANAGING THE ANESTHETIC: PREMEDICATION

Premedication is useful for controlling anxiety; reducing the risk of aspiration during induction of anesthesia; and controlling postoperative pain, nausea, and vomiting. Because outpatients go home on the day of surgery, the drugs given before anesthesia should not hinder their recovery.

A. Benzodiazepines

  1. Midazolam is the benzodiazepine most commonly used preoperatively. For children, oral midazolam in doses as small as 0.25 mg/kg produces effective sedation and reduces anxiety. With this dose, most children can be effectively separated from their parents after 10 minutes, and satisfactory sedation can be maintained for 45 minutes. Discharge may be delayed, though, when midazolam is given before a short procedure.

  2. Routine administration of supplemental oxygen with or without continuous monitoring of arterial

MANAGEMENT

oxygenation is recommended whenever benzodiazepines are given intravenously (IV).

3. The potential for anterograde amnesia after premedication is a concern, especially for patients undergoing ambulatory surgery.

B. Opioids and Nonsteroidal Analgesics

1. Opioids may be administered preoperatively to sedate patients, control hypertension during tracheal intubation, and decrease pain before surgery. Meperidine (but not morphine or fentanyl) is sometimes helpful in controlling shivering in the operating room or postanesthesia care unit (PACU).

2. Preoperative administration of opioids or nonsteroidal antiinflammatory drugs may be useful for controlling pain in the early postoperative period.

IV. INTRAOPERATIVE MANAGEMENT: CHOICE OF ANESTHETIC METHOD

A. General anesthesia, regional anesthesia, and local anesthesia are equally safe.

1. Even for experienced anesthesiologists, a failure rate is associated with regional anesthesia (Fig. 32-3).

2. Some procedures are possible only with a general anesthetic. For others, the preferences of the patient, surgeon, or anesthesiologist may determine selection.

3. Time to recovery may also influence the choice of anesthetic method (Fig. 32-4).

4. One adverse effect associated with spinal anesthesia is headache, but headaches may also be experienced by patients after general anesthesia.

B. Regional techniques commonly used for ambulatory surgery, in addition to spinal and epidural anesthesia, include local infiltration, brachial plexus and other peripheral nerve blocks, and IV regional anesthesia.

1. Performing a block takes longer than inducing general anesthesia, and the incidence of failure is higher (see Fig. 32-3).

2. Unnecessary delays can be obviated by performing the block beforehand in a preoperative holding area.

3. Postoperative pain control is best with regional techniques. Patients may still have a numb extremity (after a brachial plexus block) but otherwise meet all criteria for discharge. In such instances, the extremity must be well protected (sling for an upper extremity

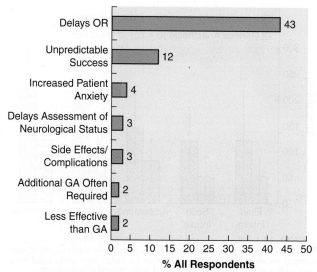

FIGURE 32-3. Operating room (OR) delays are the major reasons orthopedic surgeons do not favor regional anesthesia. GA = general anesthesia. (Reprinted with permission from Oldman M, McCartney CJ, Leung A, et al: A survey of orthopedic surgeons' attitudes and knowledge regarding regional anesthesia. *Anesth Analg* 98:1486, 2004.)

procedure), and patients must be cautioned to protect against injury because they are without normal sensations that would warn them of vulnerability. Reassurance that sensation will return should be provided.

C. **Spinal Anesthesia**

1. **Children.** Spinal anesthesia is used in some centers, particularly for children undergoing inguinal hernia repair.

2. **Adults.** The use of pencil point spinal needles with noncutting tips has prompted a resurgence of spinal anesthesia for ambulatory surgery in adults. Motor block of the legs may delay a patient's ability to walk. However, the use of a short-acting local anesthetic minimizes this problem. Nausea is much less frequent after epidural or spinal anesthesia than after general anesthesia.

3. **Lidocaine and mepivacaine** are ideal for ambulatory surgery because of their short durations of action,

MANAGEMENT

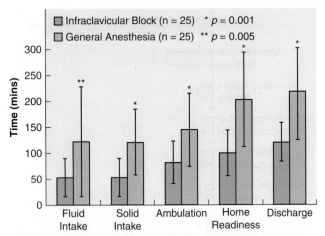

FIGURE 32-4. Recovery was faster when an infraclavicular brachial plexus block with a short-acting local anesthetic was used compared with general anesthesia and wound infiltration for outpatients undergoing hand and wrist surgery. Times are calculated from the end of anesthesia. (Reprinted with permission from Hadzic A, Arliss J, Kerimoglu B, et al: A comparison of infraclavicular nerve block versus general anesthesia for hand and wrist day-case surgeries. *Anesthesiology* 101:127, 2004.)

   although lidocaine use has been problematic because
   of transient neurologic symptoms. Although transient
   neurologic symptoms may be seen after
   administration of other local anesthetics, the risk is
   seven times higher after intrathecal lidocaine administration than after bupivacaine, prilocaine, or procaine
   administration.
   a. Chloroprocaine spinal anesthesia has a rapid onset
      and offset.
   b. Ropivacaine and bupivacaine have been used for
      ambulatory surgical procedures, but the recovery
      times are relatively long.
4. Although headache is a common complication of lumbar puncture, smaller-gauge needles result in a lower
   incidence of postdural puncture headache.
   a. For patients who receive spinal anesthesia, it is
      incumbent on the anesthesiologist and the facility
      to follow up with telephone calls to ensure no dis-
      abling symptoms of headache have developed.

   b. If the headache does not respond to bed rest, analgesics, and oral hydration, the patient must return to the hospital for a course of IV caffeine therapy or an immediate epidural blood patch.

   c. Bed rest does not reduce the frequency of headache; early ambulation may decrease the incidence.

D. Epidural and Caudal Anesthesia

 1. Epidural anesthesia takes longer to perform than spinal anesthesia. Onset with spinal anesthesia is more rapid, although recovery may be the same with either technique.

 2. Caudal anesthesia is a form of epidural anesthesia commonly used in children before surgery below the umbilicus as a supplement to general anesthesia and to control postoperative pain.

   a. Bupivacaine 0.175 to 0.25% or ropivacaine 0.2% in a volume of 0.5 to 1.0 mL/kg may be used; a safe maximal dose is 2.5 mg/kg. When added to the anesthetic solution, epinephrine 1:200,000 may allow earlier detection of IV, rather than epidural, injection.

   b. The block is usually administered while the child is anesthetized. After injection, the depth of general anesthesia can be reduced.

   c. Because of better pain control after a caudal block, children can usually ambulate earlier and be discharged sooner than without a caudal block.

E. Nerve Blocks

 1. There is widespread use of axillary and interscalene blocks for surgery in the upper extremity and ankle and femoral blocks for lower extremity surgery.

 2. Nerve blocks improve postoperative patient satisfaction because of lower levels of postoperative nausea, vomiting, and pain. Costs are also lower.

F. Sedation and Analgesia

 1. Many patients who undergo surgery with local or regional anesthesia prefer to be sedated and to have no recollection of the procedure. Sedation is important, in part, because injection with local anesthetics can be painful and lying on a hard operating room table can be uncomfortable.

 2. Levels of sedation vary from light, during which a patient's consciousness is minimally depressed, to very deep, in which protective reflexes are partially blocked and response to physical stimulation or verbal commands may not be appropriate.

MANAGEMENT

3. Children who have surgery usually will not remain immobile unless they are deeply sedated or receive general anesthesia.

G. **General Anesthesia.** Drugs selected for general anesthesia determine how long patients stay in the PACU after surgery, and for some patients, whether they can be discharged to go home.

1. **Induction**

a. The popularity of propofol as an induction agent for outpatient surgery partly relates to its half-life. (Impairment after thiopental administration may be apparent for up to 5 hours but only for 1 hour after propofol administration.) Pain on injection can be a problem with propofol. Thrombophlebitis does not appear to be a problem after IV administration of this agent, but it can be evident after thiopental administration. IV lidocaine 0.2 mg/kg may be used to decrease the incidence and severity of pain.

b. Sevoflurane has a relatively low blood–gas partition coefficient, and the speed of induction is similar to, albeit somewhat slower than, that of propofol. Induction with sevoflurane can be hastened when the patient is told to breathe out to residual volume, take a vital capacity breath through a primed anesthesia circuit, and then hold the breath.

c. For short procedures, some patients may not require neuromuscular blocking drugs, but others may need brief paralysis with succinylcholine (Sch) to facilitate tracheal intubation. Nondepolarizing drugs such as rocuronium have rapid onset times that are similar to those of Sch. Sch should be used with caution in children because of the possibility of cardiac arrest related to malignant hyperthermia or unsuspected muscular dystrophy, particularly Duchenne muscular dystrophy.

2. **Maintenance.** Although many factors affect the choice of agents for maintenance of anesthesia, two primary concerns for ambulatory anesthesia are speed of wake-up and the incidence of postoperative nausea and vomiting.

a. **Anesthesia Maintenance and Wake-Up Times.** Time to recovery may be measured by various criteria. However, actual discharge from an ambulatory center may depend on administrative issues, such as a written order from a surgeon or anesthesiologist. Sevoflurane, unlike desflurane, facilitates a smooth inhalation induction of anesthesia and is the preferred technique for ensuring rapid recovery of children in ambulatory surgery centers. It is important to distinguish between wake-up time and discharge time.

   b. **Intraoperative Management of Postoperative Nausea and Vomiting.** Nausea, with or without vomiting, is probably the most important factor contributing to a delay in discharge of patients and an increase in unanticipated admissions of both children and adults after ambulatory surgery (Table 32-2).

   c. Receptor antagonists (selective serotonin antagonists such as ondansetron, dolasetron, and granisetron) have been shown to have similar efficacy to help alleviate nausea and vomiting. Dopamine antagonists, antihistamines, and anticholinergic drugs are useful and are generally less expensive but are associated with extensive side effects.

   d. Combination therapy is probably the most effective way to control postoperative nausea and vomiting (Table 32-3).

 3. **Paralysis.** Reversal agents must be used unless there is no doubt that muscle relaxation has been fully reversed.

 4. **Intraoperative Management of Postoperative Pain**

   a. When given intraoperatively, opioids (most commonly fentanyl) are useful for supplementing both intraoperative and postoperative analgesia.

TABLE 32-2

PATIENTS AT GREATEST RISK FOR POSTOPERATIVE NAUSEA AND VOMITING

Pregnant women
History of motion sickness or postanesthetic emesis
Surgery within 1 to 7 days of the menstrual cycle
Non smokers
Specific procedures (laparoscopy; lithotripsy; major breast surgery; ear, nose, or throat surgery)
Inhalation agents
Postoperative opioid use

TABLE 32-3

APPROACHES FOR REDUCING THE INCIDENCE OF
POSTOPERATIVE NAUSEA AND VOMITING

Avoidance of nitrous oxide except for induction of anesthesia
Avoidance of inhalation agents
Avoidance of muscle relaxant reversal
Avoidance of opioids
Fluid hydration
Administration of a 5-HT$_3$ antagonist and dexamethasone
Inclusion of propofol in management of anesthesia

       b. All opioids may cause nausea, sedation, and dizziness, which may delay a patient's discharge.
       c. Nonsteroidal analgesics are not effective as supplements during general anesthesia, although they are useful in controlling postoperative pain, particularly when given before skin incision.
    5. Depth of Anesthesia. Use of bispectral index (BIS) and entropy or auditory-evoked potential monitors can decrease anesthesia requirements without sacrificing amnesia during general anesthesia.
    6. Airways. The use of a laryngeal mask airway or similar type of airway provides several advantages for allowing a patient to return quickly to baseline status (Table 32-4).

V. MANAGEMENT OF POSTANESTHESIA CARE

The three most common reasons for delay in patient discharge from the PACU are drowsiness, nausea and vomiting, and pain.
A. Reversal of Drug Effects
    1. Reversal of opioids may sometimes be necessary.
    2. Flumazenil, a benzodiazepine receptor antagonist, has primarily been used to reverse the effects of sedation after endoscopy and spinal anesthesia.

TABLE 32-4

ADVANTAGES OF LARYNGEAL MASK AIRWAYS

Muscle relaxants required for intubation can be avoided.
Coughing is less than with tracheal intubation.
Anesthetic requirements are reduced.
Hoarseness and sore throat are reduced.
There is a cost savings.

B. **Nausea and vomiting** are the most common reasons both children and adults have protracted stays in the PACU or unexpected hospital admission after anesthesia. A variety of drugs are effective in treating the problem (5-HT$_3$ antagonists seem particularly effective). Midazolam and propofol, although more commonly used for sedation, have antiemetic effects that are longer in duration than their sedative effects.

C. **Pain.** Postsurgical pain must be treated quickly and effectively. It is important for the practitioner to differentiate postsurgical pain from the discomfort of hypoxemia, hypercapnia, or a full bladder.

   1. Medications for pain control should be given in small IV doses (1 to 3 mg/70 kg of morphine or 10 to 25 μg/70 kg of fentanyl).

   2. Nonsteroidal medications, such as ketorolac or ibuprofen, can also effectively control postoperative pain and, compared with opioids, can give pain relief for a longer period and are associated with less nausea and vomiting.

D. **Preparation for Discharging the Patient**

   1. In addition to the PACU, many ambulatory surgery centers have a phase II recovery room, where patients may stay until they are able to tolerate liquids, walk, and void.

   2. Patients who undergo procedures under monitored anesthesia care can usually go straight to the phase II area from the operating room.

   3. Some criteria for discharge to home were created without scientific basis. One criterion is the ability to tolerate liquids before being discharged. Postoperative nausea may be greater if patients are required to drink liquids before discharge. Even though it is warranted after spinal or epidural anesthesia, the requirement that low-risk patients void before discharge may only lengthen the hospital stay, particularly if the patient is willing to return to a medical facility if he or she is unable to void.

   4. Patients may feel fine after they leave the hospital, but they should be advised against driving for at least 24 hours after a procedure.

   5. Patients should also be informed that they may experience pain, headache, nausea, vomiting, or dizziness and, if Sch was used, muscle aches and pains apart from the incision for at least 24 hours.

MANAGEMENT

6. Anesthesia for ambulatory surgery is a rapidly evolving specialty. Patients once believed unsuitable for ambulatory surgery are now considered to be appropriate candidates. Operations once believed unsuitable for outpatients are now routinely performed in the morning so patients can be discharged in the afternoon or evening. The availability of both shorter-acting anesthetics and longer-acting analgesics and antiemetics enables us to care effectively for patients in ambulatory centers.

CHAPTER 33 ■ OFFICE-BASED ANESTHESIA

The field of office-based anesthesia (OBA) has become an intrinsic and vital component within the field of anesthesiology (Hausman LM, Rosenblatt MA: Office-based anesthesia. In *Clinical Anesthesia*. Edited by Barash PG, Cullen BF, Stoelting RK, Cahalan MK, Stock MC. Philadelphia: Lippincott Williams & Wilkins, 2009, pp 847–860). An office-based anesthetic is one that is performed in a location, usually an office or procedure room, that is not accredited by a state agency as an ambulatory surgery center (ASC) or as a hospital and may, in some states, have no accreditation at all. It was estimated that by 2005, approximately 82% of all procedures were outpatient and of these, 24% were office based. A challenge to office-based practitioners is that presently there is little or no training in OBA within the standard anesthesia residency program.

I. ADVANTAGES AND DISADVANTAGES (Table 33-1)

II. OFFICE SAFETY

Injuries and deaths occurring in offices are often multifactorial in their causation (including overdosages of local anesthetics, prolonged surgery with occult blood loss, accumulation of multiple anesthetics, hypovolemia, hypoxemia, and the use of reversal drugs with short half-lives). Both the Anesthesia Patient Safety Foundation and the American Society of Anesthesiologists (ASA) have emerged as leaders in the field of OBA safety and have advocated that the quality of care in an office-based practice be no less than that of a hospital or ASC. Reports of morbidity and mortality within office-based practices vary dramatically. The challenge of acquiring accurate morbidity and mortality data for OBA is complicated by the fact that many offices

TABLE 33-1

ADVANTAGES AND DISADVANTAGES OF
OFFICE-BASED ANESTHESIA

Advantages
Cost containment (facility fee)
Ease of scheduling
Patient and surgeon convenience
Decreased patient exposure to nosocomial infections
Improved patient privacy
Continuity of care

Disadvantages
Issues of patient safety and peer review
May be an absence of regulations regarding certification of the
  surgeon or anesthesiologist
May be an absence of documentation, policies, and procedures
  and reporting of adverse outcomes

are not required to report adverse events. There are
reported cases of injuries to patients in offices resulting
from obsolete and malfunctioning anesthesia machines, as
well as resulting from alarms that have not been serviced or
are not functioning properly (Table 33-2). The ASA has created guidelines for defining obsolete anesthesia machines.

III. PATIENT SELECTION

Before presenting for an office-based procedure, the patient
must be medically optimized. The patient should have a
preoperative history and physical examination recorded
within 30 days, all pertinent laboratory tests performed,
and any medically indicated specialist consultation(s) done.

TABLE 33-2

CAUSES OF INJURY IN THE OFFICE

Inadequate resuscitation equipment
Inadequate monitoring (most commonly, no pulse oximetry)
Inadequate preoperative or postoperative evaluation
Human error
  Slow recognition of an event
  Slow response to an event
  Lack of experience
  Drug overdosage

TABLE 33-3

CHARACTERISTICS OF PATIENTS WHO MAY NOT BE GOOD CANDIDATES FOR OFFICE-BASED PROCEDURES

Poorly controlled diabetes mellitus
Expected significant blood loss or postoperative pain
History of substance abuse
Seizure disorder
Susceptibility to malignant hyperthermia
Potential difficult airway
 Morbid obesity
 Obstructive sleep apnea syndrome
NPO less than 8 hours
No escort
Previous adverse outcome from anesthesia
Significant drug allergies
Pulmonary aspiration risk

The ideal patient for an office-based procedure has an ASA physical status of 1 or 2. The ASA also has developed recommendations regarding patient selection. When determining whether a patient is suitable for OBA, it is important to realize that the location is often remote and the anesthesiologist may be unable to get assistance if it is required. Anticipated anesthetic problems must be avoided (Table 33-3).

A. **Obesity and Obstructive Sleep Apnea.** It is estimated that 60% to 90% of all patients with obstructive sleep apnea (OSA) are obese. The majority of the patients with OSA have not been formally diagnosed. There may be failure to intubate the trachea or ventilate the lungs, they may have respiratory distress soon after tracheal extubation, or they may suffer from respiratory arrest with preoperative sedation or postoperative analgesia. These patients tend to be exquisitely sensitive to the respiratory depressant effects of even small dosages of sedation or analgesics.

B. Pulmonary embolism from deep vein thrombosis is a significant cause of perioperative morbidity and mortality from office-based surgical procedures.

IV. SURGEON SELECTION

The relationship between the surgeon and anesthesiologist must be one of mutual trust and understanding. There have been cases reported of surgeons performing procedures for

TABLE 33-4

SENTINEL EVENTS THAT SHOULD TRIGGER A CHART REVIEW AND
BE PRESENTED AT A PERFORMANCE IMPROVEMENT QUALITY
ASSURANCE MEETING

Dental injury
Corneal abrasion
Perioperative myocardial infarction or stroke
Pulmonary aspiration
Reintubation of the trachea
Return to the operating room
Peripheral nerve injury
Adverse drug reaction
Uncontrolled pain, nausea, or vomiting
Unexpected hospital admission
Cardiac arrest
Death
Incomplete charts
Controlled substance discrepancy
Patient complaints

which they have little or no training. A system should be in
place for monitoring continuing medical education as well
as peer review and performance improvement, for both
surgeons and anesthesiologists (Table 33-4).

V. OFFICE SELECTION

The office needs to be appropriately equipped and stocked to
perform general anesthesia (Table 33-5). All equipment
described in the ASA algorithm for management of the
difficult airway should be present. Perioperative monitoring
must adhere to the ASA standards for basic anesthetic
monitoring. The office-based anesthesiologist should be
prepared to begin the initial treatment of malignant
hyperthermia, which requires having at least 12 bottles of
dantrolene. Drug accounting must be performed in
accordance with state and federal regulations. A medical
director who is responsible for overall operations should be
identified for every office.

A. **Emergencies** can occur in an office-based setting (Table
   33-6). Destinations for a patient in need of hospital
   admission must be identified with a formal written
   arrangement with a nearby hospital. Contingency plans
   must be in place in the event of a power supply interruption or electrical failure.

TABLE 33-5

EQUIPMENT NEEDED FOR SAFE DELIVERY OF
OFFICE-BASED ANESTHESIA

Monitors
  Noninvasive blood pressure with an assortment of cuff sizes
  Heart rate and electrocardiography monitors
  Pulse oximeter
  Temperature
Airway supplies
  Nasal cannulas
  Oral airways
  Face masks
  Self-inflating bag-mask ventilation device
  Laryngoscopes (multiple sizes and styles)
  Tracheal tubes (various sizes)
Intubating stylets
  Emergency airway equipment (LMAs, cricothyrotomy kit,
    means for transtracheal jet ventilation)
  Suction catheters and suction equipment
Cardiac defibrillator
Emergency drugs
  ACLS drugs
  Dantrolene and malignant hyperthermia supplies
Anesthetic drugs
Vascular cannulation equipment

TABLE 33-6

EMERGENCIES THAT MAY OCCUR WITHIN AN OFFICE THAT
REQUIRE CONTINGENCY PLANS

Fire
Bomb or bomb threat
Power loss
Equipment malfunction
Loss of oxygen supply pressure
Cardiac or respiratory arrest in the waiting room, operating room,
  or PACU
Earthquake
Hurricane
External disturbance such as a riot
Malignant hyperthermia
Massive blood loss
Emergency transfer of the patient to a hospital

PACU = postanesthesia care unit.

MANAGEMENT

TABLE 33-7

AMERICAN SOCIETY OF ANESTHESIOLOGISTS' CLASSIFICATION OF SURGICAL OFFICES ACCORDING TO THE ANESTHESIA AND SURGICAL PROCEDURES PERFORMED

Class A
Minor surgical procedures
Local, topical, or infiltration of local anesthetic
No sedation preoperatively or intraoperatively

Class B
Minor or major surgical procedures
Sedation via oral, rectal, or intravenous sedation
Analgesic or dissociative drugs

Class C
Minor or major surgical procedures
General anesthesia
Major conduction block anesthesia

B. **Accreditation** (Tables 33-7 and 33-8). The actual improvement in safety conferred by performing surgery in an accredited office has yet to be determined, and as long as there is no mandatory reporting system in place, it will be impossible to determine true morbidity rates associated with an office-based practice.

VI. PROCEDURE SELECTION

Suitable office-based procedures range from incision and drainage of abscesses to micro-laparoscopies. Very few data are available regarding procedure length and suitability for office-based procedures, but it has been recommended that procedures not exceed 6 hours in duration and be completed by 3 p.m. to allow for recovery time. In addition, when determining the suitability of a procedure, one must consider the possibility of hypothermia, blood loss, and significant fluid shifts.

A. **Specific Procedures**

1. **Liposuction** is the most commonly performed plastic surgery procedure and is accomplished by placing hollow rods into small incisions in the skin and suctioning subcutaneous fat into an aspiration canister. Superwet and tumescent techniques use large volumes (1–4 mL) of infiltrate solution that consists of 0.9%

TABLE 33-8

FACTORS CONSIDERED BY ACCREDITING AGENCIES

Physical layout of the office
Environmental safety and infection control
Patient and personnel records
Surgeon qualification
  Training
  Local hospital privileges (surgical and admission)
Office administration
Anesthesiologist requirements
Intraoperative and postoperative staffing
Intraoperative and postoperative monitoring capabilities
Ancillary care
Equipment
Drugs (emergency, controlled substances, routine medications)
BLS or ACLS/PALS certification
Temperature
Neuromuscular functioning
Patient positioning
Pre- and postanesthesia care and documentation
Quality assurance and peer review
Liability insurance
$PaCO_2$ evaluation
Discharge evaluation
Emergency procedure (fire, admission, and transfer)

saline or Ringer's lactate with epinephrine 1:1,000,000 and lidocaine 0.025% to 0.1%. Blood loss is generally 1% of the aspirate with these techniques. The peak serum levels of lidocaine occur 12 to 14 hours after injection. Liposuction is not a benign procedure and may be associated with morbidity and mortality caused by pulmonary embolism, anesthesia, myocardial infarction, infection, and hemorrhage. Risk factors include the use of multi-liter wetting solution infiltrations, large-volume aspiration causing massive third spacing, multiple concurrent procedures, anesthetic sedative effects yielding hypoventilation, and permissive discharge policies.

2. **Aesthetics.** Many facial aesthetic procedures, such as blepharoplasty, rhinoplasty, and meloplasty, are routinely performed in the office setting, usually under varying depths of monitored anesthesia care (MAC), but occasionally under general anesthesia.

MANAGEMENT

a. Facial plastic procedures that require the use of a laser pose a problem for the use of supplemental nasal oxygen to maintain adequate SpO_2. Any supplemental oxygen must be turned off during periods of laser or electrocautery use about the face.

b. The avoidance of supplemental oxygen when medically appropriate is ideal.

3. **Breast.** Procedures such as breast biopsy or augmentation, implant exchanges, and completion of transverse rectus abdominal muscle (TRAM) flaps may be performed in office settings. It is likely that patients undergoing breast surgery will require antiemetic medication and postoperative analgesics.

4. **Gastrointestinal endoscopy** includes esophageal, gastric, and duodenal endoscopies (EGD) and colonoscopies. This patient population tends to be older, with significant comorbid conditions. Insertion of the endoscope can usually be accomplished with sedation using small doses of propofol with or without midazolam.

a. Colonoscopy is painful secondary to the insertion and manipulation of the endoscope and may be associated with cardiovascular effects, including dysrhythmias, bradycardia, hypotension, hypertension, myocardial infarction, and death.

b. The gastroenterology community has sought to be able to provide moderate or even deep sedation with propofol without the assistance of an anesthesia professional. (Propofol's package insert states that it may only be administered by individuals who are trained in the administration of drugs that cause deep sedation and general anesthesia.)

5. **Dentistry and Oral and Maxillofacial Surgery.** Nitrous oxide has been used for most of the world's office-based dental anesthetics since 1884, when Horace Wells, himself a dentist, had nitrous oxide administered for a wisdom tooth extraction by a colleague. A high level of safety is attributed to the use of pulse oximetry, blood pressure, and ventilation monitoring, as well as administration of supplemental oxygen.

6. **Orthopedics and Podiatry.** The orthopedic office provides an excellent location for an anesthesiologist who

practices regional anesthesia (intra-articular local anesthesia and MAC, three-in-one block of the lumbar plexus, brachial plexus block, ankle block). Spinal anesthetics in the office-based setting must be of short duration. Lidocaine, which provides reliable short-acting analgesia, may be associated with an increased risk of transient neurologic symptoms in the ambulatory patient population.

7. **Gynecology and Genitourinary.** Many procedures, such as dilation and curettage, vasectomy, and cystoscopy have been performed in the office setting for many years, and recently there has been an increase in more invasive procedures such as mini-laparoscopies, ovum retrieval, prostate biopsies, and lithotripsy, necessitating an anesthesiologist's expertise.

8. **Ophthalmology and Otolaryngology.** Topical anesthesia or periorbital and retrobulbar blocks are frequently used to provide analgesia. Supplemental sedation may be required.

9. **Pediatrics.** Although no minimum age requirement for a child to undergo an office-based anesthetic has been established, patients older than 6 months of age and with an ASA physical status of 1 or 2 may be reasonable candidates for OBA (dental surgery, lacrimal duct probing, myringotomy) (Table 33-9).

VII. ANESTHETIC TECHNIQUES

The ASA recommends that anesthetics be provided or supervised by an anesthesiologist. The ASA has developed definitions regarding depths of anesthesia (Table 33-10). When formulating an anesthetic plan, one must consider that all agents and techniques used should be short acting, and the patient should be ready for discharge home soon after the completion of the procedure.

A. **Anesthetic Agents.** Intravenous sedation (propofol, barbiturates, midazolam, fentanyl, meperidine) is the most commonly used anesthetic technique in the OBA setting. Drugs should have a short half-life, be inexpensive, and not be associated with undesirable side effects such as nausea and vomiting.

1. **Remifentanil** is an ultra-short-acting opioid that, in combination with propofol for conscious sedation, provides discharge readiness within 15 minutes after

TABLE 33-9

GUIDELINES FOR THE PEDIATRIC PERIOPERATIVE
ANESTHESIA ENVIRONMENT

Patient Care Facility and Medical Staff Policies
Designation of operative procedures
Categorization of pediatric patients undergoing anesthesia
Annual minimal case volume to maintain clinical competence

Clinical Privileges of Anesthesiologists
Regular privileges
Special clinical privileges
Pain management

Patient Care Units
Preoperative evaluation and preparation units
Operating room
Anesthesiologists
Other health care providers involved in perioperative care
Availability and capabilities of clinical laboratory and radiologic
  services
Pediatric anesthesia equipment and drugs, including resuscitation
  cart
$PaCO_2$
Nursing staff
Anesthesiologist and physician staff

Postoperative Intensive Care Units

colonoscopy (48–80 minutes after meperidine or
midazolam administration).

  a. Remifentanil is an ideal drug for use during many
  office-based procedures (e.g., facial cosmetic surgery) that may be painful during injection of the
  local anesthetic.

  b. Disadvantages of remifentanil are possible nausea
  and vomiting, risk of drug-induced apnea, and the
  need for an infusion pump.

2. **Ketamine** functions as both an anesthetic and an analgesic. It is particularly useful because it does not depress
  respirations and is not associated with nausea and vomiting. Ketamine may cause an increase in secretions as
  well as cause hallucinations. Another advantage of ketamine is that it is relatively inexpensive.

3. **Clonidine** facilitates blood pressure control throughout the perioperative period and may decrease the
  total propofol usage.

TABLE 33-10

DEFINITIONS OF LEVELS OF SEDATION/ANALGESIA BY THE AMERICAN SOCIETY OF ANESTHESIOLOGISTS (OCTOBER 13, 1999, BY THE HOUSE OF DELEGATES)

Minimal Sedation (Anxiolysis)
Drug-induced sedation
The patient responds normally to verbal commands
Cognitive and motor function may be impaired
Ventilatory and cardiovascular function are maintained normally

Moderate Sedation/Analgesia (Conscious Sedation)
Drug-induced sedation
The patient responds purposefully to verbal commands either alone or with light tactile stimulation
The patient maintains a patent airway and spontaneous ventilation
Cardiovascular function is maintained

Deep Sedation/Analgesia
Drug-induced sedation
The patient cannot be easily aroused but can respond purposefully to repeated or painful stimulation
Ventilatory function may be impaired, requiring assistance in maintaining a patent airway, and spontaneous ventilation may be inadequate
Cardiovascular function is usually maintained

General Anesthesia
Drug-induced loss of consciousness
The patient is not arousable by painful stimulation
Ventilatory function is often impaired; the patient may require assistance in maintaining a patent airway
Spontaneous ventilation and neuromuscular functioning may be impaired
Positive-pressure ventilation is often required
Cardiovascular function may be impaired

4. It is vital that the office be adequately equipped and staffed to rescue patients from a deeper stage of anesthesia. (MAC is planned, but general anesthesia must be anticipated.)
5. Depth of anesthesia monitoring during MAC procedures has been shown to decrease the total propofol usage.

VIII. POSTANESTHESIA CARE UNIT (PACU)

After an office-based procedure, it is expected that the patient will be able to sit in a chair or ambulate to an

MANAGEMENT

examination room to dress almost immediately. A formal PACU may not be present, and the patient may recover in the surgical suite. Regardless of where the patient recovers, it is important to adhere to all ASA standards for monitoring and documentation throughout the postoperative period. Problems of postoperative nausea and vomiting (PONV) and pain may become particularly troublesome. It is imperative that every anesthetic administered is designed to maximize patient alertness and mobility and minimize the risks of the need for a prolonged PACU stay.

  A. **Pain Management.** Local anesthesia and conscious sedation supplemented by wound infiltration with local anesthetics or nerve blocks often form the basis for a multimodal strategy for postoperative pain management. Non-opioid analgesics (acetaminophen) and nonsteroidal antiinflammatory drugs (ketorolac) are routinely used. To minimize the potential for postoperative bleeding and risk of gastrointestinal complications, more specific cyclo-oxygenase-2 inhibitors are being increasingly used as non-opioid adjuvants for minimizing postoperative pain.

  B. **Postoperative Nausea and Vomiting.** An optimal antiemetic regimen for OBA has yet to be established, but because the causes of PONV are multifactorial, combination therapies may be more beneficial in high-risk patients. Many of the traditional first-line therapies are associated with sedation. Serotonin receptor antagonists and dexamethasone may be valuable.

IX. REGULATIONS

Governmental oversight of office-based surgery varies among states; regulations currently exist in many states, and others are following. It is imperative that the anesthesiologist act as a patient advocate and help educate the surgeon as to what constitutes a safe anesthetizing location.

X. BUSINESS AND LEGAL ASPECTS

It is in the anesthesia provider's best interest to seek legal counsel and create a valid business plan before embarking on a career in OBA. Billing strategies must be legal. In this complex environment of third-party payers, it is quite easy to make errors.

XI. CONCLUSIONS

OBA continues to rapidly expand and pose unique challenges to anesthesiologists. Decisions about appropriate patient and procedure selection and equipping anesthetizing locations must be made in conjunction with the surgeon.

MANAGEMENT

CHAPTER 34 ■ ANESTHESIA PROVIDED AT ALTERNATE SITES

Alternate sites may be defined as locations that are remote from the main operating room complex (radiology department or endoscopy) (Souter KJ: Anesthesia provided at alternative sites. In *Clinical Anesthesia*. Edited by Barash PG, Cullen BF, Stoelting RK, Cahalan MK, Stock MC. Philadelphia: Lippincott Williams & Wilkins, 2009, pp 861–875).

I. GENERAL PRINCIPLES

A. Standards introduced by The Joint Commission (formerly the Joint Commission on Accreditation of Healthcare Organizations, or JCAHO) require that the anesthesia service of a hospital participate with non-anesthesiology departments in setting up a uniform quality of care for patients undergoing sedation in all parts of the hospital.

B. The American Society of Anesthesiologists (ASA) has developed practice guidelines for sedation and analgesia by non-anesthesiologists.

C. Anesthesiologists undertake most of their training in the operating room surrounded by familiar equipment and staff experienced in the care of anesthetized patients. Away from the operating room, these facilities may not be taken for granted, and a simple three-step paradigm can be used to approach an anesthetic assignment in an alternate site (Table 34-1).

D. **The Environment.** The ASA has developed standards to apply to anesthesia in remote locations (Table 34-2).

1. **Anesthesia Equipment and Monitors.** Anesthesia machines and monitors that remain in an outside location need to be routinely serviced along with the anesthesia equipment used in the main operating rooms. This equipment is not often used on a daily basis, so attention should be paid to the freshness of the soda lime.

TABLE 34-1

A THREE-STEP APPROACH TO ANESTHESIA AT ALTERNATE SITES

1. **Environment**
   Anesthetic equipment
   Anesthesia monitors
   Suction
   Resuscitation equipment
   Personnel
   Technical equipment
   Radiation hazard
   Magnetic fields
   Ambient temperature

2. **Procedure**
   Diagnostic or therapeutic
   Duration
   Level of discomfort or pain
   Position of patient
   Special requirements (functional monitoring)
   Potential complications
   Surgical support

3. **Patient**
   Ability to tolerate sedation versus general anesthesia
   ASA grade and comorbidity
   Airway assessment
   Allergies (IV contrast)
   Monitoring requirements (simple versus advanced)
   Warming blankets

ASA = American Society of Anesthesiologists; IV = intravenous.

2. **Technical Equipment.** The complex technical equipment used in alternate sites, particularly in the radiology suites, is often bulky and fixed to the floor. Magnetic resonance imaging (MRI) creates its own environmental concerns related to magnetic fields.

E. **Procedures** (Table 34-3). It is vital that the anesthesiologist understands the nature of the procedure, the position the patient will be in, how painful the procedure is, and how long the procedure will last. Knowledge of these areas allows for the development of an anesthesia plan to provide safe patient care and facilitate the procedure.

F. **Patients** (Table 34-4). Children represent a special group of patients who are more likely to require sedation or anesthesia (pediatric procedural sedation) for various diagnostic and therapeutic procedures.

MANAGEMENT

TABLE 34-2

AMERICAN SOCIETY OF ANESTHESIOLOGISTS GUIDELINES FOR NON-OPERATING ROOM ANESTHETIZING LOCATIONS

1. **Oxygen**
   Reliable source
   Backup E cylinder (full)
2. **Suction**
   Adequate and reliable
3. **Scavenging system, if inhalation agents are administered**
4. **Anesthetic equipment**
   Backup self-inflating bag to deliver positive-pressure ventilation
   Adequate anesthetic drugs and supplies
   Anesthesia machine with equivalent function to those in the operating rooms and maintained to the same standards
   Adequate monitoring equipment to allow adherence to the ASA Standards for Basic Monitoring
5. **Electrical outlets**
   Sufficient for anesthesia machine and monitors
   Isolated electrical power or ground fault circuit interrupters if they are in a "wet location"
6. **Adequate illumination**
   Battery-operated backups
7. **Sufficient space**
   Personnel and equipment
   Easy and expeditious access to the patient, anesthesia machine, and monitoring
8. **Immediately available resuscitation equipment**
   Defibrillator
   Emergency drugs
   Cardiopulmonary resuscitation equipment
9. **Adequate trained staff to support the anesthesia team**
10. **Observation of all building and safety codes and facility standards**
11. **PACU facilities**
    Adequately trained staff to provide postanesthesia care
    Appropriate equipment to allow safe transport to the main PACU

ASA = American Society of Anesthesiologists; PACU = postanesthesia care unit.

II. ANESTHESIA CARE

The Joint Commission defines anesthesia care as the administration of intravenous (IV), intramuscular (IM), or inhalation agents that may result in the loss of the patient's protective reflexes.

TABLE 34-3

COMMON PROCEDURES REQUIRING ANESTHESIA AT ALTERNATE SITES

Radiology
Computed tomography (CT)
Radiofrequency ablation (RFA)
Magnetic resonance imaging (MRI)
Interventional radiology (vascular and nonvascular)
Interventional neuroradiology (INR)
Functional brain imaging

Radiotherapy
Radiation therapy
Intraoperative radiotherapy
Radiosurgery

Gastroenterology
Upper gastrointestinal endoscopy
Endoscopic retrograde cholangiopancreatography (ERCP)
Colonoscopy
Liver biopsy
Transjugular intrahepatic portosystemic shunt (TIPS)

Cardiology
Cardiac catheterization
Radiofrequency ablation
Cardioversion

Psychiatry
Electroconvulsive therapy (ECT)

TABLE 34-4

PATIENT FACTORS REQUIRING SEDATION OR GENERAL ANESTHESIA AT ALTERNATE SITES

Anxiety and panic disorders
Claustrophobia
Developmental delay and learning difficulties
Cerebral palsy
Seizure disorders
Movement disorders
Severe pain
Acute trauma with unstable cardiovascular, respiratory, or
  neurologic function
Significant comorbidity
Children

MANAGEMENT

TABLE 34-5

DEFINITION OF GENERAL ANESTHESIA AND LEVELS OF
SEDATION/ANALGESIA

	Minimal Anesthesia ("Anxiolysis")	Moderate Sedation/ Analgesia ("Conscious Sedation")	Deep Sedation/ Analgesia	General Anesthesia
Responsive-ness	Normal response to verbal stimulation	Purposeful response to verbal or tactile stimulation	Purposeful response after repeated or painful stimulation	Unarousable even with painful stimulation
Airway	Unaffected	No interventions required	Interventions may be required	Inter-ventions are often required
Spontaneous ventilation	Unaffected	Adequate	May be inadequate	Frequently inadequate
Cardio-vascular function	Unaffected	Usually maintained	Usually maintained	May be impaired

A. Patients who receive anesthesia or sedation at alternate sites should expect the same standard of care that they would receive in the operating room.

B. The ASA has published guidelines and standards and definitions of general anesthesia and levels of sedation (Table 34-5).

C. At the conclusion of the procedure, patients should recover from anesthesia or sedation in a postanesthesia care unit (PACU) or similar setting supervised by personnel who are trained to take care of unconscious patients and with appropriate monitoring and resuscitation equipment immediately at hand.

III. RADIOLOGY AND RADIATION THERAPY

Interventional radiologists now perform an increasing number of procedures that were once in the domain of surgeons. Two important aspects of the radiologic environment are the side effects of contrast media, which are commonly used to enhance radiologic images, and the hazards of ionizing radiation.

A. **Intravenous contrast agents** are iodinated compounds that are eliminated via the kidneys. Contrast-induced nephropathy is a recognized complication of their use.
   1. Contrast-induced nephropathy is the third leading cause of hospital-acquired acute renal failure, accounting for about 12% of cases.
   2. Patients with chronic renal disease, diabetes, and hypovolemia are most at risk for contrast-induced nephropathy; patients taking metformin are at risk of developing lactic acidosis.
   3. Adequate hydration, monitoring of urine output, and the use of low-osmolarity and non-ionic contrast media help reduce the risk.
   4. Contrast-induced nephropathy can be prevented by the use of adequate hydration and sodium bicarbonate infusions 1 hour before the procedure. (Dopamine and fenoldopam have not been shown to be effective.)

B. **Protection from Ionizing Radiation.** Patients, physicians, and other health care workers are frequently exposed to ionizing radiation, usually in the form of x-rays. With the routine use of a lead apron, protective goggles, and a thyroid shield, exposure to radiation can be kept to a low level.

IV. SPECIFIC RADIOLOGIC PROCEDURES

Cerebral and spinal angiography cause minimal discomfort and may be performed under local anesthesia with or without light sedation administered by non-anesthesiologists. Patients are required to remain completely motionless during these procedures.

A. **Interventional Neuroradiology.** Endovascular treatment of intracranial aneurysms with detachable platinum coils has become an acceptable alternative to surgery for reducing the risk of spontaneous recurrent hemorrhage after subarachnoid hemorrhage. Endovascular treatment avoids the need for craniotomy and reduces the cognitive impairment and frontotemporal brain damage associated with craniotomy. Patients with arteriovenous malformations (AVMs) are increasingly being treated endovascularly.
   1. **Anticoagulation** is required during and up to 24 hours after interventional radiologic procedures to prevent thromboemboli.

MANAGEMENT

TABLE 34-6

COMPLICATIONS OF INTERVENTIONAL NEURORADIOLOGIC PROCEDURES

Air embolism via femoral artery sheath
Hematoma or hemorrhage from femoral artery puncture
Pulmonary embolism
Bradycardia during carotid artery stent placement
Intracranial hemorrhage
Thromboembolic stroke

2. **Complications** (Table 34-6)
3. **Anesthetic Technique.** General anesthesia is usually conducted with endotracheal intubation and intermittent positive-pressure ventilation, although the laryngeal mask airway (LMA) is a suitable alternative to an endotracheal tube. Propofol and thiopental are the most commonly used induction agents.
   a. Invasive monitoring is used less often in patients undergoing interventional neuroradiologic techniques than in those having neurosurgical procedures.
   b. Controlled hypotension is often requested to facilitate embolization of AVMs.
   c. Certain procedures require patients to be awake for at least part of the procedure. A "sleep–awake–sleep anesthetic technique" using a propofol infusion allows the patient to be rapidly woken up for appropriate neurologic testing, and after this is complete, the patient is resedated or anesthetized while the definitive procedure is carried out.
B. **Computed Tomography, Radiofrequency Ablation, and Magnetic Resonance Imaging** are used for a wide array of diagnostic imaging procedures and an increasingly large number of therapeutic procedures, such as aspiration of masses and needle placement for nerve blockade. The procedures are similar in that they are relatively painless and most adults can tolerate them without the need for sedation or anesthesia. There is, however, an absolute requirement for the patient to remain motionless while the study is being performed. Children and adults with a variety of psychological or neurologic disorders may require sedation or anesthesia to allow them to tolerate the procedures (see Table 34-4).

1. **Computed Tomography (CT).** Modern CT scanners obtain a cross-sectional image in just a few seconds, and spiral scanners can image a slice of the body in less than 1 second, minimizing the problems associated with motion artifacts.
2. **Radiofrequency Ablation (RFA).** Percutaneous RFA is performed in the radiology suite for treatment of primary and metastatic hepatic tumors, including tumors of the lung, adrenal gland, kidney, breast, thyroid, prostate, and spleen.
   a. The majority of these procedures are tolerated without sedation. (Percutaneous RFA of pulmonary lesions requires conscious sedation or general anesthesia.)
   b. The presence of a cardiac pacemaker is an absolute contraindication to percutaneous RFA of lung lesions because surrounding tissues heat up.
3. **Magnetic Resonance Imaging.** Deaths and adverse outcomes in MRI scanners are entirely caused by the presence of ferrometallic foreign bodies such as cerebral aneurysm clips or implanted devices such as pacemakers.
   a. Before entering the vicinity of the magnet, patients and staff members must complete a rigorous checklist to make sure they have no ferrometallic objects in their bodies.
   b. Ferromagnetic anesthetic gas cylinders become potentially lethal projectiles.
   c. Standard pulse oximeters work in the MRI scanner but have been reported to produce burns. Nonferrous or fiberoptically cabled pulse oximeters should be used. The electrocardiogram is sensitive to the changing magnetic signals, and it is nearly impossible to eliminate all artifacts. Noninvasive blood pressure monitors and transducers for invasive pressure monitoring are available. In the absence of MRI-compatible monitors, long sampling tubes can be connected to standard capnographs and anesthetic agent monitors.
   d. Resuscitation attempts should take place outside the scanner because laryngoscopes, oxygen cylinders, and cardiac defibrillators cannot be taken close to the magnet.
4. **Anesthetic Techniques.** Fourteen percent of adult patients require some form of sedation to tolerate

MRI scanning. In most cases, it may be provided as either oral sedation with benzodiazepines or IV sedation administered under the supervision of a radiologist.

  a. Anesthesiologists are usually only involved in more complex cases, such as patients with obesity, obstructive sleep apnea, increased intracranial pressure, movement disorders, developmental delays, or the potential for a difficult airway.

  b. Most children younger than age 5 years and many up to the age of 11 years require sedation or general anesthesia to tolerate MRI and CT scanning.

C. **Radiation Therapy.** Two different types of radiation therapy commonly require anesthesia care: external-beam radiation treatments (usually used for children with malignancies) and intraoperative radiation of tumor masses that cannot be completely resected.

  1. Patients with central nervous system tumors should be assessed for signs of increased intracranial pressure.

  2. Many children receive cytotoxic or immunosuppressive chemotherapy as well as radiotherapy. This may result in increased risk of sepsis, thrombocytopenia, and anemia.

  3. General anesthesia or deep sedation techniques with propofol is preferable to prevent patient movement (Table 34-7).

    a. Portable monitors and methods for delivery of oxygen and agents to maintain general anesthesia during transport are all required.

    b. After treatment, patients must be transported back to the operating room for surgical closure.

TABLE 34-7

GOALS OF ANESTHETIC MANAGEMENT OF PEDIATRIC PATIENTS UNDERGOING RADIATION THERAPY

Rapid onset
Brief duration of action
Not painful to administer
Prompt recovery
Minimal interference with eating, drinking, and playing
Avoidance of tolerance to the anesthetic agents
Maintenance of a patent airway in a variety of body positions

TABLE 34-8

INTERVENTIONS IN THE CARDIAC CATHETERIZATION LABORATORY

Diagnostic cardiac catheterization
Coronary angiography and stenting
Electrophysiology studies and ablations
Placement of pacing and defibrillator devices
Balloon dilation and stenting for valvular and subvalvular lesions
Electrophysiologic studies and ablation of specific pathways
  (Wolff-Parkinson-White) or areas (atrial fibrillation)
Biventricular pacing for heart failure

V. CARDIAC CATHETERIZATION (Table 34-8)

A. Cardiac catheterization is performed in children with congenital heart disease for both hemodynamic assessment and interventional procedures. Patients often present with cyanosis, dyspnea, congestive heart failure, and intracardiac shunts.

1. Hypoxia, hypercarbia, and sympathetic stimulation as a result of anxiety may all exacerbate cardiopulmonary abnormalities.

2. In patients with a patent ductus arteriosus, high oxygen tension may lead to premature closure and should be avoided. Prostaglandin infusions are often used to maintain duct patency.

3. Meticulous attention must be paid to preventing air bubbles entering IV lines because they may cross to the arterial circulation via a right-to-left shunt.

4. General anesthesia is necessary when children cannot tolerate sedation techniques, when a child has significant cardiac or other morbidity, and when the procedure involves severe hemodynamic disturbances such as ventricular septal defect occlusion. Ketamine is useful in children with myocardial depression and can be used as an infusion together with propofol.

B. **Electrophysiologic Procedures (EPs).** EP studies and ablation of abnormal conduction pathways are performed increasingly for treatment of arrhythmias caused by aberrant conduction pathways.

1. Volatile anesthetics and propofol have been shown not to interfere with cardiac conduction during these procedures.

2. EP studies are lengthy and may be painful; children usually require general anesthesia.

MANAGEMENT

C. **Automatic implantable cardiac defibrillators** are usually implanted in the EP laboratory under general anesthesia or sedation rather than in the operating room.

VI. CARDIOVERSION

Transthoracic cardioversion is an accepted, often used treatment for atrial fibrillation (AF) and atrial flutter.

A. Two strategies are used to prevent thromboembolism after cardioversion in patients who have been in AF for longer than 48 hours. The conventional approach is to initiate anticoagulation 3 weeks before cardioversion, usually with Coumadin, and to continue it for 4 weeks after cardioversion.

B. **Transesophageal echocardiography** (TEE) has been recommended to determine whether patients are at low or high risk of thromboembolism. In low-risk patients, the dose of anticoagulants can be reduced.

C. **Anesthetic Technique.** Cardioversion is a brief but distressing procedure and should be carried out using sedation. The usual anesthetic technique for cardioversion is a small bolus of IV induction drug (propofol, etomidate, midazolam).

   1. Propofol provides a more rapid recovery than midazolam after cardioversion in elderly patients.
   2. A combination of propofol sedation together with an LMA may be used when TEE is performed before cardioversion.

VII. GASTROENTEROLOGY

Gastroenterologists are increasingly using propofol sedation techniques for upper and lower endoscopies (Table 34-9). The American Gastroenterological

---

TABLE 34-9

COMMON GASTROENTEROLOGY PROCEDURES

Upper endoscopy
Sigmoidoscopy
Colonoscopy
Endoscopic retrograde cholangiopancreatography (ERCP)
Esophageal dilatation
Esophageal stenting
Percutaneous endoscopic gastrostomy (PEG) tube placement
Transjugular intrahepatic portosystemic shunt (TIPS)

Association recommends appropriate training for endoscopists in sedation techniques and involvement of an anesthesiologist in selected patients.

A. **Upper gastrointestinal endoscopy** is tolerated without sedation in the majority of patients. In the rest of patients, conscious sedation is usually sufficient.

B. **Endoscopic retrograde cholangiopancreatography (ERCP)** is important in the diagnosis and treatment of biliary and pancreatic diseases.

   1. Patients usually experience discomfort during ERCP, particularly with instrumentation and stenting of the biliary and pancreatic ducts. Conscious or deep sedation techniques are recommended.

   2. If sphincter of Oddi manometry is being performed, opioids, glycopyrrolate, atropine, and glucagon should be avoided because they alter sphincter tone.

   3. Patients presenting for emergency ERCP may have significant comorbidities, including acute cholangitis with septicemia; jaundice with liver dysfunction; coagulopathy and bleeding from esophageal varices resulting in hypovolemia; and biliary stricture after major hepatobiliary surgery, including liver transplantation.

   4. Antispasmodics (IV hyoscyamine) decrease the incidence of spasm but may result in sinus tachycardia.

C. **Transjugular intrahepatic portosystemic shunt** (TIPS) connects the right or left portal vein through the liver parenchyma to one of the three hepatic veins. The purpose is to decompress the portal circulation in patients with portal hypertension.

   1. The TIPS procedure causes minimal stimulation, lasts between 2 to 3 hours, and may be performed under sedation or general anesthesia.

   2. Patients presenting for a TIPS procedure generally have significant hepatic dysfunction and require careful preoperative assessment (Table 34-10).

VIII. **ELECTROCONVULSIVE THERAPY (ECT)** is used to treat depression, mania, and affective disorders in patients with schizophrenia as well as a number of other psychiatric disorders. Typically, ECT is performed three times a week for six to 12 treatments followed by weekly or monthly maintenance therapy to prevent relapses.

A. **Physiologic Response to Electroconvulsive Therapy** (Table 34-11).

MANAGEMENT

TABLE 34-10

PREOPERATIVE CONSIDERATIONS IN PATIENTS PRESENTING
FOR THE TRANSJUGULAR INTRAHEPATIC PORTOSYSTEMIC
SHUNT PROCEDURE

System	Considerations
Airway (risk of aspiration)	Recent GI bleeding
	Increased intragastric pressure
	Decreased level of consciousness from hepatic encephalopathy
Respiratory system	Decreased functional residual capacity from ascites
	Pleural effusion
	Intrapulmonary shunts
	Pneumonia
Cardiovascular system	Associated alcoholic cardiomyopathy
	Altered volume status
	Acute hemorrhage from esophageal varices
	Intraperitoneal hemorrhage
Hematologic system	Coagulopathy
	Thrombocytopenia
Neurologic system	Hepatic encephalopathy

TABLE 34-11

PHYSIOLOGICAL RESPONSES TO ELECTROCONVULSIVE THERAPY

Grand mal seizure (10- to 15-second tonic phase followed by a
   30- to 60-second clonic phase)
Cardiovascular responses
   Increased cerebral blood flow
   Increased intracranial pressure
   Initial bradycardia
   Hypertension and tachycardia
   Cardiac dysrhythmias
   Myocardial ischemia
Short-term memory loss
Muscular aches
Fractures or dislocations
Emergence agitation
Status epilepticus
Sudden death

B. **Anesthetic Considerations**
1. Patients with depression presenting for ECT are often elderly with a number of coexisting conditions, so a thorough preoperative assessment and work-up should be performed before the patient begins treatment. Patients may be taking a variety of drugs (e.g., monoamine oxidase inhibitors), which can have important interactions with anesthetic agents.
2. The anesthetic requirements for ECT include amnesia; airway management; prevention of bodily injury from the seizure; control of hemodynamic changes; and a smooth, rapid emergence.
    a. Propofol is effective at attenuating the acute hemodynamic responses to ECT, and recovery is rapid. Propofol has anticonvulsant effects, although seizure duration is usually acceptable with a small dose (0.75 mg/kg).
    b. The short-acting opioids alfentanil and remifentanil can be used to decrease the dose of induction drug and prolong seizure duration without reducing the depth of anesthesia.
    c. Muscle relaxants are used to prevent musculoskeletal complications such as fractures or dislocations during the seizure. Succinylcholine 0.75 to 1.5 mg/kg is the most commonly used agent and is preferable to the longer acting nondepolarizing agents.
3. Before inducing the seizure, a bite guard is placed to protect the teeth.
4. In younger patients, 15 to 30 mg of IV ketorolac helps to reduce ECT-induced myalgia.
5. The parasympathetic effects of ECT (salivation, transient bradycardia, asystole) may be prevented by premedication with glycopyrrolate or atropine.
6. Labetalol (0.3 mg/kg) and esmolol (1 mg/kg) both ameliorate the hemodynamic responses, although esmolol has a lesser effect on seizure duration than labetalol, controlling blood pressure without affecting seizure duration. Clonidine and dexmetomidine (1 µg/kg over 10 minutes) administered just before induction of anesthesia are effective in controlling blood pressure without affecting seizure duration.

IX. DENTAL SURGERY

General anesthesia may be required during more complicated or prolonged cases and when patients are uncooperative, phobic, or mentally challenged.

A. Patients with Down syndrome are commonly
   encountered, and the anesthesia team should be aware
   of their possible cardiac abnormalities, including
   conduction abnormalities and structural defects; the risk
   of atlanto-occipital dislocation; and a variety of potential airway problems, including macroglossia, hypoplas-
   tic maxilla, palatal abnormalities, and mandibular protrusion.

B. If the patient is positioned head up in the dental chair,
   vasodilation and myocardial depressant effects of anesthetics can be pronounced, especially in patients with
   cardiovascular diseases.

C. **Anesthetic Management**
   1. Ketamine is a useful induction drug. Doses are 1 to 2
      mg/kg IV, 5 to 10 mg/kg orally, and, 2 to 4 mg/kg IM
      with an onset time of 5 to 10 minutes. Oral midazo-
      lam is popular. EMLA cream facilitates the placement
      of IV lines.
   2. Tracheal intubation, often via the nasal route, is
      required to protect the airway, although the LMA has
      recently been used successfully. The immediate post-
      operative complications include bleeding, airway
      obstruction, and laryngeal spasm.

IX. TRANSPORT OF PATIENTS

Patients who receive anesthesia or sedation at alternate
sites need to be transported to the PACU at the end of the
procedure, which may be some distance away. During
transport, the patient should be accompanied by a member
of the anesthesia team, who should continue to evaluate,
monitor, and support the patient's medical condition.

CHAPTER 35 ■ ANESTHESIA FOR THE OLDER PATIENT

All caregivers, including anesthesiologists, should be knowledge-able of at least some aspects of aging in order to provide intelligent modification of their standard practice (Rooke GA: Geriatric anesthesia. In *Clinical Anesthesia*. Edited by Barash PG, Cullen BF, Stoelting RK, Cahalan MK, Stock MC. Philadelphia: Lippincott Williams & Wilkins, 2009, pp 876–888).

I. DEMOGRAPHICS AND ECONOMICS OF AGING

A. When Social Security was initiated in 1935, only 6.1% of the U.S. population was older than 65 years old. By 2005, that percentage had more than doubled to 12.4%, and by 2035, it is expected to be more than 20% of the U.S. population.

B. Elderly patients account for more than 44% of all inpatient days. Of the 26.6 million inpatient surgical procedures in 2004, 33% were performed on elderly patients.

C. It is estimated that people older than age 65 years account for nearly half of the nation's health care costs.

II. THE PROCESS OF AGING

A. Mammalian aging clearly involves a gradual, cumulative process of damage and deterioration.

1. Protective mechanisms against aging are costly to the organism. The "disposable soma" theory of aging states that anti-aging mechanisms only need to be good enough to give the next generation the best opportunity to reproduce. In fact, most of the gains in average human lifespan have been as the result of reducing the factors that cause premature death (accidents, violence, disease).

2. The inability to completely thwart aging implies that the average human lifespan is limited and that if everyone only died of "old age," the age at death would end up being a bell-shaped curve centered at a certain value, probably around age 85 years.

3. A variety of deleterious processes continually attack DNA, proteins, and lipids (free radicals and non-enzymatic glycosylation of sugars and amines).

   a. Collagen becomes stiffer from aromatic ring cleavage and by cross-linking to other collagen molecules. In the cardiovascular system, arteries, veins, and the myocardium all stiffen with age.

   b. DNA damage occurs, and mitochondrial DNA suffers more damage than nuclear DNA.

   c. Caloric restriction, well documented to increase lifespan in small mammals, probably does so by decreasing the rate of oxidative damage.

B. **Functional Decline and the Concept of Frailty**

1. Functional reserve represents the degree to which organ function can increase above the level necessary for basal activity. For healthy individuals, reserve peaks at approximately age 30 years, gradually declines over the next several decades, and then experiences more rapid decline beginning around the eighth decade of life. Anesthesiologists often assess the patient's reserve.

   a. The ability to achieve the desired minimum of four metabolic equivalents (METs) presumably provides enough cardiovascular reserve to tolerate the stress of most surgical procedures.

   b. Even without formal assessment, an intuitive sense of reserve is often obtained through simple observation (loss of subcutaneous tissue, unsteady or slowed gait, stooped body habitus, minimal muscle mass [sarcopenia]).

2. Diminished mentation is a risk factor for postoperative delirium.

C. **Physiologic Age**

1. The rate at which a given individual ages is highly variable and is determined to a great extent by genetics and luck at avoiding illnesses, trauma, or environmental exposure that may contribute to functional loss. Nevertheless, successful aging can be promoted through avoidance of obesity, good nutrition, and regular exercise.

2. The older we get, the less likely our chronologic age reflects our physiologic status and functional reserve.

III. THE PHYSIOLOGY OF ORGAN AGING

A. Changes in Body Composition and Liver and Kidney Aging

1. Changes in body composition are primarily characterized by a gradual loss of skeletal muscle and an increase in body fat, although the latter is more prominent in women.

   a. Basal metabolism declines with age, with most of the decline accounted for by the change in body composition. A reduction in total body water reflects the reduction in cellular water that is associated with a loss of muscle and an increase in adipose tissue.

   b. Aging causes a small decrease in plasma albumin levels and a small increase in α_1-acid glycoprotein, yet the effect of these changes on drug protein binding and drug delivery appears to be minimal.

2. Liver mass decreases with age and accounts for most, but not all, of the 20% to 40% decrease in liver blood flow. Even in very old individuals, liver reserve should be more than adequate.

3. Renal cortical mass also decreases by 20% to 25% with age, but the most prominent effect of aging is the loss of up to half of the glomeruli by age 80 years.

   a. The decrease in the glomerular filtration rate (GFR) after age 40 years typically reduces renal excretion of drugs to a level so that drug dosage adjustment becomes a progressively important consideration beginning at approximately age 60 years. Nevertheless, the degree of decline in GFR is highly variable and is likely to be much less than predicted in many individuals.

   b. Aged kidneys do not eliminate excess sodium or retain sodium when necessary as effectively as kidneys in young adults. Fluid and electrolyte homeostasis is more vulnerable in older patients, particularly when the patient has acute injury or disease and eating and drinking becomes more of a chore.

4. Aging is associated with decreased insulin secretion in response to a glucose load. It is also associated with increased insulin resistance, particularly in skeletal

muscle (even healthy elderly patients may require insulin therapy more often perioperatively than young adults).

B. **Central Nervous System Aging**
   1. Brain mass begins to decrease slowly starting at approximately age 50 years and declines more rapidly later such that an 80-year-old brain has typically lost 10% of its weight.
   2. Neurotransmitter functions suffer more significantly, including dopamine, serotonin, γ-aminobutyric acid (GABA) and especially the acetylcholine system (which is connected to Alzheimer's disease). Nearly half of patients age 85 years and older demonstrate significant cognitive impairment.
   3. Some degree of atherosclerosis appears to be inevitable.
   4. Contrary to prior belief, the aged brain does make new neurons and is capable of forming new dendritic connections.
   5. There is an approximate 6% decrease in the minimum alveolar concentration (MAC) per decade after age 40 years. For many intravenous (IV) anesthetic agents, the same brain concentration produces approximately twice the effect in an older person than a young adult.
   6. Age is a major risk factor for postoperative delirium and cognitive decline.

IV. **DRUG PHARMACOLOGY AND AGING**
   (Table 35-1)

   A. Drugs often have more pronounced effects in older patients. The cause can be either pharmacodynamic, in which case the target organ (often the brain) is more sensitive to a given drug tissue level, or pharmacokinetic, in which case a given dose of drug commonly produces higher blood levels in older patients.
   B. Typically, the initial blood concentration of bolus drugs is higher in older patients, partly because of a mildly contracted blood volume. Despite the typically enhanced effect of bolus drugs on older patients, there is a general impression that bolus drugs take longer to achieve that greater effect (the reasons are unclear).
   C. The most prominent pharmacokinetic effect of aging is a decrease in drug metabolism because of both a decrease in clearance and an increase in Vd_{ss} (increase in body fat). In addition, elderly patients often take a host of

TABLE 35-1

EFFECT OF AGE ON DRUG DOSING

Drug	Bolus Administration	Multiple Boluses or Infusion	Comments
Propofol	20%–60% reduction Dose on lean body mass (1 mg/kg in very old patients)	50% reduction Infusions beyond 50 minutes progressively increase the time required to decrease the blood level by 50% (but effect site levels may decrease faster in elderly patients)	Possible increased brain sensitivity Decreased V_{cen} Slowed redistribution
Thiopental Etomidate Midazolam	20% reduction 25%–50% reduction Compared with 20-year-old patients, modest reduction at age 60 years and 75% reduction at age 90 years	20% reduction Similar to bolus	Decreased V_{cen} Slowed redistribution Increased brain sensitivity
Morphine	Probably 50% reduction Peak morphine effect is 90 minutes (half of peak effect at 5 minutes)	Long effect site equilibration time translates into a very slow reduction in the effect on termination of the infusion (4 hours for 50% reduction)	Metabolite morphine-6 glucuronide buildup requires prolonged morphine use, but its renal excretion makes it very long lasting Increased brain sensitivity
Fentanyl	50% reduction	50% reduction	Minimal change in pharmacokinetics Delayed absorption from fentanyl patch

(continued)

TABLE 35-1

EFFECT OF AGE ON DRUG DOSING *(Continued)*

Drug	Bolus Administration	Multiple Boluses or Infusion	Comments
Alfentanil	50% reduction	50% reduction	Probably increased brain sensitivity
Sufentanil	50% reduction	50% reduction	Minimal changes in pharmacokinetics
Remifentanil	50% reduction	50% reduction	Slower blood–brain equilibration, suggesting slower onset and offset
			Modest decreased V_{cen}
Meperidine	Used only for postoperative shivering	Do not use	Toxic metabolite normeperidine whose renal excretion decreases with age
Vecuronium	Slower onset	Slower recovery	Slightly greater liver metabolism than renal metabolism
			Age nearly doubles metabolic half-time
Cisatracurium	Slower onset	No significant changes with age	Mostly Hoffmann elimination
			Modest prolongation of metabolic half-time
Rocuronium	Minimally slower onset		Liver metabolism slightly greater than renal metabolism
			Modest increase in metabolic half-time

Succinylcholine	Slower onset	
Edrophonium	Similar dosing and onset	Decreased V_{cen} Primarily renal elimination Modest increase in metabolic half-time
Neostigmine	Despite pharmacokinetic changes, some studies indicate the need for an increased dose with age	Decreased V_{cen} Hepatic elimination Modest increase in metabolic half-time

V_{cen} = central volume of distribution or initial volume of distribution; a smaller V_{cen} increases initial plasma levels and enhances transfer of drug in the target organ (brain, muscle).

TABLE 35-2

THE EFFECTS OF AGING ON THE CARDIOVASCULAR SYSTEM

Decreased response to beta-receptor stimulation (decreased heart rate response to catecholamines and exercise; baroreflex control of heart rate is decreased and contributes to impaired autoregulation of blood pressure)

Stiffening of the myocardium (slows diastolic relaxation and impairs ventricular filling; maintenance of an adequate central blood volume becomes critical), arteries, and veins (postural hypotension is more likely with mild hypovolemia)

Increased sympathetic nervous system activity

Decreased parasympathetic nervous system activity

Conduction system changes (atrial fibrillation)

Defective ischemic preconditioning (the protective effect of angina is absent)

chronic medications, a setup for drug interactions as well as for inhibition of drug metabolism.

1. Drugs with primarily renal elimination experience decreased metabolism because of reductions in GFR with aging. The net effect on drug metabolism is typically a doubling of the elimination half-life between old and young adults. In the case of diazepam, the half-life in hours is roughly equal to the patient's age.

2. The concept of the context-sensitive half-time (time necessary for a 50% [or any desired percent] decrease in plasma concentration after termination of an infusion) is often increased in elderly patients.

V. CARDIOVASCULAR AGING (Table 35-2)

VI. PULMONARY AGING

A. The most prominent effects of aging on the pulmonary system are stiffening of the chest wall and a decrease in elasticity of the lung parenchyma.

1. The need for greater lung inflation to prevent small airway collapse is reflected by the increase in closing capacity with age. Closing capacity typically exceeds functional residual capacity in the mid 60s and eventually exceeds the tidal volume at some later age.

2. These changes, plus a modest reduction in alveolar surface area with age, contribute to a modest decline in resting PaO_2.

B. Changes within the nervous system further influence the respiratory system. Aging leads to an approximate 50% decrease in the ventilatory response to hypercapnia and an even greater decrease in the response to hypoxia, especially at night.

C. Generalized loss of muscle tone with age applies to the hypopharyngeal and genioglossal muscles and predisposes elderly individuals to upper airway obstruction.

   1. A high percentage, perhaps even 75%, of people older than age 65 years have sleep-disordered breathing, a phenomenon that may or may not be the same as sleep apnea, but certainly places elderly individuals at increased risk for postoperative hypoxia.

   2. Aging also results in less effective coughing and impaired swallowing. Aspiration is a significant cause of community-acquired pneumonia and may well play a role in the development of postoperative pneumonia.

VII. THERMOREGULATION AND AGING

A. Elderly individuals are prone to hypothermia when stressed by modestly cold environments that would not affect younger individuals.

B. Aging has a variable effect on vasoconstriction and shivering, with some elderly people demonstrating responses identical to young subjects and others demonstrating a near-absent response. Overall vasoconstriction and metabolic heat production are diminished in magnitude in elderly individuals.

   1. The increased risk of intraoperative hypothermia in elderly patients owing to effective vasoconstriction is compounded by decreased basal metabolism (heat production) in elderly patients. (Hypothermia has been observed more frequently in older patients than in their younger counterparts.)

   2. The risks of hypothermia include myocardial ischemia, surgical wound infection, coagulopathy with increased blood loss, and impaired drug metabolism.

VIII. CONDUCT OF ANESTHESIA

A. The Preoperative Visit

   1. The preoperative visit should begin with a detailed review of the patient's medical history, current

functional status of all vital organs, and medication list. Basic laboratory testing is not warranted for older subjects. Some additional issues more prevalent among elderly patients should also be raised. For example, whether the patient's living situation is capable of providing the support necessary for a successful recovery should be explored.

2. Elderly patients may require a long time to return to their preoperative levels of function.

3. Older patients' expectations from surgery may be much different than the expectations of their younger counterparts, and the anesthesiologist must be careful not to judge a patient's decision making based on more typical goals.

4. Polypharmacy and drug interaction are a significant problem for older patients.

5. Dehydration, elder abuse, and malnutrition (vitamin D, vitamin B_{12}, inadequate caloric intake, poor oral hygiene) are all more common in very old individuals than generally appreciated. Nutritional status is underappreciated as a risk factor for surgery. (Albumin is as sensitive an index for mortality or morbidity as any other single indicator, including the American Society of Anesthesiologists status.)

B. **Intraoperative Management**

1. Smaller doses are needed for the induction of general anesthesia in older patients. A given blood level of propofol causes a greater decrease in brain activity in older patients.

2. Although swings in blood pressure may not be desirable, there is no evidence that even major, but brief, changes in blood pressure lead to adverse outcomes.

3. Whether general or neuraxial anesthesia is used, induction and maintenance of anesthesia commonly result in a significant decrease in systemic blood pressure, more so than typically occurs in younger patients.

C. **Postoperative Care**

1. The goals of emergence and the immediate postoperative period are no different for an elderly than a young patient.

2. Analgesia is a major goal, and there is no evidence that pain is any less severe or any less detrimental in older patients than in younger ones. Elderly patients sometimes underreport their pain level and may be more tolerant of acute pain.

TABLE 35-3

ADVERSE OUTCOMES ASSOCIATED WITH INADEQUATE
POSTOPERATIVE PAIN RELIEF IN ELDERLY PATIENTS

Sleep deprivation
Respiratory impairment
Ileus
Suboptimal mobilization
Insulin resistance
Tachycardia
Systemic hypertension

      a. Older patients have more difficulty with visual
analog scoring systems than verbal or numeric
systems. If the patient is cognitively impaired,
communication of pain is further impaired;
indeed, demented patients often experience severe
pain after hip surgery, but even mild cognitive
impairment can lead to problems with pain assessment or with use of a patient-controlled analgesia
machine.

      b. Failure to achieve adequate levels of analgesia is
associated with numerous adverse outcomes (Table
35-3). The consequences include longer hospitalization and increased incidence of delirium
(meperidine should be avoided).

      c. Epidural analgesia provides analgesia that is supe-
rior to IV therapy in elderly patients.

   3. Delirium often goes undetected in older patients,
partly because older patients are less likely to exhibit
agitation than young delirious patients.

IX. PERIOPERATIVE COMPLICATIONS (Table 35-4)

  A. Older patients are at increased risk for complications
(cardiovascular, pulmonary, renal, central nervous system [CNS], wound infection, death) in the perioperative period, reflecting comorbid diseases and a reduction in organ system reserve because of the aging
process.

  B. Complications of the cardiovascular and pulmonary systems are associated with the greatest perioperative mortality. The higher incidences of the pulmonary complications suggest that greater mortality results from
pulmonary complications than cardiac complications.

MANAGEMENT

TABLE 35-4

THE EFFECTS OF AGE ON SELECTED PERIOPERATIVE
COMPLICATIONS AND ASSOCIATED MORTALITY*

	Complication Rate		Mortality Rate from the Complication	
	Age <80 Years	Age ≥ 80 Years	Age <80 Years	Age ≥80 Years
Myocardial infarction	0.4	1.0	37.1	48.0
Cardiac arrest	0.9	2.1	80.0	88.2
Pneumonia	2.3	5.6	19.8	29.2
>48 hours on ventilator	2.1	3.5	30.1	38.5
Required reintubation	1.6	2.8	32.3	44.0
Cerebrovascular accident	0.3	0.7	26.1	39.3
Coma ≥24 hours	0.2	0.3	65.9	80.9
Prolonged ileus	1.2	1.7	9.2	16.0

*All differences between patients younger than 80 years versus those 80 years and older are significant ($P < 0.001$) except for coma mortality ($P = 0.004$). Modified with permission from Hamel MD, Henderson WG, Khuri SF, Daley J: Surgical outcomes for patients aged 80 and older: Morbidity and mortality from major noncardiac surgery. *J Am Geriat Soc* 2005;53:424.

C. CNS complications are also a major source of morbidity and mortality. The incidence of stroke in the general surgical population is approximately 0.5%.
  1. Age is a risk factor, as is atrial fibrillation, and a history of a prior stroke increases the risk of perioperative stroke by as much as 10-fold.
  2. Strokes typically occur well after surgery (on average, 7 days later).
D. Postoperative cognitive decline and postoperative delirium are significant sources of debilitating morbidity. Although these two entities may prove to be related to each other, at present they appear to be distinct clinical syndromes.
  1. **Postoperative delirium** is an acute confusional state manifested by sudden onset (hours to days) and vacillating levels of attention and cognitive skill.
    Emergence delirium does not qualify as postoperative delirium.

TABLE 35-5

RISK FACTORS FOR DELIRIUM IN ELDERLY PATIENTS

Patient age
Baseline low cognitive function
Depression
General debility (dehydration, visual or auditory impairment)
Use of drugs with central nervous system effects
    Opioids (especially meperidine)
    Benzodiazepines (especially lorazepam)
    Anticholinergic drugs (except glycopyrrolate)
Sleep deprivation
Unfamiliar environment
Postoperative pain

    a. The risk of postoperative delirium after major surgery in older patients is approximately 10%. The risk varies with the surgical procedure and is highest after hip surgery, with an approximate incidence of 35%.

    b. The cause of delirium is multifactorial (Table 35-5).

    c. The choice of regional versus general anesthesia does not appear to be a factor, especially if sedation is used in conjunction with the regional technique.

    d. Delirium is associated with an increased duration of hospitalization and its attendant costs, poorer long-term functional recovery, and increased mortality.

2. **Postoperative cognitive dysfunction** is characterized by a long-term decrease in mental abilities after surgery. It is inherently more difficult to diagnose than delirium because it usually requires sophisticated neuropsychologic testing, including baseline tests before surgery.

    a. Compared with nonsurgical control subjects, the cognitive decline lessens over time, with a 25% incidence at 1 week and about a 10% incidence at 3 months.

    b. At 6 months and beyond, there may be a prevalence of 1% of subjects with cognitive decline.

    c. Anesthetic management does not appear to affect cognitive decline when comparisons are made between general versus regional anesthesia,

MANAGEMENT

controlled hypotension versus normotension, or IV versus inhalation anesthesia.

d. Patient risk factors include age, lower levels of education, and history of stroke even without residual deficit.

e. Increased mortality at 1 year is associated with patients who demonstrate cognitive decline at both hospital discharge and at 3 months after surgery.

X. THE FUTURE

A. Improvements in surgical and anesthetic techniques that reduce the overall stress to the patient are permitting more surgeries to be performed on older and sicker patients than ever before.

B. The most pressing issues are the prevention of postoperative delirium, cognitive decline, pneumonia, and respiratory failure.

C. Improved pain control techniques that also diminish side effects, especially to the brain and bowels, would be welcome.

CHAPTER 36 ■ ANESTHESIA FOR TRAUMA AND BURN PATIENTS

Approximately 75% of the hospital mortality from trauma occurs within 48 hours of admission, most commonly from thoracic, abdominal or retroperitoneal, vascular, or central nervous system injuries (Capan LM, Miller SM: Trauma and burns. In *Clinical Anesthesia*. Edited by Barash PG, Cullen BF, Stoelting RK, Cahalan MK, Stock MC. Philadelphia: Lippincott Williams & Wilkins, 2009, pp 889–926).

I. INITIAL EVALUATION AND RESUSCITATION

The general approach to evaluation of an acute trauma victim includes three sequential components: rapid overview, primary survey, and secondary survey (Fig. 36-1). During this period, the anesthesiologist identifies injuries, pre-existing conditions, and the resulting functional abnormalities that require either immediate treatment or provision for resuscitative and anesthetic management. Universal infection control precautions are the standard because many trauma victims are carriers of hepatitis B, hepatitis C, or human immunodeficiency virus.

A. **Airway Evaluation and Intervention.** The American Society of Anesthesiologists' difficult airway algorithm can be applied to trauma airway management scenarios.
1. **Airway Obstruction.** If the patient can speak, serious airway obstruction is unlikely. Signs of upper and lower airway obstruction include dyspnea, hoarseness, stridor, dysphoria, subcutaneous emphysema, and hemoptysis. Cervical deformity, edema, crepitation, tracheal deviation, or jugular venous distention may be present before the appearance of symptoms.
2. After immobilization of the cervical spine and administration of oxygen by face mask, airway management should include chin lift, jaw thrust, clearing of the

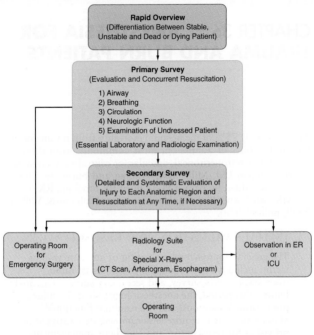

FIGURE 36-1. The general approach to evaluation of acute trauma patients includes the sequential steps of rapid overview, primary survey, and secondary survey. CT = computed tomography; ED = emergency department; ICU = intensive care unit.

oropharyngeal cavity, and placement of an oral or nasopharyngeal airway.

   a. Ventilation is supported in inadequately breathing patients with a self-inflating bag.

   b. If these measures do not provide adequate ventilation, the trachea must be intubated using either direct laryngoscopy or cricothyroidotomy.

   c. Proper placement of devices, such as a laryngeal mask airway (LMA), Combitube, or endotracheal tube, by paramedics should be confirmed by capnometry as soon as possible after the patient enters the hospital.

B. **Full stomach** is a background condition in acute trauma, and the urgency of securing the airway often does not permit time for pharmacologic measures to decrease gastric volume and acidity.

1. Excessive cricoid pressure may displace a vertebral bone fragment with potential damage to the spinal cord. Spinal cord injury may also accompany cricoid pressure and manual incline stabilization to cervical spine-injured patients.

2. The LMA may be used temporarily to maintain airway patency (a full stomach precludes its sustained use) or to facilitate intubation aided by a fiberoptic laryngoscope.

3. The presence of uncorrectable hypotension may preclude use of intravenous (IV) anesthetics. (Muscle relaxants alone may be sufficient in these patients.) If only a mild to moderate degree of hypovolemia is present, decreased doses (30% to 50%) of anesthetics should be administered.

4. There is no consensus about the extent of the airway that can be safely anesthetized with topical drugs. (Avoidance of transtracheal anesthesia preserves the cough reflex even in the presence of an impaired glottic closure reflex owing to a superior laryngeal nerve block or topical anesthesia.)

5. Agitated and uncooperative patients (topical anesthesia is not possible) may require a rapid sequence induction of anesthesia followed by direct laryngoscopy to secure the airway.

C. **Head, Open Eye, and Contained Major Vessel Injuries**

1. These conditions require deep anesthesia (opioids and IV anesthetics) and profound skeletal muscle relaxation before airway manipulation (this assumes a difficult tracheal intubation is not anticipated and the patient is not hypotensive).

2. Hypertension, coughing, and reacting to the tracheal tube may adversely increase systemic blood pressure, intracranial pressure (ICP), and intraocular pressure.

3. Hypotension dictates either reduced or no IV anesthetic administration.

D. **Cervical Spine Injury.** Immobilization of the neck in a neutral position is indicated before airway management in all acute trauma patients suspected to have cervical spine injury. Intubation may theoretically cause spinal

TABLE 36-1

FIVE CRITERIA THAT RULE OUT CERVICAL SPINE INJURY

No midline cervical tenderness
No focal neurologic deficit
Normally alert
Not intoxicated
No distracting painful injury

cord damage during manipulation of the neck, although the available literature attests to the rare, possibly non-existent occurrence of this event.

1. **Initial Evaluation.** In a conscious patient with a suspected injury, the diagnosis is relatively easy (Table 36-1). Computed tomography (CT) scanning is the primary diagnostic measure for detection of fractures; magnetic resonance imaging [MRI] is used for ligamentous injury.

2. **Airway Management.** Almost all airway maneuvers (jaw thrust, chin lift, head tilt, oral airway placement) result in some degree of cervical spine movement. Stabilization of the head, neck, and torso in a neutral position is best accomplished by manual in-line immobilization (a cervical collar does not provide absolute protection). The first operator stabilizes and aligns the head in a neutral position without applying cephalad traction, and the second operator stabilizes both shoulders by holding them against the supporting surface. Use of fiberoptic bronchoscopy in a sedated patient is a consideration when time constraints, a full stomach, and patient cooperation issues are not present.

E. **Direct Airway Injuries** (Table 36-2)

F. **Management of Breathing Abnormalities**

1. Of the several causes that may alter breathing after trauma, tension pneumothorax, flail chest, and open pneumothorax are immediate threats to life and therefore require rapid diagnosis and treatment.

2. A flail chest results from comminuted fractures of at least three adjacent ribs or rib fractures with associated costochondral separation or sternal fracture.

   a. An underlying pulmonary contusion with increased elastic recoil of the lung and work of breathing is

TABLE 36-2

MECHANISMS OF DIRECT AIRWAY INJURY

Maxillofacial Injuries

Soft tissue edema of the pharynx (hematoma or edema may expand during the 6–12 hours after injury; liberal fluid administration may contribute to edema)

Blood and debris in the oropharyngeal cavity

Mandibular condylar fractures (if bilateral, they prevent opening of the mouth)

Cervical Airway Injuries

Blunt or penetrating trauma (hoarseness, dysphagia, flattening of the thyroid cartilage protuberance)

Thoracic Airway Injuries

Blunt injury usually involves the posterior membranous portion of the trachea and the mainstem bronchi (it should be suspected when a seal around the tracheal tube cuff cannot be obtained)

the main cause of respiratory insufficiency or failure and resulting hypoxemia.

  b. Respiratory failure often develops over a 3- to 6-hour period, causing gradual deterioration seen on chest radiography and arterial blood gas analysis.

3. Tracheal intubation is often necessary in patients with pulmonary contusion or respiratory insufficiency or failure despite adequate analgesia.

  a. Positive end-expiratory pressure is used if ventilation is controlled.

  b. In intubated and spontaneously breathing patients, airway pressure release ventilation provides improved arterial oxygenation and maintenance of blood pressure, lower sedation requirements, and shorter periods of intubation.

  c. In bilateral severe contusions with life-threatening hypoxemia, high-frequency jet ventilation may enhance oxygenation as well as cardiac function, which may be compromised by concomitant myocardial contusion.

4. The definitive diagnosis of tension pneumothorax is with chest radiography. When there is no time for radiologic confirmation, a 14-gauge angiocath can be placed through the fourth intercostal space in the midaxillary line.

5. In the absence of significant gas exchange abnormalities, chest wall instability alone is not an indication

MANAGEMENT

TABLE 36-3

INDICATIONS FOR MECHANICAL VENTILATION IN PATIENTS
WITH FLAIL CHEST

Clinical evidence of respiratory failure
Progressive fatigue or deterioration
Respiratory rate >35 breaths/min
PaO_2 <60 mm Hg breathing at least 50% oxygen
$PaCO_2$ >55 mm Hg
Vital capacity <15 mL/kg
Clinical evidence of shock
Associated severe head injury with need to hyperventilate the
　patient's lungs
Severe associated injury requiring surgery
Airway obstruction
Significant pre-existing chronic pulmonary disease

for tracheal intubation and mechanical ventilation
(Table 36-3). Effective pain relief (continuous
epidural analgesia) by itself can improve respiratory
function and often prevent the need for mechanical
ventilation.

6. Hypoxia and hypercarbia result from an open pneumothorax. (Occlusive dressing is the initial
treatment.)

G. **Management of Shock.** In the initial phase of trauma,
hypotension has many causes, but hemorrhage is the
most common (Table 36-4). Evaluation of the severity of
hemorrhagic shock in the initial phase is based on a few
relatively insensitive and nonspecific clinical signs (Table
36-5).

1. Although heart rate is one of the earliest signs of
hemorrhagic shock, the heart rate does not necessarily
correlate with the blood loss. Tachycardia may be
absent in up to 30% of hypotensive trauma patients
because of increased vagal tone or chronic cocaine
use.

2. Equating a normal systemic blood pressure with nor-
movolemia during initial resuscitation may lead to
loss of valuable time for treating underlying
hypovolemia.

3. The response of the heart rate and blood pressure to
initial fluid therapy also aids in assessment of the
degree of hypovolemia (Table 36-6).

TABLE 36-4

CAUSES OF HYPOTENSION IN THE INITIAL PHASE OF TRAUMA

Hemorrhage or Extensive Tissue Injury
Tachycardia, narrow pulse pressure, peripheral vasoconstriction
Crystalloid solution should be given initially and the patient should
be transfused if 2000 mL in 15 minutes does not improve blood
pressure

Cardiac Tamponade
Tachycardia, dilated neck veins, muffled heart sounds
Pericardiocentesis

Myocardial Contusion
Tachycardia, cardiac dysrhythmias
Crystalloids, vasodilators, inotropes

Pneumothorax or Hemothorax
Tachycardia, dilated neck veins, absent breath sounds, dyspnea,
subcutaneous emphysema
Chest tube

Spinal Cord Injury
Hypotension without tachycardia, narrow pulse pressure, or
vasoconstriction
Crystalloids, vasopressor, inotropes

Sepsis
Develops typically a few hours after colon injury (in
normovolemic patients, it manifests as modest tachycardia, wide
pulse pressure, and fever)
Antibiotics, crystalloids, inotropes

4. Markers of organ perfusion to guide resuscitation
   include base deficit, blood lactate level, and sublingual
   capnometry (gut perfusion).
5. During the initial phase of treatment, serial measurements of hematocrit (which are helpful if the first
   sample is obtained before administration of large
   volumes of fluid) help to determine the need for
   transfusion.
   a. A low hemoglobin determination (<8 g/dL) imme-
      diately after injury is a strong indicator of ongoing
      blood loss and poor prognosis.
   b. During fluid infusion, a reasonable transfusion
      threshold is a hematocrit below 25 mL/dL for
      young, healthy patients and below 30 mL/dL for
      older patients and those with coronary or cere-
      brovascular disease.

MANAGEMENT

TABLE 36-5

ADVANCED TRAUMA LIFE SUPPORT CLASSIFICATION OF
HEMORRHAGIC SHOCK

	Class I	Class II	Class III	Class IV
Blood loss (mL)	≤750	750–1500	1500–2000	>2000
Blood loss (% of blood volume)	≤15	15–30	20–40	>40
Heart rate (bpm)	<100	>100	>120	>140
Systemic blood pressure	Normal	Normal	Decreased	Decreased
Pulse pressure	Normal or increased	Decreased	Decreased	Decreased
Capillary refill test	Normal	Positive	Positive	Positive
Respiratory rate (breaths/min)	14–20	20–30	30–40	<35
Urine output (mL/hr)	>30	20–30	5–15	Negligible
Mental status	Slightly anxious	Mildly anxious	Anxious and confused	Confused and lethargic
Fluid replacement	Crystalloid	Crystalloid and blood	Crystalloid and blood	Crystalloid (3:1 rule)

TABLE 36-6

ASSESSMENT OF THE DEGREE OF HYPOVOLEMIA IN
HYPOTENSIVE AND TACHYCARDIC PATIENTS

Decrease in Circulating Blood Volume Equivalent to 10%–20%
Administration of lactated Ringer's solution (2000 mL over 15 minutes
in adults or 20 mL/kg in children) should normalize blood pressure.

Decrease in Circulating Blood Volume Equivalent to 20%–40%
Administration of lactated Ringer's solution produces a transient
increase in blood pressure.
More crystalloids with or without blood transfusions are needed.

Decrease in Circulating Blood Volume Exceeds 40%
Administration of lactated Ringer's solution does not improve
blood pressure.
Rapid infusion of crystalloids, colloids, and blood is needed.
Blood typing and cross-matching requires 45 minutes versus type
specific, which can be available in about 15 minutes, versus
immediate transfusion with type O blood (Rh-negative blood
is preferred for women of child-bearing age).

    c. The control of active bleeding has a higher priority than restoration of blood volume or placement of invasive monitors in the initial resuscitation.

  6. Rapid establishment of venous access with large-bore cannulas placed in peripheral veins that drain both above and below the diaphragm is essential for adequate fluid resuscitation in severely injured patients.

II. EARLY MANAGEMENT OF SPECIFIC INJURIES

A. **Head Injury.** Approximately 40% of deaths from trauma are caused by head injury. Prevention of progression of brain injury beyond the initial area is the primary objective of early management of patients with brain trauma. Of all the possible insults to the injured brain, hypotension has the greatest detrimental impact, followed by hypoxia.

  1. **Diagnosis.** A baseline neurologic examination should be performed before any sedative or muscle relaxant drugs are administered or the trachea is intubated, and the examination should be repeated at frequent intervals because the patient's condition may change rapidly (Table 36-7).

    a. **Computed tomography scanning** is used for the diagnosis (midline shift, distortion of the ventricles, presence of a hematoma, depressed skull fractures) of most head injuries. (MRI has the advantage of being able to demonstrate ischemia but is rarely

---

TABLE 36-7

BASELINE NEUROLOGIC EXAMINATION OF TRAUMA PATIENT

Level 1—AVPU System	
A	Alert
V	Responds to verbal stimuli
P	Responds to painful stimuli (motor activity of extremities)
U	Unresponsive

Level 2—Glasgow Coma Scale	
Score 8	Deep coma, severe head injury, poor outcome
Score 9–12	Conscious patient with moderate injury
Score 13–15	Mild injury

MANAGEMENT

TABLE 36-8

UNIVERSALLY ACCEPTED ASPECTS OF TREATMENT FOR
HEAD-INJURED PATIENTS

Normalization of systemic blood pressure (mean cerebral
  perfusion pressure >60 mm Hg)
Normalization of arterial oxygenation ($SaO_2 > 95\%$)
Sedation and skeletal muscle paralysis as necessary
Mannitol and possibly a loop diuretic to shrink the brain and
  decrease ICP
Drainage of CSF
Mechanical hyperventilation of the lungs if ICP remains increased
  (otherwise, normocapnia should be maintained)
High-dose barbiturates used only for refractory intracranial
  hypertension
Immediate surgical decompression if indicated (epidural
  hematoma)

CSF = cerebrospinal fluid; ICP = intracranial pressure.

used because of its cost and impracticality in
injured patients.)

  b. Patients in a coma (Glasgow coma score <8) have
     a 40% likelihood of having an intracranial
     hematoma.
  2. **Management** includes therapeutic maneuvers intended
     to maintain cerebral perfusion pressure and oxygen
     delivery (Table 36-8).
     a. It is not known whether active normalization of
        hyperglycemia (which is common in head-injured
        patients) has any salutary effect.
     b. Measurement of jugular bulb oxygen saturation
        (<50% is considered critical desaturation) is a use-
        ful guide for treatment of head-injured patients
        (reflects demand of the brain for oxygen and its
        supply; $[AvDO_2] > 6$ is a sign of insufficient blood
        flow).
     c. Hyperventilation may enhance increased cerebral
        vascular resistance, which is responsible for the ini-
        tial cerebral hypoperfusion likely to occur during
        the first 6 hours after head trauma. Use of hyper-
        ventilation is ideally guided by monitoring ICP and
        $AvDO_2$.
     d. Mannitol (0.25–0.5 g/kg IV) produces an osmotic
        diuretic effect to decrease ICP and may improve

cerebral blood flow by decreasing blood viscosity. There is a risk of hypovolemia and hypotension when therapeutic doses of mannitol are used. Hyponatremia reflects intravascular volume expansion.

    e. Because of a synergistic action between mannitol and loop diuretics, adding furosemide may be preferred to increasing doses of mannitol when intracranial hypertension persists.

    f. Steroids are no longer viewed as a necessary part of treatment of patients with severe head injuries.

    g. Maintenance of normovolemia rather than fluid restriction is desirable.

  3. Anesthetic considerations include the likely occurrence of hypotension and the risk of administering succinylcholine to patients with spine injury.

B. Spine and Spinal Cord Injury

  1. Initial Evaluation. The objective of the evaluation is to diagnose the instability of the spine and the extent of neurologic involvement. Often the urgency of the associated injuries precludes a definitive assessment, necessitating spine protection until a satisfactory diagnosis is established.

    a. In a comatose patient, flaccid areflexia, loss of rectal sphincter tone, diaphragmatic breathing, and bradycardia suggest the diagnosis of spinal cord injury.

    b. In cervical spine trauma, an ability to flex but not to extend the elbow and response to painful stimuli above but not below the clavicle suggest neurologic injury.

    c. Neurogenic shock describes the hypotension and bradycardia caused by the loss of vasomotor tone and sympathetic innervation of the heart as a result of functional depression of the descending sympathetic pathways of the spinal cord (usually present after high thoracic and cervical spine injuries and improves within 3–5 days).

  2. Initial Management

    a. Immobilization and Intubation. If a cervical spine fracture is suspected, immobilization or manual in-line stabilization of the neck is of paramount importance.

    b. Steroids. Treatment with methylprednisolone for 24 to 48 hours is an option.

3. **Respiratory complications** are common in all phases of the care of patients with spinal cord-injuries. Accessory respiratory muscle paresis may cause a significant loss of expiratory reserve, and pulmonary edema may occur after a catecholamine surge associated with spinal cord injury. Aspiration may also occur.
   a. Paradoxical respiration in patients with quadriplegia is aggravated when the patient is placed in the upright position.
   b. Unopposed vagal activity during tracheal intubation may result in severe bradycardia and cardiac dysrhythmias (instrumentation should be preceded by oxygen and 0.4–0.6 mg IV of atropine).
4. **Hemodynamic management** may include assessment with a pulmonary artery catheter. Left ventricular dysfunction may contribute to hypotension in quadriplegic patients.
C. **Neck Injury.** Penetrating and blunt trauma may injure major structures in the neck (vessels, respiratory, digestive, nervous system).
D. **Chest Injury**
   1. **Chest wall injury** (ribs, sternum, scapula) can predict the likelihood and severity of internal injuries to a certain extent. (Patients with three or more fractured ribs have a greater likelihood of hepatic and splenic injury.)
   2. **Pleural injury** manifesting as a closed pneumothorax most commonly develops as a result of lung puncture by a displaced rib fracture. (This is diagnosed with an upright [this position may be contraindicated in hypovolemic patients or those with suspected spine or head injury] or supine chest film that is obtained routinely in evaluation of all trauma victims.) CT is more reliable for detecting a small pneumothorax and should be performed in patients who require general anesthesia or mechanical ventilation of the lungs after thoracoabdominal trauma.
      a. Subcutaneous emphysema is suggestive of a coexisting pneumothorax.
      b. After it has been diagnosed, a traumatic pneumothorax, no matter how small, should be treated with thoracostomy drainage.
      c. Bleeding intercostal vessels are responsible for most hemothoraces. Initial drainage of more than

1000 mL of blood or collection of more than 200 mL/hr is an indication for thoracotomy.

3. **Penetrating cardiac injury** may result in **pericardial tamponade,** which is diagnosed with transesophageal echocardiography (TEE).

4. **Blunt Cardiac Injury.** Diagnosis (myocardial contusion) is based on clinical history (blunt chest trauma, angina, cardiac dysrhythmias) and results of TEE (segmental wall motion abnormalities), creatine phosphokinase-MB isoenzymes, and electrocardiography.

5. **Thoracic aortic injury** is suspected in patients with a history of high-impact trauma with deceleration, especially to the chest (a widened mediastinum should prompt search for this injury). TEE, contrast-enhanced CT, and ultrasound techniques are important tools for evaluating aortic trauma.

6. **Diaphragmatic injury** is suggested on the chest radiograph when the nasogastric tube is above the diaphragm.

E. **Abdominal and Pelvic Injuries**

1. Liver and spleen lacerations are the most common abdominal injuries after both blunt and penetrating abdominal trauma, presenting most often with signs of hemorrhage.

   a. Because of the unpredictable course of bullets in the body, exploratory laparotomy or laparoscopy (in selected cases) is required after all gunshot wounds to the abdomen.

   b. Abdominal ultrasonography and CT are useful for the evaluation of abdominal and pelvic injuries.

2. **Fractures of the pelvis** may result in major hemorrhage, especially if there is disruption of the pubic symphysis.

F. **Extremity Injuries**

1. Surgical repair of extremity fractures (open or closed) should be performed as soon as possible to decrease the risk of deep vein thrombosis, fat embolism syndrome, pulmonary complications, and sepsis (likely when repair is delayed longer than 6 hours).

2. **Compartment syndrome** is suggested by severe pain in the affected extremity, swelling, and tenseness. Profound analgesia in the presence of an extremity fracture may delay the diagnosis of this syndrome.

MANAGEMENT

III. BURNS

Determination of the size of the burned area (rule of nines) and depth of the burn set the guidelines for resuscitation as well as the timing of surgical intervention. (A partial-thickness burn is red, blanches to the touch, and is painful, but a full-thickness burn does not blanche and is insensate.) Information about the mechanism of the injury (closed space is associated with airway damage; electrocution shows little external injury despite internal injury) facilitates the diagnosis of associated clinical abnormalities.

A. **Airway Complications**
   1. Singed eyebrows or eyelashes and black soot in and around the nose or mouth should increase the suspicion of airway injury.
   2. The initial chest radiography, ABG analyses, and pulmonary function test results are usually normal in the immediate post-burn period, followed by the appearance of clinical symptoms reflecting pulmonary edema.
   3. Fiberoptic bronchoscopy is the best way to evaluate large airways.
B. **Ventilation and Intensive Care.** Hypoxemia may persist despite tracheal intubation and ventilation. In the first 36 hours, hypoxemia reflects pulmonary edema; after 2 to 5 days, it reflects atelectasis and bronchial pneumonia.
C. **Carbon Monoxide Toxicity**
   1. An increased inhaled oxygen concentration promotes elimination of carbon monoxide (100% oxygen decreases the blood half-time of carboxyhemoglobin from 4 hours to <1 hour) (Table 36-9).
   2. A normal oxygen saturation from a pulse oximeter does not exclude the possibility of carbon monoxide toxicity.
   3. Increased carboxyhemoglobin levels do not cause tachypnea because the carotid bodies are sensitive to arterial PaO_2 and not arterial oxygen content.
D. **Cyanide toxicity** (which manifests as metabolic acidosis) is a possibility when cyanide or hydrocyanic acid is produced by incomplete combustion of synthetic materials. Pulse oximetry readings are accurate in the absence of carbon monoxide toxicity and nitrate therapy–induced methemoglobinemia.

TABLE 36-9

SYMPTOMS OF CARBON MONOXIDE TOXICITY

Blood Carboxyhemoglobin Level (%)	Symptoms
<15–20	Headache
	Dizziness
	Occasional confusion
20–40	Disorientation
	Visual impairment
40–60	Agitation
	Combativeness
	Hallucinations
	Coma and shock
>60	Death

E. **Fluid Replacement**
 1. Fluid resuscitation is essential in the early care of burn patients, although overaggressive resuscitation may be deleterious (causing airway edema, pulmonary edema, or abdominal edema).
 2. If fluid resuscitation is successful, edema formation stops within 18 to 24 hours.
 3. Administration of fluids during the initial phase should be titrated to specific goals such as urine output of about 0.5 mL/kg/hr, heart rate of 110 to 120 beats/min, normal blood lactate level, and mixed venous oxygen partial pressure of above 35 mm Hg. An increase in the hematocrit during the first day of the burn injury suggests inadequate fluid resuscitation.

IV. **OPERATIVE MANAGEMENT** (Tables 36-10 and 36-11)

A. **Monitoring** (Table 36-12)
 1. **Hemodynamic Monitoring**
   a. There is no effective substitute for direct intra–arterial monitoring, which permits beat-to-beat assessment of blood pressure (a hemodynamically stable patient may suddenly become hypotensive when the chest or abdomen is opened) and facilitates sampling for measurement of blood gases. During mechanical ventilation of the patient's lungs, the extent of systolic blood pressure variation can provide reliable information about the status of the intravascular fluid volume (Fig. 36-2).

TABLE 36-10

IMPLICATIONS OF PRE-EXISTING DISEASES FOR INTRAOPERATIVE
MANAGEMENT OF TRAUMA PATIENTS

Substance Abuse
Alcohol
Delayed gastric emptying
Vasodilation and myocardial depression
Potentiation of trauma-induced hypothermia
Hemostatic defect
Postoperative alcohol withdrawal
Cocaine use
Unpredictable hemodynamic response to hemorrhage
Cardiac dysrhythmias
Opioid use
Delayed gastric emptying
Vasodilation
Postoperative opioid withdrawal

Hypertension
Decreased tolerance to hypovolemia
Exaggerated hypertensive response to pain
Increased likelihood of myocardial ischemia and cardiac
   dysrhythmias

Ischemic Heart Disease
Increased likelihood of myocardial ischemia caused by trauma-
   induced changes

Anemia

Sickle Cell Disease

Coagulation Disorders

Diabetes Mellitus
Delayed gastric emptying
Decreased response to resuscitative measures in patients with
   autonomic neuropathy
Increased likelihood of ischemic heart disease
Electrolyte abnormalities

Asthma

   b. Placement of a central venous pressure or
      pulmonary artery catheter is not necessary in young
      patients in the absence of heart disease. (A reason-
      able assessment of the patient's blood volume can
      be made by repeated observation of systemic blood
      pressure, hematocrit, ABG analyses, and urine
      output.)

TABLE 36-11

SPECIALIZED EQUIPMENT, SUPPLIES, AND DRUGS THAT MAY BE
NEEDED FOR MANAGEMENT OF TRAUMA PATIENTS

Equipment
Fiberoptic bronchoscope with a light source
Mechanical ventilator that is effective in patients with decreased
  pulmonary compliance (lung contusion, aspiration)
Jet ventilator system
Positive end-expiratory pressure valves
Blood and fluid bag pressurizing systems
Fluid warming system
Rapid infusion system
Forced air warming device and heated humidifier for inspired
  gases
Calibrated infusion pumps
Transesophageal echocardiography
Pneumatic tourniquet
Cardiopulmonary bypass

Supplies
Material for special airway management
Material for arterial and pulmonary artery catheter placement

Drugs
Vasopressors
Inotropes
Calcium chloride
THAM
Sodium bicarbonate
Topical anesthetics

THAM = tris-hydroxymethyl-aminomethane.

    c. **Transesophageal echocardiography** provides valu-
    able diagnostic information in myocardial contu-
    sion, cardiac valvular dysfunction, pericardial fluid
    accumulation, intravascular fluid volume, cardiac
    output, myocardial contractility, and large vessel
    injury. (A probe should not be placed if there is a
    possibility of esophageal injury.)
2. **Urine Output**
    a. As a rough guideline, urine output should be main-
    tained at above 0.5 mL/kg/hr. (After prolonged
    shock, renal failure may already be present on the
    patient's arrival in the operating room.)
    b. Osmotic diuresis produced by preoperative
    radiopaque dye or mannitol decreases the value of
    urine output as a monitor of organ perfusion.

MANAGEMENT

TABLE 36-12

MONITORING OF TRAUMA PATIENTS

Physiologic Parameter	Degree of Importance	Monitoring Equipment	Specific Intraoperative Uses
Cardiac rate, rhythm, and ischemia	Essential	Electrocardiogram	Routine
Arterial blood pressure	Essential	Indirect (cuff, Doppler, oscillometric system)	Routine
Central venous pressure	Useful	Direct (intra-arterial catheter)	Hypovolemia Pericardial tamponade Myocardial contusion Air embolism
Pulmonary artery and capillary wedge pressure	Selected	Pulmonary artery catheter	Blunt chest injury (contusion) Blunt cardiac injury (contusion) ARDS Pulmonary edema
Cardiac output	Useful	Computer	Same as pulmonary artery catheter
Cardiac wall motion abnormalities, myocardial ischemia	Useful	TEE	Blunt cardiac injury (contusion) Major vessel injuries
Ventilation	Essential	End-tidal carbon dioxide monitor	Routine Head injury Air embolism

Arterial oxygenation	Essential	Pulse oximetry ABG analyses	Routine
Tissue oxygenation	Useful	Oximeter pulmonary artery catheter	Low perfusion states
Renal function	Essential	Foley catheter and graduated container	All major trauma patients
Temperature	Essential	Esophageal or rectal probe	Routine
Neuromuscular function	Essential	Peripheral nerve stimulator	Routine
Neurologic function	Useful	Bolt, catheter, or fiberoptic sensor	Head injury
Coagulation	Useful	Prothrombin time, partial thromboplastin time, platelets, fibrinogen Tube test Thromboelastography	Shock Massive transfusions

ABG = arterial blood gas; ARDS = acute respiratory distress syndrome; TEE = transesophageal echocardiography.

MANAGEMENT

555

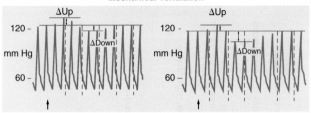

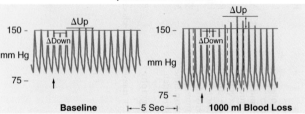

FIGURE 36-2.   The magnitude of systolic blood pressure variation may provide valuable information about the status of the intravascular fluid volume.

     c. Cola-colored urine suggests hemoglobinuria from an incompatible blood transfusion (associated with pink-stained plasma) or myoglobinuria caused by skeletal muscle destruction, as after blunt or electrical trauma. Both of these conditions may result in acute renal failure (which can be prevented with mannitol diuresis). Red-colored urine usually indicates urinary tract injury in trauma patients.

3. **Oxygenation.** Older generation pulse oximeters fail to provide accurate measurements in patients with oxygen saturations of 90% or below, hypothermia, hypotension, and decreased peripheral perfusion. Multi-wave length pulse oximeters can measure carboxyhemoglobin (acute burn injury management).

4. **Organ Perfusion and Oxygen Utilization**

     a. Occult hypoperfusion may not be detected by traditional hemodynamic monitoring such as systemic blood pressure, heart rate, and urine output.

     b. Intestinal mucosa is particularly vulnerable to occult hypoperfusion (passage of luminal microorganisms

TABLE 36-13

INFORMATION OBTAINED FROM THE "TUBE TEST"

Coagulation: Clotting factor deficiency is likely if a clot does not form or does so only after 10 to 20 minutes.

Clot Retraction: Platelet depletion or dysfunction is likely if a clot fails to contract within 1 hour.

Clot Lysis: Fibrinolysis is likely if clot lysis occurs earlier than 6 hours.

into the circulation and release of inflammatory mediators causing sepsis and multiorgan failure).
   c. Markers of organ perfusion and oxygen utilization include oxygen transport variables (oxygen delivery, oxygen consumption, oxygen extraction ratio), base deficit, and blood lactate.
5. **Coagulation**
   a. Conventional blood coagulation monitoring involves determination of prothrombin time, activated plasma thromboplastin time, platelet count, blood fibrinogen level, and fibrin degradation products.
   b. The "tube test," which involves obtaining a plain tube of blood with no anticoagulant, is a practical intraoperative method of coagulation monitoring (Table 36-13).
   c. The results of coagulation tests have little primary impact on treatment. (Platelet and factor replacement are likely to be necessary when more than one blood volume is replaced.)
B. **Anesthetic and Adjunct Drugs.** From the standpoint of anesthetic management, injuries may be placed in one of five categories.
   1. **Airway Compromise.** The primary issue is whether to manage the airway with or without the use of anesthetic drugs and muscle relaxants. As a general precaution, these drugs may be avoided if there is significant airway obstruction or if there is doubt as to whether the patient's trachea can be intubated because of anatomic limitations.
   2. **Hypovolemia.** Inhaled and IV anesthetics predictably further decrease blood pressure in the presence of hypovolemia. Two important principles in the use of anesthetic drugs are accurate estimation of the extent of

MANAGEMENT

hypovolemia and decrease of the anesthetic dose accordingly. Intraoperative use of bispectral index monitor and titrating anesthetics to levels below 60 whenever possible may prevent recall in trauma patients.

3. **Head and Open-Eye Injuries**
   a. Deep anesthesia and adequate skeletal muscle relaxation for tracheal intubation are important principles.
   b. Drugs selected for management of patients with head injury should produce the least increase in ICP, the least decrease in mean arterial pressure, and the greatest decrease in cerebral metabolic requirements for oxygen. With the exception of ketamine, all IV drugs produce similar degrees of cerebral vasoconstriction and suppression of cerebral metabolism. The disadvantage of these drugs is depression of cerebral perfusion pressure.
   c. All inhaled anesthetics have the potential to increase cerebral blood flow, cerebral blood volume, and ICP while decreasing cerebral metabolic requirements for oxygen. (The uncoupling between blood flow and metabolism is greatest for halothane and least for isoflurane.) Desflurane and sevoflurane have effects similar to those of isoflurane on cerebral hemodynamics.
   d. In patients with severe head injury with associated loss of cerebral autoregulation and responsiveness to carbon dioxide, even isoflurane may increase cerebral blood flow and ICP. In these patients, anesthesia can be maintained until the skull is open with opioids plus thiopental, propofol, midazolam, or etomidate.

4. **Cardiac Injury**
   a. **Pericardial Tamponade.** Preload, myocardial contractility, and heart rate should be maintained. If possible, the evacuation of the pericardial blood should be accomplished under local anesthesia. (All anesthetics decrease myocardial contractility and may cause peripheral vasodilation.) Ketamine is often recommended if anesthesia must be induced before evacuation of the tamponade.
   b. Blunt myocardial injury may put patients at risk for drug-induced decreases in myocardial contractility. (Use of inotropes may be necessary.)

5. **Burns**
   a. Extensive escharotomies may necessitate massive transfusions; temperature control; and management of fluid, electrolyte, and coagulation abnormalities.
   b. A hypermetabolic state necessitates increased oxygen, ventilation, and nutrition.
   c. Hypothermia is a risk in the operating room. (Room temperature should be maintained at 28°C to 32°C, fluid and blood-warming devices should be used, and inspired gases should be humidified.)
   d. After the first 24 hours, succinylcholine must be avoided for as long as 1 year because hyperkalemia may occur after its administration. (Large increases in serum potassium levels occur when the burn size exceeds 10% of the body surface area.)
   e. Resistance to nondepolarizing muscle relaxants develops in patients with more than 30% burns starting about 1 week after the burn injury and peaking in 5 to 6 weeks.
   f. For serial wound debridement, ketamine in intermittent doses, neuraxial or peripheral nerve blocks via an indwelling catheter, or sedation with opioids and IV agents may be used.

V. MANAGMENT OF INTRAOPERATIVE COMPLICATIONS

A. **Persistent hypotension** is suggestive of bleeding, tension pneumothorax, neurogenic shock, or cardiac injury.
B. **Hypothermia** that accompanies trauma is associated with increased mortality.
   1. Convective warming forced dry air (Bair Hugger) can prevent a temperature decrease in most trauma patients but cannot effectively treat those with severe hypothermia.
   2. Administration of warm IV fluids is the most effective way to prevent and treat hypothermia in trauma patients.
C. **Coagulation abnormalities** may reflect dilutional effects from transfusions, tissue thromboplastin release, and hypothermia-induced platelet dysfunction. Hypothermia may also enhance fibrinolytic activity.
   1. Prompt platelet administration should be considered when abnormal clinical bleeding is noted (assuming surgical bleeding is controlled).

MANAGEMENT

TABLE 36-14

NEEDS AND CONCERNS IN THE EARLY POSTOPERATIVE
PERIOD IN TRAUMA PATIENTS

Sedation and analgesia (improves pulmonary function)
Propofol (1.5–6 mg/kg/hr), midazolam (0.1–0.2 mg/kg/hr), or both
Morphine (0.02–0.04 mg/kg/hr) or fentanyl (1–3 µg/kg/hr)
Acute renal failure (decreased urine output is not a good indicator,
  and BUN does not increase until at least 24 hours postoperatively)
Abdominal compartment syndrome (intra-abdominal
  hypertension from edema of abdominal organs produced by
  inflammatory mediators, fluid resuscitation, or surgical
  manipulation; it should be suspected if the patient has a
  tense abdomen; its presence suggests the need to measure
  intravesical pressure)
Thromboembolism

BUN = blood urea nitrogen.

2. After the replacement with coagulation-deficient fluids
   exceeds one blood volume, clinical coagulopathy is
   likely, even in the absence of shock, hypothermia, or
   other aggravating factors.
   D. **Electrolyte and Acid–Base Disturbances**
   1. Hyperkalemia may develop as a result of shock-
      induced alteration in permeability of cell membranes,
      release from ischemic tissues, or rapid transfusion of
      blood (faster than 1 U every 4 minutes).
   2. Metabolic acidosis is caused by shock in the majority
      of patients after trauma. Treatment of metabolic
      acidosis includes correction of the underlying cause
      (hypoxemia, hypovolemia, decreased cardiac output).
      Symptomatic treatment with sodium bicarbonate has
      several disadvantages, including leftward shift of the
      oxyhemoglobin dissociation curve, hyperosmolar state,
      and alkalosis.
   3. Base deficit parallels the degree of hypovolemia.
   E. **Intraoperative death** is more likely during emergency
      trauma surgery than it is in any other operative procedure.

VI. EARLY POSTOPERATIVE CONSIDERATIONS

Re-evaluation and optimization of the circulation,
oxygenation, temperature, central nervous system function,
coagulation, electrolyte and acid–base status, and renal
function are the hallmarks of postoperative management
(Table 36-14).

CHAPTER 37 ■ EPIDURAL AND SPINAL ANESTHESIA

Spinal anesthesia and epidural anesthesia have been shown to blunt the "stress response" to surgery, decrease intraoperative blood loss, lower the incidence of postoperative thromboembolic events, possibly decrease morbidity in high-risk surgical patients, and serve as a useful method to extend analgesia into the postoperative period (better analgesia than can be achieved with parenteral opioids) (Bernards CM: Epidural and spinal anesthesia. In *Clinical Anesthesia*. Edited by Barash PG, Cullen BF, Stoelting RK, Cahalan MK, Stock MC. Philadelphia: Lippincott Williams & Wilkins, 2009, pp 927–954).

I. ANATOMY

A. Proficiency in spinal and epidural anesthesia requires a thorough understanding of the anatomy of the spine and spinal cord.

B. **Vertebrae**
   1. The spine consists of 33 vertebrae (seven cervical, 12 thoracic, five lumbar, five fused sacral, and four fused coccygeal).
   2. With the exception of C1 (which lacks a body or spinous process), the vertebrae consist of a body anteriorly; two pedicles that project posteriorly from the body; and two lamina that connect the pedicles to form the vertebral canal, which contains the spinal cord, spinal nerves, and epidural space (Fig. 37-1).
   3. The laminae give rise to the transverse processes, which project laterally, and the spinous process, which projects posteriorly (see Fig. 37-1).
   4. The fifth sacral vertebra is not fused posteriorly, giving rise to a variably shaped opening known as the sacral hiatus (opening into the sacral canal, which is the caudal termination of the epidural space). The sacral cornu are bony prominences on either side to the hiatus and aid in identifying it.

561

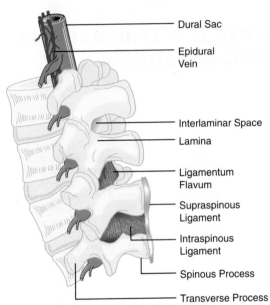

FIGURE 37-1. Anatomy of the vertebral column.

5. Identifying individual vertebrae is important for correctly locating the desired interspace for performance of epidural and spinal anesthesia (Table 37-1).

C. **Ligaments**
1. The vertebral bodies are stabilized by five ligaments that increase in size between the cervical and lumbar vertebrae (see Fig. 37-1).

TABLE 37-1

LANDMARKS FOR VERTEBRAL INTERSPACES

Spinous process of C7	First prominent spinous process in the back of the neck
Spinous process of T1	Most prominent spinous process; immediately follows C7
Spinous process of T12	Palpate the 12th rib and trace back to its attachment of T12
Spinous process of L5	Line drawn between the iliac crests crosses the body of L5 or the L4–L5 interspace

2. The **ligamentum flavum** is thickest in the midline (3–5 mm at L2–L3) and also farthest from the spinal meninges in the midline (4–6 mm at L2–L3). As a result, midline insertion of an epidural needle is least likely to result in accidental meningeal puncture.

D. **Epidural Space**
   1. The epidural space lies between the spinal meninges and the sides of the vertebral canal. It is bounded cranially by the foramen magnum, caudally by the sacrococcygeal ligament (sacral hiatus), and posteriorly by the ligamentum flavum and vertebral pedicles.
   2. The epidural space is not a closed space but communicates with the paravertebral space via the intervertebral foramina.
   3. The epidural space is composed of a series of discontinuous compartments, which become continuous when the potential space separating the compartments is opened up by injection of air or liquid.
   4. The most ubiquitous material in the epidural space is fat.
   5. Veins are present principally in the anterior and lateral portions of the epidural space with few, if any, veins present in the posterior epidural space (see Fig. 37-1). These veins anastomose freely with extradural veins (pelvic veins, azygous system, intracranial veins).

E. **Epidural fat** has important effects on the pharmacology of epidurally and intrathecally administered opioids and local anesthetics.
   1. Lipid solubility results in opioid sequestration in epidural fat with associated decreases in bioavailability.
   2. Transfer of opioids from the epidural space to the intrathecal space is greatest with poorly lipid-soluble morphine and least for the highly lipid-soluble opioids fentanyl and sufentanil.

F. **Meninges**
   1. **Dura mater** is the outermost and thickest meningeal tissue that begins at the foramen magnum (fuses with the periosteum of the skull, forming the cephalad border of the epidural space) and ends at approximately S2, where it fuses with the filum terminale. The dura mater extends laterally along the spinal nerve roots and becomes continuous with the connective tissue of

the epineurium at approximately the level of the intervertebral foramina.

a. The inner edge of the dura mater is highly vascular, which likely results in the dura mater being an
important route of drug clearance from both the
epidural and subarachnoid space.

b. The presence of a midline connective tissue band
(plica medianis dorsalis) running from the dura
mater to the ligamentum flavum is controversial
but may be invoked as an explanation for
unilateral epidural block.

c. The subdural space is a potential space between
the dura mater and arachnoid mater. Drug intended for either the epidural space or the subarachnoid space may be accidentally injected into this
space.

2. **Arachnoid Mater**

a. The arachnoid mater is an avascular membrane
that serves as the principal physiologic barrier for
drugs moving between the epidural space and the
subarachnoid space.

b. The **subarachnoid space** lies between the arachnoid
mater and pia mater and contains cerebrospinal
fluid (CSF). The spinal CSF is in continuity with
the cranial CSF and provides an avenue for drugs
in the spinal CSF to reach the brain. Spinal nerve
roots and rootlets run in the subarachnoid space.

3. **Pia mater** is adherent to the spinal cord.

4. **CSF** (100 to 160 mL in adults, produced at a rate of
20 to 25 mL/hr) is replaced roughly every 6 hours
(removed by arachnoid villi).

a. Contrary to a widely held view, CSF does not circulate through the subarachnoid space but rather
oscillates in parallel with cerebral expansion and
contraction during the cardiac cycle. (Net CSF
movement is estimated to be 0.04% per oscillation.)

b. CSF cannot be relied upon to distribute drugs in
the subarachnoid space.

c. The kinetic energy of the injection and baricity
of the solution serve to distribute drug during a
single-shot spinal.

d. The lack of significant net CSF motion explains
why drug distribution during slow infusions used
for chronic intrathecal analgesia results in limited
drug distribution.

G. Spinal Cord

1. In adults, the caudad tip of the spinal cord typically ends at the level of L1 (extends to L3 in 10% of adults).
2. The spinal cord gives rise to 31 pairs of spinal nerves, each composed of an anterior motor root and a posterior sensory root.
   a. **Dermatome** is the skin area innervated by a given spinal nerve (Fig. 37-2).
   b. The intermediolateral gray matter of T1–L12 contains the cell bodies of the preganglionic sympathetic neurons. These sympathetic neurons travel with the corresponding spinal nerve to a point just beyond the intervertebral foramen, where they exit to join the sympathetic chain ganglia.

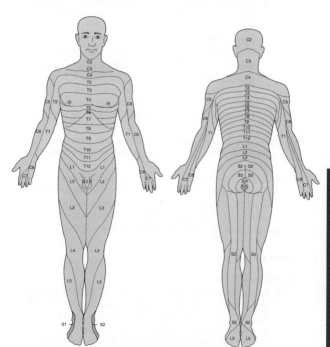

FIGURE 37-2. Human sensory dermatomes.

MANAGEMENT

    c. Because the spinal cord ends between L1 and L2, the thoracic, lumbar, and sacral nerve roots travel increasingly longer distances in the subarachnoid space (cauda equina) to reach the intervertebral foramen through which they exit.

II. TECHNIQUE

A. Spinal and epidural anesthesia should be performed only after appropriate monitors are applied in a setting where equipment for airway management and resuscitation is immediately available.

B. **Needles**
1. Spinal and epidural needles are named for the design of their tips ("pencil point," beveled tip with cutting edge) (Fig. 37-3).
    a. Epidural needles have a larger diameter than spinal needles, facilitating injection of air or fluid for the "loss of resistance" technique and passage of catheters.
    b. The outside diameters of spinal and epidural needles are used to determine their gauges. Large-gauge spinal needles (22–29 gauge) are often easier to insert if an introducer (inserted into the interspinous ligament) is used. Postdural puncture headache is less likely when small-gauge spinal needles are used.
2. All spinal and epidural needles come with a tight-fitting stylet to prevent the needle from becoming plugged with skin or fat.

C. **Sedation** before placement of the block is limited because patient cooperation (positioning, determination of level of sensory anesthesia, occurrence of paresthesias) is important. After the anesthesia is established, the patient may be sedated as deemed appropriate.

III. SPINAL ANESTHESIA

A. **Position** (Table 37-2)
1. In the lateral decubitus position, the patient lies with the operative side down when hyperbaric solutions are being used. The patient's shoulders and hips are positioned perpendicular to the bed (preventing rotation of the spine), the knees are drawn up to the chest, the neck is flexed, and the patient is asked to

Spinal Needles

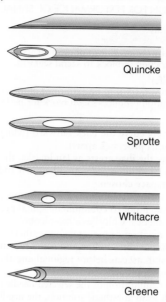

Quincke

Sprotte

Whitacre

Greene

Epidural Needles

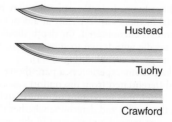

Hustead

Tuohy

Crawford

Combined Spinal/Epidural Needle

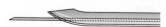

FIGURE 37-3. Examples of commercially available spinal and epidural needles. Needles are distinguished by the design of their tips.

TABLE 37-2

PATIENT POSITION FOR PERFORMANCE OF SPINAL ANESTHESIA

Lateral Decubitus
Sitting
Easier to identify the midline in obese patients
Facilitates restriction of block to sacral segments

Prone (Jackknife)
Consider when surgery is to be performed in this position
Hypobaric solution produces sacral block for perirectal surgery

---

actively curve the back outward (which spreads the spinous processes apart).

2. Using the iliac crests as landmarks, the L2–3, L3–4, and L4–5 interspaces are identified and the desired interspace chosen.

3. All antiseptic solutions are neurotoxic, and care must be taken not to contaminate spinal needles or local anesthetics. Chlorhexidine–alcohol antiseptic prevents colonization of percutaneous catheters better than 10% povidine–iodine and is the recommended prep for skin asepsis before regional anesthesia procedures.

B. **Midline Approach**

1. After infiltration of the selected needle insertion site with local anesthetic solution, the needle is advanced (subcutaneous tissue to supraspinous ligament to interspinous ligament to ligamentum flavum to epidural space to dura mater ["pop"] to arachnoid mater) until CSF is obtained (gentle aspiration may be helpful). The spinal meninges are typically at a depth of 4 to 6 cm.

2. If bone is encountered, the depth should be noted and the needle withdrawn to subcutaneous tissue and redirected more cephalad (Fig. 37-4).

3. If the patient experiences a paresthesia (which should be differentiated from discomfort caused by contacting bone), it is important to immediately stop advancing the needle and determine whether the needle tip has encountered a nerve root in the epidural space or in the subarachnoid space. (The presence of CSF confirms that the needle has encountered a cauda equina nerve root.)

4. After completing the injection of local anesthetic solution, a small volume of CSF is again aspirated to confirm that the needle tip has remained in the subarachnoid space.

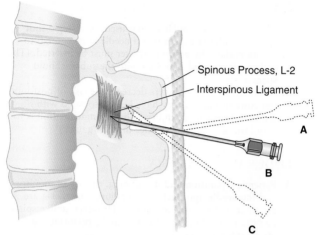

Spinous Process, L-2

Interspinous Ligament

FIGURE 37-4. Midline approach to the subarachnoid space. The spinal needle is inserted with a slight cephalad angulation and advanced in the midline (**B**). If bone is contacted, it may be either the caudad (**A**) or cephalad (**C**) spinous process. The needle should be redirected slightly, and if bone is encountered at a shallower depth, then the needle is likely walking up the cephalad spinous process. If bone is encountered at a deeper depth, then the needle is likely walking down the inferior spinous process. If bone is repeatedly contacted at the same depth, then the needle is likely off the midline and walking along the lamina.

5. After the block has been placed, strict attention must be directed to the patient's hemodynamic status with blood pressure and heart rate supported as necessary.
6. The level of anesthesia should be assessed by pinprick or temperature sensation. If the anesthesia is not rising high enough, the table may be tilted to influence spread of a hyperbaric or hypobaric local anesthetic.

C. The **paramedian approach** is used when the patient cannot flex the spine or heavily calcified interspinous ligaments. The needle is inserted 1 cm lateral to the desired interspace with advancement toward the midline. (The first significant resistance is the ligamentum flavum as the interspinous ligament is bypassed.)

D. The **lumbosacral approach** is a paramedian approach directed at the L5–S1 interspace.

MANAGEMENT

IV. CONTINUOUS SPINAL ANESTHESIA

A. The technique is similar to that used for a single-shot spinal anesthesia except that a needle large enough to accommodate the desired catheter must be inserted. (The catheter is inserted 2 to 3 cm into the subarachnoid space.)

B. Although smaller catheters decrease the risk of postdural puncture headache, they have been associated with reports of neurologic injury. (The recommendation is to avoid using a catheter smaller than 24 gauge.)

V. EPIDURAL ANESTHESIA

A. Patient preparation and positioning, the use of monitors, and the needle approaches for epidural anesthesia are the same as for spinal anesthesia. However, unlike spinal anesthesia, epidural anesthesia may be performed at any intervertebral space.

1. Using the midline approach, the epidural needle is inserted into the interspinous ligament ("gritty" feel) and then advanced slowly until the ligamentum flavum is contacted (increased resistance).

2. The epidural needle must traverse the ligamentum flavum and stop in the epidural space ("loss of resistance") before encountering the spinal meninges.

   a. A glass syringe containing 2 to 3 mL of saline and 0.1 to 0.3 mL of air is attached to the epidural needle, and the plunger is pressed. If the needle is properly placed in the ligamentum flavum, it will be possible to compress the air bubble without injecting the saline. If the air bubble cannot be compressed without injecting fluid, then the needle tip is most likely not in the ligamentum flavum but instead in the interspinous ligament or off midline in the paraspinous muscles.

   b. After the ligamentum flavum is identified, the needle is slowly advanced with the nondominant hand while the dominant hand maintains constant pressure on the syringe plunger (Fig. 37-5).

   c. As the needle enters the epidural space, there will be a sudden and dramatic loss of resistance as the saline is rapidly injected (the patient should be warned of possible pain). If the needle is advancing obliquely through the ligamentum flavum, it is

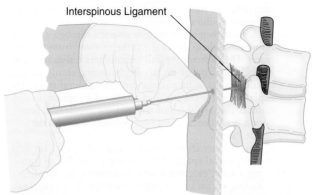

Interspinous Ligament

FIGURE 37-5. Proper hand position when using the loss of resistance technique to locate the epidural space. After placing the tip of the needle in the ligamentum flavum, a syringe containing 2 to 3 mL of saline and an air bubble is attached. The dominant hand maintains constant pressure on the syringe plunger while the nondominant hand rests against the patient's back and is used to slowly advance the needle. If the needle is properly placed in the ligamentum flavum, it will be possible to compress the air bubble without injecting the saline. As the needle tip enters the epidural space, there will be a sudden loss of resistance, and the saline will be easily ejected from the syringe.

              possible to enter into the paraspinous muscles instead of the epidural space (loss of resistance is less dramatic).

    d. When the syringe is disconnected from the needle, it is common to have a small amount of fluid flow from the needle hub (usually saline, which is at room temperature in contrast to CSF).

  3. A test dose of local anesthetic solution is injected to help detect unrecognized intravenous (IV) or subarachnoid placement of the needle. After a negative test dose, the desired volume of local anesthetic solution should be administered in 5-mL increments (this decreases the risk of pain during injection and allows early detection of adverse reactions).

VI. CONTINUOUS EPIDURAL ANESTHESIA

  A. Use of a catheter for epidural anesthesia affords greater flexibility than the single-shot technique but introduces the risk of catheter migration (subarachnoid space,

MANAGEMENT

intervertebral foramen) and increases the likelihood of a unilateral epidural block.

B. Epidural catheters are usually inserted through a curved-tip needle to help direct the catheter away from the dura mater. The catheter typically encounters resistance as it reaches the curve of the needle, but using steady pressure usually results in its passage into the epidural space. One explanation for the inability to thread an epidural catheter is that the tip of the epidural needle was bent during bony contact and now partially occludes the needle lumen.

1. The catheter should be advanced only 3 to 5 cm into the epidural space. (This minimizes the risk of forming a knot, entering a vein, puncturing dura mater, exiting via an intervertebral foramen, and wrapping around a nerve root.)

2. After the catheter is appropriately positioned, the needle is slowly withdrawn with one hand as the catheter is stabilized with the other. The length of the catheter in the epidural space is confirmed because this distance is important when trying to determine if a catheter used in the postoperative period has been dislodged.

3. A test dose of the local anesthetic solution is injected before the initial injection and any subsequent "top-up dose" (typically 50% of the initial dose at an interval equal to two thirds the expected duration of the block).

VII. EPIDURAL TEST DOSE

A. The most common test dose is 3 mL of local anesthetic solution containing 5 μg/mL of epinephrine (1:200,000).

1. This dose is sufficient to produce evidence of spinal anesthesia if accidental subarachnoid injection occurs.

2. IV injection of the epinephrine dose typically increases the heart rate an average of 30 bpm.

a. Reflex bradycardia may occur in patients being treated with α-blockers. (A increase in systolic blood pressure of 20 mm Hg or more may be a more reliable indicator of intravascular injection in these patients.)

b. The sensitivity of epinephrine as a test dose in parturients is questionable because maternal heart rate increases during contractions are often as large as those produced by epinephrine.

B. Aspirating the catheter or needle to check for blood or CSF is helpful if positive, but the incidence of false-negative aspirations is too high to rely on this technique alone.

VIII. COMBINED SPINAL–EPIDURAL ANESTHESIA

A. This technique combines the rapid onset and dense block of spinal anesthesia with the flexibility afforded by an epidural catheter.

B. After the peak spinal block height has been established, the injection of saline or a local anesthetic solution into the epidural space causes the block height to increase, presumably reflecting compression of the spinal meninges forcing CSF cephalad as well as a local anesthetic effect.

C. A potential risk of this technique is that the meningeal hole made by the spinal needle may allow high concentrations of subsequently administered epidural drugs to reach the subarachnoid space.

IX. PHARMACOLOGY

A. Interindividual variability makes it difficult to reliably predict the height and duration of central neuraxial block that will result from a particular local anesthetic dose (Table 37-3).

B. **Spinal Anesthesia**
   1. **Block Height** (Table 37-4)
      a. **Baricity and Patient Position.** Of the factors that exert significant influence on local anesthetic spread, the baricity of the local anesthetic solution relative to patient position is probably the most important.
      b. **Hyperbaric solutions** (more dense than CSF) are typically prepared by mixing the local anesthetic solution with 5% to 8% dextrose. Gravity causes hyperbaric solutions to flow downward in the CSF to the most dependent regions of the spinal column. Spinal anesthesia can be restricted to the sacral and lower lumbar dermatomes ("saddle block") by administering a hyperbaric local anesthetic solution with the patient in the sitting position.
      c. **Hyperbaric solutions** can be used to advantage for unilateral surgical procedures performed in

TABLE 37-3

REPRESENTATIVE SURGICAL PROCEDURES APPROPRIATE FOR
SPINAL ANESTHESIA

Surgical Procedure	Block Height	Suggested Technique	Comments
Perianal	L1–L2	Hyperbaric solution or sitting position	Patients must remain in relative head-up or head-down position when using hypobaric and hyperbaric solutions to maintain restricted spread during the procedure
Perirectal		Hypobaric solution or jackknife position	
		Isobaric solution or horizontal position	
Lower extremity	T10	Isobaric solution	Hypobaric and hyperbaric solutions are also suitable but may produce higher blocks than necessary
Hip			
Transurethral resection of the prostate			
Vaginal or cervical			
Herniorrhaphy	T6–T8	Hyperbaric solution or horizontal position	Isobaric solutions injected at the L2–L3 interspace may also be suitable

(continued)

TABLE 37-3

REPRESENTATIVE SURGICAL PROCEDURES APPROPRIATE FOR SPINAL ANESTHESIA (*Continued*)

Pelvic procedures		
Appendectomy	Hyperbaric solution or horizontal position	Upper abdominal procedures usually require concomitant general anesthesia to prevent vagal reflexes and pain from traction on the diaphragm and esophagus
Abdominal	T4–T6	

the supine position if the operative site is dependent during drug injection and the patient is left in the lateral position for at least 6 minutes.

d. When the patient is turned supine after hyperbaric drug injection in the lateral position, the normal

TABLE 37-4

FACTORS THAT MAY INFLUENCE THE SPREAD OF LOCAL ANESTHETIC SOLUTIONS IN THE SUBARACHNOID SPACE

Characteristics of the Local Anesthetic Solution
Baricity relative to patient position (most important of all factors)
Local anesthetic dose (little effect with isobaric solutions)
Local anesthetic concentration
Volume injected

Patient Characteristics
Age, weight, and height (poor predictors of extent of sensory blockade)
Gender
Pregnancy

Technique
Site of injection
Speed of injection
Barbotage
Direction of needle bevel
Addition of vasoconstrictors

Diffusion

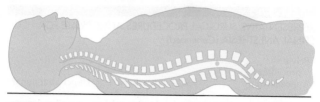

FIGURE 37-6. In the supine position, hyperbaric local anesthetic solutions injected at the height of the lumbar lordosis (*circle*) flow down the lumbar lordosis to pool in the sacrum and in the thoracic kyphosis. Pooling in the thoracic kyphosis is thought to explain the fact that hyperbaric solutions produce blocks with an average sensory level of T4–T6.

    spinal curvature influences subsequent movement of the injected solution. Hyperbaric solutions injected at the height of the lumbar lordosis tend to flow cephalad to pool in the thoracic kyphosis and caudad to pool in the sacrum (Fig. 37-6).

    e. Gravity influences the distribution of hyperbaric and hypobaric solutions only until they are sufficiently diluted in CSF so that they become isobaric (solution no longer moves in response to changes in position).

    f. **Dose, Volume, and Concentration.** Drug dose and volume appear to be relatively unimportant in predicting the spread of hyperbaric local anesthetic solutions injected in the horizontal plane (reflecting the predominate effect of baricity and patient position).

    g. **Injection site** is the same as for drug dose and volume.

    h. **Patient Characteristics.** The most important variable governing block height may be the patient's lumbosacral CSF volume. The patient's age, weight, and height have not been proven to be important predictors of block height.

2. The **onset** of spinal anesthesia is within a few minutes regardless of the drug used, although time to reach peak block is different among drugs (e.g., lidocaine sooner than bupivacaine).

3. The **duration** of spinal anesthesia is characterized by gradual waning of the block beginning with the most cephalad dermatome.

    a. When speaking about duration of block, it is necessary to distinguish between duration at the surgical

TABLE 37-5

DOSE AND DURATION OF LOCAL ANESTHETICS USED FOR SPINAL ANESTHESIA

Drug	Dose (mg)	Two-Dermatome Regression (min)	Complete Resolution (min)	Prolongation by Adrenergic Agonists (%)
Chloro-procaine	30–100	30–50	70–150	Not recommended
Lidocaine	25–100	40–100	140–240	20–50
Bupivacaine	5–20	90–140	240–380	20–50
Tetracaine	5–20	90–140	240–380	50–100

   site and the time required for anesthesia to completely resolve (which influences discharge time) (Table 37-5).
   b. A thorough understanding of the factors that govern the duration of anesthesia is necessary for the anesthesiologist to choose techniques that result in an appropriate duration (Table 37-6). Intrathecal epinephrine decreases blood flow in the dura mater without altering spinal cord blood flow, which is consistent with decreased drug clearance via the dural vasculature.
C. Epidural Anesthesia
   1. Any procedure that can be performed under spinal anesthesia can also be performed under epidural anesthesia and requires the same block height (see Table 37-3). As with spinal anesthesia, there is a great

TABLE 37-6

FACTORS THAT MAY INFLUENCE THE DURATION OF SENSORY BLOCKADE PRODUCED BY SPINAL ANESTHESIA

Local anesthetic drug (principal determinant of duration)
Drug dose
Block height (higher blocks regress faster as cephalad spread results in relatively lower drug concentration in CSF)
Adrenergic agonists (effectiveness depends on local anesthetic with which they are combined; tetracaine > bupivacaine)
   Epinephrine 0.2–0.3 mg
   Phenylephrine 2–5 mg
   Clonidine 75–150 µg

CSF = cerebrospinal fluid.

MANAGEMENT

TABLE 37-7

LOCAL ANESTHETICS USED FOR SURGICAL EPIDURAL ANESTHESIA

Drug	Two-Dermatome Regression (min)	Complete Resolution (min)	Prolongation by Epinephrine (%)
Chloroprocaine 3%	45–60	100–160	40–60
Lidocaine	60–100	160–200	40–80
Mepivacaine 2%	60–100	160–200	40–80
Ropivacaine 0.5%–1%	90–180	240–420	None
Etidocaine 1%–1.5%	120–240	300–460	None
Bupivacaine 0.5%–0.75%	120–240	300–460	None

interindividual variability in the spread and duration of epidural anesthesia (Table 37-7).

2. **Block Spread.** To choose the most appropriate local anesthetic and dose for a particular clinical situation, the anesthesiologist must be familiar with the variables that affect the spread and duration of epidural anesthesia (Table 37-8).

TABLE 37-8

FACTORS THAT MAY INFLUENCE THE SPREAD OF LOCAL ANESTHETIC SOLUTIONS IN THE EPIDURAL SPACE

Injection site (unlike spinal anesthesia, epidural anesthesia produces a segmental block that spreads both caudally and cranially from the site of injection)

Drug volume (increasing the volume results in greater spread and density of block; increases cephalad distribution)

Drug dose (important with volume in determining spread and density of block)

Drug concentration (relatively unimportant in determining block spread)

Position (does not seem to have a clinically important effect on the spread of the block from side to side)

Patient characteristics

    Age (greater spread in elderly perhaps because of less compliant epidural space and decreased likelihood of local anesthetic solution to escape via intervertebral foramina)

    Height and weight (weak correlation except at extremes)

    Pregnancy (conflicting data)

    Atherosclerosis (relationship not confirmed)

3. The **onset** of epidural anesthesia can usually be detected within 5 minutes in the dermatomes immediately surrounding the injection site.
   a. The time to peak effect is 15 to 20 minutes with shorter acting drugs and 20 to 25 minutes with longer acting drugs.
   b. Increasing the dose of local anesthetic speeds the onset of both motor and sensory block.
4. **Duration** (Table 37-9)

X. PHYSIOLOGY

A. Neurophysiology

1. The **site of action** of spinal and epidural anesthesia is not precisely known but can potentially occur at any or all points along the neural pathways extending from the site of drug administration to the interior of the spinal cord.
2. **Differential neural block** refers to the clinically important phenomenon in which nerve fibers subserving different functions display varying sensitivity to local anesthetic blockade.
   a. Sympathetic nervous system nerve fibers appear to be blocked by the lowest concentration of local anesthetic followed in order by fibers responsible for pain, touch, and motor function.
   b. Although the mechanism for differential block in spinal and epidural anesthesia is not known, it is clear that fiber diameter is not the only, nor

TABLE 37-9

FACTORS THAT INFLUENCE THE DURATION OF SENSORY
BLOCKADE PRODUCED BY EPIDURAL ANESTHESIA

Local anesthetic drug (principal determinant of duration)
Dose (increasing dose results in increased duration and density)
Age (conflicting results)
Adrenergic agonists (epinephrine 1:200,000)
  Prolongs duration of lidocaine and mepivacaine > bupivacaine
  and etidocaine
  Mechanism may reflect decreased absorption from epidural
  space or direct inhibitory effect of epinephrine on sensory and
  motor neurons

MANAGEMENT

perhaps even the most important, factor contributing to differential blockade.

c. During spinal and epidural anesthesia, differential block is manifested as a spatial separation in the modalities blocked. (Sympathetic block may extend two to six dermatomes higher than sensory block, which is two to three dermatomes higher than motor block.) This spatial separation is believed to result from a gradual decrease in local anesthetic concentration within the CSF as a function of distance from the site of injection.

d. An occasional patient has intact touch and proprioception at the surgical site despite adequate blockade of pain sensation.

e. Central neuraxial block produces sedation, potentiates the effects of sedative drugs, and markedly decreases the anesthetic requirements.

B. **Cardiovascular Physiology**

1. Understanding the homeostatic mechanisms responsible for control of blood pressure and heart rate is essential for understanding and treating the cardiovascular changes associated with spinal and epidural anesthesia (Fig. 37-7).

2. **Spinal Anesthesia.** Blockade of sympathetic nervous system efferent fibers is the principal mechanism by which spinal anesthesia produces cardiovascular derangements.

a. The incidence of significant hypotension or bradycardia is generally related to the extent of sympathetic nervous system blockade, which in turn parallels block height.

b. Hypotension during spinal anesthesia is the result of arterial (decreased systemic vascular resistance) and venous (decrease preload responsible for decreased cardiac output) dilation. An intact renin–angiotensin system helps to offset the hypotensive effects of sympathetic block. (Caution should be exercised when administering central neuraxial block to patients taking antihypertensives that impair the angiotensin system.)

c. Heart rate slows significantly in 10% to 15% of patients (because of blockade of sympathetic cardioaccelerator fibers or diminished venous return and the associated decreased stretch of intracardiac stretch receptors). Patients with unexplained severe

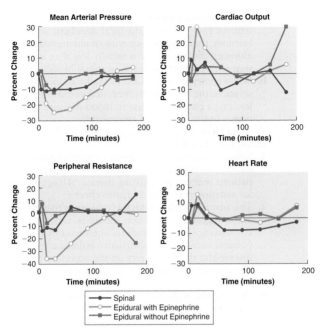

FIGURE 37-7. The cardiovascular effects of spinal and epidural anesthesia in volunteers with T5 sensory blocks. The effects of spinal anesthesia and epidural anesthesia without epinephrine were generally comparable and are both qualitatively and quantitatively different from the effects of epidural anesthesia with epinephrine added to the local anesthetic solution.

        bradycardia and asystole during spinal and epidural anesthesia may require aggressive intervention with epinephrine.

    d. Spinal anesthesia can also produce second- and third-degree heart block. Pre-existing first-degree heart block may be a risk factor for progression to higher grade heart block during spinal anesthesia.

  3. Epidural Anesthesia. The hemodynamic changes produced by epidural anesthesia are largely dependent on whether or not epinephrine is added to the local anesthetic solution (see Fig. 37-7).

    a. Hemodynamic changes of high epidural anesthesia without epinephrine in the local anesthetic solution resemble the changes seen with spinal anesthesia, although the magnitude is usually less than that seen with comparable levels of spinal block.

    b. When epinephrine is added to the local anesthetic solution, the resulting β_2-mediated vasodilation leads to a greater decrease in blood pressure than occurs in the absence of epinephrine.

  4. Treating Hemodynamic Changes (Table 37-10)

C. Respiratory Physiology

  1. Spinal and epidural anesthesia to midthoracic levels have little effect on pulmonary function in patients without pre-existing disease. (Drugs used for sedation may have a greater effect.)

  2. The adverse impact of high blocks on active exhalation suggests that caution should be exercised when using spinal or epidural anesthesia in patients with chronic obstructive pulmonary disease and those who rely on the accessory muscles of respiration to maintain adequate ventilation.

  3. Patients with high spinal or epidural anesthesia may complain of dyspnea (loss of ability to feel the chest

---

TABLE 37-10

TREATING HEMODYNAMIC CHANGES SECONDARY TO SPINAL AND EPIDURAL ANESTHESIA

Vasopressors

Ephedrine (5–10 mg IV treats causes of hypotension by increasing cardiac output [venous return] and systemic vascular resistance)

Dopamine (long-term infusion because tachyphylaxis can develop to repeated doses of ephedrine)

Phenylephrine (increase blood pressure by increasing systemic vascular resistance, which may decrease cardiac output; this may be specific treatment for hypotension during epidural anesthesia provided by epinephrine-containing local anesthetic solutions)

Fluid Administration

Prehydration with 500–1500 mL of crystalloid solution (cannot be relied on to prevent hypotension); 6% hetastarch (500 mL) may be an alternative to crystalloids move while breathing, which is usually adequately treated by reassurance). A normal speaking voice suggests that ventilation is normal (with an excessively high block, the patient will have a faint, gasping whisper).

D. **Gastrointestinal Physiology**
   1. Unopposed parasympathetic nervous system activity results in increased secretions, relaxation of sphincters, and constriction of the bowel.
   2. Nausea is a common complication of spinal and epidural anesthesia. (The cause unknown but is often associated with blocks higher than T5, hypotension, and opioid administration).
E. **Endocrine–Metabolic Physiology.** Spinal anesthesia and epidural anesthesia inhibit many of the changes associated with the stress response to surgery (presumed to reflect blockade of afferent sensory information).

XI. COMPLICATIONS

A. **Backache**
   1. Postoperative backache occurs after general anesthesia but is more common after spinal (11%) or epidural anesthesia (30%).
   2. Possible explanations for backache include needle trauma, local anesthetic irritation, and ligamentous strain secondary to muscle relaxation.
B. **Postdural Puncture Headache**
   1. Headache is characteristically mild or absent when the patient is in the supine position, but head elevation results in fronto-occipital headache. Occasionally, cranial nerve symptoms (diplopia, tinnitus) and nausea and vomiting are present.
      a. Headache is believed to result from the loss of CSF through the meningeal needle hole, resulting in decreased buoyant support for the brain.
      b. In the upright position, the brain sags in the cranial vault, putting traction on pain-sensitive structures and possibly cranial nerves.
   2. The incidence of postdural puncture headache decreases with increasing age and with the use of small-diameter spinal needles with noncutting tips.
      a. Inserting cutting needles with the bevel aligned parallel to the long axis of the meninges results in

MANAGEMENT

a meningeal opening that is likely to be pulled closed by the longitudinal tension present on the dura mater.

b. Up to 50% of young patients develop postdural puncture headache after accidental meningeal puncture with a large epidural needle.

c. If age is considered, there does not seem to be a gender difference in the incidence of postdural puncture headache.

d. Remaining supine does not decrease the incidence of postdural puncture headache.

e. Use of fluid rather than air for determining loss of resistance during attempted location of the epidural space decreases the risk of developing postdural puncture headache in the event of an accidental meningeal puncture.

3. Postdural puncture headache usually resolves spontaneously in a few days with conservative therapy (bed rest, analgesics, and caffeine).

4. **Epidural blood patch** (10–20 mL of autologous blood is aseptically injected into the epidural space near the interspace where the meningeal puncture occurred) produces relief in 85% to 95% of patients within 1 to 24 hours. (It is presumed to form a clot over the meningeal hole.)

   a. The most common side effects of blood patch are backache and radicular pain.

   b. Use of a prophylactic blood patch is effective in preventing postdural puncture headache in patients in whom the meninges are accidentally punctured during attempted epidural anesthesia.

   c. Epidural administered fibrin glue (meningeal patch) is an effective alternative to a blood patch for treatment of postdural puncture headache.

C. **Transient hearing loss** (lasting 1–3 days) is common after spinal anesthesia, especially in female patients.

D. **Systemic toxicity** manifests as central nervous system (CNS) and cardiovascular toxicity during epidural anesthesia (drug doses are too low during spinal anesthesia).

   1. CNS toxicity may result from intravascular absorption from the epidural space but is more commonly caused by accidental IV injection of the local anesthetic solution.

2. Because plasma concentrations of local anesthetic required to produce cardiovascular toxicity are high, this complication likely results only from accidental IV injection of the local anesthetic solution.

3. An adequate test dose and incremental injection of the local anesthetic solution are the most important methods for preventing systemic toxicity during epidural anesthesia.

E. **Total Spinal Anesthesia**

1. Total spinal anesthesia occurs when the local anesthetic solution spreads high enough to block the entire spinal cord and occasionally the brainstem during either spinal or epidural anesthesia.

2. Profound hypotension and bradycardia may occur secondary to sympathetic nervous system blockade. Apnea may occur as a result of respiratory muscle dysfunction or depression of brainstem control centers.

3. Management includes administration of vasopressors, atropine, fluids, and oxygen plus controlled ventilation of the lungs. If the cardiovascular and ventilatory consequences are managed appropriately, total spinal block will resolve without sequelae.

F. **Neurologic Injury**

1. Neurologic injury occurs in approximately 0.03% to 0.1% of all spinal and epidural anesthesia. (Persistent paresthesias and limited motor weakness are the most common injuries.)

2. Hyperbaric 5% lidocaine has been implicated as a cause of cauda equina syndrome after subarachnoid injection through small-bore (high-resistance) catheters during continuous spinal anesthesia. (Injection through these high-resistance catheters produces little turbulence, and undiluted local anesthetic solution tends to pool around dependent cauda equina nerve roots.)

G. **Transient neurologic symptoms** (TNS) or transient radicular irritation (TRI) is defined as pain or dysesthesia in the buttocks or legs after spinal anesthesia (Table 37-11).

1. Use of a double-orifice pencil-point needle may reduce the risk of TNS compared with the use of a single-orifice needle.

2. Pain usually resolves spontaneously in 72 hours.

MANAGEMENT

TABLE 37-11

TRANSIENT NEUROLOGIC SYMPTOMS

Risk Factors	Not Risk Factors
Lidocaine	Lidocaine dose
Addition of phenylephrine to 0.5% tetracaine	Addition of epinephrine to lidocaine
Lithotomy position	Presence of dextrose
Leg flexed (as for menisectomy)	Paresthesia or blood-tinged CSF
Outpatient status	Hypotension

CSF = cerebrospinal fluid.

3. The mechanism responsible for TRI is unknown but it is not simply a milder form of cauda equina syndrome.

H. **Chloroprocaine** (preservative free) is a short-acting spinal anesthetic and does not seem to be associated with TNS.

I. **Spinal hematoma** is a rare (estimated to occur in fewer than one in 150,000 patients) complication of spinal or epidural anesthesia manifesting as lower extremity numbness or weakness. Detection is difficult in patients receiving perioperative spinal local anesthetic solution pain control.

1. Early detection is critical because a delay of more than 8 hours in decompressing the spinal cord decreases the likelihood of neurologic recovery.

2. Coagulation defects are the principal risk factor for development of an epidural hematoma.

   a. Patients receiving nonsteroidal anti-inflammatory drugs (NSAIDs) with antiplatelet effects or subcutaneous unfractionated heparin for deep thrombosis prophylaxis are not considered to be at increased risk for development of a spinal hematoma.

   b. Patients taking antiplatelet drugs (thienopyridine derivatives such as ticlopidine and clopidogrel; glycoprotein IIb/IIIa antagonists such as abciximab) should generally not receive a neuraxial block.

   c. Patients receiving fractionated low-molecular-weight heparin (LMWH; enoxaparin, dalteparin, tinzaparin) are considered to be at increased risk for development of a spinal hematoma. Patients receiving drugs preoperatively at thromboprophy-

TABLE 37-12

CONDITIONS THAT MAY INCREASE THE RISK OF SPINAL OR
EPIDURAL ANESTHESIA

Hypovolemia
Increased intracranial pressure
Coagulopathy or thrombocytopenia (epidural hematoma)
Sepsis (increased risk of meningitis)
Infection at the puncture site
Pre-existing neurologic disease (there is no evidence that epidural
  or spinal anesthesia alters the course)
Patient refusal (absolute contraindication)

       lactic doses should have the drug held for 10 to
       12 hours before central neuraxial block.
  d. For patients in whom LMWH is begun after sur-
       gery, single-shot neuraxial blocks are not con-
       traindicated provided the first dose of heparin is
       not administered until 24 hours after surgery using
       twice-daily dosing regimens (or 6 to 8 hours if
       using once-daily dosing regimens).
  e. If an indwelling central neuraxial catheter is in
       place, it should not be removed until 10 to 12
       hours after the last dose of LMWH, and subse-
       quent doses should not be administered until at
       least 2 hours after catheter removal.
  f. Patients who are fully anticoagulated (prolonged
       prothrombin time and plasma thromboplastin

TABLE 37-13

CHOICE OF SPINAL OR EPIDURAL ANESTHESIA

Spinal Anesthesia
Less time to perform
More rapid onset
Better quality sensory and motor block
Less pain during surgery

Epidural Anesthesia
Less risk of postdural puncture headache
Less hypotension if epinephrine is not added to local anesthetic
  solution
Ability to prolong or extend block via an indwelling catheter
Option of using an epidural catheter to provide postoperative
  analgesia

MANAGEMENT

time) at the time of block placement or removal of the epidural catheter are considered to be at increased risk for the development of a spinal hematoma.

3. The risk of spinal hematoma during removal of an epidural catheter is nearly as great as with placement of the catheter. The timing for removal of the epidural catheter and the degree of anticoagulation need to be coordinated.

4. Drugs or regimens not considered to increase the risk of neuraxial bleeding when used alone (minidose unfractionated heparin, NSAIDs) may increase the risk when combined.

XII. CONTRAINDICATIONS (Table 37-12)

XIII. CHOICE OF SPINAL OR EPIDURAL ANESTHESIA (Table 37-13)

CHAPTER 38 ■ PERIPHERAL NERVE BLOCKADE

INTRODUCTION

Regional anesthesia enables site-specific, long-lasting, and effective anesthesia and analgesia (Tsui BCH, Rosenquist RW: Peripheral nerve blockade. In *Clinical Anesthesia*. Edited by Barash PG, Cullen BF, Stoelting RK, Cahalan MK, Stock MC. Philadelphia: Lippincott Williams & Wilkins, 2009, pp 955–1002). Peripheral nerve blocks (PNBs) can be used as the only anesthetic, as a supplement to provide analgesia and muscle relaxation along with general anesthesia, or as the initial step in the provision of prolonged postoperative analgesia such as with intercostal blocks or continuous peripheral nerve catheters.

I. GENERAL PRINCIPLES AND EQUIPMENT

An exciting advance in technology in relation to regional anesthesia in recent years has been the introduction of anatomically based ultrasound imaging to visualize the target nerve. In many situations, it is prudent to combine the two technologies of nerve stimulation and ultrasound imaging to achieve the goal of 100% success with all regional blocks.

- A. **Set-up and Monitoring** (Table 38-1)
- B. **Common Techniques: Nerve Stimulation**
  1. **Basics of Technique and Equipment.** A low-current electrical impulse applied to a peripheral nerve produces stimulation of motor fibers and theoretically identifies proximity to the nerve without actual needle contact of the nerve or related patient discomfort.
  2. **Practical Guidelines.** After a low threshold response is obtained, 2 to 3 mL of local anesthetic is injected, and the operator watches for disappearance of the motor twitch, which is a signal to inject the remainder of the proposed dose in divided aliquots. After nerve localization using a stimulating needle, introduction

---

TABLE 38-1

SET-UP AND MONITORING FOR REGIONAL BLOCKS

Set-up

All supplies located in this area must be readily identifiable and accessible to the anesthesiologist.

The area should be of ample size to allow block performance, monitoring, and resuscitation of patients.

There should be equipment for oxygen delivery, emergency airway management, and suction, and the area should have sufficient lighting.

A practically organized equipment storage cart is desirable and should contain all of the necessary equipment (including equipment required for emergency procedures).

A selection of sedatives, hypnotics, and intravenous anesthetics should be immediately available to prepare patients for regional anesthesia.

Emergency drugs (atropine, epinephrine, phenylephrine, ephedrine, propofol, thiopental, succinylcholine, amrinone, intralipid) should also be immediately available.

Monitoring

During the performance of regional anesthesia, it is vital to have skilled personnel monitor the patient at all times (electrocardiography, noninvasive blood pressure, pulse oximetry, and level of consciousness of the patient should be gauged frequently using verbal contact because vasovagal episodes are common with many regional procedures).

The patient should be closely observed for systematic toxicity (within 2 minutes for at least 30 minutes after the procedure).

Before performing blocks with significant sympathetic effects, a baseline blood pressure reading should be obtained.

---

of a stimulating catheter with continuous stimulation of the nerve is suitable for provision of continuous analgesia.

  C. **Common Techniques: Ultrasound Imaging**

   1. **Basics of Technique and Equipment.** Ultrasound images reflect contours, including those of anatomic structures, based on differing acoustic impedances of tissue or fluids. The Doppler effect can be very useful for identifying blood vessels during nerve localization using ultrasound guidance because many nerves are situated in close proximity to vascular structures.

   2. **Practical Guidelines**

      a. Probe sterility is paramount when performing real-time ultrasound guidance. For nerve localization during ultrasound-guided PNB, it is effective to first identify one or more reliable anatomical landmarks (bone or vessel) with a known relationship to the nerve structure (Table 38-2). The nerve structure is often placed in the center of the screen

TABLE 38-2

ANATOMICAL LANDMARKS FOR LOCALIZING NERVES DURING ULTRASOUND-GUIDED PERIPHERAL NERVE BLOCKS

Peripheral Nerve Block Location	Anatomical Landmark(s)	Approach for Ultrasound Imaging
Interscalene	Subclavian artery Scalene muscles	Locate the plexus or trunk divisions superolateral to the artery at the supraclavicular fossa and trace proximally to where the roots or trunks lie between the scalenus anterior and medius muscles.
Supraclavicular	Subclavian artery	Scan from lateral to medial on the superior aspect of the clavicle to locate the pulsatile artery. Plexus trunks or divisions lie lateral and often superior to the artery. Color Doppler is useful.
Infraclavicular	Subclavian and axillary artery Subclavian and axillary vein	Place the artery at the center of the field and locate the brachial plexus cords surrounding the artery.
Axillary	Axillary artery	Terminal nerves surround the artery.
Peripheral Nerves		
Median nerve at the antecubital fossa	Brachial artery	The large anechoic artery lies immediately lateral to the nerve.
Radial nerve at the anterior elbow	Humerus at spiral groove Deep brachial artery	Trace the nerve proximally and posteriorly toward the spiral groove of the humerus, just inferior to the deltoid muscle insertion (the nerve is adjacent to the deep brachial artery).

(continued)

MANAGEMENT

TABLE 38-2

ANATOMICAL LANDMARKS FOR LOCALIZING NERVES DURING
ULTRASOUND-GUIDED PERIPHERAL NERVE BLOCKS (*Continued*)

Ulnar nerve at the medial forearm	Ulnar artery	Scan at the anteromedial surface of the forearm approximately at the junction of its distal third and proximal two thirds to locate the ulnar nerve as it approaches the ulnar artery on its medial aspect.
Lumbar Plexus	Transverse processes	The plexus lies between and just deep to the lateral aspect (tips) of the processes.
Femoral	Femoral artery	The nerve lies lateral to the artery (vein most medial). See Fig. 38-11.
Sciatic		
Classical or labat	Ischial bone and inferior gluteal or pudendal vessels	The nerve lies lateral to the thinnest aspect of the ischial bone. The inferior gluteal artery lies medial to and at the same depth as the nerve.
Subgluteal	Greater trochanter and ischial tuberosity	The nerve lies between the two bone structures.
Popliteal	Popliteal artery	Trace the tibial and common peroneal nerves from the popliteal crease to where they form the sciatic nerve. At the crease, the tibial nerve lies adjacent to the popliteal artery. Scanning proximally to the sciatic bifurcation, the artery becomes deeper and at a greater distance from the nerve.
Ankle		
Tibial (posterior tibial)	Posterior tibial artery	The nerve lies posterior to the artery.
Deep peroneal	Anterior tibial artery	The nerve lies lateral to the artery.

to guarantee that aligning the needle puncture with the center of the probe will ensure close needle tip–nerve alignment.

b. After one observes that the needle is seen to be close to the nerve(s), a 1- to 2-mL test dose of local anesthetic or D5W can be injected to visualize the spread. The solution will be seen as a hypoechoic expansion and often illuminates the surrounding area, enabling better visibility of the nerves and block needle.

D. **Other Related Equipment**

1. **Needles** used for regional techniques are often modified from standard injection needles (continuous blocks require larger bore needles to facilitate catheter introduction).

2. **Catheters** amenable to stimulation (with an electrode placed into the catheter tip) may enable more accurate advancement of catheters for substantial distances to provide continuous analgesia.

E. **Avoiding Complications.** Despite the excellent safety record of regional anesthesia, the incidence of some complications may be higher in PNB than other regional anesthesia or analgesia techniques, and these complications can be devastating. Choosing a suitable patient and applying the right dose of local anesthetic in the correct location are the primary considerations. Follow-up before and after discharge is equally important.

II. SPECIFIC TECHNIQUES: HEAD AND NECK, UPPER EXTREMITIES, CHEST, AND ABDOMEN

A. **Head and Neck** (Figs. 38-1 to 38-4)

1. **Cervical Plexus Blocks.** Anesthesia of the deep or superficial cervical plexus or both can be used for procedures of the lateral or anterior neck such as parathyroidectomy and carotid endarterectomy. In carotid surgery, local infiltration of the carotid bifurcation may be necessary to block reflex hemodynamic changes associated with glossopharyngeal stimulation.

2. **Occipital Nerve Blocks.** The greater and lesser occipital nerves can be blocked by superficial injection at the points on the posterior skull where they emerge from below the muscles of the neck. This block is rarely used for surgical procedures; it is more often

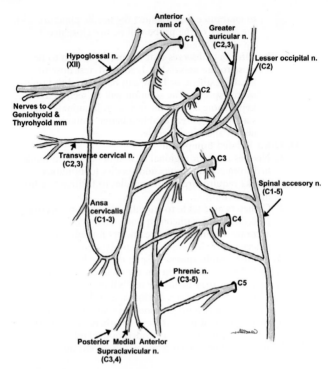

FIGURE 38-1. Schematic of the cervical plexus, which arises from the anterior primary rami of C2–C4. The motor branches (including the phrenic nerve) curl anteriorly around the anterior scalene muscle and travel caudad and medially to supply the deep muscles of the neck. The sensory branches exit at the lateral border of the sternocleidomastoid muscle to supply the skin of the neck and shoulder.

applied as a diagnostic step in evaluating complaints of head and neck pain.

B. **Upper Extremity** (Figs. 38-5 to 38-7). The four anatomic locations where local anesthetics are placed are the (1) interscalene groove near the cervical transverse processes, (2) subclavian sheath at the first rib, (3) near the coracoid process in the infraclavicular fossa, and (4) surrounding the axillary artery in the axilla. Ultrasound imaging and nerve stimulation have greatly facilitated the use of upper extremity regional anesthesia. The

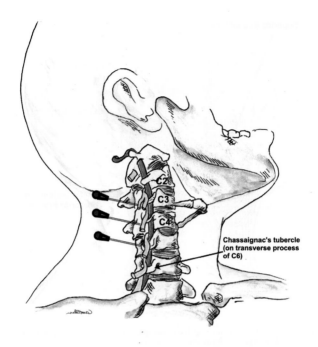

FIGURE 38-2. Needle insertion points and angles for the deep cervical plexus blockade. The nerve roots exit the vertebral column via the troughs formed by the transverse processes. The needle is inserted at each nerve roots of C2–C4 in caudad and posterior direction.

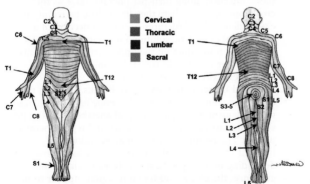

FIGURE 38-3. The cervical, thoracic, lumbar, and sacral dermatomes of the body.

MANAGEMENT

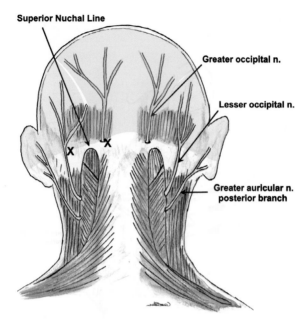

FIGURE 38-4. Greater and lesser occipital nerve distribution, supply, and block needle insertion sites.

terminal branches can also be anesthetized by local anesthetic injection along their peripheral course as they cross joint spaces, where they lie in close proximity to easily identifiable structures or by the injection of a dilute local anesthetic solution intravenously below a pneumatic tourniquet on the upper arm ("intravenous regional" or Bier block) (see Table 38-2).

C. **Brachial Plexus Blockade** (Table 38-3)

D. **Terminal Upper Extremity Nerve Blocks.** PNBs in the upper extremity are of particular value as rescue blocks to supplement incomplete surgical anesthesia and to provide long-lasting selective analgesia in the postoperative period. The peripheral nerves may be individually blocked at mid-humeral, elbow, or wrist locations, depending on the specific nerve. If using ultrasound guidance, the elbow and forearm regions appear to be the most suitable block regions, and blocks at these sites

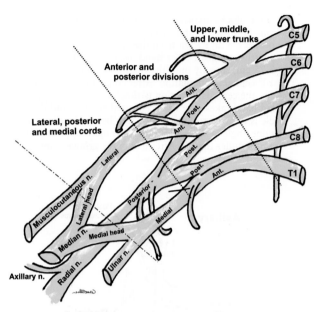

FIGURE 38-5. Schematic of the brachial plexus. Many branches, including the medial cutaneous nerves of the forearm and arm, which arise from the medial cord, are not shown here.

may improve the accuracy of nerve localization and local anesthetic spread. The wrist is highly populated with tendons and fascial tissues (flexor and extensor retinaculae), which can be difficult to distinguish from, and may obscure the images of, the nerves. Color Doppler combined with ultrasonography can be used to clearly identify the nerves at many desirable locations because they are often situated near blood vessels (see Table 38-1 and Figs. 38-7 and 38-8).

E. **Intravenous Regional Anesthesia (Bier Block).** Arm anesthesia can be provided by the injection of local anesthetic into the venous system below an occluding tourniquet without using ultrasonography or nerve stimulation (Table 38-4).

F. **Intercostal Nerve Blockade.** Anesthesia of the intercostal nerves provides both motor and sensory anesthesia of the abdominal wall from the xiphoid to the pubis. These nerve blocks involve injections along the easily palpated abrupt posterior angulation of the ribs, which occurs between 5 and 7 cm from the midline in the back. The anesthesiologist's other hand inserts a needle (22 gauge, 3.75 cm) directly onto the rib, maintaining a constant 10° cephalad angulation. After contact is made with the rib, the cephalad traction is slowly released, the cephalad hand takes over the needle and syringe, and the needle is allowed to "walk" down to below the rib at the same angle. The needle is then advanced approximately 4 mm under the rib. After it is in the groove, aspiration

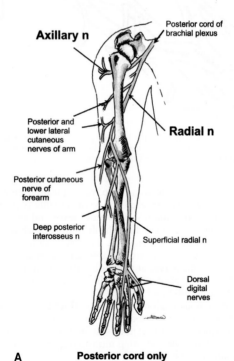

A   **Posterior cord only**

FIGURE 38-6.   Courses of the terminal nerves of the upper extremity. The posterior view (**A**) illustrates the branches from the posterior cord (axillary and radial nerves), and the anterior view.

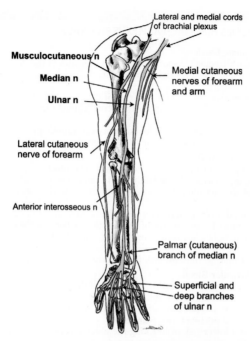

B Showing medial and lateral cords only

FIGURE 38-6. *Continued.* (B) illustrates the branches from the lateral (musculocutaneous and median nerves) and medial (median and ulnar nerves) cords.

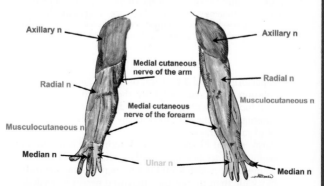

FIGURE 38-7. Cutaneous innervation of the upper extremity nerves.

TABLE 38-3

TECHNIQUES FOR BRACHIAL PLEXUS BLOCKADE

Interscalene Block

This block frequently spares the lowest branches of the plexus, the C8 and T1 fibers (which innervate the caudad [ulnar] border of the forearm).

Pneumothorax should be considered if cough or chest pain is produced while exploring for the nerve (cupola of the lung near block site).

Direct injection into the vertebral artery can rapidly produce central nervous system toxicity and convulsions.

Supraclavicular Block

The midpoint of the clavicle is identified. The subclavian artery pulse serves as a reliable landmark in thinner individuals because the plexus lies immediately cephaloposterior to the subclavian artery.

Ultrasound imaging and nerve stimulation help avoid puncturing the pleura. There is a risk of pneumothorax because the cupola of the lung lies just medial to the first rib; risk of pneumothorax is greater on the right side because the cupola of the lung is higher on that side; the risk is also greater in tall, thin patients.

Infraclavicular Block

This block provides excellent analgesia of the entire arm (blocks the musculocutaneous and axillary nerves more consistently) and allows introduction of continuous catheters to provide prolonged postoperative pain relief.

There is a lower risk of blocking the phrenic nerve or stellate ganglion.

Vessel puncture is a potential complication.

Lateral needle insertion helps avoid the risk of pneumothorax.

Axillary Block

This block is useful for surgery of the elbow, forearm, and hand (the musculocutaneous nerve may be blocked separately).

This block is associated with minimal complications (neuropathy from needle puncture or intraneural injection of local anesthetic).

is performed, and 3 to 5 mL of a local anesthetic solution is injected. Generally, the intercostal nerves are well localized with the blind landmark-based technique. Alternatively, the rib can be easily visualized with the use of ultrasonography.

G. **Paravertebral Block.** This block technique is useful for segmental anesthesia, particularly of the upper thoracic segments. It is also useful if a more proximal (central) blockade than that of the intercostal nerves is needed,

Paravertebral Block

S = Spinous process
T = Transverse process
L = Lamina

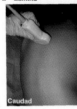

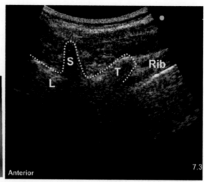

A Caudad   Anterior   7.3 B

FIGURE 38-8. Probe placement (**A**) and ultrasound image (**B**) during paravertebral block in the thoracic spine. The probe is first placed in the midline of the spine to capture a transverse view of the vertebral and costal (if thoracic spine) elements. L = lamina; S = spinous process; T = transverse process.

TABLE 38-4

INTRAVENOUS REGIONAL ANESTHESIA

A small-gauge (20- or 22-gauge) intravenous catheter is placed and taped on the dorsum of the hand in the arm to be blocked.

The arm is elevated to promote venous drainage (an Esmarch bandage is used).

After exsanguination, the tourniquet is inflated to 300 mm Hg or 2.5 times the patient's systolic blood pressure.

A 50-mL syringe with 0.5% lidocaine is attached to the previously inserted cannula, and the contents are injected slowly.

For short procedures, the cannula can be removed at this point, but if surgery may extend beyond 1 hour, the cannula can be left in place and reinjected after 90 minutes.

Beyond 45 minutes of surgery, many patients experience discomfort at the level of the tourniquet (double-cuff tourniquets alleviate this problem).

If surgery is completed in less than 20 minutes, the tourniquet is left inflated for at least that total period of time.

If 40 minutes has elapsed, the tourniquet can be deflated as a single maneuver.

Between 20 and 40 minutes, the cuff can be deflated, reinflated immediately, and finally deflated after 1 minute to delay the sudden absorption of anesthetic into the systemic circulation.

The duration of anesthesia is minimal beyond the time of tourniquet release.

MANAGEMENT

such as to relieve the pain of herpes zoster or of a proximal rib fracture.

H. **Inguinal Nerve Block.** This block is performed easily with blind technique, although ultrasound imaging may be performed to help improve the success rate. Side effects include systemic toxicity and transient femoral nerve palsy.

I. **Penile block** is used in children and adults for surgical procedures of the glans and shaft of the penis.

III. **SPECIFIC TECHNIQUES: LOWER EXTREMITY**
Combined blocks of the lumbar and sciatic plexuses provide effective surgical anesthesia to the entire lower extremity (Figs. 38-3 to 38-10).

A. **Terminal Nerves of the Lumbar Plexus** (Table 38-5)

B. **Sacral Plexus: Formation and Branches.** The anterior primary rami of S1–S4 join the lumbosacral trunk to form the sacral plexus (Fig. 38-9).
   1. **Sciatic, Tibial, and Common Peroneal Nerves.** At a variable distance within the posterior thigh (often high in the popliteal fossa), the sciatic nerve bifurcates into common peroneal and tibial nerves.
   2. **Nerves at the Ankle.** By the time the femoral, tibial, and common peroneal nerves reach the ankle, five branches cross this joint to provide innervation for the skin and muscles of the foot (Table 38-6) (Fig. 38-10).

C. **Psoas Compartment Block.** This block has the advantage of blocking the entire lumbar plexus and therefore provides anesthesia/analgesia of the anterolateral and medial thigh, the knee, and the cutaneous distribution of the saphenous nerve below the knee.

D. **Separate Blocks of the Terminal Nerves of the Lumbar Plexus.** Anesthesia can be performed for four terminal nerves (lateral femoral cutaneous, femoral, obturator, and saphenous), although a lumbar plexus block is preferable if anesthesia of all these nerves is required.
   1. Anesthesia of the lateral femoral cutaneous nerve is occasionally used to provide sensory anesthesia for obtaining a skin graft from the lateral thigh. It can also be blocked as a diagnostic tool to identify cases of meralgia paresthetica.
   2. Obturator nerve block can be effective to prevent obturator reflex during transurethral bladder tumor resections, for treatment of pain in the hip area, for

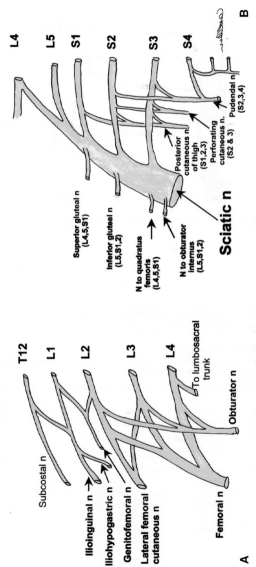

FIGURE 38-9. The lumbar (A; L1–L4) and sacral (B; L4–S4) plexuses.

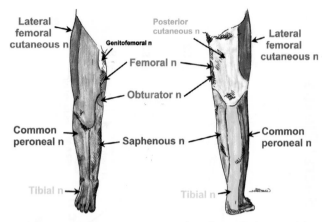

FIGURE 38-10. Cutaneous innervation from the terminal nerves of the lower extremity.

TABLE 38-5

TERMINAL NERVES OF THE LUMBAR PLEXUS

Genitofemoral Nerve (L1–L2)
Innervates the skin immediately below the crease of groin anterior to the upper part of the femoral triangle

Lateral Cutaneous Nerve of the Thigh (lateral femoral cutaneous nerve; L2–L3)
Supplies skin over the anterolateral aspect of the thigh and skin on the lateral aspect of the thigh from the greater trochanter to the mid-thigh branches

Femoral Nerve (L2–L4)
Largest nerve of the lumbar plexus, supplying muscles and skin on the anterior aspect of the thigh
Lies slightly deeper (0.5 to 1.0 cm) and lateral (approximately 1.5 cm) to the femoral artery (VAN is the mnemonic for the anatomical relationship, starting medially)

Obturator Nerve (L2–L4)
Divides into its anterior and posterior branches near the obturator foramen

TABLE 38-6

NERVES AT THE ANKLE

Deep peroneal nerve (L5–S1)
Tibial nerve (posterior tibial nerve, (S1–S3)
Superficial peroneal nerve
Sural nerve
Saphenous nerve

adductor spasm (as seen in multiple sclerosis patients), or as a diagnostic tool when studying hip mobility.

3. Procedures on the knee require anesthesia of the femoral and obturator nerves, although postoperative analgesia of the knee can usually be provided by femoral nerve block alone.

4. Femoral nerve block is used extensively for analgesia (Fig. 38-11).

E. **Sciatic Nerve Blockade Using Posterior, Anterior, and Posterior Popliteal Approaches.** A sciatic nerve block can be used with lumbar plexus block for anesthesia of the lower extremity. Together with saphenous nerve block, the block produces adequate anesthesia to the sole of the

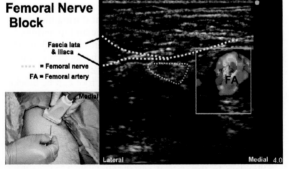

Femoral Nerve Block

Fascia lata & iliaca
····· = Femoral nerve
FA = Femoral artery

FA

Medial

A Lateral   Medial 4.0 **B**

MANAGEMENT

FIGURE 38-11.   Ultrasound-guided femoral nerve block. **A.** The probe is placed in a slightly oblique plane (at the level of and parallel to the inguinal crease) to capture the nerve in short-axis lateral to the femoral artery (FA). **B.** The needle is seen (not shown) as it transects the fascia lata and iliaca. The *dotted line* indicates the femoral nerve.

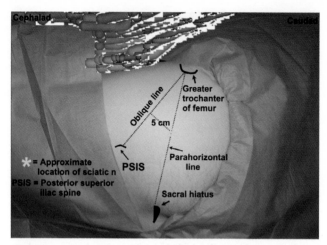

FIGURE 38-12. Landmarks for the sciatic nerve block using a posterior gluteal approach when a nerve stimulation procedure is used. This location will serve as a reference point when applying ultrasound imaging. The *asterisk* indicates the approximate location of the sciatic nerve. PSIS = posterior superior iliac spine.

foot and the lower leg. The sciatic nerve is deep within the gluteal region and may be difficult to locate blindly or with ultrasonography. Of benefit during ultrasound-guided blockade of the sciatic nerve and its terminal branches (tibial and common peroneal nerves) are the numerous bony and vascular landmarks that can be used for ease of identification (Fig. 38-12).

F. **Ankle Block.** All five nerves of the foot can be blocked at the level of the ankle. The superficial nerves (sural, superficial peroneal, and saphenous nerves) can be blocked by simple infiltration techniques. Ultrasound guidance can be useful for blocking the posterior tibial and deep peroneal (fibular) nerves because their locations can be easily identified next to reliable landmarks (bones and vessels) that are clearly visible.

CHAPTER 39 ■ ANESTHESIA FOR NEUROSURGERY

An understanding of neuroanatomy and neurophysiology is requisite knowledge for the anesthetic management of patients with disease of the central nervous system (CNS), including the brain and the spine (M Sean Kincaid, Lam AM: Anesthesia for neurosurgery. In *Clinical Anesthesia*. Edited by Barash PG, Cullen BF, Stoelting RK, Cahalan MK, Stock MC. Philadelphia: Lippincott Williams & Wilkins, 2009, pp 1003–1031).

I. NEUROANATOMY

A. The brain and spinal cord are surrounded by protective but nondistensible bony structures that surround them and provide protection.

B. The intracranial volume is fixed, thereby providing little room for anything other than the brain, cerebrospinal fluid (CSF), and blood contained in the cerebral vasculature. It is in the context of the restrictive nature of the space in which the CNS is housed that all interventions must be considered.

C. The anterior cerebral circulation originates from the carotid artery, the posterior circulation results from the vertebral arteries, and the system of collateralization is known as the circle of Willis (Fig. 39-1).

D. The spinal column is the bony structure made up of the seven cervical, 12 thoracic, and five lumbar vertebrae, as well as the sacrum.

1. The spinal cord exits the skull through the foramen magnum and enters the canal formed by the vertebral bodies. In adults, the spinal cord typically ends at the lower aspect of the first lumbar vertebral body.

2. The anterior spinal artery arises from the vertebral arteries and supplies the anterior two thirds of the spinal cord. This vessel runs the length of the cord,

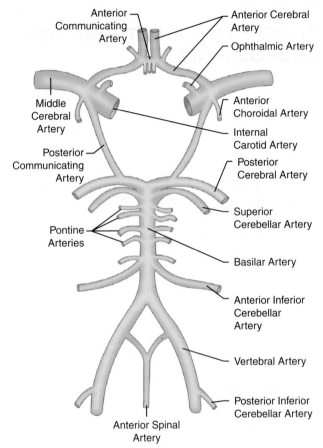

FIGURE 39-1. The circle of Willis, which supplies blood flow to the brain.

receiving contribution from radicular arteries via intercostal vessels. The artery of Adamkiewicz is the most important radicular vessel.
3. The posterior third of the cord is supplied by two posterior spinal arteries, which arise from the vertebral arteries and also receive contribution from radicular arteries.

II. NEUROPHYSIOLOGY

A. Cerebral metabolism is directly related to the number and frequency of neuron depolarizations (activity or stimulation increases the metabolic rate). Cerebral blood flow (CBF) is tightly coupled to metabolism.

B. The CSF occupies the subarachnoid space, providing a protective layer of fluid between the brain and the tissue that surrounds it. It maintains a milieu in which the brain can function by regulating pH and electrolytes, carrying away waste products, and delivering nutrients.

C. Intracranial pressure (ICP) is low except in pathologic states. The volume of blood, CSF, and brain tissue must be in equilibrium. An increase in one of these three elements, or the addition of a space-occupying lesion, can be accommodated initially through displacement of CSF into the thecal sac, but only to a small extent. Further increases, as with significant cerebral edema or accumulation of an extradural hematoma, quickly lead to a marked increase in ICP because of the low intracranial compliance (Fig. 39-2).

D. Many factors affect CBF because of their effect on metabolism. (Stimulation, arousal, nociception, and mild hyperthermia elevate metabolism and flow, and sedative-hypnotic agents and hypothermia decrease metabolism and flow.)

E. A number of other factors govern CBF directly without changing metabolism.

1. A potent determinant of CBF is $PaCO_2$. CBF changes by approximately 3% of baseline for each 1 mm Hg of change in $PaCO_2$ (Fig. 39-3).

2. As CBF changes, so does cerebral blood volume (CBV), which is the reason hyperventilation can be used for short periods of time to relax the brain or to decrease ICP. This effect is thought to be short lived (minutes to hours) because the pH of CSF normalizes over time and vessel caliber returns to baseline.

F. In contrast to $PaCO_2$, PaO_2 has little effect on CBF except at abnormally low levels (Fig. 39-4). When PaO_2 decreases below 50 mm Hg, CBF begins to increase sharply.

G. CBF remains approximately constant despite modest swings in arterial blood pressure (autoregulation) (Fig. 39-5).

1. As cerebral perfusion pressure (CPP), defined as the difference of mean arterial pressure (MAP) and ICP, changes, cerebrovascular resistance (CVR) adjusts in order to maintain stable flow.

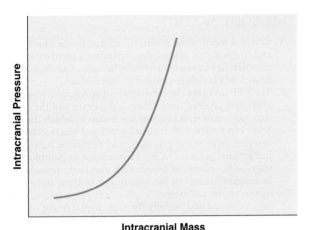

FIGURE 39-2. Intracranial compliance (elastance) curve.

2. The range of CPP over which autoregulation is maintained is termed the *autoregulatory plateau*. Although this range is frequently quoted as a MAP range of 60 to 150 mm Hg, there is significant variability between individuals, and these numbers are only approximate.

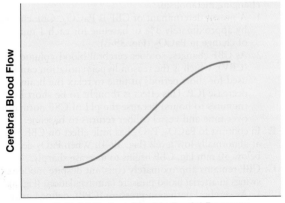

FIGURE 39-3. Cerebrovascular response to change in arterial carbon dioxide partial pressure ($PaCO_2$) from 25 to 65 mm Hg.

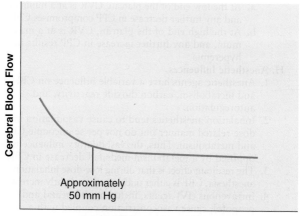

FIGURE 39-4. Cerebrovascular response to change in arterial oxygen partial pressure (PaO$_2$). The response of cerebral blood flow to change in PaO$_2$ is flat until the PaO$_2$ decreases below about 50 mm Hg.

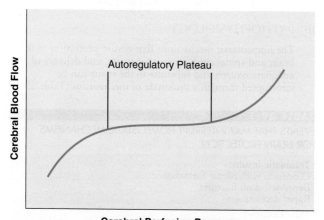

FIGURE 39-5. Cerebral autoregulation maintains cerebral blood flow constant between 60 to 160 mm Hg. These are average values, and there is considerable variation in both the lower and upper limit of cerebral autoregulation among normal individuals.

a. At the low end of the plateau, CVR is at a minimum, and any further decrease in CPP compromises CBF.
b. At the high end of the plateau, CVR is at a maximum, and any further increase in CPP results in hyperemia.

H. **Anesthetic Influences**
1. Anesthetic agents have a variable influence on CBF and metabolism, carbon dioxide reactivity, and autoregulation.
2. Inhalation anesthetics tend to cause vasodilation in a dose-related manner but do not per se uncouple CBF and metabolism. Thus, the vasodilatory influence is opposed by a metabolism-mediated decrease in CBF.
3. The resultant effect is that during low-dose inhalation anesthesia, CBF is either unchanged or slightly increased.
4. Intravenous (IV) agents, including thiopental and propofol, cause vasoconstriction coupled with a reduction in metabolism. Ketamine, on the other hand, increases CBF and metabolism.
5. Cerebrovascular carbon dioxide reactivity is a robust mechanism and is preserved under all anesthetic conditions. Cerebral autoregulation, on the other hand, is abolished by inhalation agents in a dose-related manner but is preserved during propofol anesthesia.

III. PATHOPHYSIOLOGY

The homeostatic mechanisms that ensure protection of the brain and spinal cord, removal of waste, and delivery of adequate oxygen and substrate to the tissue can be interrupted through a multitude of mechanisms (Table 39-1).

TABLE 39-1

EVENTS THAT MAY INTERRUPT HOMEOSTATIC MECHANISMS FOR BRAIN PROTECTION

Traumatic Insults
Contusion with edema formation
Depressed skull fractures
Rapid deceleration

Mass Lesions
Tumors (compress adjacent structures, increase ICP, and obstruct normal flow of CSF)

Hemorrhage (spontaneous or traumatic)

CSF = cerebrospinal fluid; ICP = intracranial pressure.

TABLE 39-2

MONITORING CENTRAL NERVOUS SYSTEM FUNCTION

Electroencephalography (depolarization of cortical neurons
  provides a pattern of electrical activity that can be measured on
  the scalp)
Evoked potential monitoring (detect signals that result from a
  specific stimuli)
  SSEP (requires intact sensory pathway, spine surgery when
    dorsal column of the spinal cord may be at risk)
  BAEP (acoustic neuroma surgery)
  VEP (difficult to record during anesthesia)
  MEP (monitors descending motor pathways, complements SSEP
    during spine surgery, signals sensitive to volatile anesthetics
    and intravenous may be preferred)
sEMG (detects injury to nerve roots in the surgical area; muscle
  relaxants must be avoided)
Electromyography (cranial nerve monitoring)

BAEP = brainstem auditory evoked potential; MEP = motor evoked
potential; sEMG = spontaneous electromyography; SSEP = somatosensory
evoked potential; VEP = visual evoked potential.

IV. MONITORING

The integrity of the CNS needs to be evaluated intraoperatively with monitors that specifically detect CNS function,
perfusion, or metabolism.
A. Central Nervous System Function (Tables 39-2 to 39-4)
B. Influence of Anesthetic Technique (Table 39-5)

TABLE 39-3

ELECTROENCEPHALOGRAM FREQUENCIES

	Frequency (Hz)	Description
Delta	0–3	Low frequency, high amplitude
		Present in deep coma, encephalopathy, deep anesthesia
Theta	4–7	Not prominent in adults
		May be seen in encephalopathy
Alpha	8–12	Prominent in the posterior region during relaxation with the eyes closed
Beta	>12	High frequency, low amplitude
		Dominant frequency during arousal

TABLE 39-4

INDICATIONS FOR ELECTROENCEPHALOGRAPHIC MONITORING

During anesthesia	Carotid endarterectomy
	Cardiopulmonary bypass
	Cerebrovascular surgery (temporary clipping, vascular bypass)
Intensive care unit	Barbiturate coma for patients with traumatic brain injury
	Subclinical seizures suspected

TABLE 39-5

INFLUENCE OF ANESTHETIC TECHNIQUE ON CENTRAL NERVOUS SYSTEM MONITORING

Inhalation agents (including nitrous oxide) generally have more depressant effects on evoked potential monitoring than IV agents.

Whereas cortical evoked potentials with long latency involving multiple synapses (SSEP, VEP) are exquisitely sensitive to the influence of anesthetic, short-latency brainstem (BAEP) and spinal components are resistant to anesthetic influence.

Monitoring of MEP and cranial nerve EMG in general preclude the use of muscle relaxants. Use of a short-acting neuromuscular blocking agent for the purpose of tracheal intubation is acceptable.

MEP is exquisitely sensitive to the depressant effects of inhalation anesthetics, including nitrous oxide. Total IV anesthesia without nitrous oxide is the recommended anesthetic technique for monitoring of MEP.

Opioids and benzodiazepines have negligible effects on recording of evoked potentials.

Propofol and thiopental attenuate the amplitude of virtually all modalities of evoked potentials but do not obliterate them.

During crucial events when part of the central neural pathway is specifically placed at risk by surgical manipulation, as in placement of a temporary clip during aneurysm surgery, change in "anesthetic depth" should be minimized to avoid misinterpretation of the changes in evoked potential.

BAEP = brainstem auditory evoked potential; IV = intravenous; MEP = motor evoked potential; SSEP = somatosensory evoked potential; VEP = visual evoked potential.

V. CEREBRAL PERFUSION

Although adequate CBF does not guarantee the well-being of the CNS, it is an essential factor in its integrity.

- A. **Laser Doppler flowmetry** requires a burr hole and measures flow in only a small region of the brain.
- B. **Transcranial Doppler ultrasonography (TCD)** is a noninvasive monitor for evaluating relative changes in flow through the large basal arteries of the brain (often flow velocity in the middle cerebral artery) (Fig. 39-6).
  1. In addition to the measurement of flow velocity, TCD is useful for detecting emboli (Fig. 39-7).
  2. Specific applications for intraoperative use of TCD include carotid endarterectomy (CEA), non-neurologic surgery in patients with traumatic brain injury (TBI), and surgical procedures requiring cardiopulmonary bypass.
- C. **Intracranial Pressure Monitoring**
  1. Although monitoring ICP does not provide direct information about CBF, it allows calculations of CPP (the difference between MAP and ICP).
  2. Within a physiologic range of CPP, CBF should remain approximately constant. A CPP that is too

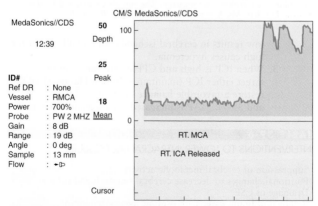

FIGURE 39-6. Transcranial Doppler tracing with release of the cross-clamp during carotid endarterectomy. The resultant hyperemia is accompanied with evidence of air embolism (*vertical streaks* in the tracing). ICA = internal carotid artery; MCA = middle cerebral artery; RT = right.

SURGICAL SUBSPECIALTIES

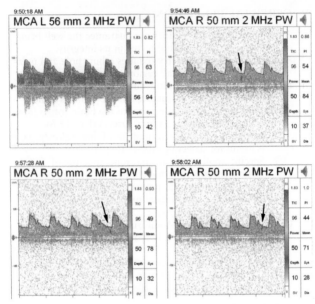

FIGURE 39-7. Particulate emboli seen on transcranial Doppler in a patient with symptoms of transient ischemic attacks consistent with right carotid artery territory embolization. The emboli are denoted by the arrows. L = left; MCA = middle cerebral artery; R = right.

low results in cerebral ischemia, and a CPP that is too high causes hyperemia.

3. When ICP is high and CPP is low, interventions can target either ICP (maintain <20 mm Hg) or MAP to restore a favorable balance of the two (Tables 39-6 and 39-7). MAP is increased via adequate intravascu-

TABLE 39-6

INTERVENTIONS TO LOWER INTRACRANIAL PRESSURE

Suppression of cerebral metabolic activity
Positional changes to decrease cerebral venous blood volume
Drainage of CSF
Removal of brain water with osmotic agents (mannitol)
Mild to moderate hyperventilation to further decrease cerebral blood volume

CSF = cerebrospinal fluid.

TABLE 39-7

INTERVENTIONS FOR MANAGEMENT OF INADEQUATE CEREBRAL PERFUSION PRESSURE

Reduce brain water	Mannitol
	Hypertonic saline
	Furosemide
Remove CSF	External ventricular drain
	Lumbar drain
Decrease CBV	Head-up tilt
	Neutral neck position
	Metabolic suppression (propofol, barbiturate)
	Mild to moderate hyperventilation
Elevate MAP	Adequate intravascular volume resuscitation
	Vasopressor

CBV = cerebral blood volume; CSF = cerebrospinal fluid; MAP = mean arterial pressure.

lar resuscitation and with a vasopressor as needed. The goal CPP in TBI is greater than 50 to 60 mm Hg.

D. **Cerebral Oxygenation and Metabolism Monitors** (Table 39-8)

VI. CEREBRAL PROTECTION

Efforts to avert neurologic insult using medications or through the manipulation of physiologic parameters have met with meager results. Although recent advances are

TABLE 39-8

MONITORS OF CEREBRAL OXYGENATION AND METABOLISM

Near-infrared spectroscopy is a noninvasive method of evaluating the oxygenation of cerebral blood and balance between flow and metabolism.

Brain tissue PO_2 probe is placed through a burr hole. It is commonly used in patients with traumatic brain injury (<15 mm Hg who warrant intervention, including treatment of anemia.)

Jugular venous oximetry provides the same information as the brain tissue PO_2 probe but over a larger portion of the brain. Normal jugular venous saturation is 65% to 75%; saturation below 50% in traumatic brain injury is associated with a poor outcome.

intriguing, no maneuver matches the cerebral protection provided by mild to moderate hypothermia. The operating room is unique in that an opportunity exists to intervene before the ischemic event occurs. (Use of a temporary aneurysm clip on the middle cerebral artery is an example of a focal ischemic insult that could be predicted; a brief period of circulatory arrest induced with adenosine to facilitate clipping of a basilar artery aneurysm is an example of a global insult.)

A. **Ischemia and Reperfusion**

1. It is reasonable to attempt to minimize ischemic insult by lowering cerebral metabolic rate, thus decreasing the likelihood of exhausting adenosine triphosphate reserves during the period of ischemia (traditional paradigm for approaching the subject of intraoperative neuroprotection).

2. Unfortunately, further damage occurs as a result of processes that are initiated during the reperfusion stage.

3. A shift in the focus of neuroprotection from metabolic suppression to targeting ischemic cascades has recently been advocated.

B. **Hypothermia**

1. Profound hypothermia is well known for its neuroprotective effects. When core body temperature decreases below 20°C, circulatory arrest of less than 30 minutes appears to be well tolerated.

2. Mild hypothermia (33° to 35°C) not only decreases cerebral metabolism but likely also modulates the immune and inflammatory response to ischemia, thus affecting the reperfusion portion of the injury as well. Although considerable evidence in rats suggests that mild hypothermia is beneficial, there is a paucity of evidence in humans. Nevertheless, hypothermia remains the most promising intervention for cerebral protection.

3. There is ample evidence that hyperthermia is associated with worse outcome in the setting of ischemic stroke, subarachnoid hemorrhage, cardiac arrest, and TBI.

4. In the operating room during neurosurgical procedures during which the brain is at risk for ischemic insult, a goal temperature of 35° to 36°C is reasonable. Mild hypothermia (33° to 35°C) may be appropriate in many patients, recognizing that there may be no benefit to this therapy.

C. **Medical Therapy for Cerebral Protection**
   1. Volatile and IV anesthetic agents decrease cerebral metabolism. Animal studies have found protective effects of volatile anesthetics, particularly isoflurane, in mitigating a mild to moderate ischemic insult, although this effect may only be short lived.
   2. Barbiturates, such as thiopental, have been shown to have at least short-term benefits on focal cerebral ischemia, but the benefit in global ischemia remain controversial. Propofol likely has similar protective effects.
   3. Current opinion is that anesthetic neuroprotection is primarily mediated through prevention of excitotoxic injury, not through termination of apoptotic pathways (it thus delays neuronal death and leaves a greater temporal window for intervention).
   4. Clinically, barbiturates and propofol are used intraoperatively to achieve burst suppression on the electroencephalogram (EEG), although its neuroprotective action does not appear to be metabolically mediated.

D. **Glucose and Cerebral Ischemia**
   1. Although considerable evidence has accumulated suggesting harm from hyperglycemia, evidence for benefit with normalization of serum glucose concentrations using insulin has been controversial.
   2. Despite a reluctance to embrace intraoperative tight glycemic control given the current literature, it is worthwhile to consider for patients undergoing cerebrovascular surgery. Given the preponderance of evidence that hyperglycemia and cerebral ischemia in combination are harmful, changing practice in these patients may be warranted. Tight glycemic control is a reasonable goal in these patients. (It cannot be stated that this intervention is neuroprotective.)

E. **A Practical Approach**
   1. For patients undergoing surgical procedures with an anticipated period of cerebral ischemia such as cerebral aneurysm surgery or cerebrovascular bypass procedures, either volatile anesthesia or an IV technique is appropriate. It is reasonable to administer additional propofol or thiopental before vessel occlusion.
   2. Euglycemia before vessel occlusion is desirable, but frequent glucose checks are essential during anesthesia

to avoid episodes of hypoglycemia if insulin is administered.

3. Hyperthermia should be avoided during this time, with the temperature kept at or below 36°C.

VII. ANESTHETIC MANAGEMENT

A. Preoperative Evaluation

1. It is prudent to consider the nature of the patient's disease that brings him or her to the operating room in the context of the patient's medical and surgical history.

2. Preoperative risk stratification for a cardiac complication is important to consider. Current guidelines include delaying surgery for at least 2 weeks after simple balloon angioplasty, 4 to 6 weeks after placement of a bare metal stent, and 1 year after placement of a drug-eluting stent.

3. Many patients presenting for spine surgery have weakness or paralysis that may present a contraindication to the use of succinylcholine (Sch).

4. Many neurosurgical patients have been exposed to antiepileptic medications. Previous allergies or reactions to these medications, especially phenytoin, should be elucidated.

B. Induction and Airway Management

1. During induction of anesthesia, three iatrogenic consequences (hypotension, hypertension, apnea) may be significant hazards for neurosurgical patients.

   a. Hypertension caused by laryngoscopy is poorly tolerated by patients after aneurysmal subarachnoid hemorrhage because systolic hypertension is thought to be a cause of recurrent hemorrhage from the aneurysm.

   b. Hypertension may worsen elevated ICP and possibly lead to herniation of cranial contents into the foramen magnum.

   c. Apnea results in a predictable increase in $PaCO_2$ and corresponding cerebral vasodilation.

2. A cervical collar for known or suspected cervical spine injury may make tracheal intubation more difficult. These patients are also particularly harmed by periods of hypotension or hypertension.

3. Because patients with subarachnoid hemorrhage are at risk for harm from hypertension, it is reasonable to

place an arterial catheter for hemodynamic monitoring before induction of anesthesia.

4. Many neurosurgical and spine surgery patients have conditions in which Sch is contraindicated.

   a. In the setting of acute stroke or spinal cord injury (SCI), it remains safe to use Sch for approximately 48 hours from the time of injury.

   b. Alternatively, a rapid-acting nondepolarizing muscle relaxant is appropriate in many neurosurgical patients to achieve acceptable intubating conditions.

C. **Maintenance of Anesthesia**

1. The primary considerations for maintenance of anesthesia include the type of monitoring planned for the procedure, brain relaxation, and the desired level of analgesia at the end of the surgical procedure.

2. Remifentanil is appropriate for neurosurgical procedures in which tracheal extubation is planned at the end of the surgery and minimal residual sedation is desired to facilitate the neurologic examination.

3. Replacement of a volatile anesthetic with a continuous infusion of propofol is desirable with motor evoked potential (MEP) monitoring and when brain relaxation is inadequate with a volatile anesthetic.

4. The use of intraoperative muscle relaxants should be avoided during MEP, spontaneous electromyography, and cranial nerve monitoring. Muscle relaxants may be used during isolated somatosensory evoked potential monitoring.

D. **Ventilation Management**

1. Hypocapnic cerebral vasoconstriction provides anesthesiologists with a powerful tool for manipulating CBF and CBV.

2. Hyperventilation is routinely used to provide brain relaxation and optimize surgical conditions.

3. Because hyperventilation decreases CBF, it has the theoretical potential for causing or exacerbating cerebral ischemia. Clinically, hyperventilation has been associated with harm only in the early period of TBI, but it is still recommended to be avoided in all patients with TBI except when necessary for a brief period to manage acute increases in ICP.

4. During neurosurgical procedures, it is reasonable to maintain the $PaCO_2$ between 30 and 35 mm Hg. Further brain relaxation should be accomplished with

other modalities, such as mannitol, hypertonic saline, or IV anesthesia. If hyperventilation to a $PaCO_2$ below 30 mm Hg is required, it is appropriate to guide this therapy with jugular venous oximetry and the arterial–jugular lactate gradient.

5. The duration of effectiveness of hyperventilation is limited. Normalization of CBF and consequently CBV has been reported to occur within minutes. Clinically, the beneficial effects of hyperventilation appear to be sustained during most neurosurgical procedures of modest duration.

E. **Fluids and Electrolytes**
1. To maintain adequate cerebral perfusion, adequate intravascular volume should be maintained (euvolemia to slight hypervolemia).
2. To minimize brain edema, it is important to maintain serum tonicity. (It is prudent to check serum sodium levels on a regular basis in prolonged surgical procedures in which mannitol has been given.)

F. **Transfusion Therapy.** The lower limit of acceptable hemoglobin or hematocrit has not been well defined. (Evidence supports avoidance of transfusion for a hematocrit above 21% except in the context of ongoing hemorrhage and possibly the early phase of resuscitation for septic patients.)

G. **Glucose Management**
1. The combination of hyperglycemia and cerebral ischemia appears to be particularly deleterious. Although a paucity of evidence addresses the topic of intraoperative glucose management, logic dictates that glucose concentrations should be normalized before periods of iatrogenic ischemia.
2. The presumed risk of tight glycemic control is inadvertent episodes of hypoglycemia.
3. A target glucose concentration above 180 mg/dL is adequate in most patients.

H. **Emergence**
1. The decisions that need to be made regarding emergence from anesthesia for neurosurgical and spine surgery patients hinge on whether the patient is an appropriate candidate for tracheal extubation.
2. For extensive spine surgeries in the prone position, significant dependent edema frequently occurs. Although the predictive value of an air leak from around the endotracheal tube cuff is poor, the

combination of pronounced facial edema and an absent cuff leak after prone surgery should make one suspicious of upper airway edema. Delaying extubation of the trachea under these circumstances may be appropriate.

3. Avoiding coughing and hemodynamic changes with emergence is important for all neurosurgical patients.

VIII. COMMON SURGICAL PROCEDURES

A. Surgery for Intracranial Tumors

1. The fundamental anesthetic considerations in tumor surgery are proper positioning of the patient to facilitate the surgical approach; providing adequate relaxation of the brain to optimize surgical conditions; and avoiding well-known devastating complications, such as venous air embolism.

2. Preoperative assessment of the level of consciousness and a review of relevant radiologic studies should be performed, and the results should be taken into consideration in the anesthetic plan.

3. Adequate brain relaxation is typically achieved with a standard anesthetic including sub-MAC volatile anesthesia, an opioid infusion, mild to moderate hyperventilation, and mannitol.

B. Pituitary Surgery

1. These patients should undergo a preoperative evaluation of their hormonal function to detect hypersecretion of pituitary hormones, which is common in patients with pituitary adenomas, as well as panhypopituitarism. Patients with panhypopituitarism need hormone replacement, including cortisol, levothyroxine, and possibly desmopressin. These medications should be continued in the perioperative period.

2. Small pituitary tumors can be resected by a transsphenoidal approach, but larger tumors may require a craniotomy.

3. Intraoperative monitoring of glucose and electrolytes is essential, particularly if the patient has pre-existing diabetes insipidus (DI) or if the patient develops signs of DI during surgery.

   a. DI is a common complication of pituitary surgery because of the loss of antidiuretic hormone production. It may be temporary or permanent and may occur either in the intraoperative or postoperative period.

   b. DI is initially suspected on the basis of copious urine output, as well as increased serum sodium concentration. A urine specific gravity 1.005 or below is confirmative.

C. Arteriovenous Malformations

1. Cerebral angiography remains the "gold standard" for diagnosis of arteriovenous malformations (AVMs).

2. Although embolization of the AVM is commonly performed, either radiosurgery or an open surgical procedure is typically required subsequent to the embolization to cure the lesion.

3. After resection of large AVMs or those in the posterior fossa, it may be appropriate to take the patient to the intensive care unit (ICU) mechanically ventilated and sedated. If the decision is made by the surgeon and anesthesiologist to allow emergence and extubation of the trachea, aggressive management of blood pressure should be instituted, and coughing should be avoided.

D. Cerebral Aneurysm Surgery and Endovascular Treatment

1. For patients who survive hemorrhage, surgical or endovascular intervention to secure the aneurysm is essential to prevent further hemorrhage.

2. Patients with aneurysmal subarachnoid hemorrhage are at risk for numerous complications that may affect the anesthetic plan. These complications include cardiac dysfunction, neurogenic or cardiogenic pulmonary edema, and hydrocephalus, as well as further hemorrhage from the aneurysm.

3. A patient presenting for the elective correction of an intracranial aneurysm typically has good brain condition, with easily achievable relaxation using mannitol (0.5–1.0 g/kg), mild to moderate hyperventilation, and administration of a low concentration of volatile anesthetic combined with an opioid infusion.

E. Carotid Surgery

1. Carotid stenosis is a common cause of transient ischemic attack and ischemic stroke. It is amenable to surgical intervention and endovascular stenting.

2. Surgery is associated with a risk of stroke, myocardial infarction, and wound infection. With recent advances in medical therapy, including more effective lipid-lowering drugs, antiplatelet agents, and

antihypertensive therapy, the margin of benefit of surgery may be even lower.

3. Both general and regional anesthesia may be used for CEA. Regional anesthesia is accomplished with a superficial cervical plexus block or a combination of superficial and deep cervical plexus block.

4. Several CNS monitors may be used during CEA under general anesthesia.

5. Rapid emergence and tracheal extubation at the end of the procedure are desirable because they allow immediate neurologic assessment.

F. **Epilepsy Surgery and the "Awake" Craniotomy**

1. Some intracranial neurosurgical procedures are performed on "awake" (sedated and pain-free yet able to respond to verbal or visual command) patients to facilitate monitoring of the region of the brain on which the surgeon is operating (epileptic focus).

2. Patients with a difficult airway, obstructive sleep apnea, or orthopnea may present a relative contraindication to an "awake" craniotomy. Patients with severe anxiety, claustrophobia, or other psychiatric disorders may be particularly inappropriate candidates for this type of procedure.

3. For suitable candidates, spontaneous ventilation with propofol anesthesia is an attractive option because it allows emergence with minimal coughing, gagging, or straining. In addition, propofol provides an acceptable anesthetic for these patients because of its low incidence of nausea and vomiting during the awake period. Benzodiazepines should be avoided because they may interfere with electrocorticography during epilepsy surgery. Allowing the patient to emerge during an infusion of low-dose remifentanil or dexmedetomidine may facilitate extubation with little movement.

IX. ANESTHESIA AND TRAUMATIC BRAIN INJURY

A. **Overview of Traumatic Brain Injury**

1. The presence of TBI is the primary determinant in quality of outcome for patients with traumatic injuries.

2. Airway and breathing are of paramount importance in any critically ill patient but even more so in patients with head injuries given the sensitivity of the brain to hypoxemia and hypercapnia.

3. Patients with TBI have a 5% to 6% incidence of an unstable cervical spine injury.
   a. Risk factors include a motor vehicle accident and Glasgow Coma Score (GCS) below 8 (Table 36-9). Therefore, all attempts at intubation should include in-line neck stabilization to decrease the chance of worsening a neurologic injury.
   b. Patients with TBI should generally be intubated orally because the potential presence of a basilar skull fracture may increase the risk associated with a nasal intubation.
4. Minimizing the risk of aspiration during airway procedures is essential. The efficacy of application of cricoid pressure has not been demonstrated, and it may displace cervical fractures; nevertheless, it may be considered the standard of care during rapid sequence intubation.
5. An important consideration is the choice of drugs to facilitate tracheal intubation. Hypotension is extremely detrimental to the injured brain.
6. Administering muscle relaxants prevents coughing and the resultant spikes of ICP. The main choice is between Sch and rocuronium. The main drawback to rocuronium is the prolonged effect when a rapid sequence dose (1.2 mg/kg) is used. The argument against Sch is the potential increase in ICP (this is not supported by clinical data).
7. The overwhelming evidence of harm from hypotension necessitates restoration of intravascular volume. The goal is to maintain CPP in the range of 50 to 70 mm Hg.
8. In the absence of ICP monitoring but with known TBI, an ICP of at least 20 mm Hg should be assumed, and MAP should be kept above 60 mm Hg.
9. Patients with TBI are typically described by their GCS (see Table 39-9). This simple test provides prognostic information and facilitates communication between providers.
10. The presence of a unilateral dilated pupil suggests brainstem compression and is a surgical emergency. The presence of bilateral dilated pupils portends a dismal prognosis.
11. Intracranial hypertension predisposes patients to poor outcomes, and elevated ICP refractory to therapy is associated with a worse prognosis.

TABLE 39-9

GLASGOW COMA SCALE

Eyes	1	No eye opening
	2	Opens to painful stimulation
	3	Open to voice
	4	Spontaneous eye opening
Verbal	1	No sounds
	2	Incomprehensible sounds
	3	Inappropriate words
	4	Confused conversation
	5	Normal speech
Motor	1	No movement
	2	Extension to painful stimulus
	3	Abnormal flexion to painful stimulus
	4	Withdrawal from painful stimulus
	5	Localization of painful stimulus
	6	Follows commands

SURGICAL SUBSPECIALTIES

12. CPP goals are 50 to 70 mm Hg.
13. Reduction of ICP in patients with head injuries can be accomplished effectively using osmotic diuretics.
    a. Mannitol is the most commonly used agent and is available for IV administration in either a 20% or 25% solution. Common doses range from 0.25 to 1 g/kg of body weight. Mannitol may be used on a repeated schedule, but the serum osmolarity should not be allowed to exceed 320 mOsm. Intravascular volume depletion should be avoided.
    b. The mechanism of ICP reduction by mannitol may be related to its osmotic effect in shifting fluid from the brain tissue compartment to the intravascular compartment as well as its ability to decrease blood viscosity.
    c. Hyperventilation is an effective way to reduce ICP. It is useful in the setting of an acutely increased ICP that needs to be controlled until more definitive therapy can be initiated. Current recommendations are that patients with TBI should be maintained at normocapnia except when hypocapnia is necessary to control acute increases in ICP. Chronic hyperventilation should be avoided if possible.
14. Given the rather limited situation in which hypothermia appears to be beneficial in patients with head injury, it is not recommended for routine use.

15. Barbiturates may be used as an adjunct to other therapy for controlling ICP. Barbiturate therapy is appropriate only in patients who are hemodynamically stable and have been adequately resuscitated. Propofol is a reasonable alternative to barbiturates for ICP management. Prolonged use of high-dose propofol is not recommended because it may cause a propofol infusion syndrome.

B. **Anesthetic Management.** Patients with TBI requiring surgery can be subdivided into those who require emergent surgery and those who require non-emergent surgery.

1. **Emergent Neurosurgical Surgery.** These patients commonly arrive in the operating room with an endotracheal tube in place. The neurologic condition of the patient can be determined rapidly by obtaining the GCS, examining the pupils, and reviewing the computed tomography (CT) scan.

   a. The patient's hemodynamic status is also extremely important. Patients may demonstrate a Cushing's response (hypertension and bradycardia), which signifies brainstem compression from increased ICP. These classic findings may be masked by hypovolemia, and their absence does not rule out brainstem compression.

   b. These patients usually do not have ICP monitors in place, but one can assume the presence of intracranial hypertension. The presence of midline shift on CT scan and pupillary abnormalities on physical examination reinforce this diagnosis.

   c. Moderate hyperventilation should be used in these patients until the dura is opened because the elevation in ICP is likely more detrimental than short-term hyperventilation.

   d. Blood pressure management is critical in these patients.

2. **Emergent Non-Neurosurgical Surgery.** Trauma patients presenting for emergent surgical management of noncranial injuries who also have a concurrent TBI are complex to manage. The most immediately life-threatening condition must take priority, but the presence of TBI should be considered, particularly in patients with a depressed level of consciousness or abnormal pupil examination results.

3. **Non-Emergent Neurosurgical Surgery.** Patients with TBI frequently have other injuries, especially fractures

requiring operative fixation. The timing of surgery in these patients remains a controversial issue. In the setting of refractory elevations in ICP or very labile ICP, only emergent surgery should be performed.

X. ANESTHESIA FOR SPINE TRAUMA AND COMPLEX SPINE SURGERY

Surgery on the spinal column has become increasingly complex and lengthy, with multilevel fusions, combined anterior and posterior approaches to the spine, and staged procedures.

A. Spinal Cord Injury

1. **Primary Injury.** SCI can occur without radiographic abnormality, and damage to the spinal column may occur without injury to the spinal cord. Unstable SCI puts the neural elements at risk and necessitates some intervention to provide stability, which may be application of a brace or surgical intervention.

2. **Secondary injury** to the spinal cord is mediated through a cascade of deleterious events similar to those seen in TBI. Secondary injury may be exacerbated by hypotension caused by hemorrhage or neurogenic shock.

3. **Central, Anterior, Brown-Séquard, and Cauda Equina Injuries.** Although a complete cord transection results in disruption of afferent and efferent signals, many injuries damage only a portion of the spinal cord.

   a. **Central cord syndrome** is characterized by greater severity of paresis in the upper extremities than the lower, as well as bladder dysfunction and variable loss of sensation below the lesion.

   b. **Anterior cord syndrome** is generally caused by disruption of blood flow through the anterior spinal artery at the level of the injury. The anterior portion of the cord becomes ischemic, disrupting motor function below the level, with a variable effect on sensation. Pain and temperature tracts are typically interrupted as well, but proprioception remains intact.

   c. **Brown-Séquard syndrome** is characterized by interruption of the lateral half of the spinal cord, typically through penetrating trauma. However, patients may not display all the classic findings of Brown-Séquard syndrome, which include loss of motor and touch sensation ipsilateral to the lesion with pain and temperature sensation lost contralateral to the lesion.

d. **Cauda equina syndrome** is the result of injury below the level of the conus, or caudal end of the cord, typically below L2. Compression of the cauda equina results in perineal anesthesia, urinary retention, fecal incontinence, and lower extremity weakness.

B. **Comorbid Injuries**

1. Cervical spine trauma is associated with blunt cerebrovascular injury, TBI, and facial fractures.

2. Thoracic trauma is also associated with vascular injury; in addition, one must consider the possibility of pneumothorax, myocardial contusion, and pulmonary contusion.

3. Lumbar spine fractures may be associated with bowel and solid viscus injury.

C. **Initial Management**

1. **Urgent Airway Management.** Endotracheal intubation can be particularly difficult in patients with SCI, especially if the lesion is in the cervical spine. Cervical spine injury should be presumed in any trauma patient requiring intubation before complete physical and radiographic evaluation. Intubation should proceed with little movement of the cervical spine. A rapid sequence induction (which may include cricoid pressure) and manual in-line stabilization are appropriate unless a difficult airway is anticipated.

2. **Hemodynamic Stabilization.** Restoration of intravascular volume is the first step in treatment of hypotension in patients with SCI. After euvolemia has been achieved, support of blood pressure with inotropic agents, vasopressors, or both may be required because of loss of sympathetic nervous system control below the level of the lesion (spinal shock).

3. **Role of Steroids.** Methylprednisolone has become a common therapy for patients with neurologic deficit after SCI, although not all practitioners agree steroids are the standard of care.

4. **Timing of Surgical Intervention.** The purpose of surgical intervention is to decompress the neural structures and stabilize the spinal column to prevent further injury to the spinal cord. Persistent hemodynamic instability or severe acute respiratory distress syndrome may impose a significant delay on surgical intervention.

D. **Intraoperative Management**
   1. **Anesthetic Induction and Airway Management.** If the patient's cervical spine has been radiographically and clinically "cleared" before arrival in the operating room, then the technique for induction of anesthesia and endotracheal intubation should be determined by the patient's other injuries, comorbidities, and airway examination results.
      a. Patients with a confirmed cervical spine injury should be immobilized in either a cervical collar or Halo device. A rapid sequence induction remains a viable option, particularly in patients who are unable to cooperate with an awake procedure.
      b. The most conservative approach to airway management in the presence of known cervical spine injury is awake fiberoptic endotracheal intubation (which requires thorough application of topical anesthesia to the airway).
   2. **Anesthetic Technique**
      a. Complex spine and trauma surgery imposes a significant risk of blood loss. An arterial catheter is essential for continuous hemodynamic monitoring and intermittent arterial blood gas and hematocrit analysis.
      b. In large thoracic or lumbar spine surgeries, particularly in the prone position, central venous access may be appropriate. The value of central venous pressure monitoring is controversial, however, because it is neither a good indicator of end-diastolic volume nor a predictor of volume responsiveness in patients with hypotension.
      c. Placement of a pulmonary artery catheter can be justified in sick patients with poor cardiac function, especially those in whom fluid management is difficult and vasopressor therapy is required.
   3. **Neuromonitoring.** The goals of spine surgery, whether for trauma or other spine disease, are typically to decompress the cord and stabilize the spinal column. These goals must be accomplished without inflicting further injury to the spinal cord. Monitoring spinal cord function is appropriate for many surgical procedures. The anesthetic plan must be tailored to accommodate these monitors.
   4. **Patient Positioning.** The prone position provides unique challenges to the anesthesiologist with respect

to achieving adequate protection of the patient from pressure points (eyes, face, breasts, genitals, knees, toes). Frequent confirmation that the eyes are free from contact is important. The slight reverse Trendelenburg position may facilitate venous drainage from the head and reduce congestion and intraocular pressure. Padding on the chest should not compress the neck because this may also obstruct venous drainage.

5. **Glucose Management.** There is little evidence to guide the management of glucose in patients with disease of the spine, particularly in the intraoperative setting.

   a. It is reasonable to continue tight glycemic control in patients who arrive in the operating room from the ICU, and it is reasonable to start tight glycemic control on patients who will be admitted to the ICU after surgery.

   b. These recommendations assume that frequent glucose monitoring is an integral part of the anesthetic procedure.

   c. In patients who are administered methylprednisolone, glucose control may be more difficult to achieve.

E. **Complications of Anesthesia for Spine Surgery**

1. **Autonomic Hyperreflexia.** Patients with chronic spinal cord lesions above T7 may develop autonomic reflexia when stimulated below the site of the lesion (intense vasoconstriction below the site of the lesion accompanied by cutaneous vasodilation above, hypertension, and bradycardia). To reduce the incidence of this complication, suppression of the afferent pathway by "deepening" anesthesia is necessary. A spinal anesthetic, if possible, may be ideal.

2. **Postoperative Visual Loss.** The visual loss is commonly bilateral and caused by ischemic optic neuropathy (which has a multifactorial etiology), although retinal artery occlusion and cortical blindness may also occur.

   a. Postoperative visual loss may occur despite the absence of pressure on the eyes from positioning errors, which would result in central retinal artery thrombosis rather than anterior or posterior ischemic optic neuropathy.

   b. Ischemic optic neuropathy is associated with blood loss and a long operative duration.

   c. Given the increasing recognition of this problem, it may be a preoperative consideration to inform high-risk patients (those in whom blood loss and long surgeries are anticipated) of this rare event.

d. There is no proven method to prevent ischemic optic neuropathy nor is there a reliable method to monitor visual function during these procedures.

e. Staging of a complex spine procedure may be the most effective means of preventing this devastating complication because limiting the duration of the procedure would also limit the risk of hypotension and blood loss.

CHAPTER 40 ■ ANESTHESIA FOR THORACIC SURGERY

The increased incidence of lung cancer has led to an increase in the amount of noncardiac thoracic surgery that is performed in the United States (Neustein SM, Eisenkraft JB, Cohen E: Anesthesia for thoracic surgery. In *Clinical Anesthesia*. Edited by Barash PG, Cullen BF, Stoelting RK, Cahalan MK, Stock MC. Philadelphia: Lippincott Williams & Wilkins, 2009, pp 1032–1072).

I. PREOPERATIVE EVALUATION

A. The preoperative evaluation should focus on the extent and severity of pulmonary disease and cardiovascular involvement. Patients undergoing thoracic surgery who are known to be at high risk for postoperative complications include elderly individuals and people with poor general health or chronic obstructive pulmonary disease (COPD).

B. **History** (Table 40-1)

C. **Physical Examination** (Table 40-2)

D. **Laboratory Studies** (Table 40-3)

1. A vital capacity at least three times the tidal volume is necessary for an effective cough. A vital capacity below 50% of predicted or below 2 L is an indicator of increased risk.

2. Thoracoscopic surgery and improved postoperative pain management have made it possible for patients with even smaller lung volumes to successfully undergo surgery.

3. The ratio of forced expiratory volume in 1 second to forced vital capacity (FEV_1/FVC) is useful in differentiating restrictive (normal ratio as both are decreased) from obstructive (low ratio as FEV_1 is decreased) disease.

TABLE 40-1

PATIENT MEDICAL HISTORY THAT SHOULD BE OBTAINED BEFORE THORACIC SURGERY

Dyspnea (quantitate as to activity required to produce it; its presence may warn of the need for postoperative ventilation)
Cough (characteristics of sputum)
Cigarette smoking
Exercise tolerance (patients have an increased risk when they are unable to climb two flights of stairs)
Risk factors for acute lung injury (alcohol abuse, high ventilatory pressures, excessive fluid administration)

TABLE 40-2

PHYSICAL EXAMINATION THAT SHOULD BE DONE BEFORE THORACIC SURGERY

Respiratory System
Cyanosis
Clubbing
Breathing rate and pattern (distinguish between obstructive and restrictive disease)
Breath sounds (wet sounds versus wheezing)

Cardiovascular System (presence of pulmonary hypertension)

TABLE 40-3

LABORATORY STUDIES THAT SHOULD BE DONE BEFORE THORACIC SURGERY

Electrocardiography (evidence of right ventricular hypertrophy)
Chest radiography
Arterial blood gas analysis ("blue bloaters" vs. "pink puffers")
Pulmonary function tests (evaluation of lung resectability; FEV_1 <35% is not considered for major lung resection)
CT and PET scan
Diffusing capacity for carbon monoxide
Maximal oxygen consumption
Maximal stair climbing

CT = computed tomography; FEV_1 = forced expiratory volume in 1 second; PET = positron emission tomography.

TABLE 40-4

FACTORS THAT PREDISPOSE PATIENTS TO COMPLICATIONS AFTER THORACIC SURGERY

Smoking (carboxyhemoglobin decreases in 48 hours; improvement of ciliary function and decrease in sputum production require 8–12 weeks)

Infection

Hypovolemia and electrolyte balance (facilitate removal of bronchial secretions)

Wheezing (sympathomimetic drugs, steroids, cromolyn, parasympatholytic drugs)

4. A 15% improvement in pulmonary function tests after bronchodilator therapy is an indication for continued preoperative therapy.
5. A mass that is seen on computed tomography is more likely to be malignant if it also demonstrates enhanced glucose uptake on the positron emission tomography scan.

II. PREOPERATIVE PREPARATION

A. Several conditions predispose patients to postoperative complications, and their preoperative treatment is associated with decreases in morbidity and mortality (Table 40-4).
B. Patients scheduled for lung resection may benefit from tests to determine the extent of resection that will be tolerated as well as cardiopulmonary function testing in the presence of unilateral pulmonary artery occlusion (Fig. 40-1).

III. INTRAOPERATIVE MONITORING

A. Invasive monitoring and pulse oximetry have improved patient care (Table 40-5).
B. An arterial catheter is essential to provide continuous recordings of blood pressure because surgical manipulations or intravascular volume shifts may cause sudden changes in blood pressure.
C. Pulse oximetry is the standard of care for noninvasive assessment of blood oxygenation (especially during one-lung ventilation).
D. Serial arterial blood gas determinations are necessary to confirm the adequacy of ventilation and

Whole-lung Function

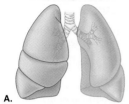

$$\begin{cases} \text{ABG (Fio}_2 = 0.21) & \text{Paco}_2 > 46 \text{ mm Hg} \\ & \text{Pao}_2 < 60 \text{ mm Hg} \\ \text{FVC} & < 50\% \text{ or } 1.5 \text{ mL/kg} \\ \text{FEV}_1 & < 50\% \\ \text{VC} & < 2 \text{ L} \\ \text{MVV} & < 50\% \text{ or } < 50 \text{ L/min} \\ \text{Lung Volume} & \text{RV/TLC} > 50\% \\ \text{DLco} & < 50\% \end{cases}$$

A.

Split-lung Function

1. Split-lung Spirometry With DLT
2. Regional Lung Radiospirometry
   Regional Perfusion (^{133}Xe, ^{131}I-MAA)
   Regional Ventilation ^{133}Xe

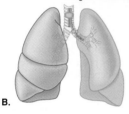

$$\begin{cases} \text{Predicted Postresection FEV}_1 < 800 \text{ mL} \\ \\ \text{Blood Flow to the Resected Lung} > 70\% \end{cases}$$

B.

**Unilateral Pulmonary
Artery Occlusion**

FIGURE 40-1. The order of tests to determine the cardiopulmonary function status of the patient and the extent of resection that will be tolerated by the patient.

    oxygenation as suggested by capnography and pulse oximetry.

  E. During thoracotomy, a radial artery catheter is often placed in the dependent arm to aid in stabilizing the catheter. This catheter can also be used to monitor for possible axillary artery compression to avoid compression of the artery and brachial plexus with placement of a chest roll (misnomer, "axillary roll") under dependent hemothorax.

IV. PHYSIOLOGY OF ONE-LUNG VENTILATION

  A. Physiology of the Lateral Decubitus Position
    1. In an open-chested, anesthetized, and paralyzed patient, the dependent lung is overperfused (gravity-dependent blood flow) and underventilated.

TABLE 40-5

INVASIVE MONITORING FOR THORACIC SURGERY

Direct arterial catheterization placed in the dependent arm for thoracotomy; right radial warns of innominate artery compression during mediastinoscopy)

Central venous pressure (acceptable in patients with good ventricular function undergoing pneumonectomy)

Pulmonary artery catheter (during one-lung ventilation, the accuracy of measurements may depend on position of the catheter)

Transesophageal echocardiography (reflects ventricular and valvular function; wall motion abnormalities may be caused by myocardial ischemia)

Noninvasive digital sensor placed on the ear lobe (continuous monitoring of $PaCO_2$, SpO_2, and heart rate)

2. Underventilation reflects minimal pressure of abdominal contents pressing against the upper diaphragm, making it easier for positive pressure ventilation to distend the nondependent lung.

V. ONE-LUNG VENTILATION

A. Indications for one-lung ventilation may be categorized as absolute and relative (Table 40-6).

B. **Double-Lumen Endobronchial Tubes**
   1. These tubes are the most widely used means of achieving lung separation and one-lung ventilation.

TABLE 40-6

INDICATIONS FOR ONE-LUNG VENTILATION

Absolute Indications
Prevent contamination of healthy lung (abscess, hemorrhage)
Control distribution of ventilation (bronchopleural fistula)
Minimally invasive cardiac procedures

Relative Indications
Surgical exposure, high priority
Thoracic aneurysm
Pneumonectomy
Upper lobe lobectomy
Surgical exposure, low priority
Esophageal resection
Middle and lower lobe lobectomy

The design of double-lumen tubes (there are many different types, but the design is similar for all) is characterized by two catheters bonded together with one lumen long enough to reach a mainstem bronchus while the other shorter catheter portion remains in the trachea above the carina.

2. Lung separation is achieved by inflation of the tracheal and bronchial cuff. The bronchial cuff on a right-sided tube is slotted to allow ventilation of the right upper lobe because the right mainstem bronchus is too short to accommodate both the right lumen tip and cuff.

3. **Robershaw tubes** are available as left- or right-sided clear plastic disposable tubes without a carinal hook. Lumina are of sufficient size to facilitate suctioning and offer low resistance to gas flow. The blue endobronchial cuff is easily recognized when fiberoptic bronchoscopy is used to confirm its position.

4. A rubber silicone left double-lumen tube (Silbonco) is especially useful if the left mainstem bronchus is angled at 90 degrees from the trachea, making it almost impossible to position a conventional double-lumen tube.

5. A left-sided double-lumen tube is preferred for both right- and left-sided procedures. (The left mainstem bronchus is longer than the right mainstem bronchus.)

   a. Typically, most women need a 37-Fr double-lumen tube, and most men are adequately managed with a 39-Fr double-lumen tube.

   b. The depth required for insertion of the double-lumen tube correlates with the patient's height (29 cm for people who are 170 to 180 cm tall, and for every 10-cm increase or decrease in height, the double-lumen tube is advanced or withdrawn 1 cm).

C. **Placement of Double-Lumen (Robershaw) Tubes**

1. Initial insertion of the tube is performed with the distal concave curvature facing anteriorly. After the tip of the tube is past the vocal cords, the stylet is removed, and the tube is rotated 90 degrees to direct the bronchial lumen appropriately toward the desired mainstem bronchus. Advancement of the tube is ended when moderate resistance to further passage is encountered (~29 cm in most adults), indicating that the tube tip has been firmly seated in the mainstem bronchus (Fig. 40-2).

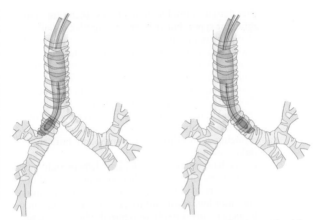

FIGURE 40-2. Schematic depiction of the proper placement of a right or left endobronchial tube.

    2. After the tube is judged to be in the proper position, a sequence of steps is performed to check the tube's location (Table 40-7).

    3. Confirmation of placement using a fiberoptic bronchoscope is recommended (Table 40-8 and Figs. 40-3 and 40-4).

  D. **Lung separation in a patient with a tracheostomy** may be achieved with a separately inserted bronchial blocker. (Standard double-lumen tubes are usually too stiff to negotiate the curve required for insertion through a tracheal stoma.)

TABLE 40-7

STEPS TO VERIFY PROPER POSITION OF A DOUBLE-LUMEN TUBE

Inflate the tracheal cuff and confirm bilateral and equal breath sounds.

Inflate the bronchial cuff (rarely >2 mL of air) and confirm bilateral and equal breath sounds (ensures that the bronchial cuff is not obstructing the contralateral hemithorax).

Selectively clamp each lumen and confirm one-lung ventilation.

Perform bronchoscopy using a fiberoptic bronchoscope. Nearly 50% of tubes thought to be properly positioned by auscultation and examination were not confirmed by bronchoscopy (see Table 40-8.)

TABLE 40-8

USE OF A FIBEROPTIC BRONCHOSCOPE TO VERIFY PROPER
PLACEMENT OF A DOUBLE-LUMEN TUBE

Left-Sided Tube
Tracheal lumen (visualize the carina and upper surface of blue
  endobronchial cuff just below the carina)
Bronchial lumen (identify the left upper lobe orifice)

Right-Sided Tube
Tracheal lumen (visualize the carina)
Bronchial lumen (identify right upper lobe orifice)

  E. **Lung separation in a patient with a difficult airway**
     may include use of a flexible fiberoptic endoscope, a
     double-lumen or Univent tube using a tube exchanger
     plus laryngoscopy, or a tube exchanger and bronchial
     blocker.

VI. MANAGEMENT OF ONE-LUNG VENTILATION

  A. A goal of one-lung ventilation is to optimize arterial
     oxygenation (Table 40-9).

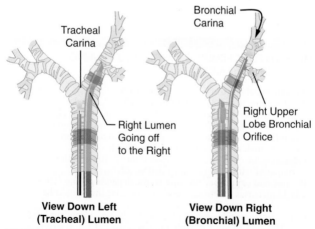

FIGURE 40-3. Use of a fiberscope to verify position of a double-lumen
tube.

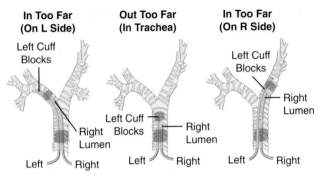

FIGURE 40-4. Examples of double-lumen tube malpositions.

B. **Clinical Approach to the Management of One-Lung Ventilation**
   1. The position of the double-lumen tube should be rechecked after the patient has been placed in the lateral decubitus position. Two-lung ventilation is maintained as long as possible.
   2. **During One-Lung Ventilation.** After initiation of one-lung ventilation, PaO_2 can continue to decrease for up to 45 minutes. (Pulse oximetry is a vital monitor.)

TABLE 40-9

METHODS FOR OPTIMIZING OXYGENATION DURING ONE-LUNG VENTILATION

Maximize delivered oxygen concentration.

Tidal volume to the dependent lung is 10 to 12 mL/kg, and the rate is adjusted to maintain the $PaCO_2$ near 35 mm Hg. The practitioner should consider decreasing the tidal volume (6 mL/kg) as necessary to avoid increase in airway pressure, thereby making acute lung injury less likely.

Pressure-controlled ventilation may improve oxygenation compared with volume-controlled ventilation.

Positive end-expiratory pressure to the dependent lung (10 cm H_2O increases functional residual capacity; this should be considered when PaO_2 is low).

Continuous positive airway pressure to the nondependent lung (5–10 cm H_2O most reliably improves the $PaCO_2$, distends alveoli, and diverts blood flow to the dependent lung).

   a. If arterial hypoxemia occurs during one-lung ventilation, it is important to verify proper positioning of the tube using a fiberscope.
   b. If arterial hypoxemia persists after verification of tube position, addition of continuous positive airway pressure or positive end-expiratory pressure should be considered.
   c. Airway pressure should be monitored because a sudden increase may reflect tube dislocation.
   3. The practitioner should never hesitate to reinstitute two-lung ventilation until a patient can be stabilized or the cause of a patient's instability (arterial hypoxemia, hypotension, cardiac dysrhythmias) has been corrected.

VII. CHOICE OF ANESTHESIA FOR THORACIC SURGERY

A. The likely presence of increased airway reactivity (cigarette smoking, chronic bronchitis, obstructive pulmonary disease) and the effect of volatile anesthetics or ketamine on bronchomotor tone should be considered.
   1. Propofol infusion in combination with remifentanil is useful for producing anesthesia associated with one-lung anesthesia and no effect on hypoxic pulmonary vasoconstriction.
   2. Lidocaine (1–2 mg/kg intravenously [IV]) has been used before airway manipulations to decrease the likelihood of reflex bronchospasm.
B. An adequate depth of anesthesia before airway manipulation is the most important goal in managing patients with increased airway reactivity.

VIII. HYPOXIC PULMONARY VASOCONSTRICTION

A. Hypoxic pulmonary vasoconstriction is a homeostatic mechanism that normally diverts blood flow away from hypoxic (atelectatic) regions of the lungs (local increases in pulmonary vascular resistance) and thereby optimizes oxygenation.
B. Inhibition of hypoxic pulmonary vasoconstriction during one-lung ventilation may accentuate arterial hypoxemia. Nevertheless, inhaled anesthetics do not seem to interfere with hypoxic pulmonary vasoconstriction.

IX. ANESTHESIA FOR DIAGNOSTIC PROCEDURES

A. **Bronchoscopy** is most often performed with a fiberoptic bronchoscope that easily passes through a tracheal tube of 8.0 to 8.5 mm internal diameter.

B. **Mediastinoscopy** (Table 40-10)

C. **Thoracoscopy**

1. Insertion of an endoscope into the thoracic cavity and pleural space is used for the diagnosis of pleural disease, effusions, and infectious diseases (especially acquired immunodeficiency syndrome) and for staging procedures and lung biopsy.

2. Anesthesia can be provided using local, regional, or general anesthesia depending on the expected duration of the procedure and the physical status of the patient.

   a. If general anesthesia is required, either a single- or a double-lumen tube may be used. Positive pressure ventilation interferes with visualization via the endoscope, so a double-lumen tube is preferred.

   b. The spontaneous partial pneumothorax that occurs when the endoscope is inserted results in improved surgical visualization. The spontaneous pneumothorax is usually well tolerated even in awake patients because the skin and chest wall form a seal around the thoracoscope and limit the degree of lung collapse.

D. **Video-assisted thoracoscopic surgery (VATS)** entails making small incisions in the chest wall, which allows the introduction of a video camera and surgical instruments into the thoracic cavity.

TABLE 40-10

ANESTHETIC CONSIDERATIONS DURING MEDIASTINOSCOPY

Signs of Eaton-Lambert syndrome
Hemorrhage
Pneumothorax
Venous air embolism
Recurrent laryngeal nerve injury
Pressure on the innominate artery (manifests as a decreased right radial pulse and necessitates repositioning of the mediastinoscope, especially in the presence of cerebrovascular disease)

1. **Anesthesia Considerations**
   a. As with traditional thoracotomy, the patient needs to be positioned in the lateral decubitus position for VATS, and lung collapse is needed for adequate surgical exposure.
   b. The need for one-lung ventilation is greater with VATS than with open thoracotomy because it is not possible to retract the lung during VATS as it is during an open thoracotomy.
   c. The operated lung should be deflated as soon as possible after tracheal intubation because it may take as long as 30 minutes for complete lung collapse to occur.
   d. Carbon dioxide insufflation into the pleural cavity is used to facilitate visualization. Insufflation pressures should be kept low (<5 mm Hg) because high pressures can cause mediastinal shift and hemodynamic compromise.
   e. Continuous positive airway pressure as commonly used to treat arterial hypoxemia during one-lung ventilation for an open thoracotomy is unacceptable during VATS (it would interfere with surgical procedure). During VATS, positive end-expiratory pressure to the non-operated (dependent) lung should be used.

2. **Postoperative Concerns**
   a. Pain after VATS is less than after an open thoracotomy.
   b. Respiratory function is better preserved after VATS.

X. ANESTHESIA FOR SPECIAL SITUATIONS

A. **High-frequency jet ventilation** techniques are often appropriate.

B. **Bronchopleural fistula and empyema** are more likely to occur after a pneumonectomy than after other types of lung resection. Management of anesthesia in such patients includes several considerations (Table 40-11).
   1. An alternative to tracheal intubation in awake patients is placement of a double-lumen tube under general anesthesia with the patient breathing spontaneously.
   2. Rapid sequence induction of anesthesia plus a muscle relaxant followed by placement of a single-lumen tracheal tube may be acceptable if the air leak is small and an empyema is not present.

TABLE 40-11

ANESTHETIC CONSIDERATIONS IN MANAGEMENT OF A PATIENT WITH A BRONCHOPLEURAL FISTULA

Drain the empyema before induction of anesthesia.

Awake tracheal intubation using a double-lumen tube (with the bronchial lumen directed to the side opposite the fistula; an outpouring of pus from the tracheal lumen should be anticipated if an empyema is present).

Instituting controlled ventilation before placement of a double-lumen tube may result in hypoventilation because of a large air leak.

The chest drainage tube should be left open to prevent tension pneumothorax.

    3. For a large bronchopleural fistula, high-frequency jet ventilation may be the nonsurgical treatment of choice.

  C. **Lung Cysts and Bullae**

    1. These disorders usually represent end-stage emphysematous destruction of the lungs associated with severe obstructive pulmonary disease and carbon dioxide retention.

    2. Positive pressure ventilation or nitrous oxide may cause bullae to expand or rupture (tension pneumothorax).

    3. Ideally, a double-lumen tube is inserted with the patient breathing spontaneously while awake or during general anesthesia.

    4. Gentle positive pressure ventilation with rapid, small tidal volumes and pressures not to exceed 10 cm H_2O may be used during the induction and maintenance of anesthesia, especially if the bullae have been shown to have no or only poor bronchial communication.

  D. **Anesthesia for resection of the trachea** may be necessary to relieve stenosis that may occur after prolonged tracheal intubation or tracheotomy (Table 40-12).

  E. **Bronchopulmonary lavage** is performed under general anesthesia using a double-lumen tube, most often for the treatment of cystic fibrosis.

XI. MYASTHENIA GRAVIS

  A. Myasthenia gravis is caused by a decrease in the number of postsynaptic acetylcholine receptors (circulating

TABLE 40-12

ANESTHETIC CONSIDERATIONS FOR TRACHEAL RESECTION

Use left radial artery cannulation (permits continuous monitoring of blood pressure during periods of innominate artery compression).

Use corticosteroids to decrease tracheal edema.

Deliver 100% oxygen to facilitate periods of apneic oxygenation.

Consider placing a small anode (wire-reinforced) tracheal tube above the stenosis, followed by distal placement of a sterile tracheal or bronchial tube after the trachea is exposed. Other options include high-frequency jet ventilation or cardiopulmonary bypass.

Postoperatively, keep the head flexed and strive for early tracheal extubation.

antibodies to the receptors), resulting in a decrease in the margin of safety of neuromuscular transmission (exercise-induced weakness).

B. **Medical Therapy**
1. Anticholinesterase drugs are administered in an attempt to prolong the duration of action of acetylcholine. Whereas anticholinesterase overdose causes a cholinergic crisis (treat with IV atropine), underdose causes a myasthenic crisis (improves with edrophonium, 2–10 mg IV).
2. Plasmapheresis decreases antibody titers, resulting in transient improvement. (It also causes a decrease in plasma cholinesterase.)

C. **Thymectomy**
1. This surgery is considered the treatment of choice in most patients with myasthenia gravis.
2. The gland is removed by a median sternotomy or transcervically using a technique similar to mediastinoscopy (there is a lower incidence of post-operative ventilatory failure).

D. **Management of General Anesthesia** (Table 40-13).

E. **Nondepolarizing Muscle Relaxants**
1. It is prudent to assume that even treated patients are sensitive to the effects of muscle relaxants, so the initial dose should be decreased. One approach is to titrate to effect using a peripheral nerve stimulator beginning with doses of muscle relaxant that are 1/10 to 1/20 the usual dose.
2. Sugammadex is designed to bind rocuronium and provide rapid, complete, and long-lasting

TABLE 40-13

ANESTHETIC CONSIDERATIONS IN MANAGEMENT OF
THYMECTOMY FOR TREATMENT OF MYASTHENIA GRAVIS

Evaluate the adequacy of drug therapy (corticosteroids,
  anticholinesterases).
Perform pulmonary function tests.
Continue anticholinesterase drugs preoperatively (controversial).
Use modest preoperative medication (benzodiazepines; avoid
  opioids).
For induction of anesthesia, use an intravenous drug followed by
  a volatile anesthetic to facilitate tracheal intubation.
Anticipate the need for postoperative support of ventilation of the
  patient's lungs.
Avoid drugs with skeletal muscle–relaxing properties
  (antiarrhythmics, diuretics, aminoglycosides).
For patients with sensitivity to nondepolarizing muscle relaxants
  avoid nonrelaxant techniques avoid risks of muscle relaxants by
  using combinations of propofol, opioids, and short-acting
  inhaled anesthetics.

TABLE 40-14

POSTOPERATIVE CONSIDERATIONS AFTER THORACIC SURGERY

Postoperative pain control (optimizes ventilation)
  Patient-controlled analgesia
  Low-dose ketamine (0.05 mg/kg/hr) as adjunct to epidural
    analgesia or added to morphine for patient-controlled
    analgesia
  Intercostal nerve blocks (2–3 mL of 0.5% bupivacaine)
  Cryoanalgesia
  Neuraxial opioids (epidural or intrathecal morphine diluted in
    saline; the intrathecal dose is about 1/10 the epidural dose; an
    opioid should be administered before surgical incision as
    "pre-emptive analgesia")
Atelectasis (rapid, shallow breathing in response to pain;
  treatment is any maneuver that increases functional residual
  capacity)
Low cardiac output syndrome (intravascular fluid volume should
  be replaced; the use of inotropes, vasodilators, or both should be
  considered)
Cardiac dysrhythmias (supraventricular tachycardias; prophylactic
  digitalis should be considered if the patient is normokalemic)
Hemorrhage (should be re-explored if blood loss >200 mL/hr)
Tension pneumothorax
Peripheral nerve injury (intercostal, brachial plexus, recurrent
  laryngeal)

antagonism of rocuronium-induced neuromuscular blockade.

F. **Depolarizing Relaxants.** Patients treated with anticholinesterases may be sensitive to succinylcholine, reflecting slowed metabolism of the muscle relaxant.

G. **Nonrelaxant Techniques.** Because of concerns over the use of muscle relaxants in patients with myasthenia gravis, there have been many reports of successful use of drug combinations (propofol with nitrous oxide and fentanyl; sevoflurane with nitrous oxide and fentanyl) that do not include paralysis.

H. **Postoperative Care.** The opioid dose should be decreased by one third because anticholinesterases may increase the analgesic effect of these drugs.

XII. POSTOPERATIVE MANAGEMENT AND COMPLICATIONS (Table 40-14)

CHAPTER 41 ■ ANESTHESIA FOR CARDIAC SURGERY

Management of anesthesia for cardiac surgery requires a thorough understanding of normal and altered cardiac physiology; knowledge of the pharmacology of anesthetic, vasoactive, and cardioactive drugs; and familiarity with the physiologic derangements associated with cardiopulmonary bypass (CPB) and specific surgical procedures (Skubas N, Lichtman AD, Sharma A, Thomas SJ: Anesthesia for cardiac surgery. In *Clinical Anesthesia*. Edited by Barash PG, Cullen BF, Stoelting RK, Cahalan MK, Stock MC. Philadelphia: Lippincott Williams & Wilkins, 2009, pp 1073–1107).

I. CORONARY ARTERY DISEASE (CAD)

Prevention or treatment of myocardial ischemia during coronary artery bypass graft (CABG) surgery decreases the incidence of perioperative myocardial infarction. Optimizing oxygen delivery to the myocardium is equally important for hemodynamic management.

A. **Myocardial Oxygen Demand.** The principal determinants of myocardial oxygen demand are wall tension and contractility. Interventions that prevent or promptly treat ventricular distention and decrease myocardial oxygen consumption decrease myocardial oxygen demand.

B. **Myocardial Oxygen Supply.** Increases in myocardial oxygen requirements can only be met by increasing coronary blood flow.

1. **Coronary Blood Flow** (Table 41-1)
   a. The left ventricular subendocardium is most vulnerable to ischemia because myocardial oxygen requirements are high and predictable perfusion can occur only during diastole. The time available for diastole decreases with an increasing heart rate.
   b. A low ventricular filling pressure is desirable for improving perfusion (higher pressure gradient)

TABLE 41-1

DETERMINANTS OF CORONARY BLOOD FLOW

Perfusion pressure
Vascular tone
Time available for perfusion (heart rate)
Severity of intraluminal obstructions
Presence of collateral circulation

and decreasing myocardial oxygen requirements (decreased ventricular volume and wall tension).

c. It is common during anesthesia for patients to exhibit signs of myocardial ischemia without any change in blood pressure, heart rate, or ventricular filling pressure.

C. **Hemodynamic Goals**

1. Although the precise relationship between intraoperative myocardial ischemia and postoperative myocardial infarction remains controversial, there is consensus that a primary goal of a successful anesthetic is the prevention of myocardial ischemia.

2. Combinations of anesthetics, sedatives, muscle relaxants, and vasoactive drugs are selected to decrease myocardial oxygen requirements and thus prevent or decrease the likelihood of myocardial ischemia.

3. Pharmacologic agents that may benefit patients with CAD include statins and angiotensin-converting enzyme (ACE) inhibitors (stabilize atherosclerotic plaques) and volatile anesthetics (anesthetic preconditioning).

D. **Monitoring for Ischemia.** The ideal monitoring technique for detecting myocardial ischemia is not yet available (Table 41-2).

E. **Selection of Anesthesia.** There is no one ideal anesthetic for patients with CAD. The choice of anesthetic depends primarily on the extent of pre-existing myocardial dysfunction and the pharmacologic properties of the specific drugs. Myocardial depression and associated decreases in myocardial oxygen requirements are only harmful in a patient whose heart cannot be further depressed without precipitating congestive heart failure.

1. Early tracheal extubation is popular for both on- and off-pump cardiac procedures. Volatile anesthetics in

TABLE 41-2

MONITORING FOR MYOCARDIAL ISCHEMIA

Electrocardiogram (ST segment analysis of leads V5 and II)
Heart rate and blood pressure (rate-pressure product is not a
  sensitive predictor of myocardial ischemia)
Pulmonary artery catheter (V waves reflect ischemia-induced
  papillary muscle dysfunction but are probably not a sensitive
  indicator of myocardial ischemia)
TEE (regional wall motion abnormalities are the most sensitive
  indicator of myocardial ischemia)

TEE = transesophageal echocardiography.

combination with low-dose opioids or total
intravenous (IV) anesthesia with short-acting drugs
(midazolam, alfentanil, propofol) has been used to
facilitate the likelihood of early tracheal extubation.
Neuraxial opioids placed before induction of anesthesia decrease postoperative pain and facilitate
early tracheal extubation.

2. **Opioids** lack myocardial depressant effects and are
useful in patients with severe myocardial
dysfunction. In critically ill patients, opioids such as
fentanyl (50–100 µg/kg IV) can be administered as
the sole anesthetic. In patients with good left
ventricular function, opioids may be inadequate to
depress sympathetic nervous system activity, requiring the addition of a volatile anesthetic or
vasoactive drug.

3. **Inhalation anesthetics** have the advantages of dose
dependency; easily reversible, titratable myocardial
depression; amnesia; and reliable suppression of
sympathetic nervous system responses to surgical
stress and CPB. Disadvantages include myocardial
depression, systemic hypotension, and lack of postoperative analgesia.

   a. Combinations of opioids and volatile anesthetics
   may produce the advantages of each with minimal undesirable side effects. It is likely that any
   volatile anesthetic could be used as a balanced
   technique.

   b. **Isoflurane** is a coronary vasodilator (more so
   than other volatile anesthetics), but this effect is
   clinically insignificant in doses below 1 MAC.

There is no evidence of an increased incidence of myocardial ischemia or worsened outcome.

   c. **Desflurane** and **sevoflurane** possess hemodynamic profiles similar to isoflurane but have the advantage of faster recovery. A sudden increase in the inspired concentration of desflurane may result in increased heart rate, systemic blood pressure, and plasma epinephrine concentration.

  4. **Intravenous Sedative Hypnotics.** An alternative adjuvant anesthetic to the low-dose opioid technique is a titratable infusion of a short-acting sedative (propofol, midazolam, dexmedetomidine) that can be continued after surgery and after discontinuation affords a predictable and fairly rapid awakening.

F. **Treatment of Ischemia.** Anesthetics or vasoactive drugs that enable the heart to return to a slower rate, smaller size, and well-perfused state are frequently essential during anesthesia (Table 41-3).

  1. **Nitrates.** Nitroglycerin is the drug of choice for the treatment of coronary vasospasm. As a venodilator, this drug decreases venous return and decreases ventricular filling pressures and thus wall tension.

TABLE 41-3

TREATMENT OF INTRAOPERATIVE MYOCARDIAL ISCHEMIA

Event Associated with Ischemia	Treatment*
Increased blood pressure and pulmonary wedge pressure	Increase anesthetic depth Nitroglycerin (0.5–3.0 µg/kg/min IV) Sodium nitroprusside (0.5–3.0 µg/kg/min IV)
Increased heart rate	β-Antagonists Calcium channel blockers
Decreased blood pressure	Decrease anesthetic depth Phenylephrine
Decreased blood pressure and increased pulmonary capillary wedge pressure	Phenylephrine Nitroglycerin Inotrope
Normal hemodynamics	Nitroglycerin Calcium channel blocker

*The goal is to return the heart to a slow, small, perfused state.
IV = intravenous.

2. **Vasoconstrictors.** Phenylephrine increases myocardial oxygen requirements, but this increase is offset by improvements in oxygen delivery produced by the increased coronary perfusion pressure.

3. **Beta-Blockers.** β-blockade improves myocardial oxygen balance by preventing or treating tachycardia and by decreasing contractility. Atenolol improves long-term survival in patients with heart disease undergoing noncardiac surgery.

4. **Calcium Channel Blockers**
   a. **Verapamil** is useful in the treatment of supraventricular tachycardia and slowing the ventricular response in atrial fibrillation and flutter. Myocardial depressant effects may limit its usefulness in some patients.
   b. **Nifedipine** and **diltiazem** are coronary vasodilators that are used as antianginal drugs and in the prevention of coronary vasospasm.

II. **VALVULAR HEART DISEASE** is characterized by pressure or volume overload of the atria or ventricles. Transesophageal echocardiography (TEE) has become a commonly used monitor in the perioperative management of patients undergoing cardiac surgery.

A. **Aortic Stenosis**
   1. The normal aortic valve is composed of three semilunar cusps attached to the wall of the aorta. The normal annular diameter is 1.9 to 2.3 cm with an aortic valve area of 2 to 4 cm^2. The normal diameter of the left ventricular outflow tract is 2.2 cm.
   2. **Pathophysiology** (Fig. 41-1). Chronic obstruction to left ventricular ejection results in concentric ventricular hypertrophy, which makes the heart susceptible to myocardial ischemia even in the absence of CAD. Because the ventricle is stiff, atrial contraction is critical for ventricular filling and stroke volume.
   3. **Anesthetic Considerations.** Maintenance of adequate ventricular volume and sinus rhythm is crucial. If hypotension develops, it must be treated early to prevent the catastrophic cycle of hypotension-induced ischemia, subsequent ventricular dysfunction, and worsening hypotension. Bradycardia is a common cause of hypotension in patients with aortic stenosis.

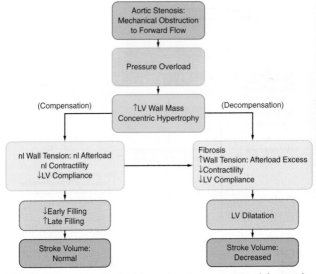

FIGURE 41-1. The pathophysiology of aortic stenosis. LV = left ventricle.

B. **Hypertrophic cardiomyopathy** is a genetically determined disease characterized by development of a hypertrophic intraventricular septum, resulting in left ventricular outflow obstruction (resembling aortic stenosis). Outflow obstruction is increased by increases in myocardial contractility or heart rate or decreases in preload or afterload. Anesthetic management is based on maintenance of left ventricular filling and controlled myocardial depression.

C. **Aortic Insufficiency**
   1. **Pathophysiology** (Fig. 41-2). Chronic volume overload of the left ventricle evokes eccentric hypertrophy but only minimal changes in filling pressures.
   2. **Anesthetic Considerations.** Maintenance of adequate ventricular volume in the presence of mild vasodilation and increases in heart rate is most likely to optimize forward left ventricular stroke volume. An incompetent aortic valve may prevent the delivery of cardioplegia to the coronary system to produce diastolic arrest of the heart. (The alternative is injecting

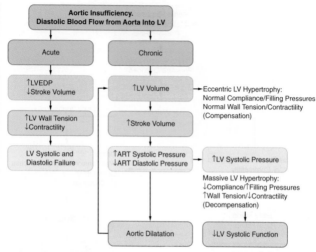

FIGURE 41-2. The pathophysiology of aortic insufficiency. ART = arterial; LV = left ventricle; LVEDP = left ventricular end-diastolic pressure.

cardioplegia directly into the coronary ostia or into the coronary sinus.)

D. **Mitral Stenosis**

1. **Pathophysiology** (Fig. 41-3). Increased left atrial pressure and volume overload are inevitable consequences of the narrowed mitral orifice. Persistent increases in left atrial pressure are reflected back through the pulmonary circulation, leading to right ventricular hypertrophy and perivascular edema in the lungs.

2. **Anesthetic Considerations.** Avoiding tachycardia is crucial for preventing inadequate left ventricular filling with concomitant hypotension. Continued preoperative administration of digitalis and β-antagonists, selection of anesthetics with minimal propensity to increase heart rate, and achievement of an anesthetic depth sufficient to suppress sympathetic nervous system responses are recommended.

E. **Mitral Regurgitation**

1. **Pathophysiology** (Fig. 41-4). Chronic volume overload of the left atrium is the cardinal feature of mitral regurgitation.

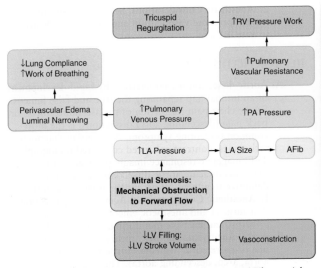

FIGURE 41-3. The pathophysiology of mitral stenosis. AFib = atrial fibrillation; LA = left atrium; LV = left ventricle; PA = pulmonary artery; RV = right ventricle.

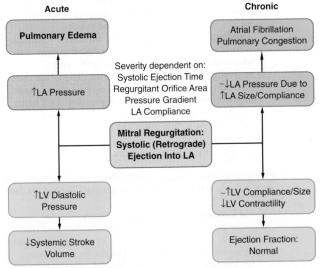

FIGURE 41-4. The pathophysiology of mitral regurgitation. LA = left atrium; LV = left ventricle.

2. **Anesthetic Considerations.** Selection of anesthetics that promote vasodilation and increase the heart rate is useful.

III. AORTIC DISEASES

A. **Aortic dissection** is characterized by rapid development of an intimal flap separating the true and false lumens. Severe chest pain (dissection of the ascending aorta) or back pain (descending aorta dissections) is the most common presenting symptom. A variety of diagnostic techniques (contrast-enhanced computed tomography, TEE, magnetic resonance imaging) are accurate in the diagnosis of acute aortic dissection. Surgery is the definitive treatment for ascending aortic dissections.
   1. **Anesthetic Considerations.** Acute aortic dissection is a surgical and anesthetic emergency necessitating IV access and invasive monitoring, including TEE.
B. **Aortic Aneurysm.** Thoracic aneurysms may involve one or more aortic segment (aortic root, ascending aorta, arch, descending aorta). The surgical replacement of an aortic arch aneurysm requires circulatory arrest and introduces the risk of global cerebral ischemia. Surgical replacement of the descending aorta is associated with postoperative paraplegia secondary to interruption of spinal cord blood supply.
   1. **Anesthetic Considerations.** The anesthetic technique is focused on preservation of cardiac function (descending thoracic aortic aneurysm) and neurologic integrity (aortic arch or descending thoracic aneurysms). Drainage of cerebral spinal fluid improves spinal cord perfusion pressure. Left heart bypass (left atrium to femoral artery) provides non-pulsatile retrograde aortic perfusion.

IV. CARDIOPULMONARY BYPASS

CPB incorporates a circuit to oxygenate venous blood and return it to the patient's arterial circulation (Table 41-4 and Fig. 41-5).
A. **Blood Conservation in Cardiac Surgery**
   1. Intraoperative autologous hemodilution involves the removal of whole blood before bypass (spared damaging effects [coagulopathy] of the bypass circuit) for reinfusion after bypass. Red blood cells may also

TABLE 41-4

COMPONENTS OF CARDIOPULMONARY BYPASS

Circuit (blood is drained from the right atrium and returned to the ascending aorta)

Oxygenator
  Bubble (time-dependent trauma to the blood)
  Membrane (less damage to the blood)

Pump (generate pressure required to return perfusate to the patient)
  Roller (nonpulsatile)
  Centrifugal
  Pulsatile (controversy exists whether this is better than standard flow)

Heat exchanger (allows production of systemic hypothermia)

Prime (decreased hematocrit offset changes in blood viscosity caused by hypothermia)

Anticoagulants (activated coagulation time >480 seconds; resistance to heparin occurs in patients with antithrombin III deficiency and is treated with fresh-frozen plasma or antithrombin III concentrate)

Myocardial protection (hypothermia to 10°C to 15°C and potassium to ensure diastolic arrest)

Aortic root (not feasible in patients with aortic insufficiency; the coronary ostia must be cannulated)

Retrograde via coronary sinus

Newly created bypass grafts

SURGICAL SUBSPECIALTIES

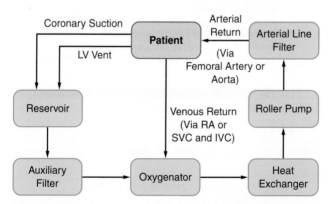

FIGURE 41-5. Diagram of a cardiopulmonary bypass circuit. IVC = inferior vena cava; LV = left ventricle; RA = right atrium; SVC = superior vena cava.

be salvaged from the surgical field and bypass tubing, washed, and retransfused (Cellsaver). Cellsaver blood may worsen coagulopathy because factors causing coagulopathy are not removed by the filtering process.

2. Pharmacologic measures include antifibrinolytics (epsilon-aminocaproic acid).

B. **Myocardial Protection.** The most common method of myocardial protection is use of intermittent hyperkalemic cold cardioplegia (diastolic electrical arrest) and moderate systemic hypothermia.

1. During CPB, the onset of left ventricular distention and lack of rapid electrical arrest may be evidence of poor myocardial protection and the possibility of difficulty in separation from bypass.

2. TEE is helpful in diagnosing ventricular distention that is relieved by venting or manual decompression.

V. PREOPERATIVE AND INTRAOPERATIVE MANAGEMENT

Data from the history, physical examination, and laboratory investigation are used to delineate the degree of left ventricular or right ventricular dysfunction (Table 41-5).

A. **Current drug therapy,** including β-adrenergic antagonists, calcium channel blockers, ACE inhibitors, and digitalis preparations (heart rate or rhythm control), is usually continued until the time of surgery.

B. **Premedication** for cardiac surgery often combines an opioid (0.1–0.2 mg/kg intramuscularly [IM] of morphine) with scopolamine (0.006 mg/kg IM) with or

---

TABLE 41-5

DATA FROM PREOPERATIVE EVALUATION

History of myocardial infarction
Signs of congestive heart failure
Evidence of myocardial ischemia or infarction on
 electrocardiography
Chest radiography
Left ventricular end-diastolic pressure >18 mm Hg
Ejection fraction <0.4
Cardiac index <2 L/min/m²
TEE (wall motion abnormalities)

TEE = transesophageal echocardiography.

without a benzodiazepine (0.05–0.1 mg/kg of diazepam or 0.05–0.07 mg/kg of lorazepam orally). Patients with valvular heart disease may be more susceptible to the ventilatory depressant effects of premedication than those with CAD who are scheduled for CABG operations.

C. **Monitoring** should emphasize the areas particularly relevant to cardiac surgery (Table 41-6). Use of specialized equipment or procedures (hypothermia, tight glucose control) have unproven benefit on neurologic outcomes.

D. **Selection of Anesthetic Drugs.** There is no single best drug, and the most critical factor governing anesthetic selection is the degree of left ventricular dysfunction. The anticipated time to tracheal extubation may influence the choice of anesthetic ("fast track"). It is useful to be able to alter the anesthetic depth to accommodate the varying intensity of the surgical stimulus (intense with tracheal intubation, sternotomy,

---

TABLE 41-6

MONITORS FOR CARDIAC SURGERY REQUIRING CARDIOPULMONARY BYPASS

Pulse oximeter (placed as the first monitor to detect unsuspected episodes of hypoxemia during catheter placement)

Electrocardiography

Temperature (gradients during cooling and rewarming should be observed)

Intra-arterial blood pressure (radial artery blood pressure may be lower than central aortic pressure early after CPB)

Central venous pressure catheter (infusion of cardioselective drugs; assumed to reflect left-sided filling pressures in the absence of left ventricular dysfunction)

Pulmonary artery catheter (awake vs asleep placement; distal migration occurs during CPB, so some recommend withdrawing the catheter a few centimeters before initiation of CPB)

TEE (provides information about cardiac structure and function that exceeds any other monitor [valve function, ventricular filling, myocardial contractility, myocardial ischemia, presence of intracardiac air, assessment of the aorta for plaques, congenital heart lesion repairs])

Central nervous system function (electroencephalography, SSEPs)

CPB = cardiopulmonary bypass; SEEP = somatosensory evoked potential; TEE = transesophageal echocardiography.

and manipulation of the aorta and minimal during hypothermic CPB).

1. Volatile anesthetics are useful as the primary anesthetic and as adjuvants to treat or prevent hypertension associated with high-dose opioid techniques. Volatile anesthetics may be administered during CPB through a vaporizer incorporated into the CPB circuit.

2. **Opioids** lack negative inotropic effects, and in high doses (50–100 μg/kg IV of fentanyl or 10–20 μg/kg IV of sufentanil) they may be used as the sole anesthetic.

   a. In patients with good left ventricular function, it is often necessary to include adjuvant drugs to provide amnesia (benzodiazepines) and control hypertension (volatile anesthetics, vasodilators).

   b. Excessive bradycardia may accompany the use of opioids, especially if nondepolarizing muscle relaxants are administered without heart rate effects.

3. **Nitrous oxide** has limited usefulness because of its myocardial depressant effects in the presence of opioids and its ability to enhance the size of air emboli, which may be present in coronary arteries after CABG operations.

4. **Neuromuscular Blocking Drugs.** The selection of muscle relaxants is influenced by the hemodynamic and pharmacokinetic properties associated with each drug, the patient's myocardial function, and the anesthetic technique used.

E. **Intraoperative Management** (Table 41-7)

   1. **Preinduction Period.** Supplemental oxygen is administered via nasal cannula after the patient is transferred to the operating table. Angina is promptly treated with oxygen and nitroglycerin (sublingual or IV). Placing a functioning pulse oximeter with the volume audible should precede line placement.

   2. **Induction and Intubation.** The dose, speed of administration, and specific drugs selected depend primarily on the patient's cardiovascular reserve and desired cardiovascular profile. A brief duration of laryngoscopy is desirable, although intubation of the trachea may be associated with myocardial ischemia, even in the absence of blood pressure or heart rate changes.

TABLE 41-7

CHECKLIST FOR MANAGEMENT OF PATIENTS UNDERGOING
CARDIOPULMONARY BYPASS

Before Cardiopulmonary Bypass
Laboratory Values
   Adequate heparinization (activated coagulation time or other
     method)
   Hematocrit
   Anesthetic
   Adequate depth using amnestics or opioids
   Nitrous oxide off
   Muscle relaxants supplemented
   Monitors
   Arterial pressure (initial hypotension and then return)
   Central venous pressure (indicates adequate venous drainage)
   Pulmonary capillary wedge pressure (elevated with left
     ventricular distention reflecting inadequate drainage, aortic
     insufficiency; the catheter should be pulled back 1 to 2 cm)
Patient and Field
   Cannulas in place (no clamps or air locks)
   Face (suffusion reflects inadequate superior vena cava drainage;
     unilateral blanching reflects innominate artery cannulation)
   Heart (signs of distention reflect ischemia or aortic insufficiency)
   Support
   Usually not necessary

During Cardiopulmonary Bypass
Laboratory Values
   Adequate heparinization
   ABG analysis (evidence of acidosis)
   Hematocrit, electrolytes, ionized calcium, glucose
   Anesthetic
   Discontinue ventilation
   Monitors
   Arterial hypotension (inadequate venous return, low pump flow,
     aortic dissection, decreased vascular tone, dampened
     waveform)
   Arterial hypertension (high pump flow, vasoconstriction)
   Venous pressure (transducer higher than atrial level, obstruction
     to chamber drainage)
   EEG
   Adequate body perfusion (acidosis, mixed venous oxygen
     saturation)
   Temperature
   Urine output
Patient and Field
   Conduct of operation (heart distention, fibrillation)
   Venous engorgement
   Signs of light anesthesia (movement, breathing)

(continued)

TABLE 41-7

CHECKLIST FOR MANAGEMENT OF PATIENTS UNDERGOING
CARDIOPULMONARY BYPASS (*Continued*)

Support
    Assist adequacy of pump flow (anesthetics or vasodilators for
      hypertension or constrictors for hypotension)
Before Separation from Cardiopulmonary Bypass
Laboratory Values
    Hematocrit and ABG analysis
    Potassium (may be elevated from cardioplegia)
    Ionized calcium
Anesthetic and Machine
    Initiate ventilation (evaluate lung compliance)
    Vaporizers off
    Alarms on
Monitors
    Normothermia (37°C nasopharyngeal; 35.5°C bladder)
    Electrocardiogram (rate, rhythm, ST wave)
    Transducers zeroed and calibrated
    Arterial and filling pressures
    Activate recorder
Patient and Field
    Look at heart (contractility, rhythm, size)
    De-aired (TEE)
    Bleeding
    Vascular resistance
Support as necessary (inotrope, vasodilator)

ABG = arterial blood gas; EEG = electroencephalography;
TEE = transesophageal echocardiography.

3. **The preincision period** between tracheal intubation
and skin incision should be one of minimal stimulation. (Blood pressure may need to be supported.)
4. **The period from incision to bypass** is characterized
by periods of intense surgical stimulation that
often require alteration in the depth of anesthesia
or administration of a vasodilator to blunt
responses (hypertension, tachycardia) that may
predispose the patient to myocardial ischemia. Any
evidence of new myocardial ischemia (ST segment
changes on the electrocardiogram) should be
treated appropriately and the surgeon notified.
5. **Cardiopulmonary bypass** is initiated after
confirmation of adequate anticoagulation with
heparin. There is no consensus about the optimal

mean arterial pressure during CPB, although pump flows of 50 to 60 mL/kg usually produce perfusion pressures of 50 to 60 mm Hg.

a. The effect of decreased viscosity (acute hemodilution) and loss of pulsatile flow may initially cause the perfusion pressure to decrease below 40 mm Hg.

b. Phenylephrine may be administered to increase perfusion pressure if it is deemed necessary for maintenance of organ blood flow.

c. After full CPB is established, there is no need to continue ventilation of the patient's lungs. There is no consensus about management of the lungs (positive end-expiratory pressure vs zero airway pressure, oxygen vs room air) during CPB.

d. Anesthetic requirements are decreased during hypothermic CPB, an effect that may offset the dilutional effect of CPB on plasma concentrations of injected drugs.

e. Continued skeletal muscle paralysis is desirable to prevent increases in oxygen requirements owing to skeletal muscle activity.

6. **Monitoring and Management During Bypass**

a. It is important to continuously observe the surgical field and cannulae to permit early detection of mechanical causes of hypotension or hypertension during CPB.

b. Maintenance of adequate depths of anesthesia is important during CPB, although clinical signs are few.

c. Maintenance of urine output with diuretics is a common practice during CPB. Nevertheless, postoperative renal failure is most likely caused by aggravation of pre-existing renal dysfunction or persistent low cardiac output after CPB.

7. **Rewarming** is begun when the surgical repair is nearly complete; the anesthesiologist should remember that patients may regain awareness as the anesthetic effects of hypothermia dissipate. (Administration of a volatile anesthetic should be considered if a smooth postbypass course is anticipated and early weaning from mechanical ventilation and extubation are planned.)

8. **Discontinuation of CPB** is considered when rewarming is adequate. A low cardiac output must

TABLE 41-8

CAUSES OF RIGHT OR LEFT VENTRICULAR DYSFUNCTION AFTER CARDIOPULMONARY BYPASS

Ischemia
Inadequate myocardial protection
Intraoperative infarction
Reperfusion injury
Coronary spasm
Coronary embolism (air, thrombus)
Technical difficulties (kinked or clotted grafts)

Uncorrected Structural Defects
Nongraftable vessels
Diffuse coronary artery disease
Residual or new valve pathology
Shunts
Pre-existing cardiac dysfunction

Cardiopulmonary Bypass–Related Factors
Excessive cardioplegia
Unrecognized cardiac distention

prompt a search for explanations (kinked grafts, air in coronary grafts, coronary artery spasm, global ischemia from inadequate myocardial protection) and consideration of pharmacologic support (inotropes, vasodilators) (Tables 41-8 and 41-9).

9. **Intra-aortic Balloon Pump** (Table 41-10). The balloon pump functions as a mechanical assist device in the thoracic aorta (25-cm balloon on a 90-cm vascular catheter) using the principle of synchronized counterpulsation to enhance left ventricular stroke volume.

   a. The balloon deflates immediately before systole to decrease afterload and myocardial oxygen requirements. Subsequently, the balloon inflates during diastole to provide diastolic augmentation that increases coronary blood flow.

   b. It is crucial to control the heart rate and to suppress cardiac dysrhythmias to ensure proper balloon timing.

   c. As cardiac function improves, the assist ratio is gradually weaned from every beat to every other beat and then removed.

10. **Ventricular Assist Device.** When the heart is unable to meet systemic metabolic demands

DIAGNOSIS AND THERAPY OF CARDIOVASCULAR DYSFUNCTION
AFTER CARDIOPULMONARY BYPASS

Blood Pressure	Filling Pressures	Cardiac Output	Diagnosis	Treatment
Increased	Increased	Increased	Hypervolemia	Remove volume Vasodilation
Increased	Increased	Decreased	Vasoconstriction Poor contractility	Vasodilation Inotrope
Increased	Decreased	Increased	Hyperdynamic	Anesthetic β-Antagonist
Increased	Decreased	Decreased	Vasoconstriction	Vasodilation Give volume
Decreased	Increased	Increased	Hypervolemia	Wait
Decreased	Increased	Decreased	Poor contractility	Inotrope Vasodilation Mechanical assist
Decreased	Decreased	Increased	Vasodilation	Vasoconstrictor
Decreased	Decreased	Decreased	Hypovolemia	Give volume

TABLE 41-10

INDICATIONS AND CONTRAINDICATIONS FOR INTRA-AORTIC
BALLOON PUMPS

Indications

Complications of Myocardial Ischemia
  Hemodynamic (cardiogenic shock)
  Mechanical (mitral regurgitation, ventricular septal defect)
  Intractable dysrhythmias
  Extension of infarct
  Acute cardiac instability
  Unstable angina
  Failed PTCA
  Cardiac contusion
  Possibly septic shock
  Open heart surgery
  Separation from cardiopulmonary bypass
  Ventricular failure
  Increasing inotropic requirements
  Progressive hemodynamic deterioration
  Refractory ischemia

Contraindications
Severe aortic insufficiency
Technical difficulties with insertion
Irreversible cardiac disease
Irreversible brain damage

PTCA = percutaneous transluminal coronary angioplasty.

TABLE 41-11

SIDE EFFECTS OF PROTAMINE

Hypotension (less likely when administered over 5 minutes)
Allergic reaction (more likely in patients receiving protamine-containing insulin preparations [NPH, PZI])
Pulmonary hypertension (mediated by release of thromboxane and C5a anaphylatoxin)

NPH = neutral protamine Hagedorn; PZI = protamine zinc insulin.

despite maximal pharmacologic therapy and insertion of the intra-aortic balloon pump, a device that pumps blood and bypasses the left or right ventricle may be useful.

11. **Postcardiopulmonary Bypass**

   a. **Reversal of Anticoagulation.** Heparin is partially reversed with protamine administered intravenously while the arterial cannula remains in place for continued transfusion of pump contents. Adequate reversal of anticoagulation with protamine is verified by measurement of the activated coagulation time. Protamine administration may be accompanied by side effects (Table 41-11). Whether protamine should be administered through the right atrium, left atrium, aorta, or a peripheral vein remains controversial.

   b. **Postbypass Bleeding.** Persistent oozing after heparin reversal is common and usually reflects inadequate surgical hemostasis or platelet dysfunction.

   c. Closure of the chest is occasionally associated with transient decreases in blood pressure. If hypotension persists despite volume replacement, the chest must be reopened to rule out cardiac tamponade or kinking of a venous graft.

VI. MINIMALLY INVASIVE CARDIAC SURGERY

The desire to avoid the complications of CPB (stroke, neurocognitive defects, renal failure, pulmonary insufficiency, coagulopathy, activation of systemic inflammatory response)

TABLE 41-12

REASONS FOR POSTOPERATIVE RE-EXPLORATION

Persistent bleeding
Excessive blood loss
Cardiac tamponade
Unexplained low cardiac output

---

as well as the complications of sternotomy led to the development of techniques not requiring CPB (minimally invasive direct coronary artery bypass [MIDCAB], off-pump coronary bypass [OPCAB], robotic surgery).

VII. POSTOPERATIVE CONSIDERATIONS

A. **Bring-backs** of the patient for postoperative re-exploration are necessary in 4% to 10% of cases, usually in the first 24 hours (Table 41-12).

B. **Tamponade** must always be included in the differential diagnosis of unexplained low cardiac output (Table 41-13). The diagnosis of tamponade is confirmed by TEE. Ketamine is useful for induction and maintenance of anesthesia in patients with cardiac tamponade because the goal is to avoid vasodilation and cardiac depression.

C. **Pain Management.** Intrathecal opioids provide analgesia that facilitates early extubation. Use of nonsteroidal anti-inflammatory drugs may play an increasing role in management of postoperative pain after cardiac surgery.

TABLE 41-13

MANIFESTATIONS OF CARDIAC TAMPONADE

Hypotension
Equalization of diastolic filling pressures (when the pericardium is no longer intact, loculated areas of clot may compress only one chamber, causing isolated increases in filling pressures)
Fixed stroke volume (cardiac output and blood pressure become dependent on heart rate)
Peripheral vasoconstriction
Tachycardia
Potential for concurrent myocardial ischemia

VIII. ANESTHESIA FOR CHILDREN WITH CONGENITAL HEART DISEASE

Congenital heart defects cause either too much blood flow to a cardiac chamber or obstruction of flow to a chamber (Table 41-14). Because "anatomy dictates physiology," the anesthetic management of children with congenital heart disease requires knowledge of anatomical defects and planned surgical procedures and comprehensive understanding of the altered physiology.

A. **Preoperative Evaluation** (Tables 41-15 and 41-16)
B. **Premedication** is intended to render the child calm but without oversedation.
C. **Monitoring** beyond the standard monitors may include peripheral and central temperature monitoring, central venous pressure monitoring (right atrial or left atrial), and TEE.
D. **Anesthetic and Intraoperative Management**
   1. Inhalation agents are useful for induction and may be continued for maintenance.

TABLE 41-14

CLASSIFICATION OF CONGENITAL HEART DEFECTS

Volume Overload of the Ventricle or Atrium Resulting in Increased Pulmonary Blood Flow
Atrial septal defect (high flow, low pressure)
Ventricular septal defect (high flow, high pressure)
Patent ductus arteriosus (high flow, high pressure)
Endocardial cushion defect (high flow, high pressure)

Cyanosis Resulting from Obstruction to Pulmonary Blood Flow
Tetralogy of Fallot
Tricuspid atresia
Pulmonary atresia

Pressure Overload on the Ventricle
Aortic stenosis
Coarctation of the aorta
Pulmonary stenosis

Cyanosis Caused By a Common Mixing Chamber
Total anomalous venous return
Truncus arteriosus
Double outlet right ventricle
Single ventricle

Cyanosis Caused By Separation of the Systemic and Pulmonary Circulations
Transposition of the great vessels

TABLE 41-15

PREOPERATIVE EVALUATION OF CHILDREN WITH CONGENITAL HEART DISEASE

History
Symptoms (poor weight gain, respiratory distress, easily exhausted, cyanosis, upper respiratory infections)
Medications (potential interactions with anesthetics)
Previous surgical procedures

Physical Examination
Evidence of cardiac failure (irritability, diaphoresis, rales, jugular venous distention, hepatomegaly)
Failure to thrive (pulmonary hypertension, poor peripheral oxygenation)
Blood pressure in the arms and legs
Auscultation of the heart (murmur reflects lesion; see Table 41-17)
Airway evaluation

Laboratory Evaluations
Hemoglobin (anemia vs polycythemia)
Coagulation profile (platelet count, prothrombin time, partial thromboplastin time)
Potassium (diuretic therapy), glucose, calcium
ABG analysis

Cardiac Evaluations
Echocardiography (delineates cardiac anatomy and permits noninvasive measurement of ventricular size, function, and cardiac output
Chest radiography (cardiac size, abnormal vessels, pneumonia)
Electrocardiography (rate and rhythm)

ABG = arterial blood gas.

TABLE 41-16

CLASSIFICATION OF CARDIAC MURMURS

Systolic
Atrial septal defect
Ventricular septal defect
Coarctation of the aorta

Diastolic
Regurgitant semilunar valves
Stenotic atrioventricular valves
Mitral flow rumble
Tricuspid flow rumble

Continuous
Patent ductus arteriosus
Arteriovenous fistula
Excessive bronchial collaterals
Aortopulmonary window
Surgical shunt
Severe pulmonic stenosis

TABLE 41-17

CHOICE OF DRUGS DURING MAINTENANCE OF ANESTHESIA FOR CORRECTION OF CONGENITAL CARDIAC DEFECTS

Intravenous Agents (fentanyl 50–100 µg/kg or remifentanil 1 µg/kg/min; bradycardia is a risk)

Inhalational Agents
Isoflurane (myocardial contractility may be better preserved than with halothane; there is a propensity for laryngospasm if it is used for induction of anesthesia)
Sevoflurane (may be used for inhalation induction and lacks significant myocardial depression because decreases in systemic blood pressure are principally caused by decreases in systemic vascular resistance)

Neuromuscular Blocking Drugs
Succinylcholine (bradycardia limits its usefulness)
Nondepolarizing relaxants (facilitate tracheal intubation and provide paralysis during surgery; pancuronium is useful when increased heart rate is desirable)

2. The choice of anesthetic drugs after induction of anesthesia is influenced by ventricular function, the use of CPB, and anticipation of controlled mechanical ventilation or tracheal extubation at the end of the operation (Table 41-17).

TABLE 41-18

MEDICATIONS ADMINISTERED BY CONTINUOUS INTRAVENOUS INFUSION

Drug	Usual Initial Dose (µg/kg/min)	Usual Dose Range (µg/kg/min)
Amrinone*	2–5	2–20
Dopamine	2–5	2–20
Dobutamine	2–5	2–20
Epinephrine	0.1	0.1–1.0
Isoproterenol	0.05–1.0[†]	0.1–1.0
Lidocaine	20	20–50
Nitroglycerin	0.5	0.5–5.0
Norepinephrine	0.1	0.1–1.0
Phentolamine	0.1–1.0	0.5–5.0
Phenylephrine	1	1–3
Prostaglandin E₁	0.05–1.00	0.05–0.20
Vasopressin	1µg (4 U)	0.0004

*Requires initial bolus of 750 µg/kg over 3 minutes before start of infusion.
[†]For chronotropic effect after cardiac transplantation, dosages of 0.005 to 0.01 µg/kg/min are used.

TABLE 41-19

CRITERIA FOR TRACHEAL EXTUBATION AFTER
COMPLEX PROCEDURES

Ability to maintain oxygenation during spontaneous respiration
Coordination of thoracic and abdominal components of
  respiration
Acceptable chest radiographs (absence of significant atelectasis,
  effusions, and infiltrates)
Short period of time without caloric support
Stable inotropic support

   3. CPB produces marked hemostatic derangements
      (dilution of clotting factors, activation of clotting
      cascade and consumption of clotting factors and
      platelets, and activation of the fibrinolytic pathway).
   4. Separation from CPB may require pharmacologic
      intervention (Table 41-18).
E. **Tracheal Extubation and Postoperative Ventilation**
   (Table 41-19)
   1. Children undergoing correction of congenital
      cardiac defects that do not require ventricular inci-
      sions (atrial septal defect, ventricular septal defect
      repaired across the tricuspid valve) can often have
      their tracheas extubated at the conclusion of
      surgery.
   2. Those with risk factors (complex surgery,
      circulatory arrest, Down syndrome, pulmonary
      hypertension, postoperative cardiovascular and pul-
      monary complications) for ventilatory failure must
      fulfill tracheal extubation criteria.

CHAPTER 42 ■ ANESTHESIA FOR VASCULAR SURGERY

The outcome after vascular surgery is principally determined by patient factors (coronary artery disease [CAD]), surgical factors, and institution-specific factors (Mantha S, Roizen MF, Katz JC, Lubarsky DA, Ellis JE: Anesthesia for vascular surgery. In *Clinical Anesthesia*. Edited by Barash PG, Cullen BF, Stoelting RK, Cahalan MK, Stock MC. Philadelphia: Lippincott Williams & Wilkins, 2009, pp 1108–1136). Low serum albumin values and high American Society of Anesthesiologists physical classification are predictors of morbidity and mortality after vascular surgery. New surgical techniques, such as angioplasty and endovascular repair with placement of stent grafts, have revolutionized vascular surgery.

I. VASCULAR DISEASE: EPIDEMIOLOGIC, MEDICAL, AND SURGICAL ASPECTS

A. **Pathophysiology of Atherosclerosis.** Atherosclerosis is a generalized inflammatory disorder of the arterial tree with associated endothelial dysfunction (Table 42-1).

B. **Natural History of Patients with Peripheral Vascular Disease.** Atherosclerosis is a systemic disease that has important sequelae in many other regional circulations (carotid artery stenosis and stroke, aortic atherosclerosis and aneurysms, claudication).

C. **Medical Therapy for Atherosclerosis**

1. Medical therapy, including the use of antihypertensives (beta-blockers, angiotensin-converting enzyme inhibitors), statin drugs, aspirin, and control of hyperglycemia [hypoglycemia or the use of insulin] may reduce perioperative morbidity and mortality in vascular surgery patients (Table 42-2). Patients with high cardiac risk undergoing vascular surgery who receive preoperative statin therapy are less likely to die. Cessation of smoking may be the most effective medical therapy.

TABLE 42-1
RISK FACTORS FOR ATHEROSCLEROSIS

Predisposing Risk Factors (aspects of the metabolic syndrome)
Abdominal obesity
Atherogenic dyslipidemia
Increased blood pressure
Insulin resistance
Proinflammatory state
Prothrombotic state

Major Risk Factors
Cigarette smoking
Elevated LDL cholesterol level
Low HDL level
Family history of premature CAD
Aging

Emerging Risk Factors
Elevated triglycerides
Small LDL particles

CAD = coronary artery disease; HDL = high-density lipoprotein;
LDL = low-density lipoprotein.

II. CHRONIC MEDICAL PROBLEMS AND MANAGMENT IN VASCULAR SURGERY PATIENTS

A. **Coronary Artery Disease in Patients with Peripheral Vascular Disease.** The presence of uncorrected CAD appears to double the 5-year mortality rate after vascular surgery.

1. Previous percutaneous transluminal coronary angioplasty (PTCA) and stenting may or may not protect against perioperative cardiac events after vascular surgery.

   a. Drug-eluting stents are slow to endothelialize, and the exposed stent material remains thrombogenic far longer than with bare-metal stents. Therefore, the duration of dual antiplatelet therapy (75 mg/day of clopidogrel and 325 mg/day of aspirin) is 1 month for bare metal stents and 12 months (perhaps forever) for drug-eluting stents.

   b. Whenever possible, noncardiac surgery should be delayed until 6 weeks after bare-metal stent placement (endotheliazation is usually complete by this time) and perhaps for 12 months after placement of a drug-eluting stent.

TABLE 42-2

MANAGEMENT OF PREOPERATIVE DRUG THERAPY

Medication	Side Effects of Potential Concern in the Perioperative Period	Recommendation for Perioperative Use
Aspirin	Platelet inhibition may increase bleeding	Continue until day of surgery, especially for carotid and peripheral vascular cases
	Decreased glomerular filtration rate	Monitor fluid status and urine output
Clopidogrel	Platelet inhibition may increase bleeding	Hold for 7 days before surgery except for CEA and severe CAD
	Rare thrombotic thrombocytopenic purpura	Consider additional cross-match of blood
		Avoid neuraxial anesthesia for at least 7 days
HMG-COA reductase inhibitors (statins)	Liver function test abnormalities	Assess liver function tests and continue through the morning of surgery
	Rhabdomyolysis	Check CPK if myalgias are present
Beta-blockers	Bronchospasm Hypotension Bradycardia Heart block	Continue through the perioperative period
ACE inhibitors	Hypotension with induction	Continue through the perioperative period
	Cough	Consider 50% the dose on the day of surgery
Diuretics	Hypovolemia	Continue through the perioperative period
	Electrolyte abnormalities	Monitor fluid status and urine output
Calcium channel blockers	Perioperative hypotension, especially with amlodipine	Continue through the perioperative period (consider withholding amlodipine on the morning of surgery)
Oral hypogly-cemics	Hypoglycemia given preoperatively and intraoperatively	When feasible, switch to insulin preoperatively
	Lactic acidosis with metformin	Monitor glucose status perioperatively

ACE = angiotensin-converting enzyme; CAD = coronary artery disease; CEA = carotid endarterectomy; CPK = creatine phosphokinase; HMG-CoA = 3-hydroxy-3-methyl-glutaryl-CoA.

TABLE 42-3

DEFINITION OF A NEW MYOCARDIAL INFARCTION

Rise and fall of a biochemical marker (troponin) of myocardial necrosis with one of the following clinical and ECG criteria:
  Ischemic symptoms
  Development of pathologic Q waves
  Ischemic ECG changes
  Coronary intervention

ECG = electrocardiogram.

    2. Perioperative myocardial infarction after vascular surgery may be early (resembling acute nonsurgical acute myocardial infarction that is most likely caused by plaque rupture and thrombosis of a coronary artery) or delayed (resembling an increase in oxygen demand in the presence of fixed coronary stenosis) (Table 42-3). Perioperative troponin screening is an effective means of surveillance for perioperative myocardial ischemia damage.

B. **Preoperative coronary revascularization** (surgical or interventional) may be of no value in preventing cardiac events except in patients in whom revascularizations is independently indicated for acute coronary syndrome. The safe time intervals between surgical revascularization and vascular surgery is 4 to 6 weeks and is 2 weeks for PTCA (longer for stents).

C. **Management of Perioperative Myocardial Ischemia and Infarction in Vascular Patients** (Table 42-4). Of the various pharmacologic risk reduction strategies, perioperative beta-blocker therapy in noncardiac surgery is useful to reduce rates of preoperative arrhythmias and myocardial ischemia but may not provide benefit regarding myocardial infarction, length of hospitalization, and mortality. Patients with few or no risk factors may not benefit from beta-blocker therapy and may have an increased risk of death, stroke, and clinically significant hypotension. Asthma, chronic obstructive airway disease, and cardiac conduction disease in the absence of a pacemaker are contraindications to beta-blocker therapy.

    1. High-dose opioid anesthetics reduce the stress response and may improve the overall outcome after major surgery.

TABLE 42-4

PHARMACOLOGIC PROPHYLAXIS AGAINST ACUTE VASCULAR
EVENTS IN PATIENTS UNDERGOING VASCULAR SURGERY

Intervention	Regimen and Comments	Recommendation*
Perioperative beta-blockade	Preoperative oral $beta_1$ selective beta-blocker (bisoprolol, metoprolol, atenolol) initiated at least 30 days before surgery and IV and postoperative period (metoprolol, atenolol, esmolol)	Class I
	• In patients with ischemia on preoperative testing, in patients with three or more clinical risk factors, and in patients receiving beta-blockers for stable cardiac symptoms	Class IIa
	• In patients with one or two clinical risk factors and no cardiac symptoms Patients with few or no risk factors may not benefit from beta blockade	
α_2-blockers	Pretreatment with oral clonidine 300 µg at least 90 minutes before surgery and therapy continued for 72 hours (oral or transdermal 0.2 mg/day) IV clonidine 300 µg/day can also be administered for 72 hours	Class IIa
Statin therapy	Typical dose of atorvastatin is 20 mg/day initiated at least 45 days before surgery Withdrawal of statin therapy for more than 4 days after vascular surgery is associated with an increased risk of cardiac complications Administration of extended-release fluvastatin preoperatively appears ideal when prolonged postoperative ileus is expected	

TABLE 42-4

PHARMACOLOGIC PROPHYLAXIS AGAINST ACUTE VASCULAR
EVENTS IN PATIENTS UNDERGOING VASCULAR SURGERY (*Continued*)

Intervention	Regimen and Comments	Recommendation*
	Use should be continued after surgery for at least 2 weeks	
	Statin use is associated with improved graft patency, limb salvage, and a decreased amputation rate in patients undergoing infrainguinal bypass	Class IIa
ACE inhibitors	Potential benefits include decreased stroke rate, limitation of ventricular remodeling that occurs after acute myocardial infarction, and decreased long-term mortality after infrainguinal bypass surgery	Class IIb
Calcium channel blockers	Reduced perioperative adverse cardiac events, including supraventricular tachycardia in patients undergoing noncardiac vascular surgery (primarily diltiazem)	Class IIb
	Evidence is limited in patients undergoing vascular surgery	
Nitroglycerin	Not indicated for prophylaxis or initial treatment of myocardial ischemia	Class III
	May be used to treat arterial hypertension, elevated filling pressures, or suspected coronary vasospasm	

*Class I: Evidence or general agreement that is useful or effective.
Class II: Conflicting evidence or a divergence of opinion regarding usefulness or efficacy.
Class IIa: Weight of evidence or opinion in favor of usefulness or efficacy.
Class IIb: Usefulness or efficacy is less well established by evidence or opinion.
Class III: Evidence that is not useful or effective.
Class I recommendations are the "dos," class II recommendations are the "maybes," and class III recommendations are the "do nots."
ACE = angiotensin-converting enzyme; IV = intravenous.

TABLE 42-5

COEXISTING MEDICAL PROBLEMS IN PATIENTS WITH PERIPHERAL VASCULAR DISEASE

Hypertension (treat with oral doses of atenolol or metoprolol if poorly controlled)
Diabetes mellitus (increased incidence of postoperative death when autonomic neuropathy is present; intraoperative euglycemia may be particularly important during thoracic and carotid surgery)
Hypercoagulability
Chronic obstructive pulmonary disease (tobacco abuse)
Renal insufficiency

2. Epidural anesthesia may reduce perioperative myocardial ischemia (reduced preload and afterload; decreased coagulation responses), but cardiac outcome has not been proven to be improved after abdominal aortic surgery, especially if heart rate is well controlled in the intensive care unit.

3. Anemia (hematocrit <28%) may increase the incidence of postoperative myocardial ischemia in high-risk patients undergoing noncardiac surgery.
(It is more likely to transfuse high-risk patients or those who demonstrate myocardial ischemia with packed red blood cells to augment the hematocrit to 30%.)

4. Hypothermia is associated with increased adrenergic tone and postoperative myocardial ischemia in patients undergoing vascular surgery. (Patients should be aggressively warmed, and heat should be conserved during and after surgery.)

5. Suctioning, tracheal extubation, and weaning from mechanical ventilation may produce myocardial ischemia (early tracheal extubation vs sedation and analgesia to permit tolerance of the tracheal tube).

D. **Other Medical Problems in Vascular Surgery Patients** (Table 42-5)

III. CAROTID ENDARTERECTOMY (CEA)

Carotid disease is primarily a problem of embolization and rarely occlusion or insufficiency. Carotid disease may manifest itself only as an asymptomatic bruit or as amaurosis fugax (transient attacks of monocular blindness) when the ophthalmic artery is embolized. Other patients may experience episodes of paresthesias, clumsiness of the extremities, or speech problems, which resolve spontaneously after a short period of time. The most common diagnostic noninvasive test is the duplex scan, which combines B-mode anatomic imaging and pulse Doppler spectral analysis of blood flow velocity. The accuracy of duplex scanning reaches 95% in experienced hands compared with angiography. Also, many surgeons use magnetic resonance angiography as the sole modality to detect disease. Combined administration of aspirin and dipyridamole, when compared with placebo, reduces the incidence of transient ischemic attacks more so than either drug alone. (Patients presenting for CEA must continue to receive aspirin, clopidogrel, or both in the perioperative period.)

SURGICAL SUBSPECIALTIES

A. **Preoperative Evaluation and Preparation.** The long-term risks of adverse cardiac events after CEA are related to progression of CAD.
B. **Monitoring and Preserving Neurologic Integrity.** The two main goals of intraoperative management are to protect the brain and heart.
   1. The rationale behind maintaining a stable, high-normal blood pressure throughout the procedure is based on the assumption that blood vessels in ischemic or hypoperfused areas of the brain have lost normal autoregulation. The judicious use of phenylephrine to increase blood pressure only in specific instances of electroencephalography (EEG)-detected reversible cerebral ischemia seems to be without detriment to the heart.
   2. Hypercapnia during CEA may be detrimental if it dilates vessels in normal areas of the brain while vessels in ischemic brain areas that are already maximally dilated cannot respond ("steal" phenomenon manifesting as a diversion of blood flow from hypoperfused brain regions to normally perfused brain regions). Most authorities recommend the maintenance of normocarbia or moderate hypocarbia.
   3. Moderate hyperglycemia may worsen ischemic brain injury, and hyperglycemia has a documented association with worse outcome after CEA (aggressive glucose control is recommended).
   4. Almost all commonly used anesthetic agents reduce cerebral metabolism, but the notion that reduced

cerebral metabolism is associated with cerebral protection has been challenged. Volatile anesthetics may provide preconditioning and neuronal protection by inducing nitric oxide synthase.

5. Barbiturates may offer a degree of brain protection during periods of regional ischemia. Thiopental decreases cerebral metabolic oxygen requirements to about 50% of baseline. These maximally achievable reductions in oxygen requirements correspond to a silent (isoelectric) EEG. Beyond this point, additional doses of barbiturates are neither necessary nor helpful. In cases of massive global ischemia in which basal cellular metabolism has already deteriorated, even high doses of barbiturates will not improve neurologic outcome.

6. The use of a shunt is beneficial only if the cause of neurologic dysfunction is inadequate blood flow. (Most neurologic deficits during CEA are caused by thromboembolic events.)

C. **Anesthetic and Monitoring Choices for Elective Surgery** (Table 42-6)

1. Often on the day of surgery, patients present with hypertension despite having taken their morning antihypertensive and antianginal medications. These

---

TABLE 42-6

ANESTHETIC AND MONITORING CHOICES FOR PATIENTS UNDERGOING ELECTIVE CAROTID ENDARTERECTOMY

Intra-arterial catheter (before surgery, blood pressure in each arm should be compared)
Electrocardiography (leads II and V5 for ST segment changes)
TEE (consider in patients at high risk for intraoperative myocardial ischemia)
Preoperatively establish range of patient's blood pressure and heart rate
Continue chronic medications to the day of surgery
Avoid intraoperative fluid overload (may contribute to postoperative hypertension)
Restrict use of opioids (sedation may confound results of early neurologic assessment)
Avoid use of continuous infusions of phenylephrine (rely on the patient's endogenous pressure-sustaining responses)
Ask the surgeon to infiltrate carotid bifurcation with 1% lidocaine
Confirm neurologic integrity before leave the operating room

TEE = transesophageal echocardiography.

patients appear to be the most prone to hypotension after the induction of general anesthesia.

2. The use of a cervical plexus block or surgeon-administered local anesthetic helps considerably in reducing to eliminating opioid requirements.

3. There is no proof that any one general anesthetic technique or general anesthesia versus regional anesthesia provides a superior outcome. The choice of anesthetic technique should take into account the preference of the surgeon and the experience and expertise of the anesthesiologist.

D. **Carotid angioplasty and stenting (CAS)** may be performed by vascular surgeons, cardiologists, or radiologists. In some cases, CAS involves sedation and monitoring provided by anesthesiologists; in other cases, no anesthesiologist will be involved. The patient needs to be arousable and responsive so that serial neurologic examinations can be conducted.

1. Both CEA and CAS may cause blood pressure to decrease immediately after reperfusion and into the postoperative period because of alterations in baroreceptor function.

2. Studies to date fail to show an outcome advantage of CAS over CEA.

E. **Postoperative Management** (Table 42-7)

1. Severe hypertension (systolic blood pressure >200 mm Hg) seems to occur more often in patients with poorly controlled preoperative hypertension.

TABLE 42-7

POSTOPERATIVE COMPLICATIONS AFTER
CAROTID ENDARTERECTOMY

New neurologic dysfunction (ability to move the extremities excludes the possibility of acute thrombosis of the endarterectomy site)
Hemodynamic instability (hypertension is more common than hypotension)
Hyperperfusion syndrome (manifests several days after surgery as ipsilateral headache that may progress to seizures; transcranial Doppler may predict susceptible patients; steroids may be used in treatment)
Respiratory insufficiency (recurrent laryngeal nerve palsy; carotid body denervation)
Wound hematomas (airway compression)

   a. Hypertension may precipitate acute myocardial ischemia (the incidence is increased in first few hours after surgery) and congestive heart failure and may lead to cerebral edema or hemorrhage. (Postoperative hypertension is associated with an increased incidence of neurologic deficits.)

   b. Causes of postoperative hypertension (pain, arterial hypoxemia, hypercarbia, and bladder distention should be ruled out) are unclear but may include denervation of the carotid sinus and overzealous administration of intravenous (IV) fluids.

   c. Hypertension usually peaks 2 to 3 hours after surgery but may persist for 24 hours in some individuals.

   d. Treatment of hypertension is with titration of short-acting drugs (nitroglycerin, labetalol, esmolol, tracheal lidocaine spray).

2. Hypotension and bradycardia after CEA are less frequent than hypertension. (Surgical removal of the atheroma again exposes the carotid sinus baroreceptors to higher levels of transmural pressure, leading to brainstem-mediated vagal responses.)

   a. Chemical denervation of the carotid sinus with local anesthetic injected by the surgeon results in fewer hypotensive patients but increases the incidence of postoperative hypertension.

   b. The baroreceptors seem to adjust over 12 to 24 hours.

   c. Treatment may not be necessary in the absence of myocardial ischemia or changes in neurologic status. Nevertheless, blood pressure is often restored to a low-normal range with IV infusion of fluids or administration of drugs (ephedrine, phenylephrine, dopamine).

F. **Management of Emergent Carotid Surgery**

1. A patient who awakens with a major new neurologic deficit or who develops a suspected stroke in the immediate postoperative period represents a surgical emergency. (Prompt removal of a carotid thrombosis may produce significant neurologic improvement.)

2. A wound hematoma occurring after CEA may be associated with airway obstruction and necessitate opening the operative site to remove pressure on the trachea before returning to the operating room.

IV. AORTIC RECONSTRUCTION

A. **Aneurysmal Disease.** Aneurysms pose an ever-present threat to life because of their unpredictable tendency to rupture or embolize. Aggressive surgical management is warranted even in the absence of symptoms.

1. **Epidemiology and Pathophysiology of Abdominal Aortic Aneurysm (AAA).** Risk factors for aneurysm include advanced age, smoking more than 40 years, hypertension, low serum high-density lipoprotein cholesterol, high level of plasma fibrinogen, and low blood platelet count. The risk of rupture of an AAA increases after the aneurysm is greater than 4.5 to 5 cm in diameter; surgical treatment is generally recommended.

B. **Pathophysiology of Aortic Occlusion and Reperfusion**

1. **Cardiovascular Changes** (Table 42-8)

2. **Renal Hemodynamics and Renal Protection.** No renal protective strategy has been proven to yield a superior outcome. However, the level of aortic clamping and the avoidance of prolonged hypotension are probably the most important factors because they markedly impact renal blood flow. Intraoperative urinary output is not predictive of postoperative renal function; rather, preoperative renal function is the most powerful predictor of postoperative renal dysfunction.

TABLE 42-8

HEMODYNAMIC CHANGES DURING AORTIC CROSS-CLAMPING AND UNCLAMPING

Increased MAP and SVR (reflecting increased afterload, activation of renin, and release of catecholamines and prostaglandins)

Decreased cardiac output in the presence of increased systemic vascular resistance (may be accompanied by increased cardiac filling pressures if underlying coronary artery disease)

Administration of a vasodilator (nitroprusside) concomitant with or immediately before placement of cross-clamp allows body to adapt

Level of clamping affects hemodynamic response (infrarenal clamping is better tolerated than suprarenal clamping)

Hypotension may accompany unclamping (pretreatment should be done with fluid loading with or without vasoconstrictors [phenylephrine] or calcium [high potassium and acid load]

Gradual unclamping is preferable

MAP = mean arterial pressure; SVR = systemic vascular resistance.

    a. Dopamine has been shown to lack specific renal hemodynamic effects and does not appear to improve postoperative renal dysfunction. Fenoldopam, despite its specific DA-1 activity, has not been shown to be of clinical benefit.

    b. One of the most important factors for preventing postoperative renal failure remains good hydration (the most important factor for maintaining renal blood flow) during clamping and postclamp release.

3. Humoral and Coagulation Profiles. Although the most evident factor contributing to hypotension after removal of the clamp is volume redistribution to the lower body, many humoral mediators are released from the underperfused areas and contribute to the hemodynamic changes.

    a. Administration of bicarbonate does not prevent immediate hypotension after unclamping. Mannitol administration before and after unclamping may be beneficial because of its function as a hydroxyl-free radical scavenger.

    b. Sequestration of microaggregates and neutrophils contributes to postoperative pulmonary dysfunction.

4. Visceral and Mesenteric Ischemia. Bowel ischemia during cross-clamping is associated with increased mortality and leads to increased gut permeability and bacterial translocation.

5. Central Nervous System and Spinal Cord Ischemia and Protection. The definitive measures for preventing spinal cord ischemia are short cross-clamping time, fast surgery, maintenance of normal cardiac function, and higher perfusion pressures. In high aortic clamping, other methods should be considered (Table 42-9)

    a. Some surgeons place a Gott shunt (heparinized tube most often from the ascending aorta to the descending aorta) that can decompress the heart and provide distal perfusion.

    b. A markedly reduced incidence of neurologic deficits has been reported when distal aortic perfusion is combined with drainage of cerebrospinal fluid (CSF).

    c. Endovascular techniques represent an alternative therapy when anatomy permits; lower paraplegia

TABLE 42-9

STRATEGIES TO PROTECT THE SPINAL CORD DURING DESCENDING THORACIC AORTIC SURGERY

Limitation of cross-clamp duration
Use of distal circulatory support (Gott shunt)
Reattachment of critical intercostal arteries
CSF drainage
Hypothermia
Maintenance of proximal blood pressure
  Pharmacotherapy
  Systemic (corticosteroids, barbiturates, calcium channel
    antagonists, oxygen free radical scavengers, NMDA antagonists,
    mannitol, magnesium, vasodilators)
  Intrathecal (papaverine, magnesium, tetracaine)
Avoidance of postoperative hypotension
Sequential aortic clamping
Enhanced monitoring for spinal cord ischemia
  SSEPs
  MEPs

CSF = cerebrospinal fluid; MEP = motor evoked potential;
NMDA = N-methyl-D-aspartic acid; SSEP = somatosensory evoked potential.

rates have been reported compared with open surgery.

C. **Traditional "Open" Surgical Procedures for Aortic Reconstruction.** Perioperative (30-day) mortality in elective aortic surgeries ranges between 0% and 12%, with a much higher probability of death in emergent surgery, especially in situations in which preoperative hypotension (systolic blood pressure <90 mm Hg) exists.

1. **Approach.** Abdominal aortic reconstruction can be performed through a transperitoneal or retroperitoneal exposure.

2. **Clamp Level.** Infrarenal aortic clamping carries the lowest risk for patients; supraceliac clamping carries the highest risk.

3. **Thoracic Aneurysm Repair** (see Table 42-9). These operations are among the most challenging for anesthesiologists. Coincident CAD and chronic obstructive pulmonary disease are common.

   a. Lung isolation (double-lumen tube, bronchial blocker) is required to facilitate surgical access to the aneurysm and to avoid an iatrogenic pulmonary contusion in the left lung.

   b. Because edema of the head and neck frequently occurs after high cross-clamping (even with distal perfusion), reintubation may be difficult at the end of the procedure.

4. **Aortomesenteric Revascularization.** Chronic mesenteric ischemia occurs because of atherosclerosis, and surgical revascularization is indicated only in patients with symptomatic disease. Partial cross-clamping of the aorta is preferred if possible and may mitigate the hemodynamic changes.

5. **Aortorenal revascularization** can be performed by several surgical techniques (endarterectomy, reimplantation, bypass, and ex vivo renal artery reconstruction).

6. **Infrarenal Operations.** Although it is generally recognized that distal ischemic complications are caused by dislodgment of atheromatous material off the diseased aorta and that the systemic use of heparin in the absence of distal occlusive disease is unnecessary, many centers still use heparin before aortic clamping.

D. **Thoracic Aortic Surgery and Endovascular Repair.** Mortality from thoracic aortic surgery may approach 20%, making endovascular thoracoabdominal aortic aneurysm repair an alternative to open surgery. Although paraplegia may still occur, its incidence seems reduced compared with open thoracic aortic aneurysm repair. One approach to attempt to lessen paraplegia after endovascular repair is to place a temporary stent under somatosensory evoked potential (SSEP) monitoring (if SSEP is unchanged, a permanent stent may be placed). However, motor evoked potential monitoring seems more appropriate for monitoring function of the anterior spinal column. Another possibility that has been shown to confer protection in animal models is intermittent aortic cross-clamping.

V. **ENDOVASCULAR ABDOMINAL AORTIC REPAIR (EVAAR)** is now being used more commonly in patients who would otherwise undergo an open repair. Patient eligibility for EVAAR depends on (1) the shape of the aneurysm, including involvement of the renal and iliac arteries and the size and shape of the neck of the aneurysm; (2) the feasibility of delivering the device through the femoral or iliac arteries; and (3) the ability of the patient to compensate for vascular exclusion (aortic branches that will not be supplied after the stent graft is in place).

A. **Outcome and Complications.** New onset or worsening of pre-existing renal failure is a significant source of perioperative morbidity and mortality in patients undergoing EVAAR. Nonperfusion of the hypogastric artery can lead to abdominal complaints. The inferior mesenteric artery is occasionally excluded, and bowel ischemia may result if flow through the superior mesenteric artery is compromised. The artery of Adamkiewicz is typically excluded, which may increase the risk of distal spinal cord ischemia, particularly in patients who have undergone thoracic aortic replacement.

B. **Anesthetic Techniques.** The selection of anesthetic technique is based on the preferences of the patient, anesthesiologist, and surgeon. Before device insertion, systemic anticoagulation is produced with heparin. Surprisingly, EVAAR has not reduced the cost of AAA repair.

C. **Conversion from EVAAR to Open Aortic Repair.** Primary conversion, or the immediate alteration of the surgical plan from an endovascular approach to an open one, occurs in the setting of aneurysm rupture, stent migration or malposition, access site disruption with arterial wall dissection, and poor anatomic parameters for endovascular repair. For anesthesiologists, the complexity of the operation increases dramatically. Hemodynamic instability may ensue with hemorrhage, aortic cross–clamping, or both.

VI. MONITORING AND ANESTHETIC CHOICES FOR AORTIC RECONSTRUCTION

A. Arterial catheters are placed in patients undergoing aortic reconstruction. In patients undergoing thoracic aortic clamping with distal perfusion, distal arterial pressure and CSF pressure may be measured. A pulmonary artery catheter is placed at the discretion of the anesthesiologist in patients undergoing suprarenal aortic cross-clamping but rarely in patients when the clamp will be infrarenal. However, recent large, randomized trials and observational studies have not been able to demonstrate any improvements in outcome with the use of pulmonary artery catheters.

B. Virtually all anesthetic techniques and drugs have been used for aortic reconstructive surgery.

1. Perhaps the most important reason to routinely include volatile anesthetics is the increasing awareness that these drugs improve preconditioning mechanisms and reduce the size of a myocardial infarction if it occurs.
2. Combined general–epidural and general–spinal anesthetics have been used successfully for aortic reconstruction. (The issue of heparinization is a consideration.) For patients requiring thoracotomy, the analgesia provided by thoracic epidural infusion of opioids or local anesthetics may be particularly helpful.

VII. MANAGEMENT OF ELECTIVE AORTIC SURGERY

A. Prehydration may limit variations in blood pressure on induction of anesthesia. The anesthetic management is planned to keep the patient's vital signs within 20% of their normal range, as long as the heart rate does not exceed 80 to 90 bpm and signs of organ ischemia are absent. Increases in blood pressure or heart rate may be treated with 10 to 50 μg of sufentanil.

B. For the half-hour immediately before cross-clamping and aortic occlusion, the patient is kept slightly hypovolemic by examining the ventricular volume by means of echocardiography or by keeping pulmonary capillary wedge pressure at 5 to 15 mm Hg. At the time of occlusion, a vasodilating drug is available for immediate use if needed. Alternatively, the concentration of volatile anesthetic may be increased or local anesthetics may be injected into the epidural catheter.

C. Immediately before removal of the cross-clamp, vasodilators are discontinued. The surgeon then opens the aorta gradually to ensure that severe hypotension or bleeding does not develop.

D. During emergence from anesthesia, infusions of nitroglycerin and esmolol or another β-adrenergic blocking agent are used if necessary to prevent hemodynamic variations outside the patient's normal range.

VIII. ANESTHESIA FOR EMERGENCY AORTIC SURGERY

The most common cause of emergency aortic reconstruction is a leaking or ruptured aortic aneurysm. (Symptoms include pain in the back or abdomen.) Ruptures most commonly occur into the retroperitoneum, resulting in a life-saving tamponade effect.

A. Shock frequently accompanies rupture. However, the absence of hypotension does not rule out the possibility of rupture, and shock may occur suddenly.
B. Rapid diagnosis with immediate laparotomy and control of the proximal aorta are the highest priorities.
C. Because of hypothermia from massive fluid resuscitation and the placement of the aortic cross-clamp above the hepatic artery, replacement blood may not pass through the liver in amounts adequate to allow for metabolism of citrate.
D. As opposed to elective aortic reconstruction, in which preserving myocardial function is the primary goal, in emergency resection, the crucial factor for patient survival is first rapid control of blood loss and reversal of hypotension and then preservation of myocardial function.

IX. LOWER EXTREMITY REVASCULARIZATION

The prevalence of intermittent claudication increases with age, affecting more than 5% of patients older than 70 years of age. The incidence of claudication doubles or triples in patients with diabetes. Advances in minimally invasive percutaneous interventions have made endovascular procedures the primary modality for revascularization in most patients.

A. The three clinical indications for elective surgery for chronic peripheral occlusive disease are claudication, ischemic rest pain or ulceration, and gangrene.
B. During surgery, tunneling of the graft may be more stimulating than other parts of the procedure and may cause hypertension or movement under general anesthesia.
C. The patient is usually given heparin during the procedure. In most cases, the heparin effect is not antagonized because bleeding problems are rare and graft reocclusion is a concern.
D. **Anesthetic Management of Elective Lower Extremity Revascularization**
   1. Morbidity and mortality after traditional distal operations approach those after infra-aortic reconstruction and are mainly of cardiac origin. Most cardiac problems arise during the postoperative

TABLE 42-10

CHOICE OF ANESTHESIA FOR LOWER
EXTREMITY REVASCULARIZATION

Anesthetic Technique	Advantages	Disadvantages
Regional	Effective blockade of stress response Postoperative analgesia Patient serves as a monitor for myocardial ischemia (angina, dyspnea) Possible prevention of postoperative hypercoagulability Improved graft blood flow	Time consuming, especially for postoperative management Sympathectomy requires volume loading Respiratory depression of block level becomes high or the patient becomes oversedated Patient discomfort while lying down during long procedures Rare neurologic sequelae Precludes thrombolytic therapy Technically difficult in patients with obesity, kyposcoliosis, or previous laminectomy
General	Hemodynamics are easily controlled during surgery No patient discomfort during long procedures Reliable	Hyperdynamic state after surgery usually must be treated Postoperative hypercoagulability not inhibited

period, and pain relief and correction of hemodynamic and fluid disequilibria are most likely to be needed.

2. The choice of anesthetic for surgical lower extremity revascularization is individualized for each patient (Table 42-10).

E. **Anesthesia for Emergency Surgery for Peripheral Vascular Insufficiency.** Emergency surgery for peripheral vascular insufficiency is required when acute arterial occlusion results in severe ischemia and threatens the viability of a limb. (The involved extremity suddenly becomes cold and pulseless, and the patient usually complains of coldness, pain, numbness, and paresthesias.)

1. Serum potassium levels can change quickly because of cell death and release of intracellular potassium into the circulation. Myoglobin may also be released into the circulation, and the development of a compartment syndrome is possible.
2. Anticoagulants are commonly administered to patients suspected of having peripheral vascular occlusion. If a patient has received anticoagulants, the appropriateness of using regional anesthesia is controversial.

CHAPTER 43 ■ OBSTETRICAL ANESTHESIA

During pregnancy, alterations occur in nearly every maternal organ system, with associated implications for anesthesiologists (Table 43-1) (Braveman FR, Scavone BM, Wong CA, Santos AC: Obstetrical anesthesia. In *Clinical Anesthesia*. Edited by Barash PG, Cullen BF, Stoelting RK, Cahalan MK, Stock MC. Philadelphia: Lippincott Williams & Wilkins, 2009, pp 1137–1170).

I. PHYSIOLOGIC CHANGES OF PREGNANCY

A. Increased alveolar ventilation along with decreased functional residual capacity enhances maternal uptake and elimination of inhaled anesthetics.

B. Decreased functional residual capacity and increased basal metabolic rate may predispose the parturient to arterial hypoxemia during periods of apnea, as associated with endotracheal intubation.

C. Vascular engorgement of the airway may predispose the patient to bleeding on insertion of nasopharyngeal airways, nasogastric tubes, or endotracheal tubes.

D. Controversy exists as to when a pregnant woman becomes at risk for aspiration. Earlier studies showing delayed emptying in the first trimester may have been a result of subjects' pain, anxiety, or opioid administration.

II. PLACENTAL TRANSFER AND FETAL EXPOSURE TO ANESTHETIC DRUGS

A. Most drugs (opioids, local anesthetics, inhaled anesthetics) readily cross the placenta.

1. Placental transfer depends on several factors (Table 43-2).

2. Rapid transfer of inhalational agents results in detectable arterial and venous concentrations after 1 minute.

TABLE 43-1

PHYSIOLOGIC CHANGES OF PREGNANCY

Hematologic Alterations
Increased total blood volume (25%–40%)
Increased plasma volume (40%–50%)
Increased fibrinogen (100%)
Decreased cholinesterase activity (20%–30%)

Cardiovascular Changes
Increased cardiac output (30%–50%)
Aortocaval compression (supine hypotensive syndrome
  occurs in about 50% of parturients)

Ventilatory Changes
Increased minute ventilation (50%)
Increased alveolar ventilation (70%)
Decreased functional residual capacity (20%)
Increased oxygen consumption (20%)
Decreased $PaCO_2$ (10 mm Hg)
Increased PaO_2 (10 mm Hg)
Airway edema

Gastrointestinal Changes
Delayed gastric emptying
Decreased lower esophageal sphincter tone (heartburn)

Altered Drug Responses
Decreased requirements (32%–40%) for inhaled anesthetics
  (MAC) by 8–12 weeks (parallels increased progesterone levels)
Decreased local anesthetic requirements (engorgement of veins
  resulting in decreased volume of the epidural and subarachnoid
  space versus progesterone-induced increased sensitivity of nerves
  to local anesthetics)

MAC = minimum alveolar concentration.

TABLE 43-2

DETERMINANTS OF DRUG PASSAGE ACROSS THE PLACENTA

Physical and Chemical Characteristics of the Drug
Molecular weight (<500)
Lipid solubility
Non-ionized vs ionized

Concentration Gradient
Dose administered
Timing of IV administration relative to uterine contraction
Use of vasoconstrictors

Hemodynamic Factors
Aortocaval compression
Hypotension from regional blockade

IV = intravenous.

TABLE 43-3

CHARACTERISTICS OF FETAL CIRCULATION THAT DELAY
DRUG EQUILIBRATION

The fetal liver is the first organ perfused by the umbilical vein
Dilution of umbilical vein blood by fetal venous blood from the
gastrointestinal tract, head, and extremities (this explains why
thiopental [4 mg/kg IV] administered to the mother does not
produce significant depressant effects in the fetus)

  B. **Fetus and Newborn.** Several characteristics of the fetal
    circulation delay equilibration between fetal arterial
    and venous blood and thus delay the onset or magni-
    tude of depressant effects of anesthetic drugs (Table
    43-3).

  C. Neurobehavioral studies in neonates born in the pres-
    ence of epidural anesthesia may reveal subtle changes
    in newborn neurologic and adaptive function. (These
    changes are minor and transient, lasting only 24 to 48
    hours.)

III. **ANESTHESIA FOR LABOR AND
    VAGINAL DELIVERY**

  Whereas analgesia for the first stage of labor (pain caused
  by uterine contractions) is provided by block of T10–L1,
  analgesia for the second stage of labor (pain caused by
  distention of the perineum) is provided by block of S2–S4.

  A. **Nonpharmacologic methods of labor analgesia** (mas-
    sage, aromatherapy, hydrotherapy, biofeedback, tran-
    scutaneous electrical nerve stimulation, acupuncture,
    hypnosis) remain unproven for efficacy.

  B. **Systemic Medication.** The time and method of admin-
    istration must be chosen carefully to avoid maternal
    and neonatal depression.

    1. Opioids

      a. **Meperidine** appears to produce less neonatal venti-
        latory depression than does morphine. Meperidine
        administered intravenously (IV) (analgesia in 5–10
        minutes) or intramuscularly (peak effect in 40–50
        minutes) rapidly crosses the placenta.

      b. **Fentanyl** (1 µg/kg IV) provides prompt pain relief
        (during forceps application) without severe
        neonatal depression. For more analgesia, fentanyl

or remifentanil may be administered with patient-controlled delivery devices.

   c. **Naloxone** (10 µg/kg IV) may be administered directly to newborns to reverse excessive opioid depression.

2. **Ketamine** (0.2–0.4 mg/kg IV) provides adequate analgesia without producing neonatal depression.

C. **Regional Anesthesia.** Regional techniques (central neuraxial blockade [spinal, epidural, combined spinal–epidural]) provide excellent analgesia with minimal depressant effects in the mother and fetus. **Hypotension** resulting from sympathectomy is the most frequent complication that occurs with central neuraxial blockade. (Maternal systemic blood pressure is typically monitored every 2 to 5 minutes for about 15 to 20 minutes after the initiation of the block and at regular intervals thereafter.) Regional analgesia may be contraindicated in the presence of coagulopathy, acute hypovolemia, or infection at the needle insertion site. (Chorioamnionitis without frank sepsis is not a contraindication.)

   1. **Epidural analgesia** may be used for pain relief during labor and vaginal delivery and may be converted to anesthesia for cesarean delivery if required.

      a. Effective analgesia during the first stage of labor may be achieved by blocking the T10–L1 dermatomes with dilute concentrations of local anesthetic with or without the use of opioids that have their effect at the opioid receptors in the dorsal horn of the spinal cord (Table 43-4). For the second stage of labor and delivery, because of pain from vaginal distention and perineal pressure, the block should be extended to include the S2–S4 segments.

TABLE 43-4

TESTS TO RULE OUT INTRATHECAL OR INTRAVASCULAR PLACEMENT OF A LUMBAR EPIDURAL CATHETER

Aspiration (may not be diagnostic)
Local anesthetic (7.5 mg of bupivacaine or 45 mg of lidocaine)
Epinephrine (15 µg; a false-positive reaction may be seen with uterine contractions; may decrease uteroplacental perfusion)

b. The first stage of labor may be slightly prolonged by epidural analgesia, but this is not clinically significant provided aortocaval compression is avoided. Epidural analgesia initiated during the latent phase of labor (2–4 cm cervical dilation) does not result in a higher incidence of dystocia or cesarean section.

c. Prolongation of the second stage of labor by epidural analgesia (presumably related to loss of the urge to push by the patient) may be minimized by the use of an ultra-dilute concentration of local anesthetic in combination with an opioid.

d. Analgesia for the first stage of labor may be achieved with 5 to 10 mL of bupivacaine, ropivacaine, or levobupivacaine (0.125%–0.25%) followed by continuous infusion (8–12 mL/hr) of 0.0625% bupivacaine or levobupivacaine or 0.1% ropivacaine. The addition of 1 to 2 µg/mL of fentanyl (or 0.3–0.5 µg/l mL of sufentanil) permits a more dilute local anesthetic solution to be administered. During delivery, the sacral dermatomes may be blocked with 10 mL of 0.5% bupivacaine or 1% lidocaine or if a rapid effect is needed, 2% chloroprocaine may be administered in the semirecumbent position.

e. Patient-controlled epidural analgesia is an alternative to bolus or infusion techniques.

2. **Spinal Analgesia**

a. A single subarachnoid injection for labor analgesia has the advantages of a reliable and rapid onset of neuraxial blockade.

b. Spinal analgesia with 10 µg of fentanyl or 2 to 5 µg of sufentanil alone or in combination with 1 mL of isobaric bupivacaine 0.25% may be appropriate in multiparous patients whose anticipated course of labor does not warrant a catheter technique.

c. Spinal anesthesia ("saddle block") is a safe and effective alternative to general anesthesia for instrumental delivery.

d. There is a risk of postdural puncture headache, and the motor block may be undesirable.

3. **Combined Spinal–Epidural Analgesia**

a. Combined spinal–epidural analgesia is an ideal analgesic technique for use during labor because it combines the rapid onset of profound analgesia (spinal injection) with the flexibility and longer duration of epidural techniques.

b. After identification of the epidural space, a long pencil-point spinal needle is advanced into the subarachnoid space through the epidural needle. After intrathecal injection (10–20 μg of fentanyl or 2.5–5 μg of sufentanil alone or in combination with 1 mL of bupivacaine 0.25% produces profound analgesia lasting 90 to 120 minutes with minimal motor block), an epidural infusion of bupivacaine 0.03% to 0.625% with added opioid is started.

c. Women with hemodynamic stability and preserved motor function who do not require continuous fetal monitoring may ambulate with assistance. (Walking has little effect on the course of labor.)

d. The most common side effects of intrathecal opioids are pruritus, nausea, vomiting, and urinary retention. The risk of postdural puncture headache does not seem to be increased. Fetal bradycardia may occur.

e. The potential exists for epidurally administered drug to leak into the subarachnoid space after dural puncture, particularly if large volumes of drug are rapidly injected.

f. This technique should be used with caution in women who may require an urgent cesarean section and women who are at most increased risk (morbidly obese, difficult airway).

4. **A paracervical block** interrupts transmission of nerve impulses from the uterus and cervix during the first stage of labor.

5. **A pudendal nerve block** may provide anesthesia for outlet forceps delivery and episiotomy repair.

IV. ANESTHESIA FOR CESAREAN DELIVERY

The choice of anesthesia is often influenced by the urgency of the operative procedure and the condition of the fetus. Most patients undergoing cesarean delivery in the United States do so under spinal or epidural anesthesia.

A. **Neuraxial anesthesia** offers the advantages of decreased risk of pulmonary aspiration of gastric contents, avoidance of depressant drugs, and fulfillment of the mother's wishes to remain awake. The risk of hypotension is greater than during vaginal delivery because the block must extend to at least the T4 dermatome. Proper positioning and prehydration with up to 20 mL/kg of crystalloid solution is recommended. If hypotension occurs despite these measures, left uterine displacement is increased, the rate of IV infusion is augmented, and 10 to 15 mg of ephedrine or 20 to 50 μg of phenylephrine is injected IV.

1. **Spinal anesthesia** is provided most often with 1.6 to 1.8 mL of hyperbaric bupivacaine 0.75% lasting approximately 120 to 180 minutes. Improved perioperative analgesia can be provided by addition of fentanyl (6.25 μg) or preservative-free morphine (100 μg) to the local anesthetic solution. It is probably not necessary to adjust the dose of local anesthetic based on the parturient's height.

   a. Despite a block extending to T4, parturients often experience visceral discomfort, particularly with exteriorization of the uterus and traction on abdominal viscera (25 μg of fentanyl IV may be useful).

   b. Oxygen should be routinely administered by face mask to optimize maternal and fetal oxygenation.

2. **Lumbar Epidural Anesthesia.** Compared with spinal anesthesia, lumbar epidural anesthesia requires more time and drug to establish an adequate sensory level, but there is a lower risk of postdural puncture headache, and the level of anesthesia can be adjusted by titration of local anesthetic solution injected through the indwelling catheter.

   a. Adequate anesthesia is usually achieved with injection through the lumbar epidural catheter of 15 to 25 mL of local anesthetic solution (Table 43-5).

TABLE 43-5

EPIDURAL ANESTHESIA FOR CESAREAN SECTION

2-Chloroprocaine 3%
Lidocaine 2% with epinephrine 1:200,000
0.5% Bupivacaine, ropivacaine, or levobupivacaine

      b. Addition of morphine (3–5 mg) to the local anesthetic solution provides postoperative analgesia.

  3. Combined spinal–epidural anesthesia for cesarean delivery provides a rapid onset of a dense block with a low anesthetic dose and the ability to extend the duration of anesthesia and perhaps to provide continuous postoperative analgesia.

B. General anesthesia may be necessary when contraindications exist to regional anesthesia or when time precludes central neuraxial blockade. Situations in which uterine relaxation facilitates delivery (multiple gestations, breech position) are most often managed with general anesthesia (Table 43-6).

TABLE 43-6

GENERAL ANESTHESIA FOR CESAREAN SECTION

Preoperative evaluation of the airway (inability to intubate is the leading cause of maternal death related to anesthesia)

Premedication with 15–30 mL of a nonparticulate antacid within 30 minutes of induction

The parturient should be maintained in the left uterine displacement position while on the operating table

Preoxygenation

A defasciculating dose of nondepolarizing muscle relaxant is not necessary

4 mg/kg IV of thiopental (2 mg/kg of propofol or 0.5 mg/kg IV of ketamine), plus 1–1.5 mg/kg IV of succinylcholine should be used during cricoid pressure (drugs should be injected at the onset of contraction if the patient is in labor)

Skin incision should be done after confirmation of tracheal tube placement

Rocuronium (0.6 mg/kg IV) is an acceptable alternative when succinylcholine is contraindicated

An LMA should be considered if tracheal intubation cannot be accomplished

Maintenance in the predelivery interval with 50% nitrous oxide and 0.5 MAC of a volatile anesthetic (temporarily increased to 2 MAC a few minutes before delivery if uterine relaxation is needed to facilitate delivery; alternatively, nitroglycerin relaxes the uterus)

Extreme hyperventilation of the lungs should be avoided because it may reduce uterine blood flow

Oxytocin is added to the infusion after delivery, and anesthesia is deepened (possibly with opioids)

The trachea is extubated when the patient awakens

IV = intravenous; LMA = laryngeal mask airway; MAC = minimum alveolar concentration.

1. A newborn's condition after cesarean section with general anesthesia is comparable to that when regional techniques are used. The uterine incision to delivery time (<180 seconds) is more important to fetal outcome than is the anesthetic technique.

2. The usual amount of blood loss during cesarean section is 750 to 1000 mL, and transfusion is rarely necessary.

3. When tracheal intubation is unexpectedly difficult, it may be prudent to permit the parturient to awaken and then to pursue alternative approaches (awake fiberoptic tracheal intubation, regional anesthesia) rather than to persist with repeated unsuccessful and traumatic attempts at tracheal intubation (Fig. 43-1).

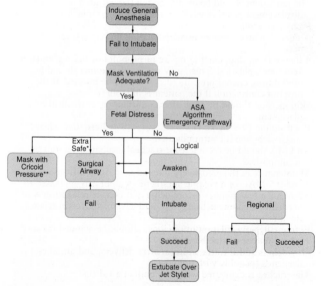

FIGURE 43-1. Management of the difficult airway in pregnancy. ASA = American Society of Anesthesiologists.

V. ANESTHETIC COMPLICATIONS (Table 43-7)

VI. MANAGEMENT OF HIGH-RISK PARTURIENTS

A. **Preeclampsia and Eclampsia.** Preeclampsia (pregnancy-induced hypertension) and eclampsia (seizures) are characterized by hypertension, proteinuria, and edema that may progress to oliguria, congestive heart failure, and seizures (eclampsia) (Table 43-8).

SURGICAL SUBSPECIALTIES

TABLE 43-7

ANESTHETIC COMPLICATIONS IN OBSTETRIC PATIENTS

Maternal Mortality
Most often related to arterial hypoxemia during airway management difficulties
Pregnancy-induced anatomic changes (decreased functional residual capacity, increased oxygen consumption, or oropharyngeal edema may expose the parturient to an increased risk of arterial oxygen desaturation during periods of apnea and hypoventilation)

Pulmonary Aspiration

Hypotension
Regional anesthesia (related to the degree and rapidity of local anesthetic-induced sympatholysis)
Prehydration (<20 mL/kg of lactated Ringer's solution) before initiation of regional anesthesia and avoidance of aortocaval compression may decrease the incidence of hypotension
Treatment is increased displacement of the uterus, rapid IV fluid infusion, titration of ephedrine (5–10 mg) or phenylephrine (20–50 µg), oxygen administration, and placement in the Trendelenburg position

Total Spinal Anesthesia

Local Anesthetic-Induced Seizures
Treatment is with IV administration of thiopental (50–100 mg) or diazepam (5–10 mg)

Postdural Puncture Headache
The incidence is lower with pencil-point needles (Whitacre or Sprotte) compared with diamond-shaped (Quincke) cutting needles
Treatment of a severe headache is with a blood patch (10–15 mL of the patient's blood is injected into the epidural space close to the site of dural puncture)

Nerve Injury
The possible role of compression of the maternal lumbosacral trunk by the fetus should be considered

IV = intravenous.

TABLE 43-8

SYMPTOMS OF SEVERE PREECLAMPSIA

Systolic blood pressure >160 mm Hg
Diastolic blood pressure >110 mm Hg
Proteinuria >5 g/24 hours
Evidence of end organ damage
   Oliguria (<400 mL/24 hours)
   Cerebral or visual disturbances
   Pulmonary edema
   Epigastric pain
   Intrauterine growth retardation
Thrombocytopenia (steroids may prevent)

1. Many of the symptoms associated with preeclampsia may result from an imbalance between the placental production of prostacyclin and thromboxane.
2. The HEELP syndrome is a form of severe preeclampsia characterized by hemolysis, elevated liver enzymes, and low platelet count. In contrast to preeclampsia, elevations in blood pressure and proteinuria may be mild.
3. **General Management** (Table 43-9)
4. **Anesthetic Management**
   a. Epidural anesthesia or combined spinal–epidural analgesia for labor and delivery is acceptable provided no clotting abnormality or plasma volume deficit is present. In volume-repleted parturients positioned with left uterine displacement, the institution of epidural anesthesia does not typically cause an unacceptable decrease in blood pressure and may result in significant improvements in placental blood flow.

TABLE 43-9

CONSIDERATIONS IN THE MANAGEMENT OF PARTURIENTS WITH PREECLAMPSIA OR ECLAMPSIA

Prevent or control seizures (magnesium sulfate potentiates muscle relaxants and may increase the severity of hypotension under regional anesthesia).
Restore intravascular fluid volume (central venous or pulmonary capillary wedge pressure, 5–10 mm Hg; urine output, 0.5–1 mL/kg/hr).
Normalize blood pressure (hydralazine, nitroprusside).
Correct coagulation abnormalities.

     b. Spinal anesthesia may produce severe alterations in cardiovascular dynamics resulting from sudden sympathetic nervous system blockade.

     c. General anesthesia is often chosen for acute emergencies, but the practitioner should keep in mind the probable exaggerated blood pressure responses to induction of anesthesia and intubation of the trachea and possible interactions of muscle relaxants with magnesium sulfate therapy.

     d. Decreased doses of ephedrine are recommended to treat patients with hypotension because parturients with preeclampsia or eclampsia may exhibit increased sensitivity to vasopressors.

B. Obstetric Hemorrhage. Life-threatening massive hemorrhage occurs in approximately one in 1000 deliveries.

    1. Placenta previa (painless, bright red bleeding after the seventh month of pregnancy) is the most common cause of postpartum hemorrhage.

    2. Abruptio placentae typically manifests as uterine hypertonia and tenderness with dark red vaginal bleeding. Maternal and fetal mortality rates are increased.

    3. General anesthesia (often with ketamine [0.75 mg/kg IV] induction of anesthesia) is used in view of the increased risk of hemorrhage and clotting disorders.

C. Heart Disease. Cardiac decompensation and death occur most commonly at the time of maximum hemodynamic stress. For example, cardiac output increases during labor, with the greatest increase immediately after delivery of the placenta. These changes in cardiac output are blunted by regional anesthesia.

    1. Congenital Heart Disease (Table 43-10)

    2. Valvular Heart Disease (Table 43-11)

TABLE 43-10

CONGENITAL HEART DISEASE AND THE PARTURIENT

Prior successful surgical repair (asymptomatic)
Uncorrected or partially corrected (may experience cardiac decompensation with pregnancy)
Eisenmenger's syndrome (pulmonary hypertension reverses flow to a right-to-left shunt; general anesthesia is often selected)

TABLE 43-11

HEMODYNAMIC GOALS WITH VALVULAR LESIONS

Lesion	Goal
Aortic stenosis	Sinus rhythm
	Maintain HR
	Avoid decreased SVR
	Maintain venous return
Aortic insufficiency	Mild increase in HR
	Avoid increased SVR
Mitral stenosis	Sinus rhythm
	Decrease HR
	Maintain SVR
	Maintain venous return
Mitral insufficiency	Sinus rhythm
	Mild increase in HR
	Avoid increased SVR
	Avoid increased venous return

HR = heart rate; SVR = systemic vascular resistance.

3. **Coarctation of the aorta** is similar to aortic stenosis and may manifest as left ventricular failure during labor and delivery.

4. **Primary pulmonary hypertension** is seen predominantly in young parturients, and pain during labor and delivery may further increase pulmonary vascular resistance. (Neuraxial analgesia is useful.)

5. **Peripartum cardiomyopathy** is a diagnosis of exclusion, and the prognosis is good if cardiac function returns to normal within 6 months of delivery.

6. **Coronary artery disease and myocardial infarction** are rare but are associated with high maternal and infant mortality.

D. **Diabetes Mellitus.** Gestational diabetes mellitus or glucose intolerance is first diagnosed during pregnancy (there is an increasing incidence with obesity).

E. **Obesity** is associated with antenatal comorbidities (hypertension, diabetes, preeclampsia) and an increasing need for cesarean delivery. Despite technical challenges, continuous neuraxial analgesia provides excellent pain relief during labor and delivery.

F. **Advanced maternal age** (older than 35 years of age) is associated with poorer outcomes and a higher incidence of maternal morbidities (gestational diabetes,

TABLE 43-12

PROBLEMS ASSOCIATED WITH PREMATURITY

Respiratory distress syndrome (glucocorticoids administered to the mother for 24–48 hours may enhance fetal lung maturity)
Intracranial hemorrhage
Hypoglycemia
Hypocalcemia
Hyperbilirubinemia

preeclampsia, placental abruption, cesarean delivery) and chronic medical conditions.

VII. PRETERM DELIVERY

Preterm labor and delivery is defined as birth before the 37th week or term weight of the infant as more than two standard deviations below the mean (small for gestational age). Such infants account for 8% to 10% of all births and nearly 80% of early neonatal deaths in the U.S.

A. Several problems are likely to develop in preterm infants (Table 43-12).
B. β_2-Agonists (ritodrine, terbutaline) used to inhibit labor may interact with anesthetic drugs or produce undesirable changes before induction of anesthesia (Table 43-13).
  1. Delay of anesthesia for at least 3 hours after the cessation of tocolysis allows β-mimetic effects of β_2-agonists to dissipate; potassium supplementation is not necessary.
  2. Preterm infants are more sensitive to the depressant effects of anesthetic drugs. Regardless of the technique or drugs selected, the most important goal is prevention of asphyxia of the fetus.

TABLE 43-13

SIDE EFFECTS OF β_2-AGONISTS ADMINISTERED TO STOP PREMATURE LABOR

Hypokalemia (cardiac dysrhythmias)
Hypotension (accentuated by regional anesthesia)
Tachycardia (atropine and pancuronium should be avoided)
Pulmonary edema (cautious prehydration)

TABLE 43-14

SUBSTANCE ABUSE AMONG WOMEN OF CHILDBEARING AGE

Tobacco abuse (intrauterine growth retardation, preterm delivery, sudden infant death syndrome)
Alcohol (fetal alcohol syndrome)
Opioids (withdrawal symptoms)
Marijuana (intrauterine growth retardation, preterm delivery)
Cocaine
Amphetamines (fetal anomalies)

VIII. HIV AND AIDS

A. Prevention of viral transmission to the fetus is based on antiretroviral therapy to decrease maternal viral load and elective cesarean delivery before rupture of membranes or labor.

B. Spread of HIV to the central nervous system occurs rapidly after initial infection, and there is no evidence linking the use of regional anesthesia to progression of the disease.

C. Using a blood patch to treat postdural puncture headache does not seem to accelerate HIV symptoms.

IX. SUBSTANCE ABUSE

Nearly 90% of women with substance abuse are of childbearing age (Table 43-14). Cocaine abuse has the greatest implications for anesthetic management (Table 43-15).

TABLE 43-15

ANESTHETIC CONSIDERATIONS ASSOCIATED WITH COCAINE OR AMPHETAMINE ABUSE

Uncontrolled hypertension
Cardiac arrhythmias (ventricular tachycardia or fibrillation)
Myocardial ischemia
Ephedrine-resistant hypotension with neuraxial blockade (a direct-acting drug should be used)
Acute use may increase the MAC of volatile drugs
Chronic use may decrease the dosage of anesthetic drugs
The patient may exhibit increased sensitivity to the arrhythmogenic effects of volatile drugs

MAC = minimum alveolar concentration.

TABLE 43-16

BIOPHYSICAL MONITORING OF THE FETUS

Baseline heart rate (normal, 120–160 bpm)
Beat-to-beat variability (reflects variations in autonomic nervous
  system tone; disappears with fetal distress, opioids, local
  anesthetics)
Fetal heart rate deceleration

X. FETAL AND MATERNAL MONITORING

A. **Biophysical Monitoring.** Ultrasonographic cardiography and measurement of uterine activity with a toco-dynamometer provide noninvasive monitoring of fetal well-being (Table 43-16 and Fig. 43-2). Prolonged

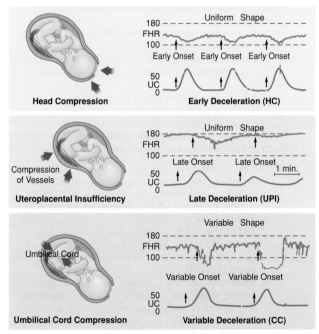

FIGURE 43-2. Relationship and significance of fetal heart rate (FHR) changes in association with uterine contractions (UCs).

TABLE 43-17

EVENTS ASSOCIATED WITH NEONATAL DEPRESSION AT BIRTH

Prematurity (80% <1500 g need resuscitation)
Drugs used during labor or delivery
Trauma or precipitated labor
Birth asphyxia (reflects interference with placental perfusion)
Tight umbilical cord
Prolapsed cord
Premature separation of placenta
Uterine hyperactivity
Maternal hypotension

deceleration is present when fetal heart rate decreases below baseline for more than 2 but less than 10 minutes. All decelerations should be quantified based on the deviation from baseline and the duration.

B. **Fetal pulse oximetry** is an adjunct to fetal heart rate monitoring as a reflection of intrapartum fetal oxygenation.

1. Fetal oxygen saturation between 30% and 70% is considered normal.

2. Saturation readings consistently below 30% for 10 to 15 minutes are suggestive of fetal acidemia.

XI. NEWBORN RESUSCITATION IN THE DELIVERY ROOM

Several factors contribute to the likelihood of depression at birth and require neonatal resuscitation (Table 43-17).

A. **Resuscitation.** Every delivery room must be equipped with appropriate resuscitation equipment and drugs for newborn and maternal resuscitation (Fig. 43-3).

1. **Initial Treatment and Evaluation of All Infants.** The pharynx is suctioned, heart rate is quantified, and ventilation is assessed. The scoring system introduced by Dr. Virginia Apgar, an anesthesiologist, is a useful method of clinically evaluating newborns (Table 43-18).

2. Meconium staining is treated by oropharyngeal suctioning at the time of delivery; tracheal intubation and airway suctioning are probably only necessary in the presence of a low Apgar score and evidence of mechanical airway obstruction.

3. **Use of cardiac massage** (chest compressions of the middle third of the sternum) should be provided if

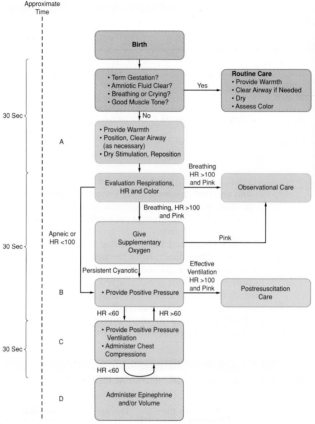

FIGURE 43-3. Algorithm for neonatal resuscitation. HR = heart rate.

heart rate is below 60 bpm despite adequate ventilation for 30 seconds. The ratio of chest compression to ventilation should be approximately 3:1 or 100 compressions to 30 breaths/min (Table 43-19).

4. **Rapid Correction of Acidosis.** Sodium bicarbonate is not recommended during brief cardiopulmonary resuscitation because hyperosmolarity and carbon dioxide generation may be detrimental to cardiac

TABLE 43-18

CALCULATION OF THE APGAR SCORE

	0	1	2
Heart rate	Absent	<100 bpm	>100 bpm
Respiratory effort	Absent	Slow and irregular	Crying
Muscle tone	Limp	Some flexion of extremities	Moving
Reflex irritability	No response	Grimace	Crying, cough
Color	Pale; blue	Body pink; extremities blue	Pink

and cerebral function. After ensuring adequate ventilation and perfusion, severe acidosis (pH <7.0) may need to be corrected promptly by infusion of sodium bicarbonate into the umbilical vein.

5. **Other Drugs and Fluids** (Table 43-20)

B. **Diagnostic Procedures.** After the neonate is successfully resuscitated and stabilized, diagnostic procedures are indicated to rule out choanal atresia (occlusion of the nostrils to confirm absence of obstruction) and esophageal atresia (aspiration of gastric contents).

1. **EXIT procedure** (ex utero intrapartum treatment) maintains uteroplacental support for a time period

TABLE 43-19

THERAPEUTIC GUIDELINES FOR NEONATAL RESUSCITATION

Drug or Volume Expander	Concentration	Dosage	Route/Rate
Epinephrine	1:10,000	0.01–0.03 mg/kg	IV or IT
Volume expanders	Packed red blood cells Normal saline Lactated Ringer's solution	10 mL/kg	Give over 5–10 minutes
Naloxone		0.1 mg/kg	IV, IM, SC, or IT given rapidly

IM = intramuscular; IT = intratracheal; IV = intravenous; SC = subcutaneous.

TABLE 43-20

OTHER DRUGS AND FLUIDS USED IN NEONATAL RESUSCITATION

Naloxone (should be avoided in infants born to opioid-addicted mothers)
Epinephrine (used to treat asystole or persistent bradycardia; administered IV or by tracheal tube)
Lactated Ringer's solution (10 mL/kg IV)
Type O-negative blood (10 mL/kg IV)

IV = intravenous.

after delivery of the fetus (large neck masses, clips placed for diaphragmatic hernia). Often two anesthesia teams are needed—one for the mother and one for the fetus or newborn).

XII. ANESTHESIA FOR NON-OBSTETRIC SURGERY IN PREGNANT WOMEN (Fig. 43-4)

A. When the necessity for surgery in a pregnant patient arises, anesthetic considerations are related to multiple factors (Table 43-21).

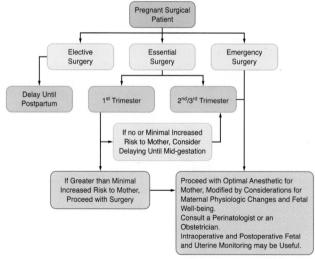

FIGURE 43-4. Recommendations for management of parturients and surgical procedures.

TABLE 43-21

CONSIDERATIONS IN THE MANAGEMENT OF ANESTHESIA FOR
NON-OBSTETRIC SURGERY IN PREGNANT WOMEN

Physiologic changes of pregnancy
Decreased requirements for local and inhaled anesthetics
Low functional residual capacity
High basal metabolic rate
Slowed gastric emptying
Aortocaval compression
Teratogenicity of anesthetic drugs (period of organogenesis is
    15–56 days; single exposure seems unlikely to cause
    abnormalities)
Adequacy of uteroplacental circulation
Initiation of premature labor

B. Only emergency surgery should be performed during
   pregnancy, especially in the first trimester. It is logical
   to select drugs with a long history of safety (opioids,
   muscle relaxants, thiopental, nitrous oxide). The fetal
   heart rate should be monitored after the 16th week.

CHAPTER 44 ■ **NEONATAL ANESTHESIA**

The first year of life is characterized by an almost miraculous growth (body weight changes by a factor of three) in size and maturity (Hall SC, Suresh S: Neonatal anesthesia. In *Clinical Anesthesia*. Edited by Barash PG, Cullen BF, Stoelting RK, Cahalan MK, Stock MC. Philadelphia: Lippincott Williams & Wilkins, 2009, pp 1171–1205).

I. PHYSIOLOGY OF THE INFANT AND THE TRANSITION PERIOD

The newborn period has been defined as the first 24 hours of life and the neonatal period as the first month. The first 72 hours are especially significant for the cardiovascular, pulmonary, and renal systems.

A. **The Cardiovascular System (Fetal Circulation)** (Fig. 44-1A
   1. **Changes at Birth** (Fig. 44-1B)
   2. Myocardial function is different in neonates because the cardiac myocytes have less organized contractile elements than in children and adults. The neonatal myocardium cannot generate as much force as in older children and is relatively noncompliant. Consequently, there is limited functional reserve in the neonatal period, and afterload increases are particularly poorly tolerated.
   3. Especially in the first 3 months of life, the influence of the parasympathetic nervous system on the heart is more mature than the influence of the sympathetic system, and the myocardium does not respond to inotropic support as well as in older children and adults.
   4. Even in the absence of stress, the neonatal heart has limited ability to increase cardiac output compared with the mature heart (Fig. 44-2).

B. **The Pulmonary System**
   1. The airways and alveoli continue to grow after birth, with the alveoli increasing in number until about 8 years of age.

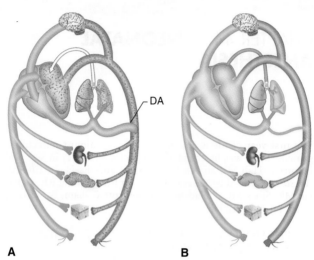

FIGURE 44-1. **A.** Schematic representation of the fetal circulation. **B.** Schematic representation of the circulation in the normal newborn. DA = ductus arteriosus.

2. With the initiation of ventilation, the alveoli transition from a fluid-filled to an air-filled state, and a normal ventilatory pattern with normal volumes develops in the first 5 to 10 minutes of life. Blood gases stabilize with the establishment of increased pulmonary blood flow (Table 44-1).

3. Tidal volume is about the same in neonates as in children and adults on a volume per kilogram body weight measure, but the respiratory rate is increased in neonates (Table 44-2 and Fig. 44-3).

   a. Increased minute ventilation mirrors the higher oxygen consumption in neonates (about double that seen in adults).

   b. The ratio of minute ventilation to functional residual capacity (FRC) is two to three times higher in newborns. As a result, anesthetic induction and emergence with a volatile anesthetic agent should be faster. In addition, the decrease in FRC relative to minute ventilation and oxygen consumption means that there is less "oxygen reserve" in the FRC than in older children and adults. There is a more rapid

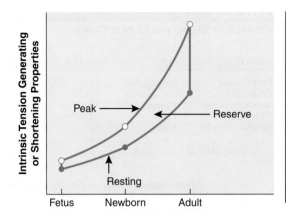

A

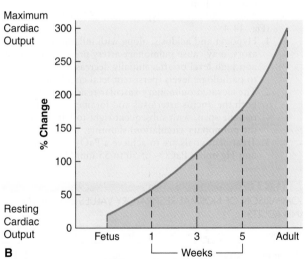

B

FIGURE 44-2. Schema of reduced cardiac reserve in fetal and newborn animal hearts compared with adult hearts.

decrease in arterial oxygen levels in newborns in the presence of apnea or hypoventilation.
4. Decreased surfactant production caused by prematurity or other conditions such as maternal diabetes can cause respiratory distress syndrome (RDS). Commercially

TABLE 44-1

NORMAL BLOOD GAS VALUES IN NEONATES

Subject	Age	PO$_2$ (mm Hg)	PCO$_2$ (mm Hg)	pH
Fetus (term)	Before labor	25	40	7.37
Fetus (term)	End of labor	10–20	55	7.25
Newborn (term)	10 min	50	48	7.20
Newborn (term)	1 hr	70	35	7.35
Newborn (term)	1 wk	75	35	7.40
Newborn (preterm, 1500 g)	1 wk	60	38	7.37

available surfactant is extraordinarily useful in treating and preventing RDS in susceptible patients.

5. Neonates do not respond as well to hypercapnia as older children.

C. **Persistent Pulmonary Hypertension of Newborns** (Fig. 44-4)

1. Hypoxia and acidosis, along with inflammatory mediators, may cause pulmonary artery pressure to persist at a high level or after initially decreasing to increase to pathologic levels (persistent fetal circulation).

2. The elevated pulmonary vascular resistance causes both the ductus arteriosus and foramen ovale to remain open, with subsequent right-to-left (bypassing the pulmonary circulation) shunting.

3. Treatment goals are to achieve a PaO$_2$ of 50 to 70 mm Hg and a PaCO$_2$ of 50 to 55 mm Hg.

TABLE 44-2

COMPARISON OF NORMAL RESPIRATORY VALUES IN INFANTS AND ADULTS

Parameter	Infant	Adult
Respiratory frequency	30–50	12–16
Tidal volume (mL/kg)	7	7
Dead space (mL/kg)	2.0–2.5	2.2
Alveolar ventilation (mL/kg/min)	100–150	60
Functional residual capacity (mL/kg)	27–30	30
Oxygen consumption (mL/kg/min)	7–9	3

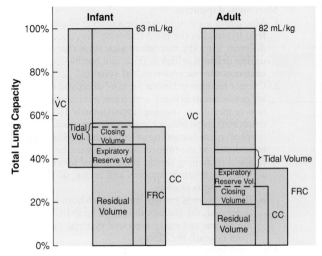

FIGURE 44-3. Static lung volumes of infants and adults. CC = closing capacity; FRC = functional residual capacity; VC = vital capacity.

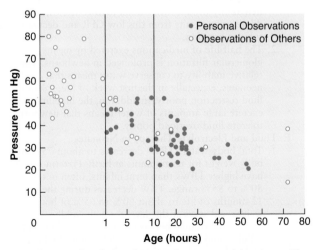

FIGURE 44-4. Correlation of mean pulmonary arterial pressure with age in 85 normal-term infants studied during the first 3 days of life.

D. **Meconium Aspiration**
1. Meconium aspiration may be a marker of chronic fetal hypoxia in the third trimester. This condition is different from the meconium aspiration that occurs during delivery, which is thick and mechanically obstructs the tracheobronchial system.
2. Current recommendations for intubation and suctioning for newborns at delivery with frank meconium aspiration or meconium staining (approximately 10% of newborns) emphasize a conservative approach. Routine oropharyngeal suctioning of meconium is recommended immediately at the time of delivery, but tracheal intubation and suctioning should be performed selectively.
   a. If the newborn is vigorous and crying, no further suctioning is needed.
   b. If meconium is present and the newborn is depressed, the trachea should be intubated and meconium and other aspirated material suctioned from beneath the glottis.
E. **The Renal System**
1. At birth, the glomerular filtration rate (GFR) is low but increases significantly in the first few days and doubles in the first 2 weeks; however, it does not reach adult levels until about 2 years of age. The limited ability of newborns' kidneys to concentrate or dilute urine results from this low GFR and decreased tubular function.
2. The half-life of medications excreted by means of glomerular filtration is prolonged in newborns. The relative inability to conserve water means that neonates, especially in the first week of life, tolerate fluid restriction poorly. In addition, the inability to excrete large amounts of water means that newborns tolerate fluid overload poorly.
F. **Fluid and Electrolyte Therapy in Neonates**
1. Total body water (TBW) decreases to about 75% of body weight for term infants at birth. Preterm infants have higher TBWs than term infants, often in the 80% to 85% range. TBW decreases during the first 12 months of life to about 60% to 65% of body weight and stays at this level through childhood.
2. TBW is distributed between two compartments, intracellular fluid (ICF) and extracellular fluid (ECF). The ECF volume is larger than the ICF volume in fetuses and newborns, usually in the 40% (ECF) and 20%

(ICF) of body weight ranges. This is the opposite of the situation in infants and children.

a. The ECF and ICF volumes (20% and 40% of body weight, respectively) approach adult values by about 1 year of age. This dramatic shift is beneficial to the child, especially in increasing the mobility of reserves in the face of dehydration.

b. Fluid can be easily mobilized from ICF volumes to replenish intravascular volume that is lost from fasting, fever, diarrhea, or other causes. This means that non-neonates are better situated to maintain intravascular volume in these situations than neonates.

3. The blood volume in normal full term newborns is approximately 85 mL/kg and approximately 90 to 100 mL/kg in the preterm newborns.

4. Maintenance fluid requirements have been estimated to be 60, 80, 100, and 120 mL/kg/24 hours for the first 4 days of life, respectively. For the rest of the neonatal period, a maintenance rate of 150 mL/kg/24 hours is appropriate.

a. Because of ongoing sodium loss secondary to the inability of the neonatal distal tubule to respond fully to aldosterone, intravenous (IV) fluids in neonates must contain some sodium (balanced salt solution such as lactated Ringer's solution or Plasmalyte).

b. The other issues for fluid choice in neonates center on appropriate glucose administration. Neonates who are scheduled for surgery and have been receiving hyperalimentation fluids or supplementary glucose must continue to receive that fluid during surgery or must have their glucose levels monitored because of concerns of hypoglycemia.

G. Blood Component Therapy in Neonates

1. The indications in the perioperative period for red blood cells are similar to those in adults, but the target values in available guidelines are higher. Transfusion is indicated for a hemoglobin less than 10 g/dL for major surgery. The hemoglobin in transfused blood is hemoglobin A as opposed to hemoglobin F in neonates at birth. An advantage of the transfused blood is better release of oxygen at the tissue level from hemoglobin A.

2. It is recommended that platelets be kept above 50,000/mL^3 for invasive procedures. These recommendations are based on expert consensus, not prospective studies.

H. The Hepatic System

1. The functional capacity of the liver is immature in newborns, especially synthetic and metabolic functions. Because of this immaturity, some drugs that undergo hepatic biotransformation, such as morphine, have prolonged elimination half-lives in newborns. Up to 85% of unmetabolized caffeine may be found in the urine in newborns compared with 1% in adults.
2. Decreased metabolism of a drug may actually increase its safety profile. Acetaminophen undergoes less biotransformation by the cytochrome P450 system in newborns, producing less reactive metabolites that are toxic.

II. ANATOMY OF THE NEONATAL AIRWAY (Fig. 44-5)

A. The majority of neonates are preferential nose breathers, and anything that obstructs the nares may compromise the neonate's ability to breathe.

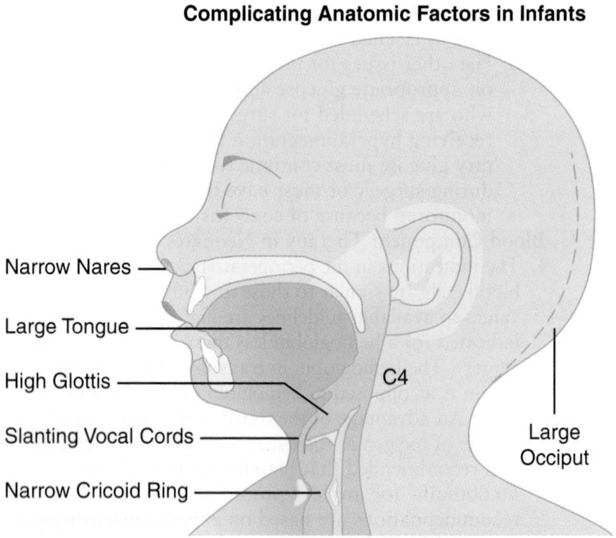

Complicating Anatomic Factors in Infants

FIGURE 44-5. Complicating anatomic factors in infants.

B. The large tongue occupies relatively more space in the infant's oropharynx, promoting both soft tissue obstruction of the upper airway and increasing the difficulty of laryngoscopic examination and intubation of the infant's trachea.

C. In adults, the narrowest aspect of the upper airway is at the vocal cords, but in neonates, there is further narrowing until the level of the cricoid ring. (This is susceptible to trauma from intubation or placement of too large an endotracheal tube.)

III. ANESTHETIC DRUGS IN NEONATES (Table 44-3)

The pharmacokinetics of drugs in neonates are different than in older children and adults. Factors affecting the metabolism of drugs in neonates include a larger volume of distribution, decreased protein binding, and decreased fat stores and immature renal and hepatic function.

IV. ANESTHETIC MANAGEMENT OF NEONATES

Effective evaluation, preparation, and anesthetic management of neonates are dependent on appropriate knowledge, clinical skills, and vigilance by the anesthesiologist. The anesthesiologist needs to develop a detailed plan that encompasses the issues of anesthetic equipment and monitoring, airway management, drug choice, fluid management, temperature control, anticipated surgical needs, pain management, and postoperative care.

A. Preoperative Considerations
   1. **Preanesthetic Evaluation: History.** The preanesthetic planning process starts with an evaluation of the course of intrauterine growth followed by labor and delivery and the immediate postpartum course.
      a. The World Health Organization definition of prematurity is less than 37 weeks gestation at birth. The greater the degree of prematurity, the more physiologic abnormalities will be expected (variability of responsiveness to anesthetic agents, fluids, cardioactive drugs, and the stress of the surgical procedure) (Table 44-4).
      b. Low birth weight is defined as a birth weight of 2500 g or less.
   2. **Preanesthetic Evaluation: Physical Examination.** Physical examination of newborns is focused by the condition requiring surgical intervention.

TABLE 44-3

ANESTHETIC DRUGS FOR USE IN NEONATES

Intravenous Agents
Anticholinergics (atropine and glycopyrrolate are used frequently in neonates to decrease secretions and the vagal response to intubation)
Midazolam (used for premedicating infants before surgery)

Sedative/Hypnotics
Thiopental (should be avoided in neonates with congenital heart disease)
Propofol
Ketamine (used frequently in neonates with congenital heart disease; based on animal data, there is a question of neurodegenerative changes)

Opioids
Fentanyl (mainstay in newborns for sedation and analgesia; even the use of small doses may result in respiratory depression)
Morphine
Remifentanil

Neuromuscular Blocking Agents
Succinylcholine (increased dose requirement; used to treat laryngospasm)
Nondepolarizing agents (variable and unpredictable duration of action)
Rocuronium (alternative to succinylcholine)
Vecuronium (long acting in infants younger than 1 year of age)

Reversal Agents
Edrophonium (rapid onset)
Neostigmine

Volatile Agents
Halothane (still used outside North America)
Isoflurane
Sevoflurane (most commonly used agent; rapid induction and awakening)
Desflurane (pungent)

Local Anesthetic Solutions
Amides
Lidocaine
Bupivacaine (most commonly used)
Ropivacaine
Levobupivacaine
Esters
Chloroprocaine
Topical Anesthesia
EMLA
LMX-4

EMLA = eutectic mixture of local anesthetic; LMX-4 = 4% liposomal lidocaine solution.

TABLE 44-4

ABNORMALITIES ASSOCIATED WITH THE PRETERM INFANTS: COMMON ANESTHETIC CONCERNS

Respiratory
Respiratory distress syndrome
Apnea
Pneumothorax, pneumomediastinum
Pneumonia
Pulmonary hemorrhage
Bronchopulmonary dysplasia

Cardiovascular
Patent ductus arteriosus
Hypotension
Bradycardia
Pulmonary hypertension
Persistent transitional circulation
Congenital heart disease

Central Nervous System
Intraventricular hemorrhage
Hypoxic-ischemic encephalopathy
Seizures
Kernicterus
Drug withdrawal

Metabolic
Hypoglycemia
Hyperglycemia
Hypocalcemia
Hypothermia
Metabolic acidosis

Renal
Hyponatremia
Hypernatremia
Hyperkalemia
Poor urine output

Gastrointestinal
Poor feeding
Necrotizing enterocolitis
Intestinal obstruction

Hematologic
Anemia
Hyperbilirubinemia
Vitamin K deficiency

Other
Retinopathy of prematurity
Sepsis and infections

SURGICAL SUBSPECIALTIES

  a. If there are clinical signs of dehydration, efforts should be made to correct the deficits before surgery except in extreme, life-threatening situations.

  b. Physical examination also focuses on the respiratory and cardiovascular systems.

 3. Preanesthetic Evaluation: Laboratory Tests

  a. Most newborns should have a blood count and glucose level drawn.

  b. Electrolyte determinations and coagulation profiles are indicated in specific patients. Unexplained hypotension, irritability, or seizures can be presenting signs of hypocalcemia.

 4. Preanesthetic Plan (Table 44-5)

 5. Premedication is not commonly used for neonatal anesthetics (atropine may be used because of the dominance of the parasympathetic nervous system and bradycardia on induction or in response to inhalational agents).

B. Intraoperative Considerations

 1. Monitoring. Neonatal patients are at a disadvantage when it comes to perioperative monitoring because of their small size. Pulse oximetry is one of the most important monitors in neonatal anesthesia. Electrocardiography is useful primarily to assess heart rate and rhythm. Blood pressure measurements are important in the management of all newborns. An effective alternative to a conventional blood pressure cuff is to use a manual cuff and place a Doppler probe over the brachial or radial artery.

 2. Anesthetic Systems. There is a long tradition in pediatric anesthesia of using semi-open, non-rebreathing systems for general anesthesia in newborns (Jackson-

---

TABLE 44-5

MAJOR FACTORS TO CONSIDER IN PLANNING THE ANESTHESIA FOR NEONATES

Need to have blood and blood products available
Need for invasive monitoring
Need for additional equipment for securing the airway or
 establishing vascular access
Need to transport the neonate to and from the operating room
Likelihood of postoperative ventilation
Plan for postoperative pain relief

Rees adaptation of the Ayre's t-piece, Bain circuit). As the use of these circuits has diminished, familiarity with their use and application has decreased in favor of the semi-closed rebreathing circle systems used in adult patients.

3. **Induction of Anesthesia.** There is no one method of induction and maintenance of anesthesia that is best for all patients.

4. **Airway Management.** Most newborns' tracheas are intubated after a rapid sequence induction. A Miller #1 blade is commonly used for full-term newborns and a Miller #0 in preterm newborns. Uncuffed tubes have traditionally been used in newborns to minimize cuff pressure on the subglottic larynx, especially at the level of the cricoid. It is prudent to use the depth markers at the end of the tube to ensure under direct vision that the tip is advanced 2 or 3 cm past the vocal cords.

5. **Anesthetic Dose Requirements of Neonates.** Neonates and premature infants have lower anesthetic requirements than older infants and children. The reasons for the lower minimum alveolar concentration (MAC) requirements are believed to be an immature nervous system, progesterone from the mother, and elevated blood levels of endorphins coupled with an immature blood–brain barrier.

6. **Regional Anesthesia** (Table 44-6)

C. **Postoperative Pain Control** (Table 44-7)

TABLE 44-6

REGIONAL ANESTHESIA TECHNIQUES THAT ARE USEFUL IN NEONATES

Central Neuraxial
Caudal
Epidural (lumbar, thoracic, caudal)
Spinal

Peripheral Nerve Blocks
Infraorbital block
Brachial plexus block (axillary, infraclavicular)
Lateral femoral cutaneous block
Penile block
Ilioinguinal block
Scalp blocks

TABLE 44-7

POSTOPERATIVE PAIN CONTROL FOR NEONATES AND INFANTS

Intravenous
Opioids: Morphine, fentanyl, methadone
NSAID: Ketorolac

Oral
Acetaminophen
Ibuprofen
Hydrocodone
Codeine

Rectal
Acetaminophen
Diclofenac

Regional and Local Anesthesia

NSAID = nonsteroidal anti-inflammatory drug.

D. **Postoperative Ventilation**
1. If the surgical procedure or the neonate's condition is such that postoperative ventilation is likely, the prolonged respiratory effects of opioids or any other drug are of little concern.
2. If the surgical procedure will be relatively short and by itself does not require postoperative ventilation, the clinician should carefully select drugs, as well as doses of anesthetic drugs and relaxants, that will not necessitate prolonged postoperative ventilation or intubation.
3. Postoperative ventilation places the neonate at added risk because of the problems associated with mechanical ventilation, trauma to the subglottic area, and potential development of postoperative subglottic stenosis or edema.

V. **SPECIAL CONSIDERATIONS**

A. **Maternal Drug Use During Pregnancy.** Maternal drug use (cocaine, marijuana) during pregnancy may result in premature birth; intrauterine growth retardation; and cardiovascular abnormalities, including low cardiac output.

B. **Temperature Control and Thermogenesis**
1. Newborns are at risk for significant metabolic derangements caused by hypothermia. (Newborns do

not shiver, increase activity, or effectively vasoconstrict like older children and adults do in response to cold.)

2. Placing the patient on a forced-air warming blanket may dramatically reduce conductive heat loss.

3. Anesthetic agents may reduce or eliminate thermogenesis, removing any ability to compensate for cold stress.

C. **Respiratory Distress Syndrome**

1. Exogenous surfactant has been widely used in premature infants of low birth weight either to prevent or to treat RDS.

2. One of the long-term consequences of RDS is bronchopulmonary dysplasia. Many patients improve as they age, but reactive airways, recurrent pulmonary infections, and prolonged oxygen requirements are seen in some patients.

   a. Anesthetic concerns in these patients include baseline oxygenation and the potential presence of active bronchoconstriction.

   b. These patients often benefit from an additional bronchodilator before induction. Although postanesthetic tracheal intubation is not usually required, a high index of suspicion should be used if there is significant clinical evidence of poor lung function before surgery.

D. **Postoperative Apnea**

1. Apnea and bradycardia are well-recognized, major complications that are possible during and after surgery in neonates. The infants at highest risk are those born prematurely, those with multiple congenital anomalies, those with a history of apnea and bradycardia, and those with chronic lung disease. Hypothermia and anemia can also contribute to the development of postoperative apnea.

2. Infants with life-threatening apnea and bradycardia before surgery may be taking central nervous system stimulants (caffeine, theophylline [metabolized to caffeine]). Administering caffeine (10 mg/kg) prophylactically to infants at risk of postoperative apnea to ensure adequate serum levels may prevent the need for prolonged periods of postoperative ventilatory support.

3. Spinal anesthesia without sedation decreases the incidence of postoperative apnea and bradycardia in

high-risk infants, but this advantage is lost if supplemental sedation is used.

E. **Retinopathy of Prematurity (ROP)**
   1. Very preterm infants, especially those weighing less than 1200 g, are at highest risk for ROP, with an incidence of significant disease of about 2%.
   2. The most common cited cause of ROP is hyperoxia from administered oxygen, but hypoxemia, hypotension, sepsis, intraventricular hemorrhage, and other stresses have also been implicated.
   3. The primary anesthetic challenge in these patients is related to their extreme prematurity and small size. Adequate monitoring, vascular access, and thermal stability are common challenges to management. Use of supplemental oxygen at pulse oximetry saturations of 96% to 99% does not cause additional progression of prethreshold ROP.

F. **Neurodevelopmental Effects of Anesthetic Agents**
   1. Studies have shown that prolonged exposure (equivalent to several weeks of continuous exposure in humans) of animal models to anesthetic agents can lead to neurodegenerative changes in the developing brain of neonatal rats.
   2. Currently, no conclusive evidence demonstrates the deleterious effect of inhaled or IV anesthetics on neurocognitive function in neonates and infants.

VI. SURGICAL PROCEDURES IN NEONATES

Surgical procedures in neonates are functionally divided into those performed in the first week and those performed in the first month of life. Emphasis of presurgical stabilization before taking the newborn to the operating room has reduced the emergent nature of newborn surgeries

---

TABLE 44-8

SURGICAL PROCEDURES PERFORMED IN THE FIRST WEEK OF LIFE

Congenital diaphragmatic hernia
Omphalocele
Gastroschisis
Tracheoesophageal fistula
Intestinal obstruction
Meningomyelocele

TABLE 44-9

SURGICAL PROCEDURES PERFORMED IN THE FIRST MONTH OF LIFE

Exploratory laparotomy for necrotizing enterocolitis
Inguinal hernia repair
Correction of pyloric stenosis
Patent ductus arteriosus ligation
Shunt procedure for hydrocephalus
Placement of a central venous catheter

SURGICAL SUBSPECIALTIES

(congenital diaphragmatic hernia, omphalocele). Exceptions include gastroschisis, which is usually attended to within 12 to 24 hours; airway lesions such webs that are causing significant airway obstruction; and acute subdural or epidural hematomas from traumatic delivery.

A. **Surgical Procedures in the First Week of Life** (Table 44-8). Two confounding factors in neonatal surgery are prematurity and associated congenital anomalies. The presence of one congenital anomaly increases the likelihood of other congenital anomalies.

B. **Surgical Procedures in the First Month of Life** (Table 44-9)

CHAPTER 45 ■ PEDIATRIC ANESTHESIA

The provision of safe anesthesia for pediatric patients requires a clear understanding of the psychological, physiologic, and pharmacologic differences between patients in different age groups from newborn to adolescent (Cravero JP, Kain ZN: Pediatric anesthesia. In *Clinical Anesthesia*. Edited by Barash PG, Cullen BF, Stoelting RK, Cahalan MK, Stock MC. Philadelphia: Lippincott Williams & Wilkins, 2009, pp 1206–1220. Numerous specific anatomic, physiologic, and psychological issues should be understood before anesthetizing pediatric patients (Table 45-1).

I. THE PREOPERATIVE EVALUATION (Table 45-2)

A. Coexisting Health Conditions

1. **Upper Respiratory Infection (URI)**
   a. A child with an URI or who is recovering from an URI is at increased risk of developing laryngospasm, bronchospasm, oxygen desaturation, and postoperative atelectasis and croup.
   b. It is unclear how long surgery should be delayed after an URI; however, bronchial hyperreactivity may exist for up to 7 weeks after an URI.
   c. The final decision should take into account the risk-to-benefit ratio of the surgical procedure.
   d. Mask anesthesia, but not a laryngeal mask airway (LMA), has been clearly shown to be associated with a significantly lower rate of perioperative complications compared with use of an endotracheal tube and thus should be used whenever possible with these children.

2. **Obstructive Sleep Apnea (OSA)**
   a. Severe adenotonsillar hypertrophy with OSA is a frequent indication for children to undergo tonsillectomy and adenoidectomy.

TABLE 45-1

ANATOMICAL AND PHYSIOLOGIC DISTINCTIONS BETWEEN ADULT AND PEDIATRIC PATIENTS

Physical or Physiologic Variable	Contrast Between Child and Adult	Anesthetic Implications
Head size	Much larger head size relative to body in children	Consider a roll under the shoulders or neck for optimal positioning
Tongue size	Larger size relative to the mouth in children	Makes the airway appear slightly anterior Oral airways are particularly useful during mask ventilation
Airway shape	In children, the narrowest diameter is below the glottis at the cricoid	Uncuffed tubes can create a seal when appropriately sized in children younger than 8 years of age
Respiratory physiology	Oxygen consumption is two to three times greater in infants than adults	Oxygen desaturation is extremely rapid after apnea
Cardiac physiology	There is a relatively fixed stroke volume in neonates and infants	Bradycardia must be treated aggressively in young patients Atropine use should be considered before airway management Heart rate <60 bpm requires circulatory support
Renal function	There is a limited GFR at birth, and it does not reach adult levels until late infancy Total body water and the percentage of ECF are increased in infants	There is a prolonged duration of action for hydrophilic drugs, particularly those that are renally excreted
Hepatic function	The P450 system not fully developed in neonates and infants Liver blood flow is decreased in newborns	There is a prolonged excretion of drugs, depending on the hepatic metabolism

(continued)

TABLE 45-1

ANATOMICAL AND PHYSIOLOGIC DISTINCTIONS BETWEEN ADULT AND PEDIATRIC PATIENTS (*Continued*)

Physical or Physiologic Variable	Contrast Between Child and Adult	Anesthetic Implications
Body surface area	There is a larger surface to body ratio in newborns, infants, and toddlers	Heat loss is more prominent for these age groups
Psychological development	0–6 months: Stress on the family 8 months–4 years: Separation anxiety 4–6 years: Misconceptions of surgical mutilation 6–13 years: Fear of not waking up 13 years and older: Fear of loss of control; body image issues	Changes the manner in which each patient and family member should be approached Issues with personal and systemic strategies should be addressed

ECF = extracellular fluid; GFR = glomerular filtration rate.

    b. Children with OSA may experience obstruction with the use of preoperative sedative medication and during the induction process, so muscle relaxants should be used carefully in these patients.

TABLE 45-2

PREOPERATIVE EVALUATION AND PREPARATION OF CHILDREN FOR SURGERY

Pertinent maternal, birth, and neonatal history
Review of systems
Physical examination (height, weight, vital signs)
Drugs (bronchodilators, steroids, chemotherapeutic drugs, herbal medicines)
Congenital malformations
Discussion of anesthetic risks, anesthetic plans, and postoperative analgesia
Address preoperative anxiety (child and parents)

c. Postoperatively, patients (especially children younger than 3 years of age) with severe OSA may exhibit worsening of their obstructive symptoms secondary to tissue edema, altered response to carbon dioxide, and residual anesthetic and analgesic agents.

d. Children with severe OSA may require postoperative observation in the hospital.

e. Obesity often accompanies OSA. (All patients with markedly increased body mass index should be questioned about sleep apnea symptoms.) Obese children have an increased incidence of difficult airway, upper airway obstruction, extended stays in the postanesthesia care unit, and postoperative nausea and vomiting.

3. **Asthma.** Children with asthma should be under optimal medical care before undergoing general anesthesia and surgery. All oral and inhaled medications, such corticosteroids and β-agonists, should be continued up to and including the day of surgery.

4. **Former Preterm Infants**

a. Three frequent problems in former preterm infants are the impact that bronchopulmonary dysplasia might have on the patient's perioperative course, the presence of anemia, and the possibility of postoperative apnea.

b. The risk of postoperative apnea is inversely related to postconceptual age, and infants with a history of apnea and bradycardia, respiratory distress, and mechanical ventilation may be at increased risk.

c. Overnight hospital monitoring should be made for any child considered to be at significant risk for postoperative apnea.

B. **Laboratory Evaluation**

1. Healthy children undergoing elective minor surgery require no laboratory evaluation (including chest radiographs and urinalysis) and thus can be spared the anxiety and pain of blood drawing.

2. Coagulation testing should only be considered in children in whom the history or medical condition suggests a possible hemostatic defect, in patients undergoing surgical procedures (cardiopulmonary

bypass) that might induce hemostatic disturbances, when the coagulation system is particularly needed for adequate hemostasis, and in patients for whom even minimal postoperative bleeding could be critical.

3. Pregnancy screening (anesthetics may be teratogenic) of female patients of childbearing age before the administration of anesthesia is a matter of policy at individual facilities.

C. **Preoperative Fasting Period**

1. Solids are prohibited within 6 to 8 hours of surgery (generally after midnight), formula within 6 hours, breast milk within 4 hours of surgery, and clear liquids within 2 hours of surgery.

2. Liquids such as apple juice and sugar water may be encouraged up to 2 hours before the induction of anesthesia.

3. Hypoglycemia with prolonged intervals of fasting is a risk in young children with smaller glycogen stores.

D. **Preoperative Sedatives** (Table 45-3). The primary goals of premedication in children are to facilitate a smooth and anxiety-free separation from the parents and induction of anesthesia.

TABLE 45-3

PREOPERATIVE SEDATIVES IN CHILDREN

Oral
Midazolam (0.5–0.75 mg/kg; onset, 30 minutes; lasts approximately 30 minutes)
Ketamine (5–6 mg/kg)
Transmucosal fentanyl (facial pruritus, nausea and vomiting, oxygen desaturation)
Clonidine (4 μg/kg)
Dexmedetomidine (1 μg/kg transmucosally or 3–4 μg/kg orally)

Nasal
Midazolam (0.2 mg/kg; rapid absorption because it avoids first-pass metabolism; a disadvantage is transient nasal irritation)

Rectal
Midazolam (0.5–1.0 mg/kg)

Intramuscular
Midazolam (0.3 mg/kg; anxiolysis in 5–10 minutes)
Ketamine (3–4 mg/kg)

II. ANESTHETIC AGENTS

A. Potent Inhalation Agents

1. **Mask Induction Pharmacology.** The incidences of bradycardia, hypotension, and cardiac arrest during inhalation induction are higher in infants younger than 1 year of age, reflecting rapid uptake of inhalation agents and high inspired concentrations used early in induction.

2. The **minimal alveolar concentration (MAC)** of anesthetic required in pediatric patients differs with age. (There are small increases in MAC between birth and 2 to 3 months; after that time, MAC slowly decreases with age.)

3. **Intracardiac Shunts.** Although intracardiac shunts can, in theory, alter the uptake of anesthetic agents and affect the speed of induction, this is rarely clinically evident.

4. **Inhaled Agents for Induction of Anesthesia.** Sevoflurane is the only potent inhalation agent available for inhalation induction. The safety and efficacy of sevoflurane for maintenance of anesthesia in children has been established in hundreds of studies. Although emergence from anesthesia is more rapid with sevoflurane than with more soluble agents such as halothane or isoflurane, a growing literature supports the fact that agitation behaviors in children on emergence are more common with this agent.

III. INTRAVENOUS AGENTS

A. **Sedative hypnotics** may be used after inhaled induction of anesthesia or as primary induction and maintenance agents in children who have intravenous lines in place.

1. Doses of IV agents used in infants and toddlers often need to be increased by 25% to 40% to obtain the same level of sedation/anesthesia in children compared with adults.

2. Propofol induction doses range from 3 to 4 mg/kg for children younger than 2 years of age to approximately 2.5 to 3.0 mg/kg for older children. Maintenance of anesthesia requires 200 to 300 μg/kg/min.

      a. Emergence from deep sedation/anesthesia is faster than that from most other sedative agents and most inhaled agents, especially after prolonged administration.

      b. Emergence from propofol is associated with less nausea and vomiting and is accompanied by less emergence agitation, so readiness for discharge is at least as rapid.

   3. Ketamine offers both hypnosis and analgesia, preserves airway reflexes, maintains respiratory drive, increases endogenous catecholamine release, and results in bronchodilation and pulmonary vasodilation.

      a. Induction doses of 1 mg/kg IV yield effective analgesia and sedation with rapid onset.

      b. Intramuscular doses of 3 to 4 mg/kg result in a similar state with significant analgesia that is appropriate for minor procedures such as IV starts or fracture manipulation.

      c. Simultaneous administration of an anticholinergic minimizes oral secretions.

      d. Emergence may be marked by diplopia, occasional disturbing dreams, and nausea or vomiting, although these are less common in children than adults.

B. Note on Toxicity of Anesthetic Agents. Animal studies involving inhalation and IV anesthetic agents (drugs that act at NMDA [N-methyl-D-aspartic acid] receptors and γ-aminobutyric acid receptors) suggest that neurodegeneration with possible cognitive sequelae is a potential long-term risk of anesthetics. At present, insufficient data suggest that operative anesthesia is harmful in humans.

C. Opioids are important elements of balanced anesthesia and sedation in children.

   1. Use of opioids for surgical anesthesia decreases the MAC of inhaled agents, smooths hemodynamics during airway management or stimulating procedures, and provides postoperative analgesia.

   2. Opioids depress central respiratory effort, and newborns and infants younger than 6 months of age are particularly susceptible to this effect because of the immature blood–brain barrier and increased levels of free drug.

TABLE 45-4

CONTRAINDICATIONS TO ADMINISTRATION OF
SUCCINYLCHOLINE TO CHILDREN

Muscular dystrophy
Recent burn injury
Spinal cord transection or immobilization
Family history of malignant hyperthermia
Relative contraindication based on FDA warning

FDA = Food and Drug Administration.

D. **Muscle Relaxants**
   1. Succinylcholine (Sch) (1.5–2.0 mg/kg IV) produces
      excellent intubating conditions in 60 seconds with
      recovery in 6 to 7 minutes.
      a. Sch can also be given intramuscularly (IM)
         (4 mg/kg) in emergencies when IV access is not
         available.
      b. Sch is contraindicated in a variety of patients
         (Table 45-4).
      c. Sch is only recommended in situations in which
         ultra-rapid onset and short duration of action are
         of paramount importance (laryngospasm), when
         relaxation is required, or when IV access is not
         available and IM administration is required.
   2. All nondepolarizing muscle relaxants used in adults
      are also effective for pediatric patients (Table 45-5).
      a. Neonates and infants have a larger percentage of
         total body water and larger extracellular fluid
         (ECF) volume and thus a larger volume of distri-
         bution for these hydrophilic drugs than older
         children and adults. On the other hand, neonates
         and infants are slightly more sensitive to these
         drugs.
      b. The result is a pharmacokinetic and pharmaco-
         dynamic profile in which the recommended doses
         of these agents are identical for children and
         adults, but the duration of action tends to be
         slightly longer.
      c. Rocuronium has the fastest onset of action in
         this class (60–90 seconds for a 1-mg/kg dose)
         and is generally the choice for rapid sequence
         intubation.
   3. Muscle twitch should be monitored and reversal
      agents (0.05 mg/kg of neostigmine with 0.015 mg/kg

TABLE 45-5

COMPARATIVE PHARMACOLOGY OF NONDEPOLARIZING NEUROMUSCULAR BLOCKING AGENTS IN CHILDREN

	Recommended Dose (μg/kg)*	Onset	Duration	Cardiovascular Effects	Cost	Special Considerations
Atracurium	500	Intermediate	Intermediate	Rare hypotension	Intermediate	Mild erythema is common
Cisatracurium	80–200	Slow to intermediate	Intermediate to long	Absent	Inexpensive to intermediate	
Mivacurium	250–400	Intermediate	Short	Rare hypotension	Intermediate	Mild erythema is common
Pancuronium	100	Intermediate	Intermediate to long	Tachycardia Occasional hypertension	Inexpensive	Effect is prolonged in renal failure
Rocuronium	500–1200	Rapid	Intermediate	Slight increase in heart rate	Intermediate	Deltoid injection facilitates tracheal intubation
Vecuronium	100–400	Intermediate (rapid with large doses)	Intermediate (long with doses >150 μg/kg)	Absent	Intermediate	

*Personal recommendations of the author.

of atropine or 0.01 mg/kg of glycopyrrolate) administered if residual weakness is detected.

IV. ANTIEMETICS

A. Postoperative nausea and vomiting (PONV) is among the most common causes of prolonged recovery stays and unanticipated hospitalization in children.

1. Ondansetron (0.05–0.15 mg/kg) is effective in tonsillectomy and strabismus models, but its effectiveness as a "rescue" medication has not been proven.
2. Dexamethasone (0.15–1.0 mg/kg) appears to be effective in limiting PONV after oral pharyngeal surgery (tonsillectomy).
3. Droperidol is effective in children as an antiemetic, but concerns regarding prolonged QT syndrome and possible torsades de pointes with its use have impacted the frequency of administration of this drug.

B. The practice of requiring patients to eat or drink before discharge increases PONV.

C. The use of pain control modalities in lieu of opioids (acetaminophen or nonsteriodal anti-inflammatory drugs [NSAIDs] and regional anesthesia) likely decreases the overall risk of PONV.

V. FLUID AND BLOOD PRODUCT MANAGEMENT

A. Perioperative fluid and blood product management for pediatric patients must take into account fluid deficits (calculated maintenance requirement times number of hours NPO), translocation of fluids and blood loss during surgery, and maintenance fluid requirements (Table 45-6).

TABLE 45-6

MAINTENANCE FLUID REQUIREMENTS FOR PEDIATRIC PATIENTS

Weight (kg)	Hourly Fluids	24-Hour Fluids
<10	4 mL/kg	100 mL/kg
11–20	40 mL + 2 mL/kg >10 kg	1000 mL + 50 mL/kg >10 kg
>20	60 mL + 1 mL/kg >20 kg	1500 mL + 20 mL/kg >20 kg

B. Immediate intravascular volume expansion may be accomplished with a 10-mL/kg bolus of isotonic fluid. The balance of the calculated fluid deficit can be given over 1 or 2 hours and is often provided in the form isotonic fluid or a 5% dextrose solution in 0.9% normal saline.

   1. Liberalized recommendations for intake of clear fluids (generally up to 2 hours before surgery) mean that hypoglycemia is unlikely in children because of fasting before surgery.

   2. Administration of 5% dextrose solutions to replace deficits or fluid losses intraoperatively may result in hyperglycemia, which is problematic for patients with intracranial injury.

   3. Intraoperative monitoring of blood glucose is appropriate for newborns, former premature infants, and all high-risk pediatric patients.

C. Surgical manipulation is associated with the isotonic transfer of fluids from the ECF compartment to the nonfunctional interstitial compartment (third-space loss).

   1. Estimated third-space loss during intra-abdominal surgery varies from 6 to 15 mL/kg/hr. In intrathoracic surgery, it is less (4–7 mL/kg/hr), and during intracranial or cutaneous surgery, it is negligible (1–2 mL/kg/hr).

   2. These third-space losses should be estimated and replaced on an hourly basis.

      a. These losses are derived from ECF, and it is important to replace them with a balanced salt solution to avoid hyponatremia that would result from using hypotonic replacement.

      b. Lactated Ringer's solution is frequently used because normal saline contains an excessive chloride and acid load for infants.

D. Indications for blood or blood component therapy in pediatric patients are based on considerations of the patient's blood volume, preoperative hematocrit, general medical condition, and ability to provide oxygen to tissues, as well as the nature of the surgical procedure and the risks versus benefits of transfusion.

   1. All blood loss should be measured as accurately as possible and accounted for with some form of volume replacement to maintain intravascular volume and perfusion.

2. If an isotonic solution is chosen to replace some element of blood loss, it should be given in a ratio of 3:1 (crystalloid:blood lost).

E. The concept of the maximum allowable blood loss takes into account the patient's total blood volume, starting hematocrit, and estimated "target" hematocrit (lowest acceptable hematocrit for the patient considering his or her age and comorbid conditions).

   1. In general, blood volume is estimated at 100 mL/kg for preterm infants, 90 mL/kg for term infants, 80 mL/kg for children 3 to 12 months old, and 70 mL/kg for patients older than 1 year of age.

   2. These estimates of blood volume may be used in calculating the individual patient's blood volume by multiplying the child's weight by the estimated blood volume per kilogram.

F. The end point of fluid and blood therapy is adequate blood pressure, tissue perfusion, and urine volume (0.5–1 mL/kg/hour).

VI. AIRWAY MANAGEMENT

The choice of airway should depend on the age of the child, the time since last oral intake, coexisting illness, and the procedure to be performed.

A. Endotracheal tubes are preferred for premature infants and most neonates because of the greater difficulty of providing effective face mask ventilation under appropriate levels of anesthesia and the risk of filling the stomach with air while providing mask ventilation.

B. LMAs come in a range of sizes and half sizes and can be used in infants, toddlers, and older children for almost any procedure that does not involve opening the abdomen or thoracic cavity.

C. Because the narrowest portion of the pediatric airway is at the level of the cricoid cartilage, uncuffed tubes can be used and create a functional seal when appropriately sized. Air should leak out at no higher than 20 to 25 cm H_2O to minimize the risk of postextubation croup.

D. Intubation in children can be safely accomplished after inhaled induction with or without the use of muscle relaxant.

VII. PEDIATRIC BREATHING CIRCUITS

Non-rebreathing circuits minimize the work of breathing because they have no valves to be opened by the patient's respiratory effort. A number of combinations of the simple T-piece tubing, reservoir bag, and sites of fresh gas entry and overflow are possible. Circle breathing systems can also be used very effectively in infants and children.

VIII. MONITORING

Pediatric patients should be monitored continuously with a precordial or esophageal stethoscope. Pulse oximetry, capnography, blood pressure (measured with appropriately sized cuffs), temperature, and the electrocardiogram should also be monitored routinely in children as in adults. Low tidal volumes, rapid respiratory rates, and changing intrapulmonary shunts make $ETCO_2$ measurements inaccurate for infants and premature neonates with respiratory distress syndrome.

A. **Awareness and Level of Consciousness Monitoring.** Monitors of depth of anesthesia that have been validated in children (bispectral index, spectral entropy, narcotrend index) track the level of sedation/anesthesia in children as they do in adults. (These monitors are not reliable in infants and neonates.) No monitors have been evaluated in term of their ability to decrease awareness in children.

IX. PAIN MANAGEMENT AND REGIONAL ANESTHESIA

Children experience pain, just like adults, regardless of their age. Younger children experience more distress and pain from procedures than older children.

A. **Pharmacologic Treatment of Pain**
 1. The most common oral analgesic used in children is acetaminophen (10–15 mg/kg orally every 4 hours). The rectal route of administration can be particularly effective for children with no IV access.
 2. Ketorolac (0.75 mg/kg IM) is effective but has the disadvantage of prolonging bleeding time because of its effect on platelet aggregation.
 3. Ibuprofen (10 mg/kg) is the most popular NSAID given orally to children.

B. **Regional Anesthesia**
  1. The ilioinguinal–iliohypogastric nerve block, ring block of the penis, or caudal block can be very useful for common pediatric surgical procedures.
  2. Use of ultrasound localization allows a lower dose or volume of local anesthetic to be used, which is particularly important in infants and children in whom total dose is limited by weight-based dosing. Strict attention must be paid to the dose of local anesthetic, dose of epinephrine, and technique of administration.
  3. **Caudal block** is the most commonly used form of regional anesthesia in children. This technique can provide postoperative analgesia after a wide variety of lower abdominal and genitourinary surgical procedures. Bupivacaine or ropivacaine produce postoperative analgesia that typically lasts 4 to 6 hours, and at concentrations used (about 0.175%), it is not associated with motor paralysis.
  4. **Spinal anesthesia** may be used for procedures involving surgical dermatomes below T6.
      a. It is important to note that the dural sac migrates cephalad during the first year of life. In neonates, it is at S3, but in children older than age 1 year, it is at the S1 level.
      b. Spinal anesthesia is an option for premature infants who undergo surgery because the incidence of postoperative apnea is reduced in these infants with the use of this technique.

X. POSTANESTHESIA CARE (Table 45-7)

TABLE 45-7

CHALLENGES DURING RECOVERY OF YOUNG CHILDREN IN THE POSTANESTHESIA CARE UNIT

Hypothermia
Nausea and vomiting (prophylactic ondansetron)
Postoperative pain (self-reported or physiologic signs, including hypertension, tachycardia, agitation, nausea and vomiting; severe pain should be treated with fentanyl or morphine IV)
Fear associated with awakening in a strange environment (parents should be permitted to be present)

IV = intravenous.

CHAPTER 46 ■
GASTROINTESTINAL DISORDERS

I. ESOPHAGUS

A. **Upper Esophageal Sphincter.** The cricopharyngeus muscle, one of the two inferior muscles of the pharynx, together with the circular fibers of the upper esophagus, acts as the functional upper esophageal sphincter (UES) at the pharyngo-esophageal junction (Ogunnaike BO, Whitten CW: Gastrointestinal disorders. In *Clinical Anesthesia*. Edited by Barash PG, Cullen BF, Stoelting RK, Cahalan MK, Stock MC. Philadelphia: Lippincott Williams & Wilkins, 2009, pp 1221–1229). The UES helps prevent aspiration by sealing off the upper esophagus from the hypopharynx in conscious, healthy patients. UES function is impaired during both normal sleep and anesthesia. Most anesthetic agents, except ketamine, reduce UES tone and increase the likelihood of regurgitation of material from the esophagus into the hypopharynx.

B. The border between the stomach and esophagus is formed by the lower esophageal sphincter (LES) (Table 46-1). The LES is the major barrier to gastroesophageal reflux. The major physiologic derangement in patients with gastroesophageal reflux is a reduction in LES pressure. The difference between the LES pressure and gastric pressure is "barrier pressure" and is more important than the LES tone in the production of gastroesophageal reflux. Anesthetic agents that may reduce the barrier pressure, thereby reducing LES pressure, include thiopental, propofol, opioids, anticholinergics, and inhaled anesthetics. Antiemetics, cholinergics, antacids, and succinylcholine (Sch) increase LES pressure. Nondepolarizing muscle relaxants and H2-receptor antagonists have no effect on LES pressure. In both conscious and

TABLE 46-1

FACTORS AFFECTING LOWER ESOPHAGEAL SPHINCTER TONE

Decrease Tone	Increase Tone	No Change in Tone
Inhaled anesthetics	Anticholinesterases (neostigmine, edrophonium)	H2-receptor antagonists (cimetidine, ranitidine)
Opioids	Cholinergics	Nondepolarizing muscle relaxants (atracurium, vecuronium)
Anticholinergics (atropine, glycopyrrolate)	Acetylcholine	
Thiopental	α-Adrenergic stimulants	Propranolol
Propofol		
Beta-blockers	Antacids	
Ganglion blockers	Metoclopramide	
Tricyclic antidepressants	Gastrin	
Secretin	Serotonin	
Glucagon	Histamine	
Cricoid pressure	Pancreatic polypeptide	
Obesity	Metoprolol	
Hiatal hernia		
Pregnancy		

unconscious patients, cricoid pressure decreases LES tone because of a significant reduction in esophageal barrier pressure while gastric pressure remains normal. The evidence that Sch increases LES tone while cricoid pressure decreases LES tone makes the necessity for application of cricoid pressure during a rapid sequence induction questionable.

II. STOMACH

The stomach is very distensible with the capacity to store large amounts of material (≤ 1.5 L of fluid) without a significant increase in intragastric pressure. There is a dose–response relationship in the severity of aspiration pneumonitis for both gastric volume and acidity that directly reaches the lung. Human breast milk predisposes individuals to an increased severity of aspiration pneumonitis when compared with other types of milk.

III. **PROTECTIVE AIRWAY REFLEXES** include apnea
   with laryngospasm, which causes closure of both the false
   and true vocal cords and coughing. Premedicated and
   anesthetized patients and elderly individuals have reduced
   airway reflexes, putting them at an increased risk for
   perioperative aspiration pneumonitis.

IV. **REDUCING PERIOPERATIVE ASPIRATION RISK**
   (Table 46-2)

   A. **Control of gastric contents** involves minimizing intake;
      increasing gastric emptying with prokinetics; and reduc-
      ing gastric volume and acidity with a nasogastric (NG)
      tube, antacids, H2-receptor antagonists, and proton
      pump inhibitors (PPIs). Clear liquids can be administered
      to children and adults up to 2 and 3 hours, respectively,
      before anesthesia without an increased risk for regurgita-
      tion and aspiration. Altered physiological states (pregnancy
      and diabetes mellitus) and gastrointestinal (GI) pathol-
      ogy (bowel obstruction and peritonitis) may adversely
      affect the rate of gastric emptying, increasing the risk of

---

TABLE 46-2

METHODS FOR REDUCING THE RISK OF REGURGITATION AND
PULMONARY ASPIRATION

Minimize Intake
Adequate preoperative fasting
Administration of clear liquids only if necessary

Increase Gastric Emptying
Prokinetics (metoclopramide)

Reduce Gastric Volume and Acidity
NG tube
Nonparticulate antacid (sodium citrate)
H2 receptor antagonists (famotidine)
PPIs (lansoprazole)

Airway Management and Protection
Cricoid pressure
Cuffed endotracheal intubation

Esophageal-Tracheal Combitube®
Proseal LMA

LMA = laryngeal mask airway; NG = nasogastric; PPI = proton pump
inhibitor.

aspiration. The extent of delayed gastric emptying with diabetes mellitus correlates well with the presence of autonomic neuropathy. The American Society of Anesthesiologists recommends a fasting period of 4 hours for breast milk and 6 hours for non-human milk; infant formula; and light, solid meals. The presence of an NG tube does not guarantee an empty stomach and may impair the function of the LES and UES, but it does not diminish the effectiveness of cricoid pressure. An NG tube also provides a direct connection to the outside for passive drainage of gastric contents and is best left in place and open to freely drain during induction of anesthesia.

B. **Prevention of Pulmonary Aspiration**
   1. **Cricoid pressure** may be recommended (its effectiveness is controversial) to occlude the upper end of the esophagus to prevent passive regurgitation of gastric contents and decrease the risk of pulmonary aspiration during a rapid-sequence induction–intubation technique.
      a. Application of cricoid pressure reduces LES tone and may cause the esophagus to be displaced to the side rather than to be compressed.
      b. The force applied to the cricoid cartilage should be sufficient to prevent aspiration but not so great as to cause airway obstruction or allow the possibility of esophageal rupture if vomiting occurs. The recommended force is estimated to range between 20 and 44 N; however, cricoid deformation occurs at 44 N with associated cricoid occlusion, vocal cord closure, and difficult ventilation. Awake patients experience pain, coughing, and retching with pressures greater than 20 N, so this amount of force should be applied only after loss of consciousness. A reasonable approach is to apply 10 N of force to the cricoid in the awake state and increase to 30 N after loss of consciousness. Cricoid pressure by itself, before laryngoscopy and intubation, increases the incidence of hypertension and tachycardia during induction of anesthesia.

C. **Airway Protection.** Use of a cuffed endotracheal intubation tube is the mainstay of prevention of regurgitated material from reaching the trachea and lungs. Of the other airway devices used, the laryngeal mask airway reduces barrier pressure at the LES with an increased incidence of reflux compared with the cuffed endotracheal tube.

V. THE INTESTINES

The small intestine (SI) is the site of most of the absorption of fluids and nutrients from the GI tract. Parasympathetic stimulation increases the activity of the SI, and antagonism decreases this activity. Whereas suppression of sympathetic activity increases SI activity, stimulation results in a decrease. Hypokalemia, peritonitis, and laparotomy all suppress intestinal activity for up to 48 hours. Neostigmine increases colonic activity, and morphine and other opioids decrease both activity and tone.

A. **Splanchnic Blood Flow.** Splanchnic blood flow is influenced predominantly by the autonomic nervous system. α-Adrenergic stimulation leads to vasoconstriction, and β_2-adrenergic stimulation causes vasodilation. Splanchnic vascular resistance increases with severe hemorrhage, which helps to divert blood flow to other vital organs. Hypocapnia significantly reduces splanchnic blood flow, and hypercapnia does the opposite. Neostigmine reduces mesenteric blood flow because of inducing exaggerated contraction. Atropine partially offsets the blood flow reduction.

B. **Postoperative Anastomotic Leakage.** Anastomotic leakage after colon surgery may be related to patient factors (anemia, comorbidity), surgical factors (bowel preparation, operative expertise), or factors related to anesthesia and pain management related (morphine, epidural analgesia, neostigmine).
   1. The theoretical mechanism by which anesthesia-related factors may increase the incidence of anastomotic dehiscence is by increasing intestinal motility and intraluminar pressure.
   2. Sugammadex, unlike neostigmine, does not stimulate bowel peristalsis.
   3. Clinical observations and animal studies have largely discounted the suggestion that neostigmine has a deleterious effect on bowel anastomosis.
   4. Prokinetics such as metoclopramide have been associated with colonic anastomotic dehiscence in animals during the early postoperative period.

C. **Postoperative Ileus.** Multiple mechanisms contribute to ileus after intestinal surgery (Table 46-3).
   1. Epidural analgesia that includes local anesthetics has been most effective in minimizing postoperative ileus.

TABLE 46-3

MECHANISMS OF ILEUS AFTER ABDOMINAL SURGERY

Abdominal pain (activates a spinal reflex that inhibits motility)
Sympathetic hyperactivity
Opioids
Electrolyte imbalance
Immobility
Intestinal wall swelling from fluid administration

Minimally invasive surgery (including laparoscopy), early enteral nutrition, and early mobilization reduce inflammatory responses, thereby reducing ileus.

2. Sham feeding by chewing gum is thought to accelerate bowel function by increasing vagal cholinergic stimulation of the gut. Gum chewing also increases gastric fluid pH and volume.

D. **Mesenteric traction syndrome** consists of sudden tachycardia, hypotension, and decreases in PaO_2. Nonsteroidal anti-inflammatory drugs and aspirin, which inhibit cyclooxygenase, significantly ameliorate these clinical features, suggesting a prostacyclin-mediated cause. Prophylactic administration of H1 and H2 antihistamines also reduce the incidence of dysrhythmias from the mesenteric traction syndrome.

E. **Nitrous Oxide and the Bowel.** Because nitrous oxide is 30 times more soluble than nitrogen in blood, nitrous oxide diffuses into gas-containing body cavities from the bloodstream faster than the nitrogen in those cavities can diffuse out into circulation. This may contribute to excessive distention of gas-containing bowels, possible bowel ischemia, and increased difficulty with surgical exposure.

1. Factors that determine the extent of distention include the amount of gas within the bowel, the duration of nitrous oxide administration, and the concentration of nitrous oxide used. Whereas use of 80% nitrous oxide may potentially result in a fivefold increase in bowel gas, use of a 50% concentration may result in no more than a doubling of bowel gas.

2. Nitrous oxide is best avoided in situations when the bowel is distended. On the other hand, it is reasonable to use low concentrations of nitrous oxide during elective abdominal operations in which no significant amount of gas is present in the bowels.

VI. **CARCINOID TUMORS** are usually asymptomatic, although nonspecific symptoms such as abdominal pain, diarrhea, intermittent intestinal obstruction, and GI bleeding are occasionally seen. Nonmetastatic carcinoid tumors secrete hormones that are usually transported to the liver through the portal vein, where they are subsequently inactivated. Carcinoid tumors, especially those arising in the midgut, secrete a variety of hormones, mediators, and biogenic amines, including large quantities of serotonin, that produce increased platelet serotonin levels and increased urinary levels of 5-hydroxy-indole-acetic-acid (5-HIAA), a metabolite of serotonin. Other secreted substances include histamine, substance P, catecholamines (including dopamine), bradykinin, tachykinin, motilin, corticotrophin, prostaglandins, kallikrein, and neurotensin. Bradykinin may produce cutaneous flushing, bronchospasm, and hypotension, and serotonin may cause hypertension or hypotension.

A. **Carcinoid Syndrome.** Metastatic carcinoid tumors release vasoactive peptides into the systemic circulation, which leads to signs and symptoms such as bronchoconstriction, hypotension, hypertension, diarrhea, and carcinoid heart disease. There is no correlation between the blood level of serotonin and the severity of symptoms.

B. **Carcinoid heart disease** is seen in up to 60% of patients with carcinoid syndrome. Cardiac involvement is usually right sided, affecting the tricuspid (tricuspid regurgitation) and pulmonary valves. The predominance of right-sided cardiac lesions suggests that the substances secreted from liver metastasis into the hepatic vein never reach the left side of the heart because of pulmonary metabolism.

C. **Perioperative Management of Carcinoid Patients.** Complete surgical excision is the most effective treatment for carcinoid tumors. Management should focus on blocking histamine and serotonin receptors and avoiding drugs that facilitate mediator release from tumor cells. Mediator release may be triggered by opioids and muscle relaxants that release histamine. Patients with carcinoid may have diarrhea and high gastric output. Therefore, fluid resuscitation may be required, and serum electrolytes and glucose should be measured at regular intervals.

1. **Somatostatin** is a GI regulatory peptide that reduces the amount of serotonin released from carcinoid tumors. Somatostatin has a very short half-life of about 3 minutes and must therefore be given as infusion.

2. **Octreotide** is a synthetic somatostatin analogue with a half-life of approximately 2.5 hours. Preoperative preparation should include 100 mg of octreotide subcutaneously three times daily in the preceding 2 weeks, and if necessary, it should be weaned slowly over 1 week postoperatively. Preoperative anxiolytics should be administered to prevent stress-triggered release of serotonin, and patients receiving octreotide preoperatively should continue with their normal dose on the morning of surgery. Octreotide also effectively treats intraoperative patients with carcinoid crises.

D. **Anesthetic Management.** Any of the currently available induction agents and muscle relaxants, including propofol, etomidate, synthetic opioids, vecuronium, cisatracurium, and rocuronium, can be used successfully. Caution should be exercised with drugs such as thiopental and Sch that can release histamine. All current inhalation agents can be used successfully, but desflurane may be the best choice in patients with liver metastasis because of its low rate of metabolism. Administration of octreotide before manipulation of the tumor attenuates adverse hemodynamic responses. The sympathetic blockade produced by epidural or spinal anesthesia may worsen hypotension, which can be minimized by dosing the epidural catheter with opioids or dilute local anesthetic solutions. Intraoperative hypotension from sympathetic blockade should be treated with volume expansion and intravenous infusion of octreotide rather than with sympathomimetics such as ephedrine, which can trigger release of vasoactive substances from carcinoid tumors. Intense hemodynamic monitoring and octreotide administration should continue into the postoperative period because secretion of vasoactive substances may still occur from residual tumor or metastasis.

CHAPTER 47 ■ ANESTHESIA AND OBESITY

Obesity, which is now at epidemic proportions worldwide, is a condition of excessive body fat with adverse health implications (Table 47-1) (Ogunnaike BO, Whitten CW: Anesthesia and obesity. In *Clinical Anesthesia*. Edited by Barash PG, Cullen BF, Stoelting RK, Cahalan MK, Stock MC. Philadelphia: Lippincott Williams & Wilkins, 2009, pp 1230–1246).

I. TYPES OF OBESITY

In android (central) obesity, adipose tissue is located predominantly in the upper body (truncal distribution) and is associated with increased oxygen consumption and increased incidence of cardiovascular disease. In gynecoid (peripheral) obesity, adipose tissue is located predominantly in the hips, buttocks, and thighs (fat is less metabolically active, so it is less closely associated with cardiovascular disease). Ideal body weight (IBW) is the weight associated with the lowest mortality rate for a given height and gender. Lean body weight (LBW) is the total body weight minus the adipose tissue. In clinical practice, body mass index (body mass index [BMI] = weight in kg/height^2 in meters) is used to estimate the degree of obesity (obesity is BMI >30 kg/m^2, and morbid obesity is BMI >40 kg/m^2). Waist circumference (>102 cm in men and >89 cm in women) strongly correlates with abdominal fat and is an independent risk predictor of disease.

II. PATHOPHYSIOLOGY OF OBESITY

A. **Respiratory System.** Fat accumulation on the thorax and abdomen decreases chest wall and lung compliance. Polycythemia from chronic hypoxemia contributes to increased

TABLE 47-1

MEDICAL CONSEQUENCES OF OBESITY

System	Consequences
Respiratory	Obstructive sleep apnea
	Obesity-hypoventilation syndrome
	Asthma
	Pulmonary hypertension
Cardiovascular	Coronary artery disease
	Systemic hypertension
	Sudden cardiac death (dysrhythmias)
	Cardiomyopathy
	Thromboembolism
Gastrointestinal	Gastroesophageal reflux disease
	Nonalcoholic fatty liver disease
	Colon cancer
	Gallbladder disease
Endocrine and Metabolic	Metabolic syndrome
	Diabetes mellitus
	Insulin resistance
	Hypothyroidism
Genitourinary	End-stage renal disease
	Urinary incontinence
	Prostate cancer
Hematology	Hypercoagulability
	Polycythemia
Musculoskeletal	Osteoarthritis
	Rheumatoid arthritis
Psychology and psychiatry	Depression
	Reduced self-esteem
	Social stigma

SURGICAL SUBSPECIALTIES

total blood volume and may lead to pulmonary hypertension and cor pulmonale. Increased elastic resistance and decreased compliance of the chest wall further reduce total respiratory compliance while the individual is in a supine position, leading to shallow and rapid breathing.

1. Decreased pulmonary compliance leads to decreased functional residual capacity (FRC), vital capacity (VC), and total lung capacity (TLC). Reduced FRC may result in lung volumes below closing capacity (CC) in the course of normal tidal ventilation, leading to small airway closure, ventilation/perfusion mismatch, right-to-left shunting, and arterial hypoxemia. (Anesthesia worsens this situation such that up to a 50%

reduction in FRC occurs in obese anesthetized patients compared with 20% in non-obese patients.)

2. Expiratory reserve volume is the most sensitive indicator of the effect of obesity on pulmonary function.

3. Obesity increases oxygen consumption and carbon dioxide production because of the metabolic activity of excess fat and the increased workload on supportive tissues. Arterial oxygen tension in morbidly obese patients breathing room air is lower than that predicted for similarly aged non-obese subjects in both sitting and supine positions.

B. **Obstructive Sleep Apnea (OSA)** (Table 47-2). Up to 5% of obese patients have clinically significant OSA that is characterized by periodic, partial, or complete obstruction of the upper airway during sleep. In addition, these individuals may have frequent episodes of apnea or hypopnea during sleep and snoring and daytime symptoms that include sleepiness, impaired concentration, memory problems, and morning headaches.

1. Apnea is defined as 10 seconds or more of total cessation of airflow five or more times per hour despite continuous respiratory effort against a closed glottis combined with a decrease in arterial oxygenation of greater than 4%.

2. Physiologic abnormalities resulting from OSA include hypoxemia, hypercapnia, secondary polycythemia, and an increased risk of ischemic heart disease and cerebrovascular disease.

C. **Obesity Hypoventilation (OHS; Pickwickian Syndrome)** (see Table 47-2). Long-term OSA may lead to OHS, which is seen in 5% to 10% of morbidly obese patients. These patients also have an increased sensitivity to the respiratory depressant effects of general anesthetics.

D. **Cardiovascular and Hematologic Systems.** Total blood volume is increased in obese individuals, but on a volume-to-weight basis, it is less than in non-obese individuals (50 mL/kg compared with 70 mL/kg). Cardiac output increases with increasing weight, with resulting left ventricular hypertrophy, reduced compliance, and impairment of left ventricular filling (diastolic dysfunction and eventual biventricular failure).

1. Obesity accelerates atherosclerosis, but symptoms such as angina and exertional dyspnea occur only occasionally because morbidly obese patients often have very limited mobility and may appear asymptomatic even when they have significant cardiovascular disease.

TABLE 47-2

COMPARISON OF OBSTRUCTIVE SLEEP APNEA AND OBESITY HYPOVENTILATION SYNDROME

	Obstructive Sleep Apnea	Obesity Hypoventilation Syndrome
Gender distribution	Males >Females	Males = Females
BMI >30	Risk increases with obesity	Yes
Ventilation pattern	Normal (except during apnea)	Hypoventilation
$PaCO_2$	Normal (increased during apnea)	Increased (>45 mm Hg)
PaO_2	Normal (decreased during apnea)	Decreased; most severe during REM sleep
SaO_2	Normal (decreased during apnea)	Decreased
Nocturnal upper airway obstruction	Yes (choking or gasping during sleep)	No (except with coexisting OSA)
Recurrent awakenings from sleep	Yes	No
Pulmonary hypertension	Uncommon	Common
Nocturnal monitoring	Five or more obstructive breathing events per hour of sleep	Increased $PaCO_2$ during sleep to >10 mm Hg from awake supine values. Oxygen desaturation during sleep not explained by apnea or hypopnea

BMI = body mass index; OSA= obstructive sleep apnea; REM = rapid eye movement.

2. Intraoperative ventricular failure may occur from rapid intravenous (IV) fluid administration. Many obese patients have mild to moderate hypertension with a 3- to 4-mm Hg increase in systolic and a 2-mm Hg increase in diastolic arterial pressure for every 10 kg of weight gained.
3. The renin–angiotensin system is important in the hypertension of obesity.
4. Obese patients are prone to cardiovascular disease because adipose tissue releases bioactive mediators

(abnormal lipids, insulin resistance, inflammation, coagulopathies).

E. **Gastrointestinal System.** Gastric volume and acidity may be increased, hepatic function altered (fatty liver infiltration, abnormal liver function tests), and drug metabolism adversely affected by obesity. Delayed gastric emptying may occur because of increased abdominal mass that causes antral distention, gastrin release, and a decrease in pH with parietal cell secretion. An increased incidence of hiatal hernia and gastroesophageal reflux may also increase the risk of aspiration.

1. Gastric emptying has been said to be actually faster in obese individuals, especially with high energy content intake such as fat emulsions, but because of the larger gastric volume (≤75% larger) in obese patients, the residual volume is larger.

2. Nonpremedicated, nondiabetic, fasting, obese surgical patients who are free from significant gastroesophageal pathology are unlikely to have high-volume, low pH gastric contents after routine preoperative fasting, so they should follow the same fasting guidelines as non-obese patients and be allowed to drink clear liquids until up to 2 hours before elective surgery.

3. A positive correlation exists between obesity and frequent symptoms of gastroesophageal reflux disease (GERD).

4. Morbidly obese patients who have undergone intestinal bypass surgery have a particularly high prevalence of hepatic dysfunction and cholelithiasis.

5. The high prevalence of non-alcoholic fatty liver disease and cirrhosis necessitates careful assessment for pre-existing inpatients with liver disease who are scheduled for surgery.

F. **Renal and Endocrine Systems.** Impaired glucose tolerance in morbidly obese individuals is reflected by a high prevalence of type II diabetes mellitus caused by resistance of peripheral fatty tissues to insulin. Exogenous insulin may be required perioperatively even in obese patients with type II diabetes mellitus to oppose the catabolic response to surgery.

1. Subclinical hypothyroidism occurs in about 25% of all morbidly obese patients.

2. With prolonged obesity, there may be a loss of nephron function, with further impairment of natriuresis and further increases in arterial pressure.

G. **Metabolic syndrome** is a cluster of metabolic abnormalities (abdominal obesity, glucose intolerance, hypertension, dyslipidemia) that is associated with an increased risk of vascular events.

III. PHARMACOLOGY

The volume of the central compartment in which drugs are first distributed remains unchanged in obese patients, but absolute body water content is decreased, and lean body and adipose tissue mass are increased, affecting lipophilic and polar drug distribution. Plasma albumin concentrations and plasma protein binding are not significantly changed by obesity. There is no significant difference in absorption and bioavailability of orally administered medication when comparing obese and normal weight subjects.

A. Histologic abnormalities of the liver are common in obese people, with concomitant deranged liver function test results, but drug clearance is not usually affected.
B. Renal clearance of drugs is increased in obesity because of increased renal blood flow and glomerular filtration rate.
C. Highly lipophilic substances, such as barbiturates and benzodiazepines, show significant increases in volume of distribution (VD) for obese individuals. Less lipophilic compounds have little or no change in VD with obesity. Drugs with weak or moderate lipophilicity can be dosed on the basis of IBW or lean body mass (LBM).
D. Adding 20% to the estimated IBW dose of hydrophilic medications (nondepolarizing muscle relaxants) is sufficient to include the extra lean mass.

IV. SPECIFIC INTRAVENOUS AGENTS (Table 47-3)

V. MEDICAL THERAPY FOR OBESITY

Medications used to treat obesity are formulated to reduce energy intake, increase energy utilization, or decrease absorption of nutrients.

A. **Sibutramine** inhibits the reuptake of norepinephrine to increase satiety after the onset of eating rather than reduce appetite. Unlike fenfluramine and dexfenfluramine, sibutramine does not promote the release of serotonin, which may explain the absence of reports of sibutramine causing cardiac valvular lesions. Sibutramine also results

TABLE 47-3

DETERMINANTS OF DOSING FOR INTRAVENOUS DRUGS
IN OBESE PATIENTS

Drug	Dosing	Comments
Propofol	Induction: LBW	Systemic clearance and VD at steady-state correlates
	Maintenance: TBW	High affinity for excess fat and other well-perfused organs
		High hepatic extraction and conjugation
Thiopental	Induction: LBW	Increased VD
		Increased blood volume, cardiac output, and muscle mass
		Increased absolute dose
		Prolonged duration of action
Succinylcholine	TBW	Pseudocholinesterase activity increases in proportion to body weight
Rocuronium	LBW	Faster onset and longer duration of action when dosed according to TBW
		Pharmacokinetics and pharmacodynamics are not altered in obese subjects
		Sugammadex encapsulates rocuronium for rapid and complete neuromuscular blockade reversal
Vecuronium	LBW	Prolonged action when dosed according to TBW
		Obesity does not alter distribution or elimination
Atracurium	LBW	Absolute clearance, VD, and elimination-half time do not change
		Unchanged dose per unit body weight without prolongation of recovery because of organ-independent elimination
Fentanyl	LBW	Dosing based on TBW overestimates the dose requirements in obese patients

(continued)

TABLE 47-3

DETERMINANTS OF DOSING FOR INTRAVENOUS DRUGS
IN OBESE PATIENTS (*Continued*)

Drug	Dosing	Comments
Sufentanil	LBW	Increased VD and prolonged elimination half-time correlate with the degree of obesity
		Clearance is similar in obese and non-obese patients
Remifentanil	LBW	Systemic clearance and VD corrected per kilogram of TBW is significantly smaller in obese patients
		Age and LBM should be considered for dosing
Dexmedetomidine	TBW	Lacks significant effects on respiration
		Good analgesic in morbidly obese patients
		Age and lean body mass should be considered for dosing

LBM = lean body mass; LBW = lean body weight; TBW = total body weight;
VD = volume of distribution.

in transient dose-related increases in systolic and
diastolic blood pressure (2–4 mm Hg) and a slight
increase in heart rate (3–5 bpm).
   B. **Orlistat** blocks the absorption and digestion of dietary
fat by binding lipases in the gastrointestinal tract.
Chronic dosing of orlistat results in an increase in
coumadin's anticoagulant effect because of decreased
absorption of vitamin K. This leads to an abnormal
prothrombin time (PT) with a normal partial thromboplastin time (PTT) because of deficiency of clotting
factors II, VII, IX, and X. The resulting coagulopathy
should be corrected 6 to 24 hours before elective surgery with a vitamin K analogue such as phytonadione
and fresh-frozen plasma for emergency surgery or
active bleeding.
   C. **Rimonabant** is a cannabinoid receptor antagonist that
decreases appetite, leading to weight loss and a
decreased incidence of the metabolic syndrome.

SURGICAL SUBSPECIALTIES

VI BARIATRIC SURGERY

Bariatric surgery encompasses a variety of surgical procedures (classified as malabsorptive, restrictive, or combined) used to treat morbid obesity.

A. Gastric restriction (gastroplasty) creates a small upper pouch (15–30 mL) in the stomach and is the most commonly performed bariatric procedure in the United States. Adjustable gastric banding is a restrictive gastric operation usually done by minimally invasive laparoscopic approach.

B. Laparoscopic bariatric surgery is minimally invasive and is associated with less postoperative pain, lower morbidity, and faster recovery.

1. Profound muscle relaxation is important during laparoscopic bariatric procedures to facilitate ventilation and maintain an adequate working space for visualization, safe manipulation of laparoscopic instruments, and extraction of excised tissues.

2. Laparoscopic bariatric surgery requires maneuvering the operating table into various surgically favorable positions (a malleable "bean bag," in addition to belts and straps, may help keep the patient secured). Anesthesia personnel may be asked to facilitate the proper placement of an intragastric balloon to help the surgeon size the gastric pouch and facilitate performance of leak tests with saline or methylene blue through a nasogastric (NG) tube. After the gastric pouch has been created, insertion of an NG tube should be aided by viewing the laparoscope monitor and carefully watching to avoid disruption of the anastomosis. Cephalad displacement of the diaphragm and carina from a pneumoperitoneum during laparoscopy may cause a firmly secured endotracheal tube to displace into a mainstem bronchus.

3. **Rhabdomyolysis** is more common in morbidly obese patients undergoing laparoscopic procedures than in those undergoing an open procedure (Table 47-4).

4. **Gastric electrical stimulation** by means of an implantable gastric stimulator (IGS) causes smooth muscles of the stomach to stop peristalsis so that the patient feels full. Possible lead dislodgment from violent stomach contractions during postoperative nausea and vomiting is a consideration for the anesthesiologist. The

TABLE 47-4

MANAGEMENT OF RHABDOMYOLYSIS

Diagnosis
Presence of risk factors (morbid obesity, prolonged operative time)
Buttock, hip, or shoulder pain in the postoperative period
Unexplained elevation in CPK levels

Prevention and Treatment
Proper positioning and padding of pressure areas
Reduced total operative time
High index of suspicion
Aggressive hydration
Stimulation of diuresis with mannitol (target urine output, 1.5
  mL/kg/hr)
Alkalinization of urine to prevent myoglobin deposition in renal
  tubules (alkalinization increases the solubility of myoglobin)
Hemofiltration may be necessary for rapid clearance of myoglobin

CPK = creatine phosphokinase.

stimulating pulses emitted by the IGS can be picked
up on the electrocardiograph, which may lead to false
readings.

VII. PREOPERATIVE CONSIDERATIONS

A. **Preoperative Evaluation** (Table 47-5)
B. **Concurrent, Preoperative, and Prophylactic Medications.**
   Patients' usual medications should be continued until the
   time of surgery with the possible exception of insulin
   and oral hypoglycemics. Antibiotic prophylaxis is important because of an increased incidence of wound
   infections in obese patients. Anxiolysis and prophylaxis
   against both aspiration pneumonitis and deep vein
   thrombosis (DVT) should be addressed at
   premedication.
   1. Morbid obesity is a major independent risk factor for
      sudden death from acute postoperative pulmonary
      embolism. Subcutaneous heparin 5000 IU
      administered before surgery and repeated every 8 to
      12 hours until the patient is fully mobile reduces the
      risk of DVT. Other risk factors include venous stasis
      disease, BMI of 60 kg/m^2 or above, truncal obesity,
      and obesity hypoventilation syndrome (OHS) or sleep
      apnea syndrome (SAS), suggesting that enoxaparin
      dosing in obese patients should be varied with age
      and LBM.

TABLE 47-5

PREOPERATIVE CONSIDERATIONS IN OBESE PATIENTS

Evaluation of cardiorespiratory systems and airway (previous anesthetic experiences)

Evaluation for systemic hypertension, pulmonary hypertension, signs of ventricular failure, and ischemic heart disease

Examination for signs of cardiac failure (elevated jugular venous pressure, added heart sounds, pulmonary crackles, hepatomegaly, peripheral edema)

Chest radiography (evidence of underlying lung disease and prominent pulmonary arteries)

Metabolic and nutritional abnormalities (scheduled for repeat bariatric surgery)

Postoperative polyneuropathy (vitamin and nutritional deficiency, known as APGARS neuropathy)

Protracted postoperative vomiting, hyporeflexia, and muscular weakness (implications for NMDBs)

Electrolyte and coagulation indices should be checked before surgery (a vitamin K analog or fresh frozen plasma may be needed)

Evidence of OSA and OHS should be sought preoperatively (OSA patients on a CPAP device at home should be instructed to bring it with them to the hospital because it may be needed postoperatively)

The possibility of invasive monitoring, prolonged intubation, and postoperative mechanical ventilation should be discussed with the patient

ABG measurement (routine pulmonary function tests and liver function tests are not cost effective in asymptomatic obese patients).

ABG = arterial blood gas; APGARS = acute postgastric reduction surgery; CPAP = continuous positive airway pressure; NMDA = neuromuscular blocking drug; OSA = obstructive sleep apnea.

2. A combination of short duration of surgery, lower extremity pneumatic compression, and routine early ambulation may preclude mandatory heparin anticoagulation except in patients with a history of DVT or a known hypercoagulable state.

VIII. AIRWAY (Table 47-6)

A. Neck circumference has been identified as the single biggest predictor of problematic intubation in morbidly obese patients. Intubation is problematic in

TABLE 47-6

ANATOMIC CHANGES ASSOCIATED WITH OBESITY THAT CONTRIBUTE TO A POTENTIALLY DIFFICULT AIRWAY

Limitation of movement of the atlantoaxial joint and cervical spine (because of upper thoracic and low cervical fat pads)
Excessive tissue folds in the mouth and pharynx
Short, thick neck
Suprasternal, presternal, and posterior cervical fat
Thick submental fat pad
Excess pharyngeal tissue in the lateral pharyngeal walls (may not be noticed during routine airway examination)

approximately 5% of patients with a 40-cm neck circumference compared with a 35% probability of those with a 60-cm neck circumference.

B. The magnitude of BMI does not seem to have much influence on the difficulty of laryngoscopy.

IX. AMBULATORY ANESTHESIA

A. There is no evidence to suggest increased morbidity in morbidly obese patients with stable concomitant diseases. Patients should not be excluded from day-case surgery based solely on absolute weight or BMI.

B. Airway surgery (uvulopalatopharyngoplasty, tonsillectomy) should not be performed on an outpatient basis.

C. Use of regional blocks (which are technically more difficult), rapidly dissipating anesthetic agents, and appropriately sized equipment and procedures for positioning and monitoring should be combined with the availability of prolonged observation and overnight admission for optimum safety.

X. INTRAOPERATIVE CONSIDERATIONS

A. **Positioning**

1. Specially designed tables or two regular operating tables may be required for safe anesthesia and surgery in obese patients. Regular operating tables have a maximum weight limit of approximately 205 kg.

2. Brachial plexus injury, ulnar neuropathy, and lower extremity nerve injuries are frequent. Carpal tunnel syndrome is the most common mononeuropathy after bariatric surgery.

3. Supine positioning causes ventilatory impairment and inferior vena cava and aortic compression in obese patients. FRC and oxygenation are further decreased with supine positioning.
   a. Trendelenburg positioning (which should be avoided, if possible), as may be required during bariatric procedures, further worsens FRC.
   b. The head-up reverse Trendelenburg position provides the longest safe apnea period during induction of anesthesia.
   c. Lateral decubitus positioning allows for better diaphragmatic excursion and should be favored over prone positioning whenever the surgical procedure permits.

B. **Monitoring.** Invasive arterial pressure monitoring may be indicated for morbidly obese patients, patients with cardiopulmonary disease, and patients in whom the noninvasive blood pressure cuff may not fit properly. Blood pressure measurements can be falsely elevated if a cuff is too small.

C. **Induction, Intubation, and Maintenance**
   1. Adequate preoxygenation is vital in obese patients because of rapid desaturation after loss of consciousness caused by increased oxygen consumption and decreased FRC.
   2. Larger doses of induction agents may be required by obese patients because blood volume, muscle mass, and cardiac output increase linearly with the degree of obesity.
   3. If a difficult intubation is anticipated, awake intubation using topical or regional anesthesia is a prudent approach. Sedation with dexmedetomidine during awake intubation provides adequate anxiolysis and analgesia without respiratory depression.
   4. Towels or folded blankets under the shoulders and head can compensate for the exaggerated flexed position of posterior cervical fat (head-elevated laryngoscopy position [HELP]).
   5. Continuous infusion of a short-acting IV agent, such as propofol, or any of the inhalational agents or a combination may be used to maintain anesthesia.
      a. Rapid elimination and analgesic properties make nitrous oxide an attractive choice for anesthesia in obese patients, but high oxygen demand in this patient population limits its use.

    b. Nitrous oxide does not cause noticeable bowel distention during short-duration laparoscopic bariatric procedures.

    c. Dexmedetomidine has no clinically significant adverse effects on respiration and is useful for sedation and analgesia in obese patients.

6. Positive end-expiratory pressure (PEEP) is the only ventilatory parameter that has consistently been shown to improve respiratory function in obese subjects. PEEP may, however, decrease venous return and cardiac output.

D. Regional anesthesia is a useful alternative to general anesthesia in morbidly obese patients because it may help avoid potential intubation difficulties. It can, however, be technically difficult because of an inability to identify the usual bony landmarks.

1. Epidural vascular engorgement and fatty infiltration reduce the volume of the space, making dose requirements of local anesthetics for epidural anesthesia 20% to 25% lower in obese patients.

2. Subarachnoid blocks are not as technically difficult as epidural blocks, but the height of a subarachnoid block in obese patients can be unpredictable.

XI. POSTOPERATIVE CONSIDERATIONS

A. Emergence

1. Prompt extubation reduces the likelihood that a morbidly obese patient who may have underlying cardiopulmonary disease will become ventilator dependent.

    a. Supplemental oxygen should be administrated after extubation. There is an increased incidence of atelectasis in morbidly obese patients after general anesthesia that persists into the postoperative period.

    b. Postoperative continuous positive airway pressure may improve oxygenation but does not facilitate carbon dioxide elimination.

B. Postoperative Analgesia. Perioperative use of regional anesthesia and analgesia reduces the incidence of postoperative respiratory complications. Potential advantages of epidural analgesia in obese patients include prevention of DVT, improved analgesia, and earlier recovery of intestinal motility. Delayed respiratory depression is one of the known complications of central neuraxial opioids.

XII. RESUSCITATION

A. The possible need for cardiopulmonary resuscitation should be considered during anesthesia for morbidly obese patients.

1. Chest compressions may not be effective, and mechanical compression devices may be required. The maximum 400 joules of energy on regular defibrillators is sufficient for morbidly obese patients because their chest walls are usually not much thicker, but the higher transthoracic impedance from the fat may obligate several attempts.

2. The laryngeal mask airway and the esophageal tracheal Combitube are temporary supraglottic airway devices that are useful during resuscitation of obese patients. Tracheostomy and percutaneous cricothyrotomy are time-consuming and technically difficult procedures in emergency situations and should be reserved as final options to be performed by experienced practitioners.

CHAPTER 48 ■ HEPATIC ANATOMY, FUNCTION AND PHYSIOLOGY

The liver provides a diverse spectrum of vital physiologic functions and plays an essential role in maintaining perioperative homeostasis (Table 48-1) (Kaufman BS, Roccaforte JD: Hepatic anatomy, function, and physiology. In *Clinical Anesthesia*. Edited by Barash PG, Cullen BF, Stoelting RK, Cahalan MK, Stock MC. Philadelphia: Lippincott Williams & Wilkins, 2009, pp 1247–1278). Normal liver function may be present in humans when as much as 80% of the organ has been resected. Insidious hepatic diseases such as chronic hepatitis C can progress silently and destroy the majority of the liver before symptoms develop. A careful preoperative history and physical examination help identify patients in whom laboratory evaluation of liver function is appropriate. These patients are often at increased risk for perioperative morbidity and mortality, including postoperative development of overt liver dysfunction, particularly after major procedures.

I. HEPATIC HOMEOSTASIS

A. Vascular Supply

1. The liver receives about 25% of the cardiac output via the hepatic artery and portal vein. The hepatic artery delivers about 25% of the total hepatic blood flow but nearly 50% of the hepatic oxygen delivery. The portal vein provides the remaining 75% of total hepatic blood flow and 50% of hepatic oxygen delivery.

    a. Because portal venous blood has already perfused the preportal organs (stomach, intestines, spleen, and pancreas), it is partially deoxygenated and enriched with nutrients and other substances absorbed from the gastrointestinal tract.

    b. When patients develop portal hypertension, connections form large portosystemic shunts, permitting

TABLE 48-1

MAJOR PHYSIOLOGIC FUNCTIONS OF THE LIVER

Blood reservoir (the liver contains nearly 25–30 mL of blood per 100 g of tissue)

Regulator of blood coagulation (synthesis of procoagulation factors and anticoagulant factors)

Endocrine organ (synthesizes insulin-like growth factor-1, angiotensinogen, and thrombopoietin; principal site of hormone biotransformation and catabolism)

Erythrocyte breakdown and bilirubin excretion (bilirubin is an end product of heme degradation).

Metabolic functions of the liver

Carbohydrate metabolism (the liver can store a maximum of approximately 75 g of glycogen; in patients with chronic liver disease, hyperglycemia commonly occurs because portosystemic shunting allows direct entry of glucose-rich portal venous blood into the systemic circulation; hypoglycemia is a late manifestation of advanced liver disease)

Lipid metabolism (fatty acids in the liver are esterified to form triglycerides, cholesterol esters, and phospholipids)

Amino acid metabolism

Synthesis of important proteins (albumin and coagulation factors and their inhibitors with the exception of factor VIII)

Immunologic function (Kupffer cells produce a variety of inflammatory mediators and cytokines)

Pharmacokinetics (by converting lipophilic substances to excretable metabolites, hepatic enzymes detoxify drugs and terminate their pharmacologic activity)

portal venous blood to return to the systemic circulation without traversing the liver (esophageal varices).

2. Hepatic arterial pressure is similar to aortic pressure, and the mean portal vein pressure is approximately 6 to 10 mm Hg.

3. Periportal hepatocytes located close to the terminal vascular branches of the portal vein and hepatic artery are the first to be supplied with oxygen and nutrients (zone 1). The perivenular (centrilobular) area, which is the most distant from these terminal vascular branches, has the least resistance to metabolic and anoxic damage (zone 3).

a. Smooth endoplasmic reticulum is more abundant in these cells. Zone 3 is a primary site for glycolysis and lipogenesis. It is also the site for general detoxification and biotransformation of drugs, chemicals, and toxins.

   b. The anaerobic milieu of zone 3, however, is also its Achilles heel because these cells are exquisitely susceptible to injury from systemic hypoperfusion and hypoxemia. Sharply defined zone 3 necrosis is also characteristic of injury resulting from accumulation of toxic products of biotransformation as seen in toxicity from hepatotoxic drugs.

B. Hepatic Blood Flow. Although the liver as a whole receives 25% of the cardiac output, regional blood flow within the organ is such that certain areas are highly prone to ischemia. The hepatic circulation is regulated by both intrinsic (regional microvascular) and extrinsic (neural and hormonal) mechanisms.

C. Innervation of the Liver. The liver is predominantly innervated by two plexuses that enter at the hilum and supply both sympathetic and parasympathetic nerve fibers.

II. PHARMACOKINETICS

A. Drug metabolism is primarily a hepatic event, and the liver influences the plasma concentration of most orally and parenterally administered drugs through its synthesis of drug-binding proteins. Albumin and α1-acid glycoprotein act as sinks to decrease plasma concentrations.

B. The goal of metabolism is to convert drugs into inactive water-soluble substances that can be excreted in the bile or urine.

   1. Patients with significant liver disease may have marked alterations of pharmacokinetics and pharmacodynamics.

   2. Portosystemic shunts allow orally administered drugs to bypass the liver.

   3. Decreases in hepatic blood flow seen in patients with liver disease may prolong the elimination half-time of high-extraction drugs.

III. ASSESSMENT OF HEPATIC FUNCTION

A. Laboratory Evaluation of Hepatic Function (Table 48-2). Liver function tests (LFTs) can be classified into several broad categories.

TABLE 48-2

LABORATORY EVALUATION OF HEPATIC FUNCTION

	Bilirubin Overload (Hemolysis)	Parenchymal Dysfunction	Cholestasis
Aminotransferases	Normal	Increased (may be normal to decreased in advanced stages)	Normal (may be increased in advanced stages)
Alkaline phosphatase	Normal	Normal	Increased
Bilirubin	Unconjugated	Conjugated	Conjugated
Serum proteins	Normal	Decreased	Normal (may be decreased in advanced stages)
Prothrombin time	Normal	Prolonged (may be normal in early stages)	Normal (may be prolonged in advanced stages)
Blood urea nitrogen	Normal	Normal (may be decreased in advanced stages)	Normal
Sulfobromophthalein or indocyanine green	Normal	Retention	Normal or retention

TABLE 48-3

CAUSES OF HYPERBILIRUBINEMIA

Unconjugated (Indirect)
Excessive bilirubin production (hemolysis)
Immaturity of enzyme systems
Physiologic jaundice of newborn
Jaundice of prematurity
Inherited defects
Gilbert's disease
Crigler-Najjar syndrome

Conjugated (Direct)
Hepatocellular disease (hepatitis, cirrhosis, drugs)
Intrahepatic cholestasis (drugs, pregnancy)
Benign postoperative jaundice, sepsis
Congenital conjugated hyperbilirubinemia
Dubin-Johnson syndrome
Rotor's syndrome
Obstructive jaundice
Extrahepatic (calculus, stricture, neoplasm)
Intrahepatic (sclerosing cholangitis, neoplasm, primary biliary
  cirrhosis)

1. **Indices of Hepatocellular Damage.** Increased serum activities of aspartate aminotransferase (AST; formerly serum glutamic oxalacetic transaminase [SGOT]) and alanine aminotransferase (ALT; formerly serum glutamic pyruvic transaminase [SGPT]) are detected when hepatocellular injury and necrosis are present.
2. **Indices of Obstructed Bile Flow.**
   a. Alkaline phosphatase (AP) elevations that are disproportionate to changes in AST and ALT occur with intrahepatic or extrahepatic obstruction to bile flow. (This is a highly sensitive test for assessing the integrity of the biliary system.)
   b. Hyperbilirubinemia is classified as either predominantly unconjugated or predominantly conjugated (Table 48-3).
3. **Indices of Hepatic Synthetic Function**
   a. Measurement of serum albumin level and assays of coagulation function are the most widely used methods for assessing hepatic synthetic function.
   b. Because the half-life in serum is as long as 20 days, the serum albumin level is not a reliable indicator of hepatic protein synthesis in patients with acute liver disease.

    c. The prothrombin time (PT) and international normalized ratio (INR) are sensitive indicators of severe hepatic dysfunction whether patients have acute or chronic liver disease because of the short half-life of factor VII. A progressively increasing PT is usually ominous in patients with acute hepatocellular disease, suggesting an increased likelihood of acute hepatic failure.

  4. **Indices of Hepatic Blood Flow and Metabolic Capacity**

    a. Elimination of the dye indocyanine green (ICG) from the blood provides an estimate of hepatic perfusion and hepatocellular function because it is highly extracted (70% to 95% by the liver after an intravenous injection).

    b. Hepatic function can also be assessed with substances that are metabolized selectively by the liver (e.g., lidocaine is metabolized by oxidative N-demethylation to monoethylglycinexylidide [MEGX]).

B. Hepatobiliary Imaging

  1. Ultrasonography is the primary screening test for hepatic disease, gallstones, and biliary tract disease.

  2. Computed tomography provides better and more complete anatomic definition than ultrasonography.

  3. Percutaneous transhepatic cholangiography may be used to determine the level and cause of biliary obstruction, confirm the presence of cholestasis without obstruction, and evaluate whether a proximal cholangiocarcinoma is surgically resectable.

  4. Endoscopic retrograde cholangiopancreatography (ERCP) uses endoscopy to visualize the ampulla of Vater and guide insertion of a guidewire and catheter through the ampulla to permit selective injection of contrast material into the pancreatic and common bile ducts, which are then imaged radiographically. ERCP is the imaging technique of choice in patients with choledocholithiasis because sphincterotomy and stone extraction can often be performed.

C. Liver biopsy has a central role in the evaluation of patients with suspected liver disease because it provides the only means of determining the precise nature of hepatic damage (necrosis, inflammation, steatosis, or fibrosis). The presence of coagulopathy (PT that is 3 seconds greater than the control or platelet count <60,000 cells/mL^3)

contraindicates percutaneous liver biopsy, although transjugular liver biopsy can be performed safely in these patients.

IV. HEPATIC AND HEPATOBILIARY DISEASES

Liver diseases are divided into parenchymal and cholestatic diseases (Table 48-4).

V. CIRRHOSIS: A PARADIGM FOR END-STAGE PARENCHYMAL LIVER DISEASE (Tables 48-5 to 48-7)

TABLE 48-4

CLASSIFICATION OF LIVER DISEASE

Parenchymal Diseases
Viral hepatitis
  Hepatitis C (accounts for 40% of chronic liver disease; because of the use of serologic testing in screening donated blood, hepatitis C has almost been eliminated as a cause of posttransfusion hepatitis)
  Cytomegalovirus
  Epstein-Barr virus
  Herpes simplex virus
Nonviral hepatitis
  Toxin and drug-induced hepatitis
    Acetaminophen
    NSAIDs
    Antibiotics
    Volatile anesthetics (metabolism to trifluoroacyl metabolites may result in cross-sensitivity between fluorinated volatile anesthetics; the exception is sevoflurane, which is not metabolized to trifluoroacyl metabolites)
    Non-opioid sedative–hypnotic agents (rare)
    Opioids (increase the tone of the common bile duct and sphincter of Oddi but are unlikely to be hepatotoxic)
Inflammation and sepsis
Hypoxia and ischemia
  Severe congestive heart failure
  Surgical stress
Chronic hepatitis
Fatty liver disease
Alcoholic liver disease

Cholestatic Diseases
Biliary obstruction

NSAID = nonsteroidal anti-inflammatory drug.

TABLE 48-5

PATHOPHYSIOLOGY OF HEPATIC CIRRHOSIS

Cardiovascular Abnormalities
Hyperdynamic circulation
Hypervolemia
Arteriovenous collateralization
Cardiomyopathy

Hepatic Circulatory Dysfunction
Portal hypertension
Ascites
Variceal hemorrhage
Sepsis and infection

Pulmonary Dysfunction
Arterial hypoxemia (intrapulmonary vascular dilations)
Hydrothorax
Portopulmonary hypertension

Ascites

Renal Dysfunction and the Hepatorenal Syndrome

Spontaneous Bacterial Peritonitis

Hematologic and Coagulation Disorders
Hyperfibrinolysis
Elevated PT and INR serve as prognostic indicators
Thrombocytopenia

Endocrine Disorders
Abnormal glucose utilization (prone to hypoglycemia)
Abnormal metabolism of sex hormones (gonadal dysfunction in
both men and women)

Hepatic Encephalopathy (treatment is orthotopic liver
transplantation)

INR = international normalized ratio; PT = prothrombin time.

VI. UNCOMMON CAUSES OF CIRRHOSIS (Table 48-8)

VII. HEPATOCELLULAR CARCINOMA

- A. Primary hepatocellular carcinoma (HCC) is one of the most common tumors in the world and is the third most frequent cause of death from cancer.
- B. HCC usually arises in a cirrhotic liver. The most common presenting complaint is abdominal pain, and the most frequent finding on physical examination is an abdominal mass.

TABLE 48-6

DIFFERENTIAL DIAGNOSIS OF ACUTE AZOTEMIA IN PATIENTS WITH LIVER DISEASE

	Prerenal Azotemia	Hepatorenal Syndrome	Acute Renal Failure (Acute Tubular Necrosis)
Urinary sodium concentration (mEq/L)	<10	<10	>30
Urine-to-plasma creatinine ratio	>30:1	>30:1	<20:1
Urinary osmolality	Exceeds plasma osmolality by at least 100 mOsm	Exceeds plasma by at least 100 mOsm	Equal to plasma osmolality
Urinary sediment	Normal	Unremarkable	Casts or cellular debris

TABLE 48-7

MODIFIED CHILD-PUGH SCORE

	Points*		
	1	2	3
Albumin (g/dL)	>3.5	2.8–3.5	<2.8
Prothrombin time			
Seconds prolonged	<4	4–6	>6
INR	<1.7	1.7–2.3	>2.3
Bilirubin (mg/dL)	<2	2–3	>3
Ascites	Absent	Slight to moderate	Tense
Encephalopathy	None	Grades I–II	Grades III–IV

*Class A, 5 to 6 points; class B, 7 to 9 points; class C, 10 to 15 points.
INR = international normalized ratio.

TABLE 48-8

UNCOMMON CAUSES OF CIRRHOSIS

Wilson's disease (characterized by hepatic copper accumulation)
Hemochromatosis (characterized by excessive iron absorption)
Primary biliary cirrhosis (positive antimitochondrial antibody test result)
α_1-Antitrypsin deficiency
Budd-Chiari syndrome (venous outflow obstruction from the liver)

VIII. PREGNANCY-RELATED DISORDERS

A. **Acute fatty liver of pregnancy** occurs in the late stages of pregnancy.
   1. Affected women usually present in the third trimester with symptoms related to hepatic failure.
   2. When acute fatty liver is diagnosed, delivery of the fetus is expedited. (The disease usually improves in response to termination of pregnancy.)
B. **Preeclampsia and HELLP Syndrome** (increased liver transaminases, thrombocytopenia, and hyperbilirubinemia). Prompt delivery of the fetus is indicated if the syndrome develops beyond 34 weeks of gestation or earlier if life-threatening morbidity develops in the mother.
C. **Hepatic Rupture, Hematoma, and Infarct.** These conditions occur in women with preeclampsia and may be the extreme end of the spectrum of HELLP syndrome.

IX. CHOLESTATIC DISEASE

A. **Cardiovascular Dysfunction.** The presence of bile salts in circulating blood (cholemia) can impair myocardial contractility.
B. **Coagulation Disorders.** Cholestatic disease predisposes the patient toward development of coagulopathy primarily related to vitamin K deficiency. The coagulation disorders are usually moderate, and parenteral vitamin K corrects the problem. If such patients need urgent surgery, the coagulopathy requires immediate treatment with fresh-frozen plasma.

X. PERIOPERATIVE MANAGEMENT (Table 48-9)

XI. CAUSES OF POSTOPERATIVE LIVER DYSFUNCTION UNRELATED TO PERIOPERATIVE FACTORS

A. **Asymptomatic and Pre-Existing Hepatic Injury.**
   Although postoperative liver dysfunction may result from anesthetic or surgical interventions, it is often unrelated to perioperative factors (pre-existing liver disease).
B. **Congenital Disorders**
   1. **Gilbert's syndrome** (familial unconjugated hyperbilirubinemia) is the most common cause of jaundice. It is

TABLE 48-9
PERIOPERATIVE MANAGEMENT OF PATIENTS WITH LIVER DISEASE

Preoperative
Hepatic evaluation and preparation (prior episodes of jaundice, use of alcohol, current medications, easy bruising, episodes of gastrointestinal bleeding; liver function tests should be performed only if there is a suspicion of liver dysfunction based on history and physical examination; surgical morbidity and mortality are increased; these patients are sensitive to all sedatives)

Intraoperative
Monitoring and vascular access (arterial cannula, central venous, assessment of coagulation status)
Selection of anesthetic technique (regional anesthesia for peripheral procedures without coagulation abnormalities)
Induction of general anesthesia (all IV induction drugs are acceptable; decreased cholinesterase activity because of liver disease is rarely a problem)
Maintenance of anesthesia (the adequacy of blood flow and oxygen supply to the liver should be considered; opioids are useful; clearance mechanisms of muscle relaxants should be considered)
Fluids and blood products
Vasopressors (peripheral vasodilation may be resistant to vasopressors)

Postoperative
Liver dysfunction and management (postoperative dysfunction is usually transient; jaundice is the earliest sign of significant dysfunction)
Hemolysis and transfusion (reabsorption of surgical hematomas and transfusions are sources of jaundice in the absence of hepatocellular dysfunction)

IV = intravenous.

a benign metabolic disorder characterized by a decrease in the activity of the hepatic enzyme bilirubin glucuronyltransferase, which is required for hepatocyte uptake of unconjugated bilirubin.

2. Patients with **Crigler-Najjar syndrome** (congenital nonhemolytic jaundice) exhibit either an absence (type 1) or marked decrease (type 2) of bilirubin glucuronyltransferase, producing unconjugated hyperbilirubinemia.

3. Surgical and anesthesia-related problems are apparently minimal in patients with Gilbert's and Crigler-Najjar syndromes.

XII. CONCLUSION: PREVENTION AND TREATMENT OF POSTOPERATIVE LIVER DYSFUNCTION

A. Identifying patients at high risk for developing liver dysfunction or for having an exacerbation of pre-existing liver disease is of utmost importance for minimizing the morbidity and mortality in such patients (careful preoperative evaluation).

1. When liver abnormalities are recognized preoperatively, it is prudent to defer elective procedures until the course of the disease can be determined.

2. For operations that cannot be deferred, clinically significant pathophysiologic changes associated with the liver disease (coagulopathy, fluid and electrolyte abnormalities) should be corrected.

B. The choice of anesthesia is usually an insignificant issue for peripheral or minor surgery (operations that do not affect splanchnic blood flow).

1. The selection of pharmacologic anesthetic agents may have important implications in patients undergoing major operations.

2. A primary goal during the maintenance of anesthesia is to ensure the adequacy of splanchnic, hepatic, and renal perfusion, especially in patients with severe liver disease who undergo major abdominal operations.

TABLE 48-10
CAUSES OF POSTOPERATIVE LIVER DYSFUNCTION

Hepatocellular	Drugs
	Anesthetics
	Ischemia
	Shock, hypotension, iatrogenic injury
	Viral hepatitis
Cholestasis	Benign postoperative cholestasis
	Sepsis
	Bile duct injury
	Drugs
	Antibiotics, antiemetics
	Choledocholithiasis or pancreatitis
	Cholecystitis
	Gilbert syndrome

C. When postoperative hepatic injury occurs, the mainstay of therapy is supportive (Table 48-10).
   1. The hepatotoxic potentials of all medications merit consideration. Any medication that is suspect should be discontinued.
   2. Extrahepatic biliary obstruction should be considered in the differential diagnosis because it may require prompt surgical intervention.

CHAPTER 49 ■ ENDOCRINE FUNCTION

An understanding of the pathophysiology of endocrine function is important in the management of anesthesia for patients with disorders of the hormone-producing glands (Schwartz JJ, Akhtar S, Rosenbaum SH: Endocrine function. In *Clinical Anesthesia*. Edited by Barash PG, Cullen BF, Stoelting RK, Cahalan MK, Stock MC. Philadelphia: Lippincott Williams & Wilkins, 2009, pp 1279–1304).

I. THYROID GLAND

A. **Thyroid Metabolism and Function.** Thyroxine (T_4) and triiodothyronine (T_3) are the major regulators of cellular metabolic activity. The thyroid gland is solely responsible for the daily secretion of T_4 (80–100 µg/day; elimination half-time, 6–7 days). About 80% of T_3 is produced by extrathyroidal deiodination of T_4 (elimination half-time, 24–30 hours). Thyroid hormone synthesis occurs in four stages (Fig. 49-1). Most of the excess effects of thyroid hormones (hyperadrenergic state) are mediated by T_3 (Table 49-1).

B. **Tests of Thyroid Function** (Table 49-2)

C. **Hyperthyroidism**

1. **Treatment and Anesthetic Considerations** (Table 49-3)

a. A combination of propranolol (effective in attenuating the manifestations of excessive sympathetic nervous system activity, as evidenced by a heart rate <90 bpm) and potassium iodide (inhibits hormone release) is effective in rendering patients "euthyroid" before anesthesia and surgery. Esmolol may be administered as a continuous intravenous (IV) infusion to maintain the heart rate below 90 bpm.

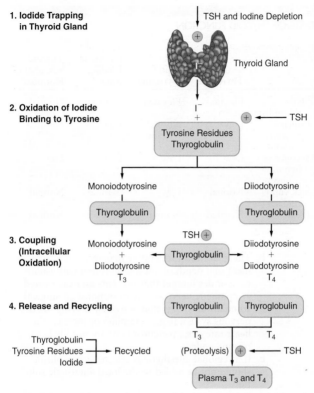

1. **Iodide Trapping in Thyroid Gland**

TSH and Iodine Depletion

Thyroid Gland

2. **Oxidation of Iodide Binding to Tyrosine**

I⁻ + → TSH

Tyrosine Residues
Thyroglobulin

Monoiodotyrosine

Thyroglobulin

Diiodotyrosine

Thyroglobulin

3. **Coupling (Intracellular Oxidation)**

Monoiodotyrosine
+
Diiodotyrosine
T_3

TSH Thyroglobulin

Diiodotyrosine
+
Diiodotyrosine
T_4

4. **Release and Recycling**

Thyroglobulin   Thyroglobulin

T_3 T_4

(Proteolysis) ← TSH

Thyroglobulin
Tyrosine Residues → Recycled
Iodide

Plasma T_3 and T_4

FIGURE 49-1. Schematic depiction of the four stages of synthesis and release of thyroid hormone. T_3 = triiodothyronine; T_4 = thyroxine; TSH = thyroid-stimulating hormone.

TABLE 49-1

EFFECTS OF TRIIODOTHYRONINE ON RECEPTOR CONCENTRATIONS

Increased number of β-receptors
Decreased number of cardiac cholinergic receptors

TABLE 49-2

TESTS OF THYROID FUNCTION

	Serum Thyroxine	Serum Triiodo-thyronine	Thyroid Hormone Binding Rate	Thyroid Stimulating Hormone
Hyper-thyroidism	Elevated	Elevated	Elevated	Normal to low
Primary hypothy-roidism	Low	Normal to low	Low	Elevated
Secondary hypothy-roidism	Low	Low	Low	Low
Sick euthy-roidism	Normal	Low	Normal	Normal
Pregnancy	Elevated	Normal	Low	Normal

    b. The goal of intraoperative management is achievement of a depth of anesthesia (often with isoflurane or desflurane) that prevents an exaggerated sympathetic nervous system response to surgical stimulation. Drugs that activate the sympathetic nervous system (e.g., ketamine) or increase the heart rate (e.g., pancuronium) are not likely to be recommended.

    c. If a regional anesthetic is selected, epinephrine should not be added to the local anesthetic solution.

TABLE 49-3

PREPARATION OF HYPERTHYROID PATIENTS

Propylthiouracil (inhibits synthesis and decreases peripheral conversion of T_4 to T_3)

Inorganic iodide (inhibits hormone release)

β-Adrenergic antagonists (propranolol administered over 12 to 24 hours decreases the heart rate to <90 bpm)

Iopanoic acid (radiographic contrast agent that decreases peripheral conversion of T_4 to T_3)

Glucocorticoids (decrease hormone release and peripheral conversion of T_4 to T_3)

T_3 = triiodothyronine; T_4 = thyroxine.

TABLE 49-4

POSSIBLE COMPLICATIONS OF THYROID SURGERY

Thyroid storm (should be distinguished from malignant hyperthermia, pheochromocytoma, and inadequate anesthesia; it most often develops in undiagnosed or untreated hyperthyroid patients because of the stress of surgery)

Airway obstruction (diagnosed with CT of the neck)

Recurrent laryngeal nerve damage (hoarseness may be present if the damage is unilateral, and aphonia may be present if the damage is bilateral)

Hypoparathyroidism (symptoms of hypocalcemia develop within 24 to 48 hours and include laryngospasm)

CT = computed tomography.

2. **Anesthesia for thyroid surgery** (subtotal thyroidectomy) is an alternative to prolonged medical therapy. Complications associated with surgery occur more frequently when preoperative preparation is inadequate (Tables 49-4 and 49-5).

   a. It is useful to evaluate vocal cord function in the early postoperative period by asking patients to say the letter "e."

   b. Unexpected difficult intubation is increased in the presence of goiter. (Inhalation induction or awake fiberoptic intubation should be considered if there is evidence of significant airway obstruction or tracheal deviation or narrowing.)

TABLE 49-5

MANAGEMENT OF THYROID STORM

IV fluids

Sodium iodide (250 mg orally or IV every 6 hr)

Propylthiouracil (200–400 mg orally or via a nasogastric tube every 6 hr)

Hydrocortisone (50–100 mg IV every 6 hr)

Propranolol (10–40 mg orally every 4–6 hr) or esmolol (titrate)

Cooling blankets and acetaminophen (12.5 mg IV of meperidine every 4–6 hr may be used to treat or prevent shivering)

Digoxin (congestive heart failure with atrial fibrillation and rapid ventricular response)

IV = intravenous.

TABLE 49-6

MANIFESTATIONS OF HYPOTHYROIDISM

Lethargy
Cold intolerance
Decreased cardiac output and heart rate
Peripheral vasoconstriction
Heart failure (unlikely unless coexisting cardiac disease is present)
Decreased platelet adhesiveness
Anemia (GI bleeding)
Impaired renal concentrating ability
Adrenal cortex suppression
Decreased GI motility (may compound the effects of postoperative
    ileus)

GI = gastrointestinal.

    c. Postoperative airway obstruction caused by
        hematoma or tracheomalacia may require urgent
        reintubation of the trachea.
    d. Operating on an acutely hyperthyroid patient may
        provoke thyroid storm.
D. Hypothyroidism
    1. Hypothyroidism is a relatively common disease
        (0.5%–0.8% of the adult population) that results
        from inadequate circulating levels of T_4, T_3, or both
        (Table 49–6).
    2. Treatment and Anesthetic Considerations
        a. No evidence supports postponement of elective
            surgery (including coronary artery bypass graft
            surgery) in the presence of mild to moderate
            hypothyroidism.
        b. No evidence supports the choice of a specific anes-
            thetic technique or selection of drugs for hypothy-
            roid patients, although opioids and volatile anes-
            thetics are often considered to have increased
            depressant effects in these patients. There appears
            to be little, if any, decrease in anesthetic require-
            ments as reflected by the minimum alveolar con-
            centration.
        c. Meticulous attention must be paid to maintaining
            body temperature.
    3. Myxedema coma is a medical emergency that requires
        aggressive therapy (Table 49-7).

TABLE 49-7
MANAGEMENT OF MYXEDEMA COMA

Tracheal intubation and controlled ventilation of the lungs as needed
Levothyroxine (200–300 mg IV over 5–10 min)
Cortisol (100 mg IV and then 25 mg IV every 6 hr)
Fluid and electrolyte therapy as guided by serum electrolyte measurements
Warm environment to conserve body heat

IV = intravenous.

II. PARATHYROID GLANDS

A. **Calcium Physiology.** Parathyroid hormone secretion is regulated by the serum ionized calcium concentration (negative feedback mechanism) to maintain calcium levels in a normal range (8.8–10.4 mg/dL).

B. **Hyperparathyroidism**
   1. Hypercalcemia is responsible for a broad spectrum of signs and symptoms (e.g., nephrolithiasis, confusion).
   2. **Treatment and Anesthetic Considerations.** Preoperative IV administration of normal saline and furosemide may lower serum calcium concentrations. There is no evidence that a specific anesthetic drug or technique is preferred. A cautious approach to the use of muscle relaxants is suggested by the unpredictable effect of hypercalcemia at the neuromuscular junction. Careful positioning of osteopenic patients during surgery is necessary to minimize the likelihood of pathologic bone fractures.

C. **Hypoparathyroidism.** Clinical features are manifestations of hypocalcemia, and treatment is with calcium gluconate (10–20 mL of 10% solution IV) (Table 49–8).

TABLE 49-8
MANIFESTATIONS OF HYPOCALCEMIA

Neuronal irritability
Skeletal muscle spasms
Congestive heart failure
Prolonged Q-T interval on the electrocardiogram

TABLE 49-9

COMPARATIVE PHARMACOLOGY OF CORTICOSTEROIDS*

	Anti-inflammatory*	Mineralo-corticoid*	Approximate Equivalent Dose (mg)
Short Acting			
Cortisol (hydrocortisone)	1.0	1.0	20
Cortisone	0.8	0.8	25
Prednisone	4.0	0.25	5.0
Prednisolone	4.0	+/−	5.0
Methylprednisolone	5.0	+/−	4.0
Intermediate Acting			
Triamcinolone	5.0	+/−	4.0
Long Acting			
Dexamethasone	30	+/−	0.75

*The glucocorticoid and mineralocorticoid properties of cortisol are considered to be equivalent to 1.

III. ADRENAL CORTEX

A. The biologic effects of adrenal cortex dysfunction reflect cortisol or aldosterone excess or deficiency (Table 49-9).

B. **Glucocorticoid Excess (Cushing's Syndrome)** (Table 49-10)

1. The diagnosis of hyperadrenocorticism is established by failure of the exogenous administration of dexamethasone to suppress endogenous cortisol secretion.

2. **Anesthetic Management** (Table 49-11). Etomidate has been used for temporizing medical treatment of severe Cushing's disease because of its inhibition of steroid synthesis.

TABLE 49-10

MANIFESTATIONS OF GLUCOCORTICOID EXCESS

Truncal obesity and thin extremities (reflects redistribution of fat and skeletal muscle wasting)
Osteopenia
Hyperglycemia
Hypertension (fluid retention)
Emotional changes
Susceptibility to infection

TABLE 49-11

MANAGEMENT OF PATIENTS UNDERGOING ADRENALECTOMY

Regulate hypertension
Control diabetes
Normalize intravascular fluid volume (diuresis with
   spironolactone helps mobilize fluid and normalize the potassium
   concentration)
Glucocorticoid replacement (cortisol 100 mg IV every 8 hr)
Careful patient positioning on the operating table (osteopenic)
Decrease the initial dose of muscle relaxant if skeletal muscle
   weakness is present

IV = intravenous.

   C. **Mineralocorticoid excess** should be considered in
      nonedematous hypertensive patients who have persistent
      hypokalemia and are not receiving potassium-wasting
      diuretics.
   D. **Adrenal Insufficiency (Addison's Disease)**
      1. Clinically, primary adrenal insufficiency is usually not
         apparent until at least 90% of the adrenal cortex has
         been destroyed.
      2. **Clinical presentation** almost always includes hypoten-
         sion. (A high degree of suspicion should be
         maintained for patients who demonstrate cardiovas-
         cular instability without a defined cause.)
      3. **Treatment and Anesthetic Considerations.** Immediate
         therapy consists of electrolyte resuscitation (glucose in
         normal saline) and steroid replacement (100 mg IV
         every 6 hours for 24 hours). Inotropic support is indi-
         cated if hemodynamic instability persists despite ade-
         quate fluid resuscitation.
   E. **Steroid Replacement During the Perioperative Period**
      1. Patients with adrenal insufficiency and those with
         hypothalamic–pituitary adrenal (HPA) axis suppres-
         sion from chronic steroid use require additional corti-
         costeroids to mimic the increased output of the nor-
         mal adrenal gland during stress.
         a. Normal adrenal gland can secrete up to 200
            mg/day of cortisol and may secrete between 200
            and 500 mg/day during stress.
         b. The HPA axis is considered to be intact if plasma
            cortisol levels are greater than 22 µg/dL during
            acute stress.
         c. Regional anesthesia postpones the elevation in
            plasma cortisol levels evoked by surgery, and deep

general anesthesia suppresses the elevation of stress hormones.

    d. Despite symptoms of clinically significant adrenal insufficiency during the perioperative period, these findings have rarely been documented in direct association with glucocorticoid deficiency.

2. Identifying patients who require steroid supplementation is not practical. (Provocative testing with adrenocorticotrophic hormone [ACTH] stimulation is too costly compared with the risk of brief steroid supplementation.)

    a. HPA axis suppression may occur after five daily doses of prednisone of 20 mg or more. Suppression may also occur with topical, regional, and inhaled steroids. (Alternate-day therapy decreases the risk of suppression.)

    b. Recovery of HPA axis function occurs gradually and can take up to 9 to 12 months.

3. There is no proven optimal regimen for perioperative steroid replacement (low-dose vs high-dose replacement) (Table 49-12). Patients who are using steroids at the time of surgery should receive their usual dose on the morning of surgery and are supplemented at a level that is at least equivalent to the usual daily replacement. Cortisol coverage is rapidly tapered to the patient's normal maintenance dosage during the postoperative period.

4. Although no conclusive evidence supports an increased incidence of infection or abnormal wound healing when supraphysiologic doses of supplemental steroids are used acutely, the goal of therapy is to use the minimal drug dosage necessary to adequately protect the patient.

  F. Exogenous Glucocorticoid Therapy (see Table 49-9)

TABLE 49-12

SUPPLEMENTAL STEROID COVERAGE REGIMENS

Physiologic (low-dose approach)
Cortisol 25 mg IV before induction of anesthesia followed by a continuous infusion (100 mg IV over 24 hr)

Supraphysiologic
Cortisol 200–300 mg IV in divided doses on the day of surgery

IV = intravenous.

TABLE 49-13

MANIFESTATIONS OF PHEOCHROMOCYTOMA

Sustained (occasionally paroxysmal) hypertension (headaches)
Masquerade as malignant hyperthermia
Cardiac dysrhythmias
Orthostatic hypotension (decreased blood volume)
Congestive heart failure
Cardiomyopathy

IV. ADRENAL MEDULLA

The adrenal medulla is analogous to a postganglionic neuron, although the catecholamines it secretes function as hormones, not as neurotransmitters.

A. **Pheochromocytoma.** These tumors produce, store, and secrete catecholamines that may result in life-threatening cardiovascular effects (Table 49-13).

1. **Diagnosis** of pheochromocytoma is based on measurement of catecholamines in the plasma and catecholamine metabolites (vanillylmandelic acid) in the urine. Excess production of catecholamines is diagnostic for pheochromocytoma. Computed tomography or magnetic resonance imaging may be used to localize these tumors.

2. **Anesthetic Considerations**
   a. **Preoperative preparation** consists of α blockade (phentolamine, prazosin) initiated before surgery, if possible, and restoration of intravascular fluid volume. β blockade is indicated only if cardiac dysrhythmias or tachycardia persists after institution of α blockade. The goals of medical therapy are to control heart rate, suppress cardiac dysrhythmias, and prevent paroxysmal increases in blood pressure.
   b. **Perioperative Anesthetic Management** (Table 49-14)
   c. Postoperatively, plasma catecholamine levels return to normal over several days, and about 75% of patients become normotensive within 10 days.

V. DIABETES MELLITUS

Diabetes mellitus is the most common endocrine disease present in surgical patients (25% to 50% of diabetics require surgery). It is a disease with a broad range of severity, and its manifestations can be altered (unmasked for the first time) in response to stress as produced by surgery.

TABLE 49-14

ANESTHETIC MANAGEMENT OF PATIENTS
WITH PHEOCHROMOCYTOMA

Continue preoperative medical therapy.
Perform invasive monitoring (arterial and pulmonary artery catheters, TEE).
Ensure an adequate depth of anesthesia before initiating direct laryngoscopy for tracheal intubation.
Maintain anesthesia with opioids and a volatile anesthetic that does not sensitize the heart to catecholamines.
Select muscle relaxants with minimal cardiovascular effects.
Control systemic blood pressure with nitroprusside or phentolamine (magnesium, nitroglycerin, and calcium channel blockers may be alternative vasodilator drugs).
Control tachydysrhythmias with propranolol, esmolol, or labetalol.
Anticipate hypotension with ligation of the tumor's venous blood supply. (initially treat with IV fluids and vasopressors; continuous infusion of norepinephrine is an option if necessary).

IV = intravenous; TEE = transesophageal echocardiography.

    A. **Classification** (Table 49-15)
    B. **Treatment** (Table 49-16)
    C. **Anesthetic Management**
       1. **Preoperative** (Table 49-17). It is axiomatic that the patient should be in the best state of metabolic control that is possible preoperatively.
       2. **Intraoperative.** The details of the anesthetic plan depend ultimately on the presence of end-organ

TABLE 49-15

CLASSIFICATION OF DIABETES MELLITUS

Type I (Insulin Dependent)
Childhood onset
Thin
Prone to ketoacidosis
Always requires exogenous insulin

Type II (Non–Insulin Dependent)
Maturity onset
Obese
Not prone to ketoacidosis
May be controlled by diet or oral hypoglycemic drugs

Gestational Diabetes
May presage future type II diabetes mellitus

TABLE 49-16

TREATMENT OF DIABETES MELLITUS

Type	Treatment
I	Insulin
II	Diet and exercise
	Sulfonylureas (enhances insulin secretion by β cells)
	Metformin (enhances sensitivity of hepatic and peripheral tissues to insulin)
	Thiazolidinediones (increase insulin sensitivity)
	α-Glucosidase inhibitors (decrease postprandial glucose absorption)

disease. Invasive monitoring may be indicated for the patient with heart disease. Fluid management and drug selection may be influenced by renal function, and aspiration considerations may be affected by the presence of gastroparesis.

   a. Blood glucose levels should be measured preoperatively and postoperatively. The need for additional measurements is determined by the duration and magnitude of surgery and the stability of the patient's diabetes.

   b. Dehydration may be present on the patient's arrival in the operating room based on osmotic diuresis.

TABLE 49-17

PREOPERATIVE EVALUATION OF PATIENTS WITH DIABETES MELLITUS

History and physical examination (detect symptoms of cerebrovascular disease, coronary artery disease, peripheral neuropathy)

Laboratory tests (electrocardiography; blood glucose, creatinine, and potassium levels; urinalysis [glucose, ketones, albumin])

Evidence of stiff joint syndrome (difficult-to-perform laryngoscopy)

Evidence of cardiac autonomic nervous system neuropathy (resting tachycardia, orthostatic hypotension)

Evidence of vagal autonomic nervous system neuropathy (gastroparesis slows emptying of solids [metoclopramide may be useful] but probably not clear fluids)

Autonomic neuropathy predisposes the patient to intraoperative hypothermia

    c. It is important to note the amount of glucose administered IV to avoid an overdose. (The standard glucose dose for adults is 5–10 g/hr or 100–200 mL of 5% glucose/hr.)

    d. Another area of patient monitoring that is extremely important in patients with diabetes is positioning on the operating table. These patients' peripheral nerves may already be partly ischemic and are therefore uniquely susceptible to pressure or stretch injuries.

  3. Glycemic Goals (Table 49-18). Although the association between perioperative hyperglycemia and poor outcomes is strong, the value of controlling glucose levels tightly intraoperatively has not been proven conclusively. It may be prudent to maintain glucose levels at 180 mg/dL or below, especially in the perioperative period.

 D. Management of Perioperative Hyperglycemia. Many factors influence glucose levels in the perioperative period and the regimen selected to control hyperglycemia (Table 49-19). The goal of any regimen is to minimize metabolic derangements and avoid hypoglycemia (Table 49-20).

 E. Emergencies

  1. Hyperosmolar Nonketotic Coma (Table 49-21)

  2. Diabetic Ketoacidosis. Manifestations of diabetic ketoacidosis reflect insufficient insulin to block the

---

TABLE 49-18

CURRENT RECOMMENDATIONS FOR GLYCEMIC CONTROL

Location	American College of Endocrinology (2004)	Canadian Diabetic Association (2003)	American Diabetic Association (2007)	AHA/ACC (2007)
ICU	Close to 110 mg/dL Generally ≤180 mg/dL	≤110 mg/dL	≤100 mg/dL	110–180 mg/dL
Intraoperative	≤150 mg/dL	90–190 mg/dL	Unknown	110–180 mg/dL
Perioperative	Noncritically ill (90–130 mg/dL)	90–180 mg/dL	Unknown	110–180 mg/dL

AHA = American Heart Association; ACC = American College of Cardiology; ICU = intensive care unit.

TABLE 49-19

FACTORS THAT INFLUENCE THE SELECTION OF DIABETIC
MANAGEMENT REGIMEN

Type of diabetes mellitus
How aggressively euglycemia will be sought
Whether the patient takes insulin
Whether surgery is minor and in an ambulatory unit
Whether surgery is elective or emergency
The ability of hospital resources to administer a complex regimen
   plan

metabolism of fatty acids, resulting in the
accumulation of acetoacetate and β-hydroxybutyrate
(Table 49-22). Because leukocytosis, abdominal pain,
ileus, and mildly elevated amylase levels are common
in the presence of diabetic ketoacidosis, an occasional

TABLE 49-20

INTRAOPERATIVE MANAGEMENT REGIMENS FOR PATIENTS WITH
DIABETES MELLITUS

Type 1 Diabetes Mellitus
Administer two thirds of the patient's usual intermediate-acting
   insulin subcutaneously on the morning of surgery.
Titrate regular insulin (sliding scale) based on blood glucose
   measurement or infuse insulin (0.5–2.0 U/hr or 100 U of regular
   insulin in 1000 mL of normal saline at 5–20 mL/hr) adjusted to
   maintain blood glucose at the desired level.
Infuse glucose (5% at 75–125 mL/hr) to prevent hypoglycemia
   while fasting.

Type II Diabetes Mellitus
Hold sulfonylureas while the patient is NPO (this decreases the
   risk of hypoglycemia; these drugs interfere with the
   cardioprotective effect of ischemic preconditioning).
Hold metformin (especially if the patient is at risk for decreased renal
   function perioperatively and associated risk of lactic acidosis).
Continue thiazolidinediones (these do not predispose patients to
   hypoglycemia).
Hold α-glucosidase inhibitors (these only work with meals).
Treat patients receiving insulin as type I diabetics.

Postoperative
Transition the patient to a chronic regimen as he or she resumes
   oral intake.
Type II diabetics who undergo gastric bypass surgery may have
   rapid resolution of glucose intolerance (the need for oral agents
   or insulin is reduced).

TABLE 49-21

MANIFESTATIONS OF HYPEROSMOLAR NONKETOTIC COMA

Elderly patients with impaired thirst mechanism
Minimal or mild diabetes
Profound hyperglycemia (>600 mg/dL)
Absence of ketoacidosis
Hyperosmolarity (seizures, coma, venous thrombosis)

patient is misdiagnosed as having an intra-abdominal surgical problem. Treatment of diabetic ketoacidosis includes insulin administration and fluid and electrolyte evaluation and management (Table 49-23).

3. **Hypoglycemia** produces signs of sympathetic nervous systemic stimulation (tachycardia, hypertension, diaphoresis), which may be masked or misdiagnosed in an anesthetized patient as an inadequate level of anesthesia relative to surgical stimulation.

   a. Diabetic surgical patients are more likely to develop hypoglycemia if insulin or sulfonylureas are given without supplemental glucose.

   b. Renal insufficiency prolongs the action of insulin and oral hypoglycemic drugs.

VI. PITUITARY GLAND

The pituitary gland is divided into the anterior pituitary (thyroid-stimulating hormone, ACTH, gonadotropins, growth hormone) and posterior pituitary (vasopressin, oxytocin). Both are under the control of the hypothalamus.

A. **Anterior Pituitary.** Acromegaly poses several problems for anesthesiologists (Table 49-24).

B. **Diabetes insipidus** reflects a relative or absolute deficiency of antidiuretic hormone (ADH), resulting in

TABLE 49-22

MANIFESTATIONS OF DIABETIC KETOACIDOSIS

Metabolic acidosis
Hyperglycemia (300–500 mg/dL)
Dehydration (osmotic diuresis and vomiting)
Hypokalemia (manifests when acidosis is corrected)
Skeletal muscle weakness (hypophosphatemia with correction of acidosis)

TABLE 49-23

MANAGEMENT OF DIABETIC KETOACIDOSIS

10 U IV of regular insulin followed by a continuous IV infusion (insulin in U/hr = blood glucose/150)

IV fluids (isotonic) as guided by vital signs and urine output (anticipate a 4- to 10-L deficit)

10–40 mEq/hr IV of potassium chloride when urine output exceeds 0.5 mL/kg/hr

Glucose 5% 100 mL/hr when serum glucose concentration decreases below 250 mg/dL

Consider IV sodium bicarbonate to correct pH below 6.9

IV = intravenous.

SURGICAL SUBSPECIALTIES

hypovolemia (inability to concentrate urine) and hypernatremia. ADH is also used in vasodilatory shock as an adjuvant to other pressors.

C. **Inappropriate secretion of antidiuretic hormone** manifests as dilutional hyponatremia and decreased serum osmolarity. These changes typically occur in the presence of head injury or an intracranial tumor. Initial treatment is restriction of daily fluid intake to 800 mL.

VII. ENDOCRINE RESPONSES TO SURGICAL STRESS

Anesthesia, surgery, and trauma elicit a generalized endocrine metabolic response (increased plasma levels of cortisol, ADH, renin, catecholamines, endorphins) and metabolic changes (hyperglycemia, negative nitrogen balance). Regional anesthesia may block part of the metabolic stress response during surgery (blockade of neural communications from the surgical area).

TABLE 49-24

ANESTHETIC PROBLEMS ASSOCIATED WITH ACROMEGALY

Hypertrophy of skeletal, connective, and soft tissues

Enlarged tongue and epiglottis (upper airway obstruction)

Increased incidence of difficult intubation

Thickening of the vocal cords (hoarseness; consider awake tracheal intubation)

Paralysis of the recurrent laryngeal nerve (stretching)

Dyspnea or stridor (subglottic narrowing)

Peripheral nerve or artery entrapment

Hypertension

Diabetes mellitus

CHAPTER 50 ■ ANESTHESIA FOR OTOLARYNGOLOGIC SURGERY

Significant obstruction and anatomic distortion caused by tumor, infection, or trauma may be present in a patient with minimal evidence of disease because clinically evident upper airway obstruction is a late sign (Ferrari LR, Gotta AW: Anesthesia for otolaryngologic surgery. In *Clinical Anesthesia*. Edited by Barash PG, Cullen BF, Stoelting RK, Cahalan MK, Stock MC. Philadelphia: Lippincott Williams & Wilkins, 2009, pp 1305–1320). In the presence of tumor or infection in the airway, radiologic evaluation may be useful.

I. ANESTHESIA FOR PEDIATRIC EAR, NOSE, AND THROAT SURGERY

A. **Tonsillectomy and Adenoidectomy.** Patients with cardiac valvular disease are at risk for endocarditis from recurrent streptococcal bacteremia secondary to infected tonsils. Tonsillar hyperplasia may lead to chronic airway obstruction, resulting in obstructive sleep apnea (OSA) syndrome, carbon dioxide retention, and cor pulmonale.

1. **Preoperative evaluation** includes a thorough history (antibiotics, aspirin-containing medications, sleep apnea) and physical examination (wheezing, stridor, mouth breathing, tonsillar size). In children with a history of cardiac abnormalities, an echocardiogram may be indicated.

2. **Anesthetic Management** (Table 50-1)
   a. Sedative premedication should be avoided in children with OSA. Premedication often includes an antisialagogue.
   b. Induction of anesthesia is usually with a volatile anesthetic and nitrous oxide (parental presence is a consideration, especially with an anxious child) followed by administration of a nondepolarizing muscle relaxant to facilitate tracheal intubation.

TABLE 50-1

GOALS OF ANESTHESIA FOR TONSILLECTOMY
AND ADENOIDECTOMY

Render the patient unconscious in the most atraumatic manner
  possible.
Provide the surgeon with optimal operating conditions.
Establish IV access for volume expansion (when necessary) and
  medications.
Ensure rapid emergence (ability to protect the recently
  instrumented airway).

IV = intravenous.

    c. A specially designated laryngeal mask airway
      (LMA) that easily fits under the mouth gag per-
      mits surgical access while the lower airway is
      protected from exposure to blood during the
      procedure. Positive pressure ventilation should be
      avoided, although gentle assisted ventilation is
      both safe and effective if peak inspiratory pres-
      sure is kept below 20 cm H_2O.

    d. **Emergence** should be rapid, and the child should
      be able to clear blood or secretions from the
      oropharynx. (Maintenance of a patent upper air-
      way and pharyngeal reflexes is important in the
      prevention of aspiration, laryngospasm, and air-
      way obstruction.)

    e. It is recommended that patients be observed for
      early hemorrhage for the first 6 hours and be free
      from significant nausea, vomiting, and pain before
      discharge.

3. **Complications** (Table 50-2)

    a. Preoperative preparation of the patient who
      requires return to the operating room for surgical
      hemostasis includes hydration. (The practitioner
      should check for orthostatic changes.)

    b. A rapid sequence induction of anesthesia with a
      styletted endotracheal tube is often recommended.

    c. Dependable suction is mandatory because blood
      in the pharynx may impair visualization.

4. **Hospital Discharge.** Patients undergoing adenoidec-
    tomy may be safely discharged on the same day
    after recovering from anesthesia. The trend is also
    to discharge patients undergoing tonsillectomy on
    the day of surgery.

TABLE 50-2

POSTOPERATIVE COMPLICATIONS OF TONSILLECTOMY

Emesis (occurs in 30%–65% of patients; mechanism unknown but may include the presence of irritant blood in the stomach)

Dehydration

Hemorrhage (75% occurs in first 6 hours after surgery; if surgical hemostasis is required, a full stomach and hypovolemia should be considered)

Pain (minimal after adenoidectomy and severe after tonsillectomy)

Postobstructive pulmonary edema (rare but possible if the patient has had a prior acute upper airway obstruction; treatment may include supplemental oxygen and administration of diuretics)

    a. After tonsillectomy, patients should be observed (for 4 to 6 hours) for early hemorrhage and be free from significant nausea, vomiting, and pain before discharge. The ability to take fluid by mouth is not a requirement for discharge. Excessive somnolence and severe vomiting are indications for hospital admission.

    b. Examples of patients in whom early discharge is not advised after tonsillectomy include those younger than 3 years of age and those with abnormal coagulation values, evidence of obstructive sleep disorder or apnea, presence of a peritonsillar abscess, and conditions (distance, weather, social conditions) that would prevent close observation or prompt return to the hospital.

B. Peritonsillar abscess (Quinsy tonsil) may interfere with swallowing and breathing. (Symptoms and signs include fever, pain, and trismus.)

    1. Treatment consists of surgical drainage and intravenous (IV) antibiotic therapy.

    2. Although the upper airway seems compromised, the abscess is usually in a fixed location in the lateral pharynx (visualization of the vocal cords should not be impaired because the pathology is supraglottic and well above the laryngeal inlet) and does not interfere with ventilation of the patient's lungs by mask after induction of general anesthesia.

    3. Direct laryngoscopy must be carefully performed to minimize the risk of rupture of the abscess and spillage of purulent material into the patient's trachea.

TABLE 50-3

ANESTHETIC CONSIDERATIONS FOR TYMPANOPLASTY
AND MASTOIDECTOMY

Place the head in a head rest and laterally rotate it. (avoid tension of heads of the sternocleidomastoid muscles.)

Ensure preservation of facial nerve (30% response should be preserved on the twitch monitor if muscle relaxants are administered)

Minimize bleeding (relative hypotension [MAP 25% below baseline] and local injection of epinephrine [1:1000]).

Discontinue nitrous oxide during placement of the tympanic membrane graft.

MAP = mean arterial pressure.

SURGICAL SUBSPECIALTIES

II. EAR SURGERY

A. Myringotomy and Tube Insertion

1. Anesthesia may be provided with a volatile anesthetic and nitrous oxide.

2. Recurrent upper respiratory infections (URIs) may not resolve until middle ear fluid is eradicated. Because tracheal intubation is not required, the presence of symptoms of an URI may not mandate a delay of surgery.

B. Middle Ear and Mastoid

1. Tympanoplasty and mastoidectomy are two of the most common procedures performed on the middle ear.

2. **Anesthetic Considerations** (Table 50-3)

III. AIRWAY SURGERY

A. **Stridor** is noisy breathing caused by airway obstruction (Table 50-4).

1. Inspiratory stridor results from upper airway obstruction, expiratory stridor results from lower airway obstruction, and biphasic stridor is present with midtracheal lesions.

   a. Information indicating positions that make the stridor better or worse are helpful for positioning the patient to take advantage of gravity in decreasing airway obstruction during induction of anesthesia.

TABLE 50-4

CAUSES OF STRIDOR

Supraglottic Airway	Larynx	Subglottic Airway
Laryngomalacia	Laryngocele	Tracheomalacia
Vocal cord paralysis	Infection (tonsillitis, peritonsillar abscess)	Vascular ring
Subglottic stenosis	Foreign body	Infection (croup, epiglottitis)
Foreign body		
Hemangiomas	Cysts	
Choanal atresia	Mass	
Cysts	Large tonsils	
	Large adenoids	
	Craniofacial abnormalities	

  b. Laryngomalacia caused by a long epiglottis that prolapses posteriorly is the most common cause of stridor in infants.

  2. Signs and Symptoms (Table 50-5)

 B. Bronchoscopy

  1. Goals of anesthesia include a quiet surgical field (coughing or straining during instrumentation with a rigid bronchoscope may result in damage to the patient's airway), use of an antisialagogue to decrease secretions that may obscure the view through the bronchoscope, and rapid return to consciousness with intact upper airway reflexes.

  2. In children, an inhalation induction of anesthesia is common, but IV drugs are usually administered to adults. Maintenance of anesthesia often includes a volatile anesthetic and muscle relaxant.

TABLE 50-5

SIGNS AND SYMPTOMS SPECIFICALLY EXAMINED IN PATIENTS WITH STRIDOR

Breathing rate
Heart rate
Wheezing
Cyanosis
Chest retractions
Nasal flaring
Level of consciousness

    a. Because ventilation of the lungs may be intermittent, it is recommended that 100% oxygen be used as the carrier gas during bronchoscopic examination.

    b. If a rigid bronchoscope is used, ventilation of the lungs is accomplished through a side port (manual vs Sander's jet ventilation).

    c. At the conclusion of rigid bronchoscopy, an endotracheal tube is usually placed to control the patient's airway during recovery of anesthesia.

IV. PEDIATRIC AIRWAY EMERGENCIES

  A. Epiglottitis is an infectious disease (caused by *Haemophilus influenzae*) of children (usually 2–7 years of age) and adults that can progress rapidly from a sore throat to total upper airway obstruction.

    1. Characteristic signs and symptoms include sudden onset of fever, dysphagia, and preference for the sitting position.

    2. Direct visualization of the epiglottis and sedation outside the operating room should not be attempted because total upper airway obstruction may result.

    3. If the clinical situation allows, oxygen should be administered by mask, and lateral radiographs of the soft tissues in the neck may be obtained.

    4. Children with severe airway compromise should proceed from the emergency room to the operating room accompanied by the anesthesiologist and surgeon.

    5. In all cases of epiglottitis, an artificial airway is established by means of tracheal intubation (Table 50-6).

  B. Laryngotracheobronchitis (LTB; Croup)

    1. LTB is usually a viral illness that occurs most often in children age 6 months to 6 years.

    2. The onset of LTB is more insidious than the onset of epiglottitis, with the child presenting with a low-grade fever, inspiratory stridor, and a barking cough.

    3. Treatment includes a cool, humid mist and oxygen, and in severe cases, nebulized racemic epinephrine and a short course of steroids.

  C. Foreign Body Aspiration

    1. This diagnosis should be suspected in any patient who presents with wheezing and a history of coughing or choking while eating.

TABLE 50-6

ESTABLISHMENT OF AN ARTIFICIAL AIRWAY IN THE PRESENCE
OF EPIGLOTTITIS

Bring the patient to the operating room (child may be
  accompanied by a parent).
Place monitors (child may remain seated).
Induce anesthesia by mask (sevoflurane in oxygen).
IV access may be accomplished after loss of consciousness.
Place an orotracheal tube with use of muscle relaxants (select a
  tube size at least one size smaller than normal).
Replace the orotracheal tube with a nasotracheal tube after the
  surgeon has examined the larynx.
Extubation of the trachea is usually possible after 48–72 hours
  (leak develops around the tracheal tube).

IV = intravenous.

2. Most foreign bodies are radiolucent, and the only
   findings on radiography are air trapping, infiltrate,
   and atelectasis.
3. Aspirated foreign bodies are considered an
   emergency requiring removal in the operating room.
   a. Inhalation induction of anesthesia with
      halothane (sevoflurane is an alternative) in oxy-
      gen may be prolonged secondary to obstruction
      of the airway.
   b. Nitrous oxide may be avoided to decrease the
      likelihood of air trapping distal to the obstruction.
   c. Spontaneous ventilation may be preserved until
      the location and nature of the foreign body have
      been determined.
   d. Respiratory compromise secondary to airway
      edema or infection is a possible complication in
      the postoperative period.

V. ANESTHESIA FOR PEDIATRIC AND
   ADULT SURGERY

   A. Laser Surgery of the Airway
      1. Lasers provide precision in targeting lesions, mini-
         mal bleeding, and edema as well as preservation of
         surrounding structures and rapid healing.
         a. The carbon dioxide laser has particular applica-
            tion in the treatment of laryngeal or vocal cord
            papillomas and coagulation of hemangiomas.

TABLE 50-7

ANESTHESIA FOR LASER SURGERY

The primary gas for anesthetic maintenance should be delivered with the lowest safe concentration of oxygen (nitrous oxide and oxygen support combustion).

Recognize that polyvinylchloride tracheal tubes can ignite and vaporize when in contact with a laser beam (reflective tape or specially designed tubes can be used).

Inflate the tracheal tube cuff with saline to which methylene blue has been added (detect cuff rupture from a misdirected laser beam).

Apneic oxygenation techniques or jet ventilation are alternatives to tracheal intubation.

    b. Misdirected laser beams may cause injury to the patient or to unprotected operating room personnel. (Eye goggles with side protectors should be used.)

    c. Laser smoke plumes may cause damage to the lungs or serve as a vehicle for spread of viral particles (possibly human immunodeficiency virus).

  2. Anesthetic Management (Table 50-7)

B. Nasal Surgery

  1. Regardless of the anesthetic technique selected (general anesthesia or conscious sedation), it is likely that local vasoconstriction (topical local anesthetics, cocaine, and epinephrine) will be used.

  2. A moderate degree of controlled hypotension combined with head elevation serves to decrease bleeding at the surgical site.

C. Maxillofacial Trauma

  1. Challenges to the anesthesiologist in caring for patients with maxillofacial trauma include securing the upper airway in the presence of unknown anatomic alterations, sharing the airway with the surgeon, and determining when it is safe to extubate the patient's trachea.

    a. In any patient with severe midfacial trauma, a fracture of the base of the skull must be considered.

    b. The mandible has a unique horseshoe shape that causes forces to occur at points often distant from the point of impact.

  2. The LeFort classification of fractures (LeFort I, II, and III) depicts the common lines of fracture of the midface.

VI. TUMORS

A. Neoplastic growths may occur anywhere within the airway and may achieve significant size with little evidence of airway obstruction.

B. Attempted tracheal intubation may produce hemorrhage and edema, leading to airway obstruction.

VII. UPPER AIRWAY INFECTION

A. Ludwig's angina is a septic cellulitis of the submandibular region that typically occurs in a patient who has undergone dental extraction of the second or third mandibular molars.

B. Soft tissue edema coupled with upward and posterior displacement of the tongue and the frequent presence of laryngeal edema may result in upper airway obstruction.

VIII. TEMPOROMANDIBULAR JOINT ARTHROSCOPY

A. Temporomandibular joint (TMJ) pathology is often caused by spasm of the muscles of mastication secondary to chronic tension of these muscles (as an involuntary mental tension-relieving mechanism).

B. Many patients with chronic TMJ dysfunction have significant psychopathology (depression, preoccupation with facial pain) and use mood-altering or tension-abating drugs.

C. Nasotracheal intubation is usually chosen.

D. Extracapsular extravasation of fluid used to irrigate the joint during arthroscopy may compromise the patency of the airway that manifests on tracheal extubation.

IX. PATIENT EVALUATION

A. Patients who have sustained facial trauma should be evaluated for other injuries (cervical spine fractures, cranial fractures, intracranial injury).

B. Patients with Ludwig's angina are often septic and poorly hydrated.

C. Tumors of the head and neck are usually associated with cigarette and alcohol abuse with associated abnormalities of pulmonary and hepatic function.

X. SECURING THE AIRWAY

A. Awake tracheal intubation or tracheostomy may be indicated in patients with upper airway tumor, infection, or trauma.

B. The technique of an "awake look" before a decision to induce anesthesia and administer a muscle relaxant may be misleading because skeletal muscle tone in the awake state that helps identify anatomic structures is absent after anesthesia and skeletal muscle paralysis are produced.

C. After maxillofacial trauma, the ability to open the mouth may be limited because of pain, trismus, edema, or mechanical dysfunction of the TMJ.

1. Pain does not influence mouth opening in an anesthetized and paralyzed patient.

2. Trismus succumbs to an anesthetic and muscle relaxant unless there is fibrosis of the masseter muscles, which is possible if trismus has been present for 2 weeks or longer.

XI. AWAKE INTUBATION

A. The airway must be anesthetized using a combination of topical anesthesia and superior laryngeal nerve block.

B. **Superior Laryngeal Nerve Block**

1. The external branch of the superior laryngeal nerve innervates the cricothyroid muscle (tensor of the vocal cords), and the internal branch provides sensory innervation from the base of the tongue to the vocal cords.

2. With the patient lying supine, a 22-gauge needle attached to a syringe containing 2 mL of 2% lidocaine is introduced until it contacts the hyoid bone.

   a. When the needle contacts the hyoid bone, it is redirected caudad until it just steps off the bone penetrating the thyrohyoid membrane.

   b. After negative aspiration, the local anesthetic is injected, and the block is repeated on the opposite side.

   c. Complications of superior laryngeal nerve block include intravascular injection of local anesthetic solution. (The carotid artery lies just posterior to the site of needle placement for performance of the block.)

C. Topical anesthesia includes local anesthetic instilled into the nose (a vasoconstrictor such as 0.5% phenylephrine should be added to shrink the nasal mucosa), mouth (nebulized in a hand-held nebulizer and inhaled by the patient), or both.
   1. Topical anesthesia may be applied below the level of the vocal cords by introducing a 22-gauge needle through the cricothyroid membrane and rapidly injecting 4 mL of 2% lidocaine.
   2. The resulting cough reflex distributes the local anesthetic along the tracheal mucosa and inferior surface of the vocal cords.
D. An LMA may be useful in temporarily securing a compromised airway, and a tracheal tube (guide over a bronchoscope inserted through an LMA) is necessary to protect the airway from aspiration of blood. The LMA-Fastrach is a modification of the intubating LMA that was designed specifically for anatomically difficult airways.

XII. LEFORT III FRACTURES

A. This type of fracture may involve the cribriform plate of the ethmoid bone and cause separation of the nasopharynx from the base of the skull.
B. Nasotracheal intubation introduces the risk of delivering foreign material from the nasopharynx into the subarachnoid space.
   1. Even positive pressure ventilation of the patient's lungs can increase pressure in the nasopharynx and force foreign material or air into the skull.
   2. The problems of securing the airway in a patient with a LeFort III fracture are usually obviated by performing a preliminary tracheostomy.

XIII. ANESTHETIC MANAGEMENT FOR THE TRAUMATIZED UPPER AIRWAY

A. After tracheal intubation or tracheostomy has been performed, general or IV drugs may be administered.
B. Because a significant incidence of intracranial injury is associated with maxillofacial trauma, the brain must be protected from increases in intracranial pressure.
C. When awake fiberoptic intubation is the preferred method of securing the airway (as in patients with

cervical spine injury), dexmedetomidine (1 µg/kg over 10 minutes followed by 0.2–0.7 µg/kg/hr) provides a moderate level of conscious sedation without causing respiratory depression or hemodynamic instability.

XIV. EXTUBATION

A. When a tracheostomy has been performed, the decision at the conclusion of surgery is whether to allow spontaneous breathing or to create suitable conditions (opioids, muscle relaxants) for continued mechanical ventilation of the patient's lungs.

B. After trauma, infection, or extensive oral resection for tumor, the endotracheal tube must not be removed until there is subsidence of edema (especially submandibular edema) or infection that might compromise the unprotected airway.

C. An orotracheal tube may be removed over a tube changer.

CHAPTER 51 ■ ANESTHESIA FOR OPHTHALMOLOGIC SURGERY

Anesthesia for ophthalmic surgery presents unique anesthetic challenges and requirements (Table 51-1) (McGoldrick KE, Gayer SI: Anesthesia for ophthalmologic surgery. In *Clinical Anesthesia*. Edited by Barash PG, Cullen BF, Stoelting RK, Cahalan MK, Stock MC. Philadelphia: Lippincott Williams & Wilkins, 2009, pp 1321–1345). Patients undergoing ophthalmic surgery may represent extremes of age (macular degeneration is the leading cause of blindness in individuals older than 65 years of age) and coexisting medical diseases.

I. OCULAR ANATOMY

A. The supraorbital notch, infraorbital foramen, and lacrimal fossa are clinically palpable and function as important landmarks for performance of regional anesthesia (Fig. 51-1).

B. The coat of the eye is composed of three layers: the sclera, uveal tract, and retina.

1. Whereas the fibrous outer layer of the sclera is protective, providing sufficient rigidity to maintain the shape of the eye, the anterior portion of the sclera, the **cornea,** is transparent, permitting light to enter the internal ocular structures.

2. The uveal tract consists of the iris, ciliary body, and choroid.

a. The pupil is part of the iris that controls the amount of light that enters by dilation (sympathetic innervation) or constriction (parasympathetic innervation).

b. The ciliary body produces aqueous humor.

3. The retina is a neurosensory membrane that converts light impulses to neural impulses that travel via the optic nerve to the brain.

TABLE 51-1
REQUIREMENTS FOR OPHTHALMIC SURGERY

Akinesia
Profound analgesia
Minimal bleeding
Avoidance of the oculocardiac reflex
Control of IOP
Awareness of possible drug interactions
Awakening without coughing, straining, or vomiting

IOP = intraocular pressure.

C. Six intraocular muscles move the eye within the orbit.
D. The **conjunctiva** is a mucous membrane (where topical ophthalmic drugs are administered) that covers the globe and serves as a lining of the eyelids.

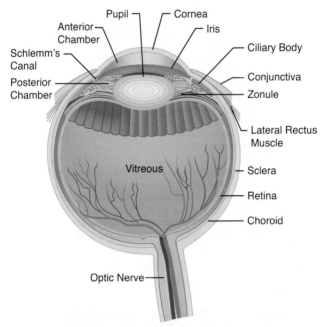

FIGURE 51-1. Diagram of the ocular anatomy.

E. Blood supply to the eye is from branches of the internal and external carotid arteries.

II. OCULAR PHYSIOLOGY

A. **Formation and Drainage of Aqueous Humor**
   1. Aqueous humor is formed in the posterior chamber by the ciliary body in an active secretory process involving carbonic anhydrase as well as by passive filtration from the vessels on the anterior surface of the iris.
   2. **Drainage** of aqueous humor is via a network of connecting venous channels (including Schlemm's canal) that empty into the superior vena cava. (Any obstruction between the eye and right atrium impedes aqueous drainage and increases intraocular pressure [IOP].)

B. **Maintenance of Intraocular Pressure**
   1. IOP normally varies between 10 and 21.7 mm Hg but becomes atmospheric when the globe is opened. The major determinant of IOP is the volume of aqueous humor.
   2. Any sudden increase in IOP when the globe is open may lead to prolapse of the iris and lens, extrusion of the vitreous, and blindness.
   3. Straining, vomiting, or coughing (as during laryngoscopy and tracheal intubation) greatly increases venous pressure and IOP.

C. **Glaucoma** is characterized by increased IOP, resulting in impairment of capillary blood flow to the optic nerve.
   1. Treatment consists of topical medication to produce miosis and trabecular stretching.
   2. Atropine premedication in the dose range used clinically has no effect on IOP in patients with glaucoma. Scopolamine may have a greater mydriatic effect, and its use may be avoided.

III. EFFECTS OF ANESTHESIA AND ADJUVANT DRUGS ON INTRAOCULAR PRESSURE (Table 51-2)

A. Intravenous (IV) injection of succinylcholine (SCh) transiently increases IOP by about 8 mm Hg with

TABLE 51-2

EVENTS THAT ALTER INTRAOCULAR PRESSURE

Decreased	Increased
Volatile anesthetics	Increased venous pressure owing to coughing or vomiting
Injected anesthetics (possibly ketamine)	Direct laryngoscopy
Hyperventilation	Hypoventilation
Hypothermia	Arterial hypoxemia
Mannitol	Succinylcholine
Glycerin	
Nondepolarizing muscle relaxants	
Timolol	
Betaxolol	

return to baseline in 5 to 7 minutes. This reflects the cycloplegic action of SCh and is not reliably prevented by pretreatment with nondepolarizing muscle relaxants or IV administration of lidocaine.

B. Etomidate-induced myoclonus may be hazardous in the setting of an open globe.

IV. OCULOCARDIAC REFLEX

A. This reflex manifests as bradycardia (and occasionally cardiac dysrhythmias) that is elicited by pressure on the globe and by traction on the extraocular muscles (strabismus surgery), especially the medial rectus.

B. Monitoring of the electrocardiogram is useful for early recognition of this reflex.

C. Atropine given IV within 30 minutes of surgery is thought to lead to a reduced incidence of the reflex (controversial). Atropine as administered intramuscularly for preoperative medication is not effective for preventing this reflex.

V. ANESTHETIC RAMIFICATIONS OF OPHTHALMIC DRUGS

A. **Echothiophate** is a long-acting anticholinesterase miotic that decreases IOP and prolongs the duration of action of SCh.

B. **Cyclopentolate** is a mydriatic that may produce central nervous system toxicity.

C. **Phenylephrine** is a mydriatic that may produce cardio-vascular effects.

D. **Acetazolamide,** when administered chronically to lower IOP, may be associated with renal loss of bicarbonate and potassium ions.

E. **Timolol** lowers IOP, but systemic absorption may result in cardiac depression and increased airway resistance. Betaxolol may be more oculo specific and has minimal systemic effects.

F. **Sulfur hexafluoride (SF_6)** is injected into the vitreous to mechanically facilitate retinal reattachment. Nitrous oxide (N_2O) (blood/gas solubility, 0.47) should be avoided for 10 days after intravitreous injection of SF_6 (blood/gas solubility, 0.004). A Medic-Alert bracelet may be helpful to identify patients at risk.

VI. PREOPERATIVE EVALUATION

A. **Establishing Rapport and Assessing Medical Conditions**
   1. Preoperative testing should be based on the history and physical examination.
      a. Many elderly adult candidates for ophthalmic surgery are on antiplatelet or anticoagulant therapy owing to a history of coronary or vascular pathology.
      b. Despite the possibility of eye injury from patient movement in the event of implanted cardiac defibrillator activation, there are no reports of activation during ophthalmic surgery, and magnets to inactivate the device before surgery are rarely used.
      c. Perioperative movement is a possible cause of patient eye injury and potential anesthesiologist liability. Inadequate sedation during monitored anesthesia care (MAC) may be associated with unpredictable movement that results in blindness or poor visual outcome. Intraoperative movement during general anesthesia may also result in adverse visual consequences.
   2. **Anesthesia Options.** A commonly selected regional anesthetic technique for cataract surgery is peribulbar block, which has a better safety profile than retrobulbar block. Topical anesthesia is also effective for cataract surgery.

TABLE 51-3

FACTORS THAT INFLUENCE THE CHOICE OF ANESTHESIA

Nature and duration of procedure
Coagulation status
The patient's ability to communicate and cooperate
Personal preference of the anesthesiologist

3. **Side Effects of Anesthesia and Surgery.** Ophthalmologic surgery and regional anesthesia confer greater risk than many other surgical procedures because of the potential for laterality errors.

VII. ANESTHESIA TECHNIQUES

Most ophthalmic procedures in adults can be performed with either local or general anesthesia. Data have failed to demonstrate a difference in complications between local and general anesthesia for cataract surgery (Table 51-3).

A. **Retrobulbar and Peribulbar Blocks.** Retrobulbar block may be associated with significant complications, emphasizing that local anesthesia does not necessarily involve less physiologic trespass than general anesthesia (Table 51-4). Elevations of IOP after a retrobulbar block can be minimized by application of gentle non-continuous digital pressure or use of an ocular decompressive device. Akinesia of the eyelids is obtained by blocking the branches of the facial nerve supplying the orbicularis muscle.

TABLE 51-4

COMPLICATIONS OF NEEDLE-BASED OPHTHALMIC ANESTHESIA

Stimulation of the oculocardiac reflex arc
Superficial hemorrhage or circumorbital hematoma
Retrobulbar hemorrhage
Retinal perfusion compromise (loss of vision)
Globe penetration and intraocular injection (retinal detachment, loss of vision)
Trauma to the optic nerve or orbital cranial nerves (loss of vision)
Optic nerve sheath injection (orbital epidural anesthesia)
Extraocular muscle injury (postoperative strabismus, diplopia)
Intra-arterial injection (immediate convulsions)
Central retinal artery occlusion
Accidental brainstem anesthesia (apnea, hypotension, coma)

TABLE 51-5
GENERAL PRINCIPLES OF MONITORED ANESTHESIA CARE
Avoid combinations of local anesthetics with heavy sedation (opioids, benzodiazepines, hypnotics).
After placement of block, the patient should be relaxed but awake to avoid head movement.
Maintain airway patency.
Avoid undersedation and associated hypertension and tachycardia (especially in patients with coronary artery disease).
Provide adequate ventilation about the face to avoid carbon dioxide accumulation.
Provide continuous monitoring of the electrocardiogram (oculocardiac reflex) and oxygen saturation.

B. **Topical analgesia** can be achieved with local anesthetic drops or gels.

C. **Choice of Local Anesthetics, Block Adjuvants, and Adjuncts.** Anesthetics for ocular surgery are selected based on the onset and duration needed (local anesthetics should be mixed to obtain the desired onset and duration). Osmotic agents (mannitol, glycerin, carbonic anhydrase) may be administered intravenously to reduce vitreous volume and IOP.

D. **General Principles of Monitored Anesthesia Care (MAC)** (Table 51-5). Cataract surgery, which is the top Medicare expenditure, is most commonly performed with the patient under some form of regional anesthesia plus monitoring equipment and often with the presence of an anesthesiologist with MAC. MAC should reflect "maximum anesthesia caution" rather than "minimal anesthesiology care."

VIII. **ANESTHETIC MANAGEMENT OF SPECIFIC SITUATIONS**

A. **Open Eye, Full Stomach.** Anesthesiologists must balance the risk of aspiration against the risk of blindness in an injured eye that may result from an acute increase in IOP and extrusion of ocular contents.

1. Rocuronium (1.2 mg/kg IV) may be useful for rapid control of the airway, but its intermediate duration of action is a disadvantage compared with succinylcholine. Sugammadex may provide a solution.

TABLE 51-6

CONSIDERATIONS FOR STRABISMUS SURGERY

Oculocardiac reflex
Increased incidence of malignant hyperthermia
Interference by succinylcholine in interpretation of forced duction test
Increased incidence of postoperative nausea and vomiting

2. When confronted with a patient whose airway anatomy or anesthetic history suggests potential difficulties, the anesthesiologist should consult with the ophthalmologist concerning the probability of saving the injured eye.

B. **Strabismus surgery** is the most common pediatric ocular operation and may introduce unique concerns (Table 51-6).
   1. The laryngeal mask airway has the potential advantage of not requiring the use of muscle relaxants and being associated with less straining or coughing with its removal.
   2. The incidence of postoperative nausea and vomiting may be decreased by use of an IV anesthetic technique with propofol, avoidance of opioids (ketorolac 750 µg/kg IV an alternative), and prophylactic administration of an antiemetic (250 µg/kg IV of metoclopramide or 150 µg/kg IV of ondansetron) immediately after induction of anesthesia.

C. **Intraocular surgery** (glaucoma drainage surgery, open-eye vitrectomy, corneal transplants, cataract extraction) introduces unique concerns and requirements (Table 51-7).
   1. Epinephrine 1:200,000 may be infused into the anterior chamber of the eye to produce mydriasis.

TABLE 51-7

CONSIDERATIONS FOR INTRAOCULAR SURGERY

Control of intraocular pressure
Continuation of miotics in glaucoma patients
Need for complete akinesia
Provide an antiemetic effect

Systemic absorption and the resulting cardiac dysrhythmias in the presence of volatile anesthetics have not been recognized as problems.

2. Nondepolarizing muscle relaxants administered to provide akinesia and facilitate performance and interpretation of the forced duction test (which can be used to differentiate between a paretic muscle and a restrictive force preventing ocular motion) can be safely antagonized, even in patients with glaucoma, because in conventional doses, the combination of anticholinesterase and anticholinergic drugs has minimal effects on pupil size and IOP.

D. **Retinal Detachment Surgery**

1. Internal tamponade of the retinal break may be accomplished by injecting the expandable gas SF_6 into the vitreous. Owing to the blood/gas partition coefficient differences, the concomitant administration of N_2O may enhance the internal tamponade effect of SF_6 intraoperatively, resulting in increases in IOP and interference with retinal circulation. For this reason, N_2O probably should be discontinued for at least 15 minutes before injection of SF_6, and likewise N_2O probably should not be administered for 10 days after the injection.

2. Decrease in IOP is often provided by IV administration of acetazolamide or mannitol.

3. Akinesia is not critical, and inhalation anesthetics need not be accompanied intraoperatively by nondepolarizing muscle relaxants.

IX. PRINCIPLES OF LASER THERAPY

A. Lasers are used to treat a wide spectrum of eye conditions, including three of the most common causes of visual loss: diabetic retinopathy, glaucoma, and macular degeneration.

B. An excimer laser is a form of high-power ultraviolet chemical laser used in refractive surgery (LASIK).

X. POSTOPERATIVE OCULAR COMPLICATIONS
(Table 51-8).

The incidence of eye injuries associated with nonocular surgery is very low (0.056%). Certain types of surgery, including complex spinal surgery in the prone position, operations involving extracorporeal circulation, and nasal

TABLE 51-8

POSTOPERATIVE OCULAR COMPLICATIONS

Corneal abrasion

Chemical injury (Hibiclens)

Photic injury (laser beams; the eyes should be protected with moist gauze pads and metal shields)

Mild visual symptoms

Photophobia

Diplopia

Blurred vision (residual effects of petroleum-based ophthalmic ointment or ocular effects of anticholinergic drugs)

Hemorrhagic retinopathy

Retinal ischemia (external pressure on the globe, increased ocular venous pressure associated with a steep head-down position combined with the prone position, deliberate hypotension and infusion of large amounts of crystalloid solution)

Central retinal arterial occlusion

Branch retinal arterial occlusion

Ischemic optic neuropathy (anterior ischemic optic neuropathy or posterior ischemic optic neuropathy)

Cortical blindness (reflects brain injury rostral to the optic nerve; emboli and profound hypotension are common causes; the differential diagnosis includes a normal optic disc on funduscopy and normal pupillary responses; CT and MRI are helpful in delineating the extent of brain infarction associated with cortical blindness)

Acute glaucoma

Postcataract ptosis

CT = computed tomography; MRI = magnetic resonance imaging.

SURGICAL SUBSPECIALTIES

or sinus surgery may increase the risk of serious postoperative visual complications. Injuries associated with regional anesthesia for ophthalmic surgery are typically permanent and related to the block technique.

A. **Corneal abrasion** is the most common ocular complication after general anesthesia. Patients complain of pain and a foreign body sensation that is exacerbated by blinking. An ophthalmology consultation is appropriate, and treatment is prophylactic topical application of antibiotic ointment and patching of the injured eye. Healing usually occurs within 24 to 48 hours.

B. **Ischemic optic neuropathy** is the most common cause of visual loss in patients older than 50 years of age. The incidence of postoperative vision loss after spine surgery performed in the prone position may be as high as 1%. (It is prudent to discuss this potential complication before surgery as part of the informed consent process.)

1. **Anterior ischemic optic neuropathy** is thought to reflect temporary hypoperfusion or nonperfusion of the vessels supplying the anterior portion of the optic nerve.

   a. Male patients undergoing prolonged spine surgery in the prone position and operations requiring cardiopulmonary bypass may be at increased risk for development of anterior ischemic optic neuropathy.

   b. The cause is very likely multifactorial, although intraoperative anemia, controlled hypotension, and increased IOP or orbital venous pressure (in the prone and head-down positions) may contribute to the ischemia of the optic nerve.

   c. Patients typically experience painless visual loss in the early postoperative period that is associated with an afferent pupillary defect and optic disc edema or pallor. Magnetic resonance imaging initially shows enlargement of the optic nerve followed by optic atrophy. Visual loss is usually permanent.

2. **Posterior ischemic optic neuropathy** is produced by decreased oxygen delivery to the optic nerve.

   a. Male patients undergoing surgery involving the neck, nose, or spine may be at increased risk for development of posterior ischemic optic neuropathy.

   b. Patients typically experience a symptom-free period that often precedes the loss of vision associated with a nonreactive pupil. Bilateral blindness is more common than after anterior ischemic optic neuropathy. Disc edema is not a feature of posterior ischemic optic neuropathy because of its retrobulbar location.

   c. Patients undergoing spinal surgery who are at greatest risk for ischemic optic neuropathy include those undergoing surgery exceeding 6 hours and those with blood loss greater than 1 L. Based on current information, there is no established "transfusion threshold," and deliberate intraoperative hypotension during surgery has not been proven as contributory to postoperative vision loss.

CHAPTER 52 ■ THE RENAL SYSTEM AND ANESTHESIA FOR UROLOGIC SURGERY

The kidney plays a central role in implementing and controlling a variety of homeostatic functions, including excreting metabolic waste products in the urine while keeping extracellular fluid (ECF) volume and composition constant (Stafford-Smith M, Shaw A, George R, Muir HL: Anesthesia for urologic surgery. In *Clinical Anesthesia*. Edited by Barash PG, Cullen BF, Stoelting RK, Cahalan MK, Stock MC. Philadelphia: Lippincott Williams & Wilkins, 2009, pp 1346–1374). Renal dysfunction may occur as a direct result of surgical or medical disease, prolonged reduction in renal oxygen delivery, nephrotoxin insult, or a combination of the three.

I. RENAL ANATOMY AND PHYSIOLOGY

A. Gross Anatomy (Fig. 52-1A)

1. Renal pain sensation is conveyed back to spinal cord segments T10–L1 by sympathetic fibers. Sympathetic innervation is supplied by preganglionic fibers from T8–L1. The vagus nerve provides parasympathetic innervation to the kidney, and the S2–S4 spinal segments supply the ureters.

2. The bladder is located in the retropubic space and receives its innervation from sympathetic nerves originating from T11–L2, which conduct pain, touch, and temperature sensations. Bladder stretch sensation is transmitted via parasympathetic fibers from segments S2–S4. Parasympathetics also provide the bladder with most of its motor innervation.

3. The prostate, penile urethra, and penis also receive sympathetic and parasympathetic fibers from the T11–L2 and S2–S4 segments. The pudendal nerve provides pain sensation to the penis via the dorsal nerve of the penis.

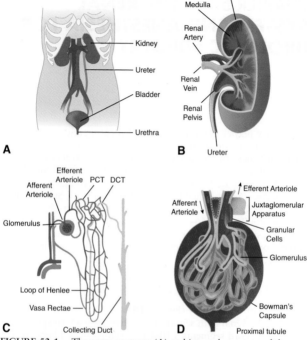

FIGURE 52-1. The gross anatomy (**A**) and internal structure of the genitourinary system and kidney. Internal organization of the kidney includes the cortex and medulla regions and the vasculature (**B**). The nephron is the functional unit of the kidney (**C**). Plasma filtration occurs in the glomerulus (**D**); 20% of plasma that enters the glomerulus passes through the specialized capillary wall into Bowman's capsule and enters the tubule to be processed and generate urine.

B. Ultrastructure (Fig. 52-1B-D)
   1. The parenchyma of each kidney contains approximately 1×10^{6} tightly packed nephrons (structural units of the kidneys), each one consisting of a tuft of capillaries (glomerulus) invaginated into the blind, expanded end (glomerular corpuscle) of a long tubule that leaves the renal corpuscle to form the proximal convoluted tubule in the cortex.

2. The distal convoluted tubule comes into very close contact with the afferent glomerular arteriole, and the cells of each are modified to form the juxtaglomerular apparatus, a complex physiological feedback control mechanism contributing in part to the precise control of intra- and extrarenal hemodynamics that is a hallmark feature of normally functioning kidneys.

C. Correlation of Structure and Function
   1. Renal tissue makes up only 0.4% of body weight but receives 25% of cardiac output, making the kidneys the most highly perfused major organs in the body, and this facilitates plasma filtration at rates as high as 125 to 140 mL/min in adults.
   2. The kidney fulfills its dual roles of waste excretion and body fluid management by filtering large amounts of fluid and solutes from the blood and secreting waste products into the tubular fluid.

D. Glomerular Filtration
   1. Production of urine begins with water and solute filtration from plasma flowing into the glomerulus via the afferent arteriole. The glomerular filtration rate (GFR) is a measure of glomerular function expressed as milliliters of plasma filtered per minute and is heavily influenced by arteriolar tone at points upstream (afferent) and downstream (efferent) from the glomerulus.
   2. An increase in afferent arteriolar tone, as occurs with intense sympathetic or angiotensin II stimulation, causes filtration pressure and GFR to decrease.

E. Autoregulation of Renal Blood Flow and Glomerular Filtration Rate
   1. Renal blood flow (RBF) autoregulation maintains relatively constant rates of RBF and glomerular filtration over a wide range of arterial blood pressure (Fig. 52-2).
   2. Autoregulation of urine flow does not occur, and above a mean arterial pressure (MAP) of 50 mm Hg, there is a linear relationship between and MAP and urine output.

F. Tubular Reabsorption of Sodium and Water
   1. Active, energy-dependent reabsorption of sodium begins almost immediately as the glomerular filtrate enters the proximal tubule. (An adenosine

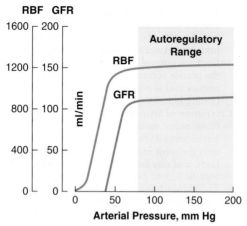

FIGURE 52-2. Renal blood flow (RBF) autoregulation. RBF and glomerular filtration rate (GFR) are relatively constant with changes in systolic blood pressure from about 80 to 200 mm Hg.

triphosphatase pump drives the sodium into tubular cells while chloride ions passively follow.)
   2. At the loop of Henle in the collecting duct, water reabsorption is controlled entirely by antidiuretic hormone secreted by the pituitary gland.
G. **The Renin–Angiotensin–Aldosterone System**
   1. Renin release by the afferent arteriole may be triggered by hypotension, increased tubular chloride concentration, or sympathetic stimulation.
   2. Aldosterone stimulates the distal tubule and collecting duct to reabsorb sodium (and water), resulting in intravascular volume expansion.
H. **Renal Vasodilator Mechanisms**
   1. Opposing the saline retention and vasoconstriction observed in stress states are the actions of atrial natriuretic peptide (ANP), nitric oxide, and the renal prostaglandin system. ANP is released by the cardiac atria in response to increased stretch under conditions of volume expansion.
   2. Nitric oxide produced in the kidney opposes the renal vasoconstrictor effects of angiotensin II and the sympathetic nervous system, promotes sodium

TABLE 52-1

CLINICAL ASSESSMENT OF THE KIDNEY

Serum creatinine (GFR should be assessed)
BUN (not ideal as influenced by dehydration and postoperative catabolic states)
Urinalysis and urine characteristics (inspection for cloudiness, color, odors)
Urine specific gravity (>1.018 implies preserved renal concentrating ability)
Urine output (<400 mL urine/24 hr) may reflect hypovolemia or impending "prerenal" renal failure (perioperative renal failure often develops in the absence of oliguria

BUN = blood urea nitrogen; GFR = glomerular filtration rate.

and water excretion, and participates in tubuloglomerular feedback.

II. CLINICAL ASSESSMENT OF THE KIDNEY

Measures such as urine output correlate only poorly with perioperative renal function, but much about the kidneys can be learned from knowing how effectively they clear circulating substances and from inspection of the urine (Table 52-1).

III. PERIOPERATIVE NEPHROLOGY

A. **Pathophysiology.** Altered renal function can be thought of as a clinical continuum ranging from normal compensatory changes seen during stress to frank renal failure.
   1. The net result of modest activity of the stress response system is a shift of blood flow from the renal cortex to the medulla, avid sodium and water reabsorption, and decreased urine output.
   2. A more intense stress response may induce a decrease in RBF and GFR by causing afferent arteriolar constriction. If this extreme situation is not reversed, ischemic damage to the kidney may result, and acute renal failure (ARF) may become clinically manifest.
B. **Electrolyte Disorders** (Table 52-2)

TABLE 52-2

ELECTROLYTE DISORDERS

Hyponatremia (most common electrolyte disorder; symptoms are rare unless sodium values are <125 mmol/L)
Hypernatremia (sodium gain or water loss; serum sodium >145 mmol/L)
Disorders of potassium balance (skeletal muscle weakness, ileus, myocardial depression)
Hypocalcemia (laryngospasm)
Hypercalcemia (primary hyperparathyroidism, malignancy)
Hypomagnesemia (<1.6 mg/dL)
Hypermagnesemia (>4 to 6 mg/dL)

C. **Acid–Base Disorders.** Acid–base homeostasis involves tight regulation of HCO_3^- and $PaCO_2$ (Table 52-3).
D. **Acute Kidney Conditions**
   1. **Acute kidney injury (AKI)** is the preferred term for an acute deterioration in renal function. It is associated with a decline in glomerular filtration and results in an inability of the kidneys to excrete nitrogenous and other wastes. AKI frequently occurs in the setting of critical illness with multiple organ failure, and the mortality rate is alarmingly high (≤90%).
   2. **Prerenal azotemia** is an increase in blood urea nitrogen associated with renal hypoperfusion or ischemia that has not yet caused renal parenchymal damage.
   3. **Intrinsic AKI** includes injury caused by ischemia, nephrotoxins, and renal parenchymal diseases.

TABLE 52-3

ACID–BASE DISORDERS

Metabolic acidosis (to determine the cause, the anion gap should be calculated)
Metabolic alkalosis (gastrointestinal acid loss)
Respiratory acidosis (acute and chronic causes can be differentiated by examining arterial pH, $PaCO_2$, and HCO_3^- values)
Respiratory alkalosis (increased minute ventilation)
Mixed acid–base disorders (common in intensive care unit patients)

TABLE 52-4

NEPHROTOXINS COMMONLY FOUND IN THE HOSPITAL SETTING

Exogenous	Endogenous
Antibiotics (aminoglycosides, cephalosporins, amphotericin B, sulfonamide, tetracyclines, vancomycin)	Calcium (hypercalcemia)
Myoglobin (rhabdomyolysis)	Uric acid (hyperuricemia and hyperuricemia)
Anesthetic agents (methoxyflurane, enflurane)	Hemoglobin (hemolysis)
NSAIDs (aspirin, ibuprofen, naproxen, indomethacin, ketorolac)	Bilirubin (obstructive jaundice)
Chemotherapeutic–immunosuppressive agents (cisplatinum, cyclosporin A, methotrexate, mitomycin, nitrosoureas, tacrolimus)	Oxalate crystals
Contrast media	Paraproteins

NSAID = nonsteroidal anti-inflammatory drug.

4. **Postrenal AKI (Obstructive Uropathy).** Downstream obstruction of the urinary collecting system is the least common pathway to established AKI, accounting for fewer than 5% of cases.

5. **Nephrotoxins and Perioperative AKI** (Table 52-4)

E. **Chronic Kidney Disease (CKD).** Patients with nondialysis-dependent CKD are at increased risk of developing end-stage renal disease (ESRD). These patients have GFRs below 25% of normal. Patients with decreased renal reserve are often asymptomatic and frequently do not have elevated blood levels of creatinine or urea.

1. The uremic syndrome represents an extreme form of CRF, which occurs as the surviving nephron population and GFR decrease below 10% of normal. It results in an inability of the kidneys to perform their two major functions: regulation of the volume and composition of the ECF and excretion of waste products.

2. Water balance in ESRD becomes difficult to manage because the number of functioning nephrons is too small either to concentrate or to fully dilute the

---

TABLE 52-5

FACTORS CONTRIBUTING TO HYPERKALEMIA IN CHRONIC
RENAL FAILURE

Potassium Intake
Increased dietary intake
Exogenous IV supplementation
Potassium salts of drugs
Sodium substitutes
Blood transfusion
GI hemorrhage

Potassium Release from Intracellular Stores
Increased catabolism or sepsis
Metabolic acidosis
β-Adrenergic blocking drugs
Digitalis intoxication
Insulin deficiency
Sch

Potassium Excretion
Acute decrease in GFR
Constipation
Potassium-sparing diuretics
ACE inhibitors (decreased aldosterone secretion)
Heparin (decreased aldosterone effect)

ACE = angiotensin-converting enzyme; GFR = glomerular filtration rate;
GI = gastrointestinal; IV = intravenous; Sch = succinylcholine.

---

urine. This results in failure both to conserve water
and to excrete excess water.

3. Patients with uremic syndrome often require
   frequent or continuous dialysis.

4. Life-threatening hyperkalemia may occur in patients
   with CKD because of slower-than-normal
   potassium clearance (Table 52-5). Derangements in
   calcium, magnesium, and phosphorus metabolism
   are also commonly seen in patients with CKD.

5. Metabolic acidosis occurs in two forms in ESRD
   (hyperchloremic, normal anion gap acidosis and a
   high anion gap acidosis caused by an inability to
   excrete titratable acids).

6. **Complications of the Uremic Syndrome** (Table 52-6)

F. **Drug Prescribing in Renal Failure.** Clearance of most
   medications involves a complex combination of both
   hepatic and renal function, and drug level

TABLE 52-6

THE UREMIC SYNDROME

Water Homeostasis
ECF expansion

Electrolyte and Acid–Base
Hyponatremia
Hyperkalemia
Hypercalcemia or hypocalcemia
Hyperphosphatemia
Hypermagnesemia
Metabolic acidosis

Cardiovascular
Heart failure
Hypertension
Pericarditis
Myocardial dysfunction
Dysrhythmias

Respiratory
Pulmonary edema
Central hyperventilation

Hematologic
Anemia
Platelet hemostatic defect

Immunologic
Cell-mediated and humoral immunity defects

Gastrointestinal
Delayed gastric emptying, anorexia, nausea, vomiting, hiccups,
   upper GI tract inflammation or hemorrhage

Neuromuscular
Encephalopathy, seizures, tremors, myoclonus
Sensory and motor polyneuropathy
Autonomic dysfunction, decreased baroreceptor responsiveness,
   dialysis-associated hypotension

Endocrine-Metabolism
Renal osteodystrophy
Glucose intolerance
Hypertriglyceridemia

ECF = extracellular fluid; GI = gastrointestinal.

SURGICAL SUBSPECIALTIES

measurement or algorithms for specific drugs are often
recommended.
   G. **Anesthetic Agents in Renal Failure.** With the possible
      exception of enflurane, anesthetic agents do not
      directly cause renal dysfunction or interfere with the

normal compensatory mechanisms activated by the stress response.

1. If the chosen anesthetic technique causes a protracted reduction in cardiac output or sustained hypotension that coincides with a period of intense renal vasoconstriction, renal dysfunction or failure may result.

2. Significant renal impairment may affect the disposition, metabolism, and excretion of commonly used anesthetic agents (with the exception of the inhalational anesthetics).

3. **Induction Agents and Sedatives**
   a. Ketamine is less extensively protein bound than thiopental, and renal failure appears to have less influence on its free fraction.
   b. Propofol undergoes extensive, rapid hepatic biotransformation to inactive metabolites that are renally excreted.
   c. AKI appears to slow the plasma clearance of midazolam.

4. **Opioids**
   a. Chronic morphine administration results in accumulation of its 6-glucuronide metabolite, which has potent analgesic and sedative effects.
   b. Meperidine is remarkable for its neurotoxic, renally excreted metabolite (normeperidine) and is not recommended for use in patients with poor renal function.
   c. Hydromorphone is metabolized to hydromorphone-3-glucuronide, which is excreted by the kidneys. This active metabolite accumulates in patients with renal failure and may cause cognitive dysfunction and myoclonus.
   d. Codeine has the potential for causing prolonged narcosis in patients with renal failure and is not recommended for long-term use.
   e. Fentanyl appears to be an acceptable choice in patients with ESRD because of its lack of active metabolites, unchanged free fraction, and short redistribution phase. Small to moderate doses, titrated to effect, are well tolerated by uremic patients.
   f. Remifentanil is rapidly metabolized by blood and tissue esterases, and renal failure has no effect on the clearance of remifentanil.

TABLE 52-7

NONDEPOLARIZING MUSCLE RELAXANTS IN RENAL FAILURE

Drug	% Renal Excretion	Half-Life (hr) Normal/ ESRD	Renally Excreted Active Metabolite	Use in ESRD
Pancuronium	30	2.3/4–8	+	Avoid
Pipecuronium	37	1.8–2.3/4.4	+	Avoid
Doxacurium	30	1.7/3.7	−	Avoid
Vecuronium	30	0.9/1.4	+	Avoid infusion
Rocuronium	30	1.2–1.6/ 1.6–1.7	−	Variable duration
Atracurium/ cis-atracurium	<5	0.3/0.4	−	Normal

ESRD = end-stage renal disease.

SURGICAL SUBSPECIALTIES

5. **Muscle relaxants** are the most likely group of drugs used in anesthetic practice to produce prolonged effects in ESRD because of their dependence on renal excretion (Table 52-7).
    a. Provided the serum potassium concentration is not dangerously elevated, succinylcholine (Sch) use can be justified as part of a rapid sequence induction technique because its duration of action in patients with ESRD is not significantly prolonged.
    b. Concern about the increase in serum potassium levels after Sch administration (0.5 mEq/L in normal subjects) implies that the serum potassium level should be normalized to the extent possible in patients with renal failure, but clinical experience has shown that the acute, small increase in potassium after administration of Sch is generally well tolerated in patients with chronically elevated serum potassium levels.
6. **Anticholinesterase and Anticholinergic Drugs**
    a. Anticholinesterases have a prolonged duration of action in patients with ESRD because of their heavy reliance on renal excretion.
    b. Atropine and glycopyrrolate, used in conjunction with the anticholinesterases, are similarly excreted by the kidney. Therefore, no dosage alteration

of the anticholinesterases is required when antagonizing neuromuscular blockade in patients with reduced renal function.

IV. DIURETIC DRUGS: EFFECTS AND MECHANISMS

A. The Physiologic Basis of Diuretic Action (Fig. 52-3)

1. **Proximal Tubule Diuretics.** Carbonic anhydrase inhibitors are drugs that inhibit this enzyme; the net effect of these agents is that sodium and bicarbonate, which would otherwise have been reabsorbed, remain in the urine, resulting in an alkaline diuresis. Specific uses for carbonic anhydrase inhibitors include the treatment of mountain sickness and open-angle glaucoma and to increase respiratory drive in patients with central sleep apnea.

2. **Osmotic Diuretics.** Substances such as mannitol that are freely filtered at the glomerulus but poorly reabsorbed by the renal tubule cause an osmotic diuresis. Mannitol also draws water from cells into the plasma and effectively increases RBF. Mannitol has been widely used, especially for the prophylaxis of ARF. There is no clear evidence that mannitol is effective either for the prevention or treatment of ARF.

3. **Loop Diuretics.** Loop diuretics (furosemide, bumetanide, torsemide) directly inhibit the electroneutral transporter (Na^+/K^+ ATPase in the loop of Henle), preventing salt reabsorption from occurring.

   a. Loop diuretics are a first-line therapeutic modality for treatment of acute decompensated congestive heart failure.

   b. Adverse effects of loop diuretics include hypokalemia, hyponatremia, and acute kidney dysfunction. Loop diuretics, especially furosemide, may cause ototoxicity, particularly in patients with renal insufficiency.

4. **Distal Convoluted Tubule Diuretics**

   a. Clinically, distal convoluted tubule diuretics are used for the treatment of hypertension (often as sole therapy) and volume overload disorders and to relieve the symptoms of edema in pregnancy.

   b. Adverse reactions associated with distal tubule diuretics include electrolyte disturbances and volume depletion.

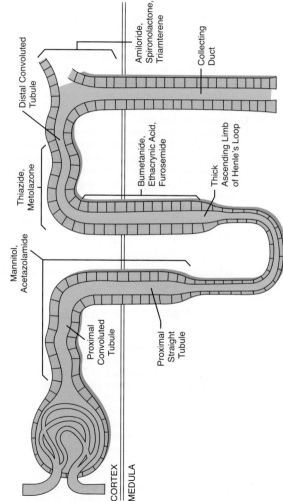

Diuretic Sites of Action

Distal Convoluted Tubule

Amiloride, Spironolactone, Triamterene

Collecting Duct

Thiazide, Metolazone

Bumetanide, Ethacrynic Acid, Furosemide

Thick Ascending Limb of Henle's Loop

Mannitol, Acetazolamide

Proximal Convoluted Tubule

Proximal Straight Tubule

CORTEX

MEDULA

FIGURE 52-3. Site of action of commonly available diuretics.

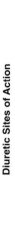

SURGICAL SUBSPECIALTIES

833

5. **Distal (collecting duct) acting diuretics** inhibit luminal sodium entry with a resulting potassium-sparing effect. A second class of distal-acting potassium-sparing diuretics is the competitive aldosterone antagonists (spironolactone and eplerenone).

a. These drugs are used primarily for potassium-sparing diuresis and in treating patients with disorders involving secondary hyperaldosteronism, such as cirrhosis with ascites.

b. Spironolactone treatment has been shown to improve survival with volume overload and left ventricular dysfunction or heart failure.

B. **Dopaminergic Agonists**

1. Intravenous (IV) infusion of low-dose dopamine (1–3 μg/kg/min) is natriuretic owing primarily to a modest increase in the GFR and reduction in proximal sodium reabsorption mediated by dopamine type 1 (DA1) receptors. Fenoldopam is a selective DA1 receptor agonist with little cardiac stimulation.

2. At higher doses, the pressor response to dopamine is beneficial in patients with hypotension, but it has little or no renal effect in critically ill or septic patients.

3. Renal-dose dopamine for the treatment of AKI, although widely used, has not been demonstrated to have significant renoprotective properties.

V. HIGH-RISK SURGICAL PROCEDURES

A. **Cardiac Surgery**

1. Cardiac operations requiring cardiopulmonary bypass can be expected to result in renal dysfunction or failure in up to 7% of patients. Renal ischemia–reperfusion and toxin exposure are considered to be the two primary pathogenetic mechanisms involved in AKI.

2. Numerous agents (mannitol, dopamine, dopexamine) have been used intraoperatively without success in attempts to protect the kidney during cardiac surgery.

B. **Noncardiac Surgery**

1. Several common noncardiac surgical procedures (emergency surgery, trauma surgery, multiple organ failure) can compromise previously normal renal function.

2. Preventing AKI in patients presenting for emergency surgery begins with restoring intravascular volume and managing shock.
   a. Invasive hemodynamic monitoring may be required to guide intraoperative management of ongoing cardiovascular instability caused by surgical manipulation, blood loss, fluid shifts, and anesthetic effects. Intraoperative transesophageal echocardiography provides excellent assessment of left and right ventricular function, as well as guidance of fluid resuscitation.
   b. There is no place for either furosemide or mannitol therapy in the early, resuscitative phase of trauma management, except in the case of head injury with elevated intracranial pressure or when massive rhabdomyolysis is suspected.
   c. Vascular surgery requiring aortic clamping has deleterious effects on renal function regardless of the level of clamp placement.
   d. Although hemodynamic changes during endovascular procedures on the aorta may be less dramatic than those accompanying open repair, the prevalence of renal complications appears to be similar. During endovascular procedures, patients may be exposed to substantial amounts of radiocontrast dye, which may exacerbate postoperative renal dysfunction, especially in those with pre-existing renal insufficiency.

VI. ANESTHESIA FOR URINARY TRACT DISEASE

A. **Cystourethroscopy and Ureteral Procedures.**
   Ureteroscopy, a simple extension of cystoscopy into the upper urinary tract using a flexible or rigid scope, can facilitate treatment of upper urinary tract malignancies and strictures and aid in diagnostic endoscopy and biopsy.

B. **Transurethral Resection of Bladder Tumors**
   1. Superficial transitional cell carcinoma accounts for approximately 90% of bladder cancers.
   2. In diagnosing and treating this cancer, most patients undergo endoscopic transurethral resection. This procedure can be performed with topical, regional, or general anesthesia.

TABLE 52-8
SAFETY ISSUES DURING USE OF LASERS
Retinal or corneal damage (protective goggles or lenses should be used) Thermal injuries Inadvertent ignition of surgical drapes Vaporization of *Condyloma acuminatum* tissue (plume of smoke that contains active human papilloma virus particles; a smoke evacuation system should be used in the operating room)

    a. If a neuraxial regional block is used, an anesthetic level to T10 is required to prevent the pain associated with bladder distention.

    b. Patient movement caused by obturator nerve stimulation during resection of an inferior lateral tumor is associated with an increased likelihood of bladder perforation. A conscious patient who experiences bladder perforation often describes sudden abdominal pain with referred shoulder pain from diaphragmatic irritation.

VII. LASERS IN UROLOGY (Table 52-8)

VIII. EXTRACORPOREAL SHOCK WAVE LITHOTRIPY (SWL)

Since 1980, when extracorporeal SWL became available, it has been the leading modality for the treatment of urinary calculi. SWL has the advantages of being a minimally invasive technique that is performed on an outpatient basis and is associated with minimal perioperative morbidity and a significant reduction in anesthetic needs.

A. **Complications of Shock Wave Lithotripsy** (Table 52-9)
B. **Anesthetic Techniques for Shock Wave Lithotripsy.** The majority of second- and third-generation lithotriptors require monitored anesthesia care with IV sedation and analgesia. The exception to this rule is pediatric patients, who usually require a general anesthetic.

TABLE 52-9

CONTRAINDICATIONS TO EXTRACORPOREAL SHOCK
WAVE LITHOTRIPSY

Absolute Contraindications
Bleeding disorder or anticoagulation
Pregnancy

Relative Contraindications
Large calcified aortic or renal artery aneurysms
Untreated UTI
Obstruction distal to the renal calculi
Pacemaker, AICD, or neurostimulation implant
Morbid obesity

AICD = automatic implantable cardioverter-defibrillator; UTI = urinary tract
infection.

IX. ANESTHESIA FOR PROSTATIC SURGERY

A. **Benign prostatic hyperplasia (BPH)** is a frequent cause of lower urinary tract symptoms in older men. The clinical symptoms are not simply attributable to mechanical obstruction of urine flow because age-related detrusor dysfunction (an androgen-related phenomenon) plays an additional significant role. The hypertrophied prostate surrounds and compresses the prostatic (proximal) urethra, causing obstruction that often produces urinary retention.

B. **Transurethral resection of the prostate (TURP)** is the surgical treatment for BPH. To facilitate clear vision of the surgical field, continuous irrigation is required. The irrigation fluid serves to distend the operative site and removes dissected tissue and blood. If the irrigating fluid infusion pressure exceeds venous pressure during a TURP procedure, the lush venous plexus of the prostate may allow intravascular absorption of irrigating fluid.

C. **Irrigating Solutions for Transurethral Resection of the Prostate** (Table 52-10). Glycine has also been attributed a role in negative hemodynamic changes.

D. **Transurethral Resection of the Prostate Syndrome** (Table 52-11)

1. Factors that predict the amount of irrigation fluid absorption during a TURP procedure include the number and size of open venous sinuses (blood loss implies potential for irrigation absorption), duration

TABLE 52-10

PROPERTIES OF COMMONLY USED IRRIGATING SOLUTIONS FOR TRANSURETHERAL RESECTION PROCEDURES

Solution	Osmolality (mOsm/L)	Advantages	Disadvantages
Distilled water	0	Improved visibility	Hemolysis Hemoglobinemia Hemoglobinuria Hyponatremia
Glycine (1.5%)	200	Less likelihood of TURP syndrome	Transient postoperative visual syndrome Hyperammonemia Hyperoxaluria
Sorbitol (3.3%)	165	Same as glycine	Hyperglycemia, possible lactic acidosis Osmotic diuresis
Mannitol (5%)	275	Isosmolar solution Not metabolized	Osmotic diuresis Possibility of acute intravascular volume expansion

TURP = transurethral resection of the prostate.

of resection, hydrostatic pressure of the irrigating fluid, and venous pressure at the irrigant–blood interface.
2. When neurologic or cardiovascular complications of TURP procedures are recognized, prompt intervention is necessary (Table 52-12).

TABLE 52-11

SIGNS AND SYMPTOMS OF ACUTE HYPONATREMIA

Serum Sodium (mEq/L)	Central Nervous System Changes	Electrocardiographic Changes
120	Confusion Restlessness	Possible widening of QRS complex
115	Somnolence Nausea	Widened QRS complex Elevated ST segment
110	Seizures Coma	Ventricular tachycardia or fibrillation

SURGICAL SUBSPECIALTIES

TABLE 52-12

TREATMENT OF THE TRANSURETHRAL RESECTION SYNDROME

Ensure oxygenation and circulatory support.
Notify the surgeon and terminate the procedure as soon as possible.
Consider insertion of invasive monitors if cardiovascular instability occurs.
Send blood to the laboratory for electrolytes, creatinine, glucose, and ABG analysis.
Obtain a 12-lead electrocardiogram.
Treat mild symptoms (with serum sodium concentration >120 mEq/L) with fluid restriction and a loop diuretic (furosemide).
Treat severe symptoms (serum sodium <120 mEq/L) with 3% sodium chloride IV at a rate <100 mL/hr.
Discontinue 3% sodium chloride when serum sodium is >120 mEq/L.

ABG = arterial blood gas; IV = intravenous.

3. Other complications of TURP include blood loss (2 mL/min) and abnormal bleeding after surgery (<1% of resections). Fever suggests bacteremia secondary to spread of bacteria through open prostatic venous sinuses and hypothermia.

E. **Anesthetic Techniques for Transurethral Resection of the Prostate**
   1. Regional anesthesia, most commonly spinal block, has long been considered the anesthetic technique of choice for TURP.
   2. Because many patients having prostate surgery are elderly, consideration should be given to prevention of postoperative cognitive dysfunction. A prospective study comparing cognitive function after TURP using general versus spinal anesthesia found a significant impairment in both groups at 6 hours after surgery but no differences between approaches at any time in the first 30 days after surgery.
   3. The incidence of perioperative myocardial ischemia in patients undergoing TURP surgery, assessed by Holter monitoring, increases after surgery, but this also appears unaffected by the choice of anesthesia.

F. **Morbidity and Mortality after Transurethral Resection of the Prostate.** The majority of patients undergoing TURP are elderly and have numerous comorbidities.

Mortality after TURP surgery is most commonly related to cardiac and respiratory comorbidities.

G. **The Future of Transurethral Resection of the Prostate**

1. The rate of TURP procedures has declined, largely because of the development of non-operative strategies for BPH management (α_1-adrenergic antagonists that reduce dynamic urethral obstruction or 5-α reductase inhibitors that block conversion of testosterone to reduce prostate hypertrophy).

2. Less invasive surgical treatments for BPH have also been developed and include balloon dilatation, intraprostatic stents, transurethral incision, needle ablation, vaporization of the prostate, and laser prostatectomy.

3. Despite these other surgical options, TURP has not been displaced as the best treatment for BPH, particularly in highly symptomatic patients and those with recurrent urinary tract infections related to incomplete bladder emptying.

X. SURGERY FOR PROSTATE CANCER

A. **Radical Retropubic Prostatectomy.** Prostate cancer is the most common cancer in men. Advances in surgical techniques for radical prostatectomy continue to improve outcomes and reduce the complexity of the anesthetic care for these procedures.

1. The traditional approach has been open radical retropubic prostatectomy (ORRP). This procedure, involving a transverse abdominal incision, is often associated with blood loss exceeding 1000 mL. Anesthetic technique and monitor selection need to be tailored toward intravascular volume assessment and using adjuncts that may help limit the volume of blood loss and reduce the need for blood transfusion.

2. Monitoring for radical prostatectomy should be dictated by patient comorbidities and anticipated blood loss. Notably, urine flow, a traditional monitor of intravascular volume, is interrupted. Central venous pressure monitoring may be helpful, both to follow intravascular volume changes and to provide access for rapid transfusion. An arterial line provides continuous blood pressure monitoring and the possibility of serial hemoglobin assessment.

3. Optimal patient positioning for this procedure is a hyperextended supine position, which may theoretically increase the risk of nerve injury and rhabdomyolysis. The patient's iliac crests are positioned over the break in the operating table, which is then extended to create a maximal distance between the iliac crest and rib cage. The patient is then tilted to a head-down (Trendelenburg) position to achieve an operative field parallel to the floor.

4. Improved postoperative pain management can also lead to better patient outcomes and overall satisfaction.

B. **Radical perineal prostatectomy** is an alternate open surgical approach to prostatectomy. Positioning for this approach poses a significant anesthetic challenge because patients are in an exaggerated lithotomy position, so ventilatory mechanics may be compromised. Although the surgical site for this approach would be ideally amenable to spinal or epidural anesthesia, the position is so poorly tolerated by patients and the ventilatory alterations are so profound that general anesthesia is often indicated.

C. **Laparoscopic and Robotic Prostatectomy (LRP)**

1. A major impetus in the development of minimally invasive prostate cancer techniques has been patient satisfaction and quality of life. Shorter convalescence with a more rapid return to normal activity and shorter urinary catheter duration can be achieved with LRP.

2. Anesthetic complications for LRP include extended surgical times coupled with high abdominal insufflation pressures and the head-down position can sometimes compromise ventilation. Because blood loss with LRP is minimal, monitoring decisions based on hemorrhage concerns with ORRP are replaced by selection of monitors focused primarily on patient comorbidities.

3. Specific considerations include attention to temperature control (forced-air warming and warming insufflated gas to maintain normothermia), use of short-acting anesthetic agents, minimizing opioid administration, addressing postoperative nausea and vomiting, and reducing insufflation pressures from 15 to 12 mm Hg (to facilitate earlier return of bowel function).

4. Pain associated with the ORRP and LRP approaches to radical prostatectomy is similar, with the overall analgesic needs for both approaches being short lived.

XI. ANESTHESIA FOR OTHER UROLOGIC CANCER SURGERY

A. **Radical nephrectomy** remains the mainstay of treatment for renal cell carcinoma. Surgery is associated with significant postoperative pain and specific risks (pneumothorax, tumor extension into the inferior vena cava and right atrium).
  1. **A primary concern** in the anesthetic management is attention to fluid management and the potential for significant blood loss.
  2. When planning for postoperative epidural analgesia, it is important to know what is planned for postoperative deep venous thrombosis (DVT) prophylaxis because all patients with cancer are at a high risk for DVT and pulmonary embolus.

B. **Radical cystectomy** with pelvic node dissection is the "gold standard" for treatment of muscle-invasive bladder carcinoma.
  1. Anesthetic care for radical cystectomy should focus on preoperative assessment and patient optimization because these patients are often elderly and have multiple comorbidities. Significant blood loss and the need for transfusion are possible. An arterial line offers the advantage of easy blood pressure monitoring in high-risk patients and a method for obtaining serial samples for hematocrit measurement.
  2. Although there is no contraindication to the use of regional anesthesia, radical cystectomy is usually performed under general anesthesia because of the long duration of surgery.

CHAPTER 53 ■ ANESTHESIA FOR ORTHOPAEDIC SURGERY

Many orthopaedic surgical procedures lend themselves to the use of regional anesthesia (intraoperative anesthesia and postoperative analgesia) (Horlocker TT, Wedel DJ: Anesthesia for orthopaedic surgery. In *Clinical Anesthesia*. Edited by Barash PG, Cullen BF, Stoelting RK, Cahalan MK, Stock MC. Philadelphia: Lippincott Williams & Wilkins, 2009, pp 1375–1392). Anesthesia for orthopaedic surgery requires an understanding of special positioning requirements (risk of peripheral nerve injury), appreciation of the possibility of large intraoperative blood loss and techniques to limit the impact of this occurrence (intraoperative hypotension, salvage techniques), and the risk of venous thromboembolism (emphasizing the need for the anesthesiologist to consider the interaction of anticoagulants and antiplatelet drugs with anesthetic drugs or techniques, especially regional anesthesia).

I. PREOPERATIVE ASSESSMENT (Table 53-1)

A brief neurologic examination with documentation of any pre-existing deficits is recommended.

II. CHOICE OF ANESTHETIC TECHNIQUE (Table 53-2)

III. SURGERY TO THE SPINE

A. **Spinal Cord Injuries.** Spinal cord injuries must be considered in any patient who has experienced trauma. (Cervical spine injuries are associated with head and thoracic injuries, and lumbar spine injuries are associated with abdominal injuries and long bone fractures.)

TABLE 53-1

PREOPERATIVE ASSESSMENT OF ORTHOPAEDIC SURGICAL PATIENTS

Pre-Existing Medical Problems
Coronary artery disease (perioperative β blockade should be considered)
Rheumatoid arthritis (steroid therapy, airway management)

Physical Examination
Mouth opening or neck extension
Evidence of infection and anatomic abnormalities at proposed sites for introduction of regional anesthesia (peripheral techniques may be acceptable if a regional technique is contraindicated)
Arthritic changes and limitations to positioning

1. **Tracheal Intubation**
   a. Airway management is critical because the most common cause of death with acute cervical spinal cord injury is respiratory failure.
   b. All patients with severe trauma or head injuries should be assumed to have an unstable cervical fracture until proven otherwise radiographically.
   c. Awake fiberoptic-assisted intubation may be necessary, with general anesthesia induced only after voluntary upper and lower extremity movement is confirmed.
   d. In a truly emergent situation, oral intubation of the trachea with direct laryngoscopy (minimal flexion or extension of the neck) is the usual approach.

TABLE 53-2

ADVANTAGES OF REGIONAL VERSUS GENERAL ANESTHESIA FOR ORTHOPAEDIC SURGICAL PROCEDURES

Improved postoperative analgesia
Decreased incidence of nausea and vomiting
Less respiratory and cardiac depression
Improved perfusion because of sympathetic nervous system block
Decreased intraoperative blood loss
Decreased blood pressure
Blood flow redistribution to large caliber vessels
Locally decreased venous pressure

2. **Respiratory considerations** include an inability to cough and clear secretions, which may result in atelectasis and infection.
3. **Cardiovascular considerations** are based on loss of sympathetic nervous system innervation ("spinal shock") below the level of spinal cord transection. (Cardioaccelerator fiber [T1–T4] loss results in bradycardia and possible absence of compensatory tachycardia if blood loss occurs.)
4. **Succinylcholine-Induced Hyperkalemia.** It is usually safe to administer succinylcholine (Sch) within the first 48 hours after spinal cord injury. It should be avoided after 48 hours in all patients with spinal cord injuries.
5. **Temperature Control.** Loss of vasoconstriction below the level of spinal cord transection causes patients to become poikilothermic. (Body temperature should be maintained by increasing ambient air temperature and warming intravenous [IV] fluids and inhaled gases.)
6. **Maintaining Spinal Cord Integrity.** An important component of anesthetic management is preservation of spinal cord blood flow. (Perfusion pressure should be maintained, and extreme hyperventilation of the lungs should be avoided.) Neurophysiologic monitoring (somatosensory or motor evoked potentials), a "wake-up test," or both are used to recognize neurologic ischemia before it becomes irreversible.
7. **Autonomic Hyperreflexia** (Table 53-3).
B. Scoliosis
1. **Pulmonary Considerations.** Postoperative ventilation of the patient's lungs is likely to be necessary if

TABLE 53-3

CHARACTERISTICS OF AUTONOMIC HYPERREFLEXIA

Occurs in 85% of patients with spinal cord transection above T5
Paroxysmal hypertension with bradycardia (baroreceptor reflex)
Cardiac dysrhythmias
Cutaneous vasoconstriction below and vasodilation above the level of transection
Precipitated by any noxious stimulus (distention of a hollow viscus)
Treatment is removal of stimulus, deepening of anesthesia, and administration of a vasodilator

the vital capacity is below 40% of the predicted value. Prolonged arterial hypoxemia, hypercapnia, and pulmonary vascular constriction may result in right ventricular hypertrophy and irreversible pulmonary hypertension.

2. **Cardiovascular Considerations.** Prolonged alveolar hypoxia caused by hypoventilation and ventilation/perfusion mismatch eventually causes irreversible vasoconstriction and pulmonary hypertension.

3. **Surgical Approach and Positioning.**
   a. The prone position is used for the posterior approach to the spine. (The hazards of the prone position, including brachial plexus stretch injury [the head should be rotated toward the abducted arm and the eyes taped closed], should be considered.)
   b. The anterior approach is achieved with the patient in the lateral position, usually with the convexity of the curve uppermost. Removal of a rib may be necessary. A double-lumen endotracheal tube is used to collapse the lung on the operative side.
   c. A combined anterior and posterior approach in one or two stages yields higher union rates but is associated with increased morbidity, including blood loss and nutritional deficits.

4. **Anesthetic Management**
   a. Respiratory reserve is assessed by exercise tolerance, vital capacity measurement, and arterial blood gas analysis. Autologous blood donation is often recommended (usually ≥4 U can be collected in the month before surgery).
   b. There are specific anesthetic considerations for surgical correction of scoliosis by spinal fusion and instrumentation (Table 53-4).
   c. Adequate hemodynamic monitoring and venous access are essential in the management of patients undergoing spinal fusion and instrumentation (Table 53-5).

C. **Degenerative Vertebral Column Disease.** Spinal stenosis, spondylosis, and spondylolisthesis are forms of degenerative vertebral column disease that may lead to neurologic deficits necessitating surgical intervention.

1. **Surgical Approach and Positioning**

TABLE 53-4

ANESTHETIC CONSIDERATIONS FOR SURGICAL CORRECTION OF SCOLIOSIS

Management of the prone position
Hypothermia (long procedure and extensive exposed area)
Extensive blood and fluid losses
Maintenance of spinal cord integrity
Prevention and treatment of venous air embolism
Reduction of blood loss through hypotensive anesthetic techniques

a. Cervical laminectomy is most often performed with patients in the prone position (Fig. 53-1).
b. Fiberoptic-assisted intubation may be necessary in patients with severely limited cervical movement.
c. The anterior approach places the surgical incision (anterior border of the sternocleidomastoid muscle) near critical structures (carotid artery, esophagus, trachea [edema and recurrent nerve injury are possible]).
d. The use of the sitting position for cervical laminectomy allows a more blood-free surgical field but introduces the risk of venous air embolism. The incidence is less than for sitting posterior fossa craniotomy, but the patient still needs to be monitored with precordial Doppler.

2. **Anesthetic Management**
a. General anesthesia is most often selected for spinal surgery because it ensures airway access

TABLE 53-5

MONITORING FOR PATIENTS UNDERGOING SCOLIOSIS SURGERY

Cannulation of radial artery (direct blood pressure measurement and assessment of blood gases)
Central venous catheter (evaluates blood and fluid management and aspirate air if venous air embolism occurs)
Pulmonary artery catheter (pulmonary hypertension)
Neurophysiologic monitoring (prompt diagnosis of neurologic changes and early intervention)
Somatosensory evoked potentials
Motor evoked potentials
Wake-up test

SURGICAL SUBSPECIALTIES

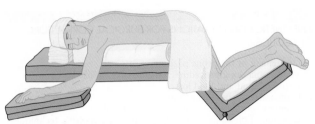

FIGURE 53-1. Prone position with the patient's head turned and the dependent ear and eye protected from pressure. Chest rolls are in place, the arms are extended forward without hyperextension, and the knees are flexed.

and is acceptable for prolonged operations. Patients undergoing cervical laminectomy should be assessed preoperatively for cervical range of motion and the presence of neurologic symptoms during flexion, extension, and rotation of the head. (Awake fiberoptic intubation of the trachea may be necessary.)

  b. Sch should be avoided if there is evidence of a progressive neurologic deficit.

D. Spinal Cord Monitoring. Paraplegia is a feared complication of major spine surgery. The incidence of neurologic injuries associated with scoliosis correction is 1.2%. When patients awaken with paraplegia, neurologic recovery is unlikely, although immediate removal of instrumentation improves the prognosis. It is therefore essential that any intraoperative compromise of spinal cord function be detected as early as possible and reversed immediately. The two methods for detecting intraoperative compromise of spinal cord function are the "wake-up test" and neurophysiologic monitoring.

  1. The **wake-up** test consists of intraoperative awakening of patients after completion of spinal instrumentation. Surgical anesthesia (often including opioids) and neuromuscular blockers are allowed to dissipate, and the patient is asked to move the hands and feet before anesthesia is re-established. Recall may occur but is rarely viewed as unpleasant, especially if the patient is fully informed before surgery.

  2. Neurophysiologic monitoring (as an adjunct or an alternative to the wake-up test) includes

somatosensory evoked potentials (SSEPs)
(waveforms may be altered by volatile anesthetics,
hypotension, hypothermia, hypercarbia), motor
evoked potentials (MEPs) (neuromuscular blocking
drugs cannot be used), and electromyography.

   a. SSEPs reflect the dorsal columns of the spinal
   cord (proprioception and vibration) supplied by
   the posterior spinal artery.
   b. MEPs reflect the motor pathways and the portion of the spinal cord supplied by the anterior
   spinal artery.
   c. The combined use of SSEPs and MEPs may
   increase the early detection of intraoperative
   spinal cord ischemia.
   d. If both SSEPs and MEPs are to be monitored
   during major spine surgery, one might consider
   providing anesthesia with an ultrashort-acting
   opioid infusion with a low dose of inhaled anesthetic and monitoring the electroencephalogram
   to minimize the potential for intraoperative
   awareness.

E. Blood Loss
   1. A combination of IV hypotensive agents and
   volatile anesthetics is frequently used in an attempt
   to decrease blood loss during surgery.
   2. Perioperative coagulopathy from dilution of coagulation factors, platelets, or fibrinolysis may be predicted from measurement of either the prothrombin
   time or activated partial thromboplastin time.

F. Visual Loss After Spine Surgery. Most cases are associated with complex instrumented fusions often associated with prolonged intraoperative hypotension, anemia, large intraoperative blood loss, and prolonged
   surgery (also present in patients who do not develop
   blindness). The American Society of Anesthesiologists'
   Closed Claims Registry concludes that patients at high
   risk for postoperative visual loss after major spine surgery are those in whom blood loss is 1000 mL or
   greater or undergoing surgery lasting 6 hours or
   longer.

G. Venous Air Embolus. Venous air embolism can occur
   in all positions used for laminectomies because the
   operative site is above the heart level. Presenting signs
   are usually unexplained hypotension and an increase
   in the end-tidal nitrogen concentration.

TABLE 53-6

CHANGES AFTER MAJOR SPINE SURGERY THAT MAY INFLUENCE
THE ABILITY TO PERFORM EPIDURAL OR SPINAL ANESTHESIA

Degenerative changes (spondylothesis below level of fusion) that
increase the chance of spinal cord ischemia and neurologic
complications with regional anesthesia

Ligamentum flavum injury from prior surgery results in adhesions
and possible obliteration of the epidural space or interference
with spread of local anesthetic solution ("patchy block")

Increased incidence of accidental dural puncture if the epidural
space is altered by prior surgery (blood patch is difficult to
perform if needed)

Prior bone grafting or fusion may prevent midline insertion of the
needle

H. Postoperative Care

1. Most patients' tracheas can be extubated
   immediately after posterior spinal fusion operations
   if the procedure was relatively uneventful and preoperative vital capacity values were acceptable. The
   presence of severe facial edema may prevent prompt
   tracheal extubation.
2. Aggressive postoperative pulmonary care, including
   incentive spirometry, is necessary to avoid atelectasis and pneumonia.
3. Continued hemorrhage in the postoperative period
   is a concern.

I. Epidural and Spinal Anesthesia After Major Spine Surgery

1. Postoperative anatomic changes make needle or
   catheter placement more difficult after major spine
   surgery (Table 53-6).
2. Spinal anesthesia may be a more reliable technique
   than epidural anesthesia if a regional technique is
   selected.
3. The presence of postoperative spinal stenosis or
   other degenerative changes in the spine or pre-existing neurologic symptoms may preclude the use of
   regional anesthesia in these patients.

IV. SURGERY TO THE UPPER EXTREMITIES

Orthopaedic surgical procedures to the upper extremities
are well suited to regional anesthetic techniques (Table
53-7). Upper extremity peripheral nerve blocks may be

TABLE 53-7

REGIONAL ANESTHETIC TECHNIQUES FOR UPPER EXTREMITY SURGERY

Brachial Plexus Technique	Level of Blockade	Peripheral Nerves Blocked	Surgical Applications	Comments
Axillary	Peripheral nerve	Radial Ulnar Median Musculocutaneous not reliably blocked	Forearm Hand Less often used for procedures about the elbow	Unsuitable for proximal humerus or shoulder surgery The patient must be able to abduct the arm for the block to be performed
Infraclavicular	Cords	Radial Ulnar Median Musculocutaneous Axillary	Elbow Forearm Hand	The catheter site (near coracoid process) is easy to maintain There is no risk of hemothorax or pneumothorax
Supraclavicular	Distal trunk (proximal spinal cord)	Radial Ulnar Median Musculocutaneous Axillary	Mid-humerus Elbow Forearm Hand	There is a risk of pneumothorax, so it is unsuitable for outpatient procedures Phrenic nerve paresis in 30% of patients
Interscalene	Upper and middle trunks	The entire brachial plexus (inferior trunk [ulnar nerve]) is not blocked in 15% to 20% of cases	Shoulder Proximal to mid-humerus	Phrenic nerve paresis is seen in 100% of patients for duration of the block, so it is unsuitable for patients unable to tolerate a 25% reduction in pulmonary function

The duration of the block performed with long-acting local anesthetic (bupivacaine, ropivacaine) is 12 to 20 hours; intermediate-acting agents (lidocaine, mepivacaine) resolve after 4 to 6 hours.

used in the treatment and prevention of reflex sympathetic dystrophy. Continuous catheter techniques provide postoperative analgesia and facilitate early limb mobilization. The patient should be examined preoperatively to document any neurologic deficits because orthopaedic surgical procedures often involve peripheral nerves with pre-existing deficits (ulnar nerve transposition at the elbow, carpal tunnel release of the median nerve at the wrist) or may be adjacent to neural structures (total shoulder arthroplasty or fractures of the proximal humerus). Improper surgical positioning, the use of a tourniquet, and the use of constrictive casts or dressings may also result in perioperative neurologic ischemia. Local anesthetic selection should be based on the duration and degree of sensory or motor block required. (Prolonged anesthesia in the upper extremity in contrast to the lower extremity is not a contraindication to hospital discharge.)

A. **Surgery to the Shoulder and Upper Arm**
  1. A significant incidence of neurologic deficits in patients undergoing this type of surgery demonstrates the importance of clinical examination before regional anesthetic techniques are performed.
     a. **Total shoulder arthroplasty** may be associated with a postoperative neurologic deficit (brachial plexus injury) that is at the same level of the nerve trunks at which an interscalene block is performed. It is impossible to determine a surgical or anesthetic cause. Most of these injuries represent neurapraxia and resolve in 3 to 4 months.
     b. **Radial nerve palsy** is associated with humeral shaft fractures, and **axillary nerve injury** is associated with proximal humeral shaft fractures.
  2. **Surgical Approach and Positioning**
     a. Typically, the patient is flexed at the hips and knees ("beach chair position") and placed near the edge of the operating table to allow unrestricted access by the surgeon to the upper extremity.
     b. The head and neck are maintained in a neutral position because excessive rotation or flexion of the head away from the side of surgery may result in stretch injury to the brachial plexus.
  3. **Anesthetic Management.** Surgery to the shoulder and humerus may be performed under regional

(interscalene or supraclavicular brachial plexus block) or general anesthesia. The ipsilateral diaphragmatic paresis and 25% loss of pulmonary function produced by interscalene block mean that this block is contraindicated in patients with severe pulmonary disease.

B. **Surgery to the Elbow.** Surgical procedures to the distal humerus, elbow, and forearm are suited to regional anesthetic techniques. Supraclavicular block of the brachial plexus is more reliable than the axillary approach (which may miss the musculocutaneous nerve) but introduces the risk of pneumothorax (typically manifests 6–12 hours after hospital discharge such that postoperative chest radiography may not be useful).

C. **Surgery of the Wrist and Hand**
   1. Brachial plexus block (axillary approach) is most commonly used for surgical procedures of the forearm, wrist, and hand. The interscalene approach is seldom used for wrist and hand procedures because of possible incomplete block of the ulnar nerve (15%–30% of patients), and the supraclavicular approach introduces the risk of pneumothorax.
   2. IV regional anesthesia ("Bier block") permits the use of a tourniquet but has disadvantages of limited duration (90–120 minutes), possible local anesthetic systemic toxicity, and rapid termination of anesthesia (and postoperative analgesia) on tourniquet deflation.

D. **Continuous Brachial Plexus Anesthesia**
   1. Catheters placed in the sheath surrounding the brachial plexus permit continuous infusion of local anesthetic solution. (Bupivacaine 0.125% prevents vasospasm and improves circulation after limb reimplantation or vascular repair.)
   2. Indwelling catheters may be left in place for 4 to 7 days after surgery.

V. SURGERY TO THE LOWER EXTREMITIES

Orthopaedic procedures to the lower extremity may be performed under general or regional anesthesia, although regional anesthesia may provide some unique advantages (Table 53-8).

A. **Surgery to the Hip**

TABLE 53-8

LUMBOSACRAL TECHNIQUES FOR MAJOR LOWER EXTREMITY SURGERY

Peripheral Technique	Area of Blockade	Duration of Blockade*	Perioperative Outcomes†
Lumbar Plexus			
Femoral	Femoral	12–18 hours	Improved analgesia and joint range of motion
	Partial lateral femoral cutaneous		Decreased hospital stay compared with PCA
	Obturator		Fewer technical problems
			Lower incidence of urinary retention
			Less hypotension than with epidural analgesia (TKA)
Fascia iliaca	Femoral		Improved analgesia and joint range of motion compared with PCA (TKA)
	Partial lateral femoral cutaneous		
	Obturator		
	Sciatic (S1)		
Psoas compartment	Complete lumbar plexus		Reduced morphine consumption and pain at rest compared with PCA (TKA)
	Occasional spread to sacral plexus or neuraxis		Reduced blood loss (THA)
			Analgesia equivalent to continuous femoral block (TKA)
Sciatic	Posterior thigh and leg (except saphenous area)	18–30 hours	Supplemental sciatic block is required (TKA)
			The proximal approach allows block of posterior femoral cutaneous nerve (TKA)

*The duration of the block performed with long-acting anesthetic (bupivacaine, ropivacaine); intermediate-acting agents (lidocaine, mepivacaine) resolve in 4 to 6 hours

†Outcomes are most marked in patients who receive a continuous lumbar plexus catheter with infusion of 0.1% to 0.2% bupivacaine or ropivacaine at 6 to 12 mL/hr for 48 to 72 hours.

PCA = patient-controlled analgesia; THA = total hip arthroplasty; TKA = total knee arthroplasty.

1. **Surgical Approach and Positioning.** The lateral decubitus position is frequently used to facilitate surgical exposure for total hip arthroplasty, and a fracture table is often used for repair of femur fractures. The patient must be carefully monitored for hemodynamic changes during positioning when under general or regional anesthesia. (Adequate hydration and gradual movement minimize blood pressure decreases.) Care should be taken to pad and position the arms and to avoid compression of the brachial plexus. (A "chest roll" is placed caudad to the axilla to support the upper part of the dependent thorax.)

2. **Anesthetic Technique.** Spinal or epidural anesthesia is well suited to procedures involving the hip. Deliberate hypotension can also be used with general anesthesia as a means of decreasing surgical blood loss.

B. **Total Knee Arthroplasty (TKA)**

1. Patients undergoing TKA experience significant postoperative pain, which impedes physical therapy and rehabilitation.

2. Regional anesthetic techniques that can be used for surgical procedures on the knee include epidural, spinal, and peripheral leg blocks. Spinal anesthesia is often selected, but an advantage of a continuous epidural is postoperative pain management. (Aggressive postoperative regional analgesic techniques for 48–72 hours shorten the rehabilitation period more than systemic opioids.)

3. Patients undergoing amputation of a lower limb often benefit from the use of regional anesthesia, although adequate sedation is imperative.

C. **Postoperative Analgesia after Major Joint Replacement.** Pain after total joint replacement, particularly total knee replacement, is severe. Single-dose and continuous peripheral nerve techniques that block the lumbar plexus (femoral nerve block) with or without sciatic nerve block provide excellent postoperative analgesia.

D. **Knee Arthroscopy and Anterior Cruciate Ligament (ACL) Repair.** Diagnostic knee arthroscopy may be performed under local anesthesia with sedation. (A single dose or continuous lower extremity block is not warranted in most patients.) ACL repair requires postoperative analgesia (femoral nerve blocks should be considered).

 1. **Intra-articular injection** of local anesthetics (bupivacaine), opioids (morphine), or both has become routine for perioperative management after arthroscopic knee surgery.

E. **Surgery to the Ankle and Foot**
 1. The selection of a regional technique is based on the surgical site, use of a tourniquet (use of a high tourniquet for longer than 15–20 minutes necessitates a neuraxial or general anesthetic), and need for postoperative analgesia.
 2. Peripheral nerve blocks (femoral and sciatic nerve) provide acceptable anesthesia for surgery on the foot and ankle.

VI. MICROVASCULAR SURGERY (Table 53-9)

TABLE 53-9

ANESTHETIC CONSIDERATIONS FOR MICROVASCULAR SURGERY FOR LIMB REPLANTATION

Maintain blood flow through microvascular anastomoses (critical for graft viability).

Prevent hypothermia (increase temperature of operating room to 21°C; warm IV solutions and inhaled gases).

Maintain perfusion pressure.

Avoid vasopressors.

Use vasodilators (volatile anesthetics, nitroprusside) and sympathetic nervous system block (regional anesthesia).

Consider normovolemic hemodilution.

Administer antithrombotics (heparin) with or without fibrinolytics (low-molecular-weight dextran).

Remember positioning considerations associated with long surgical procedures.

Replace blood and fluid losses.

Consider the choice of anesthesia (often a combination of regional and general anesthesia)

Sympathectomy is helpful, but the long duration of surgery may limit use of single-shot techniques (another option is a continuous technique)

Ensure airway access and patient immobility.

IV = intravenous.

VII. PEDIATRIC ORTHOPAEDIC SURGERY

A. Regional anesthetic techniques are adaptable to pediatric patients, especially in those older than 7 years of age.
B. IV regional anesthesia is particularly useful in pediatric patients for minor procedures such as closed reduction of forearm fractures.
   1. The use of local anesthetic creams minimizes patient discomfort during placement of an IV catheter.
   2. The size of the upper arm often precludes the use of a double tourniquet in pediatric patients, thus limiting the duration of the surgical procedure to 45 to 60 minutes (tourniquet pain typically develops by this time).

VIII. OTHER CONSIDERATIONS

A. **Anesthesia for Nonsurgical "Closed" Orthopaedic Procedures.** Some minor procedures (cast and dressing changes in pediatric patients, pin removal) require only light sedation, but procedures involving bone and joint manipulation (hip and shoulder relocation, closed reduction of fractures) usually require a general or regional anesthetic.
B. **Tourniquets**
   1. Opinions differ as to the pressure required in tourniquets to prevent bleeding (usually 100 mm Hg above patient's systolic blood pressure for the leg and 50 mm Hg above systolic blood pressure for the arm). Before the tourniquet is inflated, the limb should be elevated for about 1 minute and tightly wrapped with an elastic bandage distally to proximally. Oozing despite tourniquet inflation is most likely caused by intramedullary blood flow in long bones.
   2. The duration of safe tourniquet inflation is unknown (1–2 hours is not associated with irreversible changes). Five minutes of intermittent perfusion between 1 and 2 hours may allow more extended use.
   3. Transient systemic metabolic acidosis and increased $PaCO_2$ (1–8 mm Hg) may occur after tourniquet deflation.
   4. Tourniquet pain despite adequate operative anesthesia typically appears after about 45 minutes (may

reflect more rapid recovery of C fibers as the block wanes). During surgery, this pain is managed with opioids and hypnotics.

C. **Fat Embolus Syndrome**

1. Patients at risk include those with multiple traumatic injuries and surgery involving long bone fractures, intramedullary instrumentation or cementing, or total knee surgery. The incidence of fat embolism syndrome in isolated long bone fractures is 3% to 4%, and the mortality rate is 10% to 20%.

2. Clinical and laboratory signs usually occur 12 to 40 hours after injury and may range from mild dyspnea to coma (Table 53-10).

3. Treatment includes early stabilization of fractures and support of oxygenation. Steroid therapy may be instituted.

D. **Methyl Methacrylate**

1. Insertion of this cement may be associated with hypotension, which has been attributed to absorption of the volatile monomer of methyl methacrylate or embolization of air (nitrous oxide should be discontinued before cement is placed) and bone marrow during femoral reaming.

2. Adequate hydration and maximizing oxygenation minimize the hypotension and arterial hypoxemia that may accompany cementing of the prosthesis.

TABLE 53-10

CRITERIA FOR DIAGNOSIS OF FAT EMBOLISM SYNDROME

Major Criteria	Minor Criteria
Axillary or subconjunctival petechiae	Tachycardia (>100 bpm)
Hypoxemia ($PaO_2 < 60$ mm Hg)	Hyperthermia
CNS depression (disproportionate to hypoxemia)	Retinal fat emboli
Pulmonary edema	Urinary fat globules
	Decreased platelets
	Increased ESR
	DIC

CNS = central nervous system; DIC = disseminated intravascular coagulation; ESR = erythrocyte sedimentation rate.

TABLE 53-11

ANTITHROMBOTIC REGIMENS TO PREVENT THROMBOEMBOLISM
IN ORTHOPEDIC SURGICAL PATIENTS

Hip and Knee Arthroplasty and Hip Fracture Surgery
LMWH* started 12 hours before surgery or 12 to 24 hours after
    surgery or 4 to 6 hours after surgery at half the usual dose and
    then increasing to the usual high-risk dose the following day
Fondaparinux (2.5 mg started 6 to 8 hours after surgery)
Adjusted-dose warfarin started preoperatively or the evening after
    surgery (INR target, 2.5; range, 2.0–3.0)
Intermittent pneumatic compression is an alternative option to
    anticoagulant prophylaxis in patients undergoing total knee (but
    not hip) replacement.

Spinal Cord Injury
LMWH after primary hemostasis is evident
Intermittent pneumatic compression is an alternative when
    anticoagulation is contraindicated early after surgery.
During the rehabilitation phase, conversion to adjusted-dose
    warfarin (INR target, 2.5; range, 2.0–3.0).

Elective Spine Surgery
Routine use of thromboprophylaxis, apart from early and
    persistent mobilization, is not recommended.

Knee Arthroscopy
Routine use of thromboprophylaxis, apart from early and
    persistent mobilization, is not recommended.

*Use with caution in patients receiving neuraxial anesthesia/analgesia.
INR = international normalized ratio; LMWH = low-molecular-weight
heparin.

SURGICAL SUBSPECIALTIES

E. **Venous thromboembolism** is a major cause of death
after surgery or trauma to the lower extremities. Without prophylaxis, 40% to 80% of orthopaedic patients
develop venous thrombosis. (The incidence of fatal
pulmonary embolism is highest in patients who have
undergone surgery for hip fracture.)

F. **Antithrombotic prophylaxis** is based on identification
of risk factors (Table 53-11). Several studies show a
deceased incidence of deep vein thrombosis (DVT) and
pulmonary embolism in patients undergoing hip
surgery and knee surgery under epidural and spinal
anesthesia (Table 53-12).

G. **Neuraxial Anesthesia and Analgesia in Patients Receiving Antithrombotic Therapy**

TABLE 53-12

POSSIBLE EXPLANATIONS FOR DECREASED INCIDENCE OF
DEEP VEIN THROMBOSIS IN PATIENTS RECEIVING
REGIONAL ANESTHESIA

Rheologic changes resulting in hyperkinetic lower extremity blood
  flow and associated decrease in venous stasis and thrombus
  formation
Beneficial circulatory effects from epinephrine added to local
  anesthetic solution
Altered coagulation and fibrinolytic responses to surgery under
  neural blockade, resulting in decreased tendency for blood to clot
Absence of positive pressure ventilation and its effects on circulation
Direct local anesthetic effects (decreased platelet aggregation)

TABLE 53-13

NEURAXIAL ANESTHESIA AND ANALGESIA IN ORTHOPEDIC
PATIENTS RECEIVING ANTITHROMBOTIC THERAPY

Low-Molecular-Weight Heparin
Needle placement should occur 10 to 12 hours after a dose.
Indwelling neuraxial catheters are allowed with once-daily (but
  not twice-daily) dosing of LMWH.
It is optimal to place and remove indwelling catheters in the morning
  and administer LMWH in the evening to allow normalization of
  hemostasis to occur before catheter manipulation.

Warfarin
Adequate levels of all vitamin K–dependent factors should be
  present during catheter placement and removal.
Patients chronically on warfarin should have a normal INR before
  performance of the regional technique.
PT and INR should be monitored daily.
The catheter should be removed when INR <1.5.

Fondaparinux
Neuraxial techniques are not advised in patients who are
  anticipated to receive fondaparinux.

Nonsteroidal Anti-Inflammatory Drugs
No significant risk of regional anesthesia-related bleeding is
  associated with aspirin-type drugs.
For patients receiving warfarin or LMWH, the combined
  anticoagulant and antiplatelet effects may increase the risk of
  perioperative bleeding.
Other medications affecting platelet function (thienopyridine
  derivatives and glycoprotein IIb/IIIa platelet receptor inhibitors)
  should be avoided.

INR = international normalized ratio; LMWH = low molecular weight
heparin; PT = prothrombin time.

1. Despite perceived advantages of neuraxial techniques for hip and knee surgery (including a decreased incidence of DVT), patients receiving perioperative anticoagulants and antiplatelet medications are often not considered candidates for spinal or epidural anesthesia because of the risk of neurologic deficit from a spinal or epidural hematoma (Table 53-13).

2. The patient should be closely monitored in the perioperative period for signs of paralysis. If a spinal hematoma is suspected, the treatment is immediate decompressive laminectomy. (Recovery of neurologic function is unlikely if >10–12 hours elapse.)

CHAPTER 54 ■ TRANSPLANT ANESTHESIA

To optimize organ allocation, the United States is divided into 11 regions for purposes of organ distribution, each with its own regional review board (Ceste M, Glas K: Transplant anesthesia. In *Clinical Anesthesia*. Edited by Barash PG, Cullen BF, Stoelting RK, Cahalan MK, Stock MC. Philadelphia: Lippincott Williams & Wilkins, 2009, pp 1393–1418).

I. ANESTHETIC MANAGEMENT OF ORGAN DONORS

A. **Brain-Dead Donor.** Legal and medical brain death criteria differ from state to state, but all require cessation of both cerebral and brainstem function. Potentially reversible causes of coma or unresponsiveness (hypothermia, hypotension, drugs, toxins) must be ruled out before declaration of brain death. A flat electroencephalogram is consistent with brain death. Transcranial Doppler and traditional or isotope angiography are used to confirm the clinical examination and lack of blood flow to the brain.

1. Brain-dead patients may have intact spinal reflexes, so they may require neuromuscular blockade during organ procurement.

2. Brain death is associated with hemodynamic instability, hormonal chaos, systemic inflammation, and oxidant stress, all of which may negatively impact donor organ function. After pituitary failure ensues, hormone therapy may help stabilize patients hemodynamically. Cardiac graft function is likely improved by donor hormone therapy (tri-iodothyronine, methylprednisolone, desmopressin, insulin).

3. The mainstay of donor management is maintenance of euvolemia, so central venous pressure (CVP)

monitoring is standard. (CVP is maintained at 6 to 12 mm Hg.)

4. Efforts should be made to maintain serum sodium below 155 mmol/L. Packed cells are used to maintain hematocrit of 30%, and fresh-frozen plasma (FFP) is used to maintain the international normalized ratio (INR) below 1.5.

5. The anesthesiologist is responsible for maintaining donor oxygenation, perfusion, and normothermia.

6. Donor lungs are more susceptible to injury in brain-dead patients before procurement than are other organs, likely from contusion, aspiration, or edema with fluid resuscitation (Table 54-1). In selected recipients, these kinds of marginal donors can be used without increasing the incidence of primary graft dysfunction (PGD).

B. **Donation After Cardiac Death (DCD)**

1. The criteria for death of DCD donors (previously called non–heart-beating donors) are distinct from those of brain-dead donors. DCD donors typically have severe whole brain dysfunction but have electrical activity in the brain. Death is defined by cessation of circulation and respiration. Life support measures are used to control the timing of death and organ procurement to maximize the function of organs from these donors.

2. Anesthesiologists do not necessarily have to be involved in DCD donor management. Circulation and respiration must be absent for 2 minutes before the start of organ recovery.

TABLE 54-1

CHARACTERISTICS OF THE IDEAL DECEASED LUNG DONOR

Age younger than 55 years
ABO compatibility
Clear chest radiographs
$PaO_2 > 300$ on F_1O2 1.0, PEEP 5 cm H_2O
Tobacco history <20 pack-years
Absence of chest trauma
No evidence of aspiration or sepsis
Negative sputum Gram stain
Absence of purulent secretions at bronchoscopy

PEEP = positive end-expiratory pressure.

II. LIVING KIDNEY DONORS

Safety and comfort are the primary considerations in the care of living donors. Open nephrectomy is being progressively replaced by laparoscopic donor nephrectomy.

A. Both anesthetics and insufflation of the peritoneum with CO_2 decrease renal blood flow, so fluid repletion is important to maintaining renal perfusion.

B. Nitrous oxide is contraindicated for laparoscopic donor nephrectomy because bowel distention can impede surgery.

III. LIVING LIVER DONORS

Left lobe liver donation is usually done in the context of parent-to-child donation. Donor right lobectomy is needed for adult-to-adult liver transplantation.

A. Large liver resections may require virtually complete hepatic venous exclusion (cross-clamping of the hepatic pedicle, usually without cava clamping).

B. Transesophageal echocardiography is ideal and may obviate placement of central lines.

C. INR increases significantly after right lobe surgery, peaking a few days after surgery along with a decrease in platelet counts, just when an epidural catheter for postoperative pain management is usually removed.

IV. IMMUNOSUPPRESSIVE DRUGS (Table 54-2)

Pharmacologic suppression of the immune response to allografts is associated with major side effects (Table 54-3). Immune-suppressed patients coming to the operating room deserve special attention to sterile technique and

---

TABLE 54-2

IMMUNOSUPPRESSIVE DRUGS

Calcineurin inhibitors (cyclosporine, tacrolimus)
Corticosteroids (maintenance immunosuppression)
Monoclonal and polyclonal antibodies
mTOR inhibitors
Azathioprine
Mycophenolate mofetil

mTOR = mammalian target of rapamycin.

TABLE 54-3

COMPLICATIONS OF CHRONIC IMMUNE SUPPRESSION

System	Complication
Central nervous system	Lowered seizure threshold
Cardiovascular	Hypertension
	Hyperlipidemia
	Atherosclerosis
Renal and electrolyte	Decreased GFR
	Hyperkalemia
	Hypomagnesemia
Hematologic and immune	Increased risk of infections
	Increased risk of malignancy
	Pancytopenia
	Diabetes
Endocrine or other	Osteoporosis
	Poor wound healing

GFR = glomerular filtration rate.

maintenance of antibiotic, antifungal, and antiviral regimens during the perioperative period.

V. RENAL TRANSPLANTATION

A. **Preoperative Considerations.** An enormous variety of diseases are treated with renal transplants (Table 54-4). About half the mortality of patients on dialysis is

TABLE 54-4

COMMON CAUSES OF RENAL FAILURE IN ADULT RENAL TRANSPLANT RECIPIENTS

Diagnosis	% of Patients on List
Type 2 diabetes	21.7
Hypertensive nephrosclerosis	19.4
Retransplant or graft failure	8.7
Polycystic kidney disease	5.9
Type 1 diabetes	5.0
Focal glomerular sclerosis	4.7
Systemic lupus erythematosus	2.9
Chronic glomerulonephritis	2.9
Malignant hypertension	2.6
IgA nephropathy	2.4

SURGICAL SUBSPECIALTIES

caused by heart failure. Hypercoagulable states are common in patients with renal disease. All solid organ transplant patients are screened for tumors (mammography, Pap test, colonoscopy, prostate specific antigen) and infection (dental evaluation, viral serologies).

B. **Intraoperative Protocols.** Renal transplantation is generally done under general anesthesia. Before incision, antibiotics are given. A central venous catheter (usually triple lumen) is placed for CVP monitoring and drug administration, and a bladder catheter is placed.

1. The major anesthetic consideration is maintenance of renal blood flow.
2. Typical hemodynamic goals during renal transplant surgery are systolic pressure above 90 mm Hg, mean systemic pressure above 60 mm Hg, and CVP above 10 mm.
3. After the first anastomosis is started, a diuresis is initiated (mannitol and furosemide are often both given). Dopamine does not reliably improve renal function in this setting.

VI. LIVER TRANSPLANTATION

A. **Preoperative Considerations.** Patients with end-stage liver disease (ESLD) have multisystem dysfunction with cardiac, pulmonary, and renal compromise because of their liver disease, and multiorgan dysfunction at the time of transplantation is common (Table 54-5).

1. Patients with ESLD generally have very low systemic vascular resistance, high cardiac index, and increased mixed venous oxygen saturation. Echocardiography is also used to screen patients for portopulmonary hypertension and intracardiac shunts.
2. There is general agreement that mean pulmonary artery pressure above 50 mm Hg is an absolute contraindication to liver transplantation.

B. **Intraoperative Procedures**

1. Rapid sequence induction of general anesthesia is indicated because patients with ESLD often have gastroparesis in addition to increased intra-abdominal pressure from ascites.
2. A rapid infusion system with the ability to deliver at least 500 mL/min of warmed blood is primed and

TABLE 54-5

MULTISYSTEM COMPLICATIONS OF END-STAGE LIVER DISEASE

System	Consequences
Central Nervous System	Fatigue
Encephalopathy (confusion to coma)	Blood–brain barrier disruption and intracranial hypertension (acute liver failure)
Pulmonary	Hypoxemia or hepatopulmonary syndrome
Respiratory alkalosis	
Pulmonary hypertension	Reduced right heart function
Cardiovascular	
Reduced SVR	Hyperdynamic circulation
Diastolic dysfunction	
Prolonged QT interval	
Blunted responses to inotropes	
Blunted responses to vasopressors	
Diabetes	
Gastrointestinal	
GI bleeding from varices	
Ascites	
Delayed gastric emptying	
Hematologic	
Decreased synthesis of clotting factors	Risk of massive surgical bleeding
Hypersplenism (pancytopenia)	
Impaired fibrinolytic mechanisms	
Renal	
Hepatorenal syndrome	Impaired renal excretion of drugs
Hyponatremia	
Endocrine	
Glucose intolerance	
Osteoporosis	Fracture susceptibility
Nutritional or metabolic	Muscle wasting and weakness
Other	
Poor skin integrity	
Increased volume of distribution for drugs	
Decreased citrate metabolism	Calcium requirement with rapid FFP infusion

FFP = fresh-frozen plasma; GI = gastrointestinal; SVR = systemic vascular resistance.

in the room. Normothermia, which is essential for optimal hemostasis, is maintained with fluid warmers and convective air blankets over the legs and upper body.

3. Liver transplantation is traditionally described in three phases: the dissection, anhepatic, and neohepatic phases, with reperfusion of the graft marking the start of the neohepatic phase.

C. **Coagulation Management**

1. FFP is used to maintain INR at 1.5 or below in patients with anticipated or ongoing bleeding.

2. Maintaining fibrinogen above 150 mg/dL with cryoprecipitate is critical for hemostasis.

3. Perioperative renal dysfunction, with hypovolemia and anesthetic-induced reduction of renal blood flow, is a major challenge in liver transplantation. Hepatorenal syndrome is a functional renal disorder that is associated with liver disease.

D. **Pediatric Liver Transplantation.** Indications for pediatric liver transplantation differ considerably from those in adults, with biliary atresia the most common indication. Portopulmonary hypertension is rare in children, but biliary atresia is associated with atrial septal defects and situs inversus.

E. **Acute Liver Failure.** Anesthetic considerations for both adults and children with acute liver failure are focused on protection of the brain. Patients with acute or fulminant hepatic failure may have a rapidly progressive course of elevated intracranial pressure (ICP), leading to herniation and death. Mannitol is used for osmotherapy to an end point of 310 mOsm/L, and hyperventilation is commonly used to manage ICP. Hypothermia is also considered brain protective in patients with acute liver failure.

VII. PANCREAS AND ISLET TRANSPLANTATION

A. The majority of pancreas transplants (~75%) are done as simultaneous pancreas and kidney transplants from a single deceased donor.

B. The major difference between pancreas transplantation and other procedures is that strict attention to control of blood glucose is indicated to protect newly transplanted β cells from hyperglycemic damage.

VIII. SMALL BOWEL AND MULTIVISCERAL TRANSPLANTATION

A. In general, intestinal transplantation should only be considered in patients with life-threatening complications from intestinal failure.

B. For anesthesiologists, a major hurdle for these transplants is line placement that is adequate for transfusion of blood products and fluids, which may be substantial during these long procedures. Ultrasound devices are helpful in identifying the known patent vessels for cannulation, but surgical cutdowns for venous access may be necessary.

C. Nitrous oxide, as in liver transplantation, should be avoided.

D. Common complications of intestinal failure include dehydration and electrolyte abnormalities, gastric acid hypersecretion, pancreatic insufficiency, bone disease, and total parenteral nutrition–induced liver failure.

IX. LUNG TRANSPLANTATION

Chronic obstructive pulmonary disease, idiopathic pulmonary fibrosis, cystic fibrosis, and α_1-antitrypsin deficiency are the most common indications for lung transplantation. Surgical options for lung transplantation are single-lung transplant, en bloc double-lung transplants, sequential double-lung transplants, and heart–lung transplantation.

A. **Recipient Selection** (Table 54-6). Pulmonary function tests, left and right heart catheterization, and transthoracic echocardiography are routinely used for evaluating recipients.

B. **Preanesthetic Considerations**

1. By definition, lung transplant candidates have poor pulmonary status and are frequently receiving multiple therapies, including oxygen, inhaled bronchodilators, steroids, and vasodilators.

2. After determining oxygen saturation, slow, incremental dosing of a short-acting benzodiazepine (0.25–1.0 mg midazolam) is used for anxiolysis.

C. **Intraoperative Management: Single-Lung Transplantation**

1. Lung transplant recipients tend to be chronically intravascularly volume depleted, and anesthetic induction can be associated with hypotension.

TABLE 54-6

LUNG RECIPIENT SELECTION GUIDELINES

General Indications
End-stage lung disease
Failed maximal medical treatment of lung disease
Age within limits for planned transplant
Life expectancy <2–3 yr
Ability to walk and undergo rehabilitation
Sound nutritional status (70%–130% of ideal body weight)
Stable psychosocial profile
No significant comorbid disease

Disease-Specific Indications
COPD
  FEV_1 <25% of predicted value after bronchodilators
  $PaCO_2$ > 55 mm Hg
  Pulmonary hypertension (especially with cor pulmonale)
  Chronic oxygen therapy
Cystic fibrosis
  FEV_1 <30% predicted
  Hypoxemia, hypercapnia, or rapidly declining lung function
  Weight loss and hemoptysis
  Frequent exacerbations, especially in young women
  Absence of antibiotic-resistant organisms
  Idiopathic pulmonary fibrosis
  Vital capacity <60%–65% of predicted
  Resting hypoxemia
  Progression of disease despite therapy (steroids)
Pulmonary hypertension
  NYHA functional status class III or IV despite prostacyclin
    therapy
  Mean right atrial pressure <15 mm Hg
  Mean pulmonary artery pressure <55 mm Hg
  Cardiac index <2 L/min per m²
Eisenmenger's syndrome
  NYHA class III or IV despite optimal therapy
Pediatric
  NYHA class III or IV
  Disease unresponsive to maximal therapy
  Cor pulmonale, cyanosis, low cardiac output

COPD = chronic obstructive pulmonary disease; FEV_1 = forced expiratory volume in 1 second; NYHA = New York Heart Association.

2. Nitrous oxide is rarely an anesthetic option because of bullous emphysematous disease, pulmonary hypertension, or intraoperative hypoxemia.
3. Lung isolation, preferably with a double-lumen endotracheal tube, is necessary for single and bilateral sequential lung transplantation.

4. Lung recipients are susceptible to development of pulmonary hypertension and right ventricular dysfunction or failure during one-lung ventilation. Vasodilator or inotropic support may be required. Inhaled nitric oxide is another option for improving respiratory and right ventricular status.

5. During one-lung ventilation, hypoxemia is common.

D. **Double-Lung Transplantation**

1. En bloc double-lung transplant requires cardiopulmonary bypass (CPB), and a single-lumen endotracheal tube is sufficient. Bilateral sequential transplant is now the preferred procedure because a tracheal anastomosis is unnecessary and surgical bleeding is less.

2. The clamshell incision is extensive and can cause significant postoperative pain. Thoracic epidurals are often used to provide pain relief.

E. **Pediatric Lung Transplantation.** The most common diagnoses are cystic fibrosis, congenital heart disease, and primary pulmonary hypertension. Most pediatric patients receive double-lung transplantation with CPB.

F. **Primary Graft Dysfunction (PGD)**

1. The cause of PGD is not yet clearly defined and is certainly multifactorial. The diagnosis is not applicable for dysfunction starting more than 72 hours after reperfusion.

2. Anesthetic management does not appear to be a risk factor for PGD.

3. Severe, life-threatening PGD has been successfully managed with extracorporeal membrane oxygenation.

G. **Inhaled nitric oxide** is used to decrease pulmonary vascular resistance and improve oxygenation.

X. HEART TRANSPLANTATION

Overall 1-year survival has improved from 74% in the early 1980s to 87% currently.

A. **Left Ventricular Assist Devices (LVADs)**

1. LVADs differ with respect to flow pattern (pulsatile or nonpulsatile), requirements for anticoagulation (none, aspirin, coumadin), filling pattern (fill-to-empty or various other modes), power source (battery or alternating current), potential for electromagnetic interference, and impact of arrhythmias and defibrillation on the device.

2. Failure to maintain adequate preload or normal afterload results in decreased LVAD flow and hypotension from low functional cardiac output.
3. Patients presenting for initial device placement are in various stages of decompensated heart failure and need invasive monitoring with an arterial line and either a pulmonary artery catheter or central venous line.

B. Recipient Selection

1. Medical therapy for patients with congestive heart failure has improved dramatically over the past decade. Pharmacologic options now include angiotensin-converting enzyme inhibitors, beta-blockers, diuretics, and digoxin.
2. Pulmonary hypertension is associated with increased perioperative mortality, so severe, irreversible pulmonary hypertension is a contraindication to transplant.

C. Preanesthetic Considerations

1. Donor heart function worsens with donor cold ischemia times above 6 hours. Preoperative evaluation and preparation of the patient must be expeditious.
2. Induction of anesthesia and surgical incision of the recipient begin when the donor team has evaluated the donor and made the final determination that the organ is acceptable. There must be strict attention to sterility. Inotropes (dobutamine, vasopressin) should be readily available before induction (Table 54-7).

D. Intraoperative Management. Anesthetic induction in patients with poor ventricular function can be complicated by hemodynamic instability. High-dose opioid techniques have been used for induction and management of cardiac transplant patients with good results.

XI. MANAGMENT OF TRANSPLANT PATIENTS FOR NONTRANSPLANT SURGERY

A. For solid organ recipients, evaluation of patients is centered on function of the grafted organ.
B. A major consideration for renal transplant recipients is maintenance of renal perfusion with adequate volume replacement. Thus, CVP monitoring is useful for preventing prerenal damage to transplanted kidneys, but

TABLE 54-7

EFFECT OF DENERVATION ON CARDIAC PHARMACOLOGY

Substance	Recipient	Mechanism
Digitalis	Normal increase of contractility	Direct myocardial effect
	Minimal effect on atrioventricular node	Denervation
Atropine	None	Denervation
Adrenaline	Increased contractility	Denervation hypersensitivity
	Increased chronotropy	
Noradrenaline	Increased contractility	Denervation
	Increased chronotropy	No neuronal uptake
Isoproterenol	Normal increase in contractility	
	Normal increase in chronotropy	
Quinidine	No vagolytic effect	Denervation
Verapamil	Atrioventricular block	Direct effect
Nifedipine	No reflex tachycardia	Denervation
Hydralazine	No reflex tachycardia	Denervation
Beta-blocker	Increased antagonist effect	Denervation

central venous lines must be placed using strict aseptic technique.

C. For all transplant recipients, antibiotic, antiviral, antifungal, and immune suppression regimens should be disrupted as little as possible in the perioperative period.

D. Transplanted hearts are denervated and cannot respond to indirect-acting agents, such as ephedrine and even dopamine. Dobutamine can also be helpful, but norepinephrine and epinephrine should be reserved for refractory cardiogenic shock.

CHAPTER 55 ■ POST ANESTHESIA RECOVERY

Each patient recovering from an anesthetic has circumstances that require an individualized problem-oriented approach (Fowler MA, Spiess BD: Postoperative recovery. In *Clinical Anesthesia*. Edited by Barash PG, Cullen BF, Stoelting RK, Cahalan MK, Stock MC. Philadelphia: Lippincott Williams & Wilkins, 2009, pp 1419–1443). Dissemination of anesthesia services beyond the perisurgical arena has brought changes and greater demands on recovery units.

I. VALUE AND ECONOMICS OF THE POSTANESTHESIA CARE UNIT (PACU)

PACU resources are efficiently utilized by having trained staff that routinely care for postsurgical patients, thereby recognizing and preventing complications and by having physicians institute appropriate and timely therapies. Routine testing and therapies may unnecessarily add to staffing resources required per patient without widespread demonstrated benefit to patient care.

A. Communication is perhaps the least expensive tool in medicine and the one that is most universally proven to be involved in human error events.

B. Having patients bypass the PACU creates a savings opportunity only if paid nursing hours are reduced or if more surgical cases are covered with the same hours.

II. LEVELS OF POSTOPERATIVE AND POSTANESTHESIA CARE

A. Using a less intensive postanesthesia setting for selected patients may reduce costs for a surgical procedure and allow the facility to divert scarce PACU resources to patients with greater needs.

B. Creation of separate PACUs for inpatients, ambulatory patients, or offsite patients is one possible way to streamline PACU care for appropriately triaged patients. Phase I recovery would be reserved for more intense recovery and would require more one-on-one care for patients. Phase II recovery would be less intensive and would be appropriate for patients after less invasive procedures requiring less nursing attention while recovering.

III. **POSTANESTHETIC TRIAGE** should be based on clinical condition, length and type of procedure and anesthetic, and the potential for complications that require intervention.
A. An individual patient undergoing a specific procedure or anesthetic should receive the same appropriate level of postoperative care whether the procedure is performed in a hospital operating room, ambulatory surgical center, endoscopy room, invasive radiology suite, or outpatient office.
B. After superficial procedures using local infiltration, minor blocks, or sedation, patients can almost always recover with less intensive monitoring and coverage (bypass phase I recovery to phase II).

IV. **SAFETY IN THE POSTANESTHESIA CARE UNIT**

A. The PACU medical director must ensure that the PACU environment is as safe as possible for both patients and staff.
B. Observance of procedures for hand washing, sterility, and infection control should be strictly enforced.
C. Compulsive documentation and clear delineation of responsibility protect staff against unnecessary medicolegal exposure.

V. **ADMISSION TO THE POSTANESTHESIA CARE UNIT**

A. Every patient admitted to a PACU should have their heart rate, rhythm, systemic blood pressure, airway patency, peripheral oxygen saturation, ventilatory rate and character, and level of pain recorded and periodically monitored. Assessment with periodic recording every 5 minutes for the first 15 minutes and every 15 minutes thereafter is a minimum.

B. Documenting temperature, level of consciousness, mental status, neuromuscular function, hydration status, and degree of nausea on admission and discharge and more frequently if appropriate are also minimum standards of care.

C. Every patient should be continuously monitored with a pulse oximeter and at least a single-lead electrocardiogram. Capnography is necessary for patients receiving mechanical ventilation and those at risk for compromised ventilatory function.

D. Anesthesiology personnel should manage the patient until a PACU nurse secures admission vital signs and attaches appropriate monitors. Care should be transferred with a complete report to the nursing staff (Table 55-1).

VI. POSTOPERATIVE PAIN MANAGEMENT

Relief of surgical pain with minimal side effects is a major goal during PACU care and is a top priority for patients.

A. In addition to improving comfort, analgesia reduces sympathetic nervous system response, avoiding hypertension, tachycardia, and dysrhythmias. In hypovolemic patients, the sympathetic nervous system activity may well mask relative hypovolemia.

B. Administration of analgesics may precipitate hypotension in an apparently stable patient, especially if direct or histamine-induced vasodilation occurs. Before giving analgesics that might precipitate or accentuate hypotension, it is important to carefully assess a tachycardic patient with low or normal blood pressure who complains of pain.

C. The best measure of analgesia is the patient's perception. Heart rate, respiratory rate and depth, sweating, and nausea and vomiting may be signs of pain, but their absence or presence is not in itself reliable as a measure of the presence of pain.

D. Surgical pain can be effectively treated with intravenous (IV) opioids as part of a planned analgesic continuum that begins before the induction of surgical anesthesia and continues throughout the postoperative course.

TABLE 55-1

COMPONENTS OF A POSTANESTHESIA CARE UNIT ADMISSION REPORT

Preoperative History and Procedures
Medication allergies or reactions
Pertinent earlier surgical procedures
Underlying medical illness
Chronic medications
Acute problems (ischemia, acid–base status, dehydration)
Premedications (antibiotics and time given, beta-adrenergic blockers, antiemetics)
Preoperative pain control (nerve blocks, adjunct medications, narcotics)
Preoperative pain assessment (chronic and acute pain scores)
NPO status

Intraoperative Factors
Surgical procedure
Type of anesthetic
Type and difficulty of airway management
Relaxant and reversal status
Time and amount of opioids administered
Type and amount of IV fluids administered
Estimated blood loss
Urine output
Unexpected surgical or anesthetic events
Intraoperative vital sign ranges
Intraoperative laboratory findings
Drugs given (steroids, diuretics, antibiotics, vasoactive medications, antiemetics)

Assessment and Report of Current Status
Airway patency
Ventilatory adequacy
Level of consciousness
Level of pain
Heart rate and heart rhythm
Endotracheal tube position
Systemic pressure
Intravascular volume status
Function of invasive monitors
Size and location of intravenous catheters
Anesthetic equipment (epidural catheters, peripheral nerve catheters)
Overall impression

PERIOPERATIVE

(continued)

TABLE 55-1

COMPONENTS OF A POSTANESTHESIA CARE UNIT ADMISSION
REPORT (*Continued*)

Postoperative Instructions
Expected airway and ventilatory status
Acceptable vital sign ranges
Acceptable urine output and blood loss
Surgical instructions (positioning, wound care)
Anticipated cardiovascular problems
Orders for therapeutic interventions
Diagnostic tests to be secured
Therapeutic goals and end points before discharge
Location of responsible physician

IV = intravenous.

1. Short-acting opioids are useful to expedite discharge
   and minimize nausea in ambulatory settings,
   although the duration of analgesia can be a
   problem. Other analgesic modalities provide pain
   relief in and beyond the PACU.
2. IV opioid loading in the PACU is important for
   smooth transition to IV patient-controlled analgesia.
3. Injection of opioids into the epidural or subarachnoid
   space during anesthesia or in the PACU yields
   prolonged postoperative analgesia in selected patients.
   Nausea and pruritus are troubling side effects, and
   immediate or delayed ventilatory depression may
   occur related to vascular uptake and cephalad spread
   in cerebrospinal fluid. Nausea should resolve with
   antiemetics, and pruritus and ventilatory depression
   often respond to naloxone infusion.
4. Placement of long-acting regional analgesic blocks
   reduces pain, controls sympathetic nervous system
   activity, and often improves ventilation.
   a. After shoulder procedures, interscalene block yields
      almost complete pain relief with only moderate
      inconvenience from motor impairment. Paralysis of
      the ipsilateral diaphragm may impair postoperative
      ventilation in patients with marginal reserve,
      although the impact is small in most patients.
   b. Suprascapular nerve block might be an alterna-
      tive to avoid this potentially serious side effect.
   c. Caudal analgesia is effective in children after
      inguinal or genital procedures. Infiltration of
      local anesthetic into joints, soft tissues, or inci-
      sions decreases the intensity of pain.

VII. DISCHARGE CRITERIA (Table 55-2)

TABLE 55-2

THE TWO MOST COMMONLY USED POSTANESTHESIA CARE UNIT DISCHARGE CRITERIA SYSTEMS

Modified Aldrete Scoring System	Postanesthetic Discharge Scoring System
Respiration 2 = Able to take deep breath and cough 1 = Dyspnea or shallow breathing 0 = Apnea	**Vital Signs** 2 = BP and pulse within 20% of preoperative baseline 1 = BP and pulse within 20%–40% of preoperative baseline 0 = BP and pulse >40% of preoperative baseline
O_2 Saturation 2 = Maintains Spo_2 >92% on room air 1 = Needs O_2 inhalation to maintain O_2 saturation >90% 0 = O_2 saturation <90% even with supplemental O_2	**Activity** 2 = Steady gait, no dizziness, or meets preoperative level 1 = Requires assistance 0 = Unable to ambulate
Consciousness 2 = Fully awake 1 = Arousable on calling 0 = Not responding	**Nausea and Vomiting** 2 = Minimal; treated with PO medication 1 = Moderate; treated with parenteral medication 0 = Severe; continues despite treatment
Circulation 2 = BP ± 20 mm Hg preoperative 1 = BP ± 20–50 mm Hg preoperative 0 = BP ± 50 mm Hg pre	**Pain** Controlled with oral analgesics and acceptable to patient: 2 = Yes 1 = No
Activity 2 = Able to move four extremities voluntarily or on command 1 = Able to move two extremities 0 = Unable to move extremities	**Surgical Bleeding** 2 = Minimal or no dressing changes 1 = Moderate or ≤2 dressing changes required 0 = Severe or >3 dressing changes required
Score ≥9 for discharge	**Score ≥9 for discharge**

BP = blood pressure; PO = per os.

VIII. STANDARDS FOR POSTANESTHESIA CARE

The American Society of Anesthesiologists (ASA) House of Delegates approved Standards for Postanesthesia Care on October 12, 1988, and last amended them on October 27, 2004.

IX. CARDIOVASCULAR COMPLICATIONS

A. The first sign of myocardial ischemia may well be hypotension, and the most common sign of myocardial ischemia is tachycardia. Early intervention with nitrates, opioids, beta-blockers, and even anticoagulants may save lives. Cardiology should be involved to gain immediate and timely access to the cardiac catheterization laboratory or for anxiolytic drug therapy.

B. Congestive heart failure is epidemic in our ever-aging population. Echocardiography allows rapid viewing of myocardial contractility, regional wall motion, volume status, and valvular dysfunction.

X. POSTOPERATIVE PULMONARY DYSFUNCTION

A. **Inadequate postoperative ventilation** should be suspected when (1) respiratory acidemia occurs coincident with tachypnea, anxiety, dyspnea, labored ventilation, or increased sympathetic nervous system activity; (2) hypercarbia reduces the arterial pH below 7.30; or (3) $PaCO_2$ progressively increases with a progressive decrease in arterial pH.

B. **Inadequate Respiratory Drive**

1. During early recovery from anesthesia, residual effects of IV and inhalational anesthetics blunt the ventilatory responses to both hypercarbia and hypoxemia. Sedatives augment depression from opioids or anesthetics and reduce the conscious desire to ventilate.

2. Hypoventilation and hypercarbia may evolve insidiously during transfer and admission to the PACU. Although the effects of intraoperative medications are usually waning, the peak depressant effect of IV opioid given just before transfer occurs in the PACU.

3. Patients may communicate lucidly and even complain of pain while experiencing significant opioid-induced

hypoventilation. A balance must be struck between an acceptable level of postoperative ventilatory depression and a tolerable level of pain or agitation.

4. Patients with abnormal CO_2/pH responses from morbid obesity, chronic airway obstruction, or sleep apnea are more sensitive to respiratory depressants.

5. The abrupt diminution of a noxious stimulus (tracheal extubation, placement of a postoperative block) may promote hypoventilation or airway obstruction by altering the balance between arousal from discomfort and depression from medication.

C. **Increased airway resistance** increases the work of breathing and CO_2 production.

1. In postoperative patients, increased upper airway resistance is caused by obstruction in the pharynx, larynx (laryngospasm, laryngeal edema), or large airways (extrinsic compression from hematoma).

2. Weakness from residual neuromuscular relaxation may contribute but is seldom the primary cause of airway compromise.

3. Laryngospasm can usually be overcome by providing gentle positive pressure (10–20 mm Hg continuous) in the oropharynx by mask with 100% oxygen. Prolonged laryngospasm is relieved with a small dose of succinylcholine (0.1 mg/kg) or deepening sedation with propofol.

D. **Decreased compliance** accentuates the work of breathing. Obesity affects pulmonary compliance, especially when adipose tissue compresses the thoracic cage or increases intra-abdominal pressure in the supine or lateral positions. Allowing patients to recover in a semi-sitting (semi-Fowler's) position reduces the work of breathing.

E. **Neuromuscular and Skeletal Problems**

1. Postoperative airway obstruction and hypoventilation are accentuated by incomplete reversal of neuromuscular relaxation. Residual paralysis compromises airway patency, the ability to overcome airway resistance, airway protection, and the ability to clear secretions.

2. PACU staff should be aware of patients who have received nondepolarizing muscle relaxants but have not received reversal agents because these patients often exhibit low levels of residual paralysis, and in the presence of severe kyphosis or scoliosis may cause postoperative ventilatory insufficiency.

PERIOPERATIVE

3. Simple tests help assess the patient's mechanical ability to ventilate. The ability to sustain head elevation in a supine position, a forced vital capacity of 10 to 12 mL/kg, an inspiratory pressure that is lower than −25 cm H_2O, and tactile train-of-four assessment imply that the strength of ventilatory muscles is adequate to sustain ventilation and to take a large enough breath to cough. However, none of these clinical end points reliably predicts the recovery of airway protective reflexes, and failure on these tests does not necessarily indicate the need for assisted ventilation.

F. **Inadequate Postoperative Oxygenation**

1. Systemic arterial partial pressure of oxygen (PaO_2) is the best indicator of pulmonary oxygen transfer from alveolar gas to pulmonary capillary blood.

2. Arterial hemoglobin saturation monitored by pulse oximetry yields less information on alveolar–arterial gradients and is not helpful in assessing the impact of hemoglobin dissociation curve shifts or carboxyhemoglobin.

3. In postoperative patients, the acceptable lower limit for PaO_2 varies with individual patient characteristics. Maintaining PaO_2 between 80 and 100 mm Hg (saturation, 93% to 97%) ensures adequate oxygen availability. Little benefit is derived from elevating PaO_2 above 110 mm Hg because hemoglobin is saturated, and the amount of additional oxygen dissolved in plasma is negligible.

4. During mechanical ventilation, a PaO_2 above 80 mm Hg with 0.4 fraction of inspired oxygen (FIO_2) and 5 cm H_2O positive end-expiratory pressure (PEEP), continuous positive airway pressure (CPAP), or a spontaneous breathing trial usually predicts sustained adequate oxygenation after tracheal extubation.

G. **Obstructive sleep apnea** (OSA) is a syndrome in which patients exhibit a period of partial or complete obstruction of the upper airway (Table 55-3).

1. In May 2003, the ASA Task Force on Perioperative Management of Patients with Obstructive Sleep Apnea issued guidelines for patients with OSA.

2. The perioperative management of a patient with OSA must start preoperatively with a well-planned anesthetic, taking into account the type, location, and recovery of surgery.

TABLE 55-3

MANIFESTATIONS OF OBSTRUCTIVE SLEEP APNEA

Daytime hypersomnolence
Decreased ability to concentrate
Increased irritability
Episodic oxygen desaturation
Hypercarbia

    a. Postoperative management concerns include analgesia, oxygenation, patient positioning, and monitoring.

    b. Regional anesthesia with minimal sedation (rather than increased use of opioids) is best for recovery.

    c. Patients who use CPAP or noninvasive positive-pressure ventilation should continue to use these therapies.

    d. Pulse oximetry should be used until the patient's oxygen saturation remains above 90% on room air while sleeping.

H. Anemia

    1. Patients with vascular disease are at increased risk of vital organ ischemia as hematocrit decreases.

    2. It is now well accepted that patients who are stable, not bleeding, and euvolemic can tolerate a hemoglobin level of 6.0 g/dL. Transfusion may be of some benefit between 6 and 8 g/dL but is rarely of use above 10 g/dL.

I. Supplemental Oxygen

    1. Clinical observation and assessment of cognitive function do not accurately screen for hypoxemia, so monitoring with oximetry is essential throughout the PACU admission.

    2. One cannot predict which patients will develop hypoxemia or when hypoxemia will occur. However, patients with lung disease or obesity, those recovering from thoracic or upper abdominal procedures, and those with preoperative hypoxemia are at increased risk.

    3. Supplemental oxygen does not address the underlying causes of hypoxemia in postoperative patients, its use does not guarantee that hypoxemia will not occur, and it is likely to mask hypoventilation.

PERIOPERATIVE

J. **Perioperative Aspiration.** During anesthesia, depression of airway reflexes places patients at risk for intraoperative pulmonary aspiration that may manifest in the PACU or for aspiration during recovery.

1. Aspiration of acidic gastric contents during vomiting or regurgitation causes chemical pneumonitis initially characterized by diffuse bronchospasm, hypoxemia, and atelectasis.

2. The incidence of serious aspiration is relatively low in PACU patients, but the risk is still significant. Hypotension, hypoxemia, or acidemia cause both emesis and obtundation, increasing the risk of aspiration.

3. Suspicion that aspiration has occurred mandates 24 to 48 hours of monitoring for development of aspiration pneumonitis. If the likelihood of aspiration is small in an ambulatory patient, outpatient follow-up can be done, assuming hypoxemia, cough, wheezing, and radiographic abnormalities do not appear within 4 to 6 hours. The patient should receive explicit instructions to contact a medical facility at the first appearance of malaise, fever, cough, chest pain, or other symptoms of pneumonitis. If likelihood of aspiration is high, the patient should be admitted to the hospital.

XI. POSTOPERATIVE RENAL COMPLICATIONS

A. The **ability to void** should be assessed because opioids and autonomic side effects of regional anesthesia interfere with sphincter relaxation and promote urine retention. An ultrasonic bladder scan helps assess bladder volume before discharge.

B. **Oliguria** (≤ 0.5 mL/kg/hr) occurs frequently during recovery and usually reflects an appropriate renal response to hypovolemia. The stress response of surgery also increases antidiuretic hormone (ADH), which may lead to decreased urine output. Decreased urine output may also indicate abnormal renal function. Systemic blood pressure must be adequate for renal perfusion based on preoperative pressures.

1. After urine is sent for electrolyte and osmolarity determinations, a 300- to 500-mL IV crystalloid bolus helps assess whether oliguria represents a renal response to hypovolemia. If output does not

improve, a larger bolus or a diagnostic trial of furosemide (5 mg IV) should be considered.

2. The persistence of oliguria despite hydration, adequate perfusion pressure, and a furosemide challenge increases the likelihood of acute tubular necrosis, ureteral obstruction, renal artery or vein occlusion, and inappropriate ADH secretion. Consultation with a nephrologist is prudent.

XII. METABOLIC COMPLICATIONS

A. **Postoperative Acid–Base Disorders.** Categorization of postoperative acid–base abnormalities into primary and compensatory disorders is difficult because rapidly changing pathophysiology can often generate multiple primary disorders.

B. **Respiratory acidemia** is frequently encountered in PACU patients because anesthetics, opioids, and sedatives promote hypoventilation by depressing central nervous system (CNS) sensitivity to pH and $PaCO_2$.

1. Symptoms of respiratory acidemia include agitation, confusion, and tachypnea. Sympathetic nervous system response to low pH causes hypertension, tachycardia, and dysrhythmias.

2. Treatment consists of correcting the imbalance between CO_2 production and alveolar ventilation. Increasing the level of consciousness by the judicious reversal of opioids or benzodiazepines improves ventilatory drive. It is important to ensure that the patient does not have increased airway resistance or residual neuromuscular blockade. If spontaneous ventilation cannot maintain CO_2 excretion, tracheal intubation and mechanical ventilation are necessary.

C. **Metabolic Acidemia** (Table 55-4)

1. Large volumes of saline infusions during surgery can generate a mild hyperchloremic, metabolic acidemia, but use of lactated Ringer's solution avoids this problem.

2. Postoperative metabolic acidemia almost always represents lactic acidemia secondary to insufficient delivery or utilization of oxygen in peripheral tissues. Peripheral hypoperfusion is often caused by low cardiac output (hypovolemia, cardiac failure, dysrhythmia) or peripheral vasodilation (sepsis, catecholamine depletion, sympathectomy).

PERIOPERATIVE

TABLE 55-4
CAUSES OF ACIDEMIA

Normal Anion Gap Acidosis
GI loss of bicarbonate
  Diarrhea
  Urinary diversion
  GI fistulas or drains
Renal loss of bicarbonate
  Renal tubular acidosis
  Renal insufficiency
  Recovery phase of ketoacidosis

Increased Anion Gap Acidosis
Ketoacidosis (diabetic, alcoholic, severe cachexia)
Lactic acidosis (seizures, neuroleptic malignant syndrome, MH,
  severe asthma, pheochromocytoma, cardiogenic shock,
  hypovolemia, severe anemia, regional ischemia, sepsis,
  hypoglycemia)

Respiratory Acidosis

GI = gastrointestinal; MH = malignant hyperthermia.

3. A spontaneously breathing patient will increase minute ventilation in response to metabolic acidemia and quickly generate a respiratory alkalosis to compensate for metabolic acidemia (general anesthetics and analgesics suppress this ventilatory response).

D. Respiratory Alkalemia

1. Pain or anxiety during emergence causes hyperventilation and acute respiratory alkalemia. Excessive mechanical ventilation also generates respiratory alkalemia, especially if hypothermia or paralysis has decreased CO_2 production.

2. Acute respiratory alkalemia may lead to confusion, dizziness, atrial dysrhythmias, and abnormal cardiac conduction. Alkalemia decreases cerebral blood flow. If the alkalemia is severe, reduced serum ionized calcium concentration precipitates muscle fasciculation or hypocalcemic tetany.

3. Metabolic compensation for acute respiratory alkalemia is limited because time constants for bicarbonate excretion are large.

4. Treatment necessitates reducing alveolar ventilation, usually by administering analgesics and sedatives for pain and anxiety. Rebreathing of CO_2 has little application in the PACU.

E. **Metabolic alkalemia** is rare in PACU patients unless vomiting, gastric suctioning, dehydration, alkaline ingestion, or potassium-wasting diuretics have caused an alkalemia that existed before surgery. Respiratory compensation through retention of CO_2 is rapid but limited because hypoventilation eventually causes hypoxemia. Hydration and correction of hypochloremia and hypokalemia allow the kidney to excrete excess bicarbonate.

XIII. GLUCOSE DISORDERS AND CONTROL

Tight glucose control has been recommended to reduce morbidity in a variety of postsurgical patients. The potential for hypoglycemia and coma should not be discounted.

A. **Hyperglycemia.** Glucose infusions and stress responses commonly elevate serum glucose levels after surgery. For most patients, glucose should not be included in maintenance IV solutions during anesthesia.

1. Moderate postoperative hyperglycemia (150–250 mg/dL) resolves spontaneously and has little adverse effect in nondiabetic patients.

2. Higher glucose levels cause glycosuria with osmotic diuresis and interfere with serum electrolyte determinations. Severe hyperglycemia increases serum osmolality to a point that cerebral disequilibrium and hyperosmolar coma occur.

B. **Hypoglycemia** in the PACU is rare and easily treated with IV 50% dextrose followed by glucose infusion. Either sedation or excessive sympathetic nervous system activity masks the signs and symptoms of hypoglycemia after anesthesia. Diabetic patients and especially patients who have received insulin therapy intraoperatively must have serum glucose levels measured to avoid the serious problems related to hypoglycemia.

XIV. ELECTROLYTE DISORDERS

A. **Hyponatremia.** Postoperative hyponatremia occurs if free water is infused IV during surgery or if sodium-free irrigating solution is absorbed during transurethral prostatic resection or hysteroscopy.

1. Symptoms of moderate hyponatremia include agitation, disorientation, visual disturbances, and

nausea. Severe hyponatremia causes unconsciousness, impaired airway reflexes, and CNS irritability that progress to grand mal seizures.

2. Therapy includes IV normal saline and IV furosemide to promote free water excretion.

B. **Hypokalemia**

1. A potassium deficit caused by chronic diuretic therapy, nasogastric suctioning, or vomiting often underlies hypokalemia.

2. Potassium is an intracellular ion, and a plasma potassium deficit is indicative of a far greater intracellular deficit. The intracellular to extracellular ratio may well be important, and rapid changes may contribute to as many dysrhythmias as can mild hypokalemia alone.

C. **Hyperkalemia**

1. A high serum potassium level raises the suspicion of spurious hyperkalemia from a hemolyzed specimen

---

TABLE 55-5

MISCELLANEOUS COMPLICATIONS IN THE POSTANESTHESIA CARE UNIT

Incidental trauma (should be documented and the physician notified)

Ocular injuries and visual changes (corneal abrasion caused by dry or inadvertent eye contact)

Hearing impairment (after dural puncture for spinal anesthesia)

Oral, pharyngeal, and laryngeal injuries (dental injury, sore throat, hoarseness)

Nerve injuries (malpositioning, compression, postspinal anesthesia, idiopathic)

Soft tissue and joint injuries

Skeletal muscle pain (succinylcholine, immobility)

Hypothermia and shivering (complicates and prolongs care in the PACU)

Persistent sedation (approximately 90% of patients regain consciousness within 15 minutes of admission to the PACU; unconsciousness persisting for a greater period is considered prolonged, and pharmacologic reversal should be considered; if the condition is persistent, a neurologist should be consulted)

Altered mental status (combativeness, disorientation)

Emergence reactions (evaluate oxygenation and ventilation)

Delirium and cognitive decline (especially elderly patients)

PACU = postanesthesia care unit.

or from sampling near an IV catheter containing potassium or banked blood. Acute acidemia exacerbates hyperkalemia.

2. Treatment with IV insulin and glucose acutely lowers potassium, and treatment with IV calcium counters myocardial effects.

XV. MISCELLANEOUS COMPLICATIONS (Table 55-5)

CHAPTER 56 ■ **CRITICAL CARE MEDICINE**

In North America, anesthesiologists were integral to the development of critical care medicine as a specialty (Treggiari MA, Deem S: Critical care medicine. In *Clinical Anesthesia*. Edited by Barash PG, Cullen BF, Stoelting RK, Cahalan MK, Stock MC. Philadelphia: Lippincott Williams & Wilkins, 2009, pp 1444–1472). However, in contrast to other countries, in the United States, anesthesiologists have played an ever-diminishing role in the specialty, and today they make up a minority of the intensivist workforce. The driving forces behind intensive care unit (ICU) development included advances in surgical techniques, polio epidemics that resulted in widespread respiratory failure, and later the recognition of the acute respiratory distress syndrome (ARDS). In the late 1960s, a group including Dr. Safar and another anesthesiologist, Ake Grenvik, were instrumental in inaugurating the Society of Critical Care Medicine (SCCM). Anesthesiologists working through SCCM were instrumental in developing the board certification process for critical care medicine, and in 1986, the first Critical Care Medicine Certification examination was administered by the American Board of Anesthesiology.

I. ANESTHESIOLOGY AND CRITICAL CARE MEDICINE: THE FUTURE

Forces that will shape the evolution of the specialty of critical care medicine and the contribution that anesthesiologists will make to this evolution include quality of care issues and the contribution of intensivists to improved ICU outcomes, business and economic factors, and the aging population and increasing demand for critical care services. Mortality and other intermediate end points such as ICU length of stay can be reduced when "high-intensity" physician staffing models that mandate management or co-management by intensivists are used.

TABLE 56-1

EVALUATING EVIDENCE FOR MEDICAL THERAPIES

Levels of Evidence
Large, randomized trials with clear-cut results; low risk of false-positive (α) or false-negative (β) errors
Small, randomized trials with uncertain results; moderate to high risk of false-positive (α) or false-negative (β) errors
Non-randomized, contemporaneous controls
Non-randomized, historical controls, and expert opinion
Case series, uncontrolled studies, and expert opinion

Grades of Recommendation Based on Expert Consensus*
Supported by two or more level I studies
Supported by only one level I study
Supported by level II studies
Supported by level III studies
Supported by level IV or V studies

II. CRITICAL CARE MEDICINE: A SYSTEM AND EVIDENCE-BASED APPROACH (Table 56-1)

A. Process of Care in the Intensive Care Unit

1. Implementation of evidence-based practices in the ICU could save up to 200,000 lives per year in the United States.

2. **The Leapfrog Group** is a coalition of more than 150 purchasers and providers of health care benefits with the stated goal of improving healthcare, particularly by reducing deaths caused by medical errors. To accomplish this aim, the Group formulated the Leapfrog Initiative, which includes a series of "safety standards" that health care providers (largely hospitals) should strive for if they are to provide care for Leapfrog.

III. NEUROLOGIC AND NEUROSURGICAL CRITICAL CARE

A. **Neuromonitoring** devices used in the ICU setting may help in assessing pathophysiologic processes and adjusting therapy.

1. **Transcranial Doppler (TCD) ultrasonography** measures mean, peak systolic, and end-diastolic flow velocities and indirectly estimates cerebral blood

PERIOPERATIVE

flow. In patients with subarachnoid hemorrhage (SAH) or traumatic brain injury (TBI), TCD can be used as a tool to identify vasospasm. In patients with TBI, flow velocities are depressed, and impaired autoregulation and vascular reactivity are common. In these patients, monitoring of TCD and jugular venous oxygen saturation (SjO_2) may be used to define the optimum cerebral perfusion pressure (CPP) level.

2. **Brain tissue oxygenation** ($PbrO_2$) measurements are performed by introducing a small, oxygen-sensitive catheter into the brain tissue (normal $PbrO_2$ values, 25–30 mm Hg). An increase in intracranial pressure (ICP) and a decrease in CPP or arterial oxygenation along with hyperventilation may result in decreased $PbrO_2$. CPP above 60 mm Hg has been identified as the most important factor determining sufficient brain tissue oxygenation.

3. **Microdialysis** uses a probe as an interface to the brain to continuously monitor the chemistry of a small focal volume of the cerebral extracellular space. (This allows measurement of chemical substances such as lactate, pyruvate, glucose, glutamate, glycerol, metabolites of several biochemical pathways, and electrolytes and thus provides insight into the bioenergetic status of the brain.) Increased lactate, decreased glucose, and an elevated lactate/glucose ratio indicate accelerated anaerobic glycolysis. This metabolic pattern commonly occurs with cerebral ischemia or hypoxia, and increased glycolysis in this setting is associated with a poor outcome.

B. **Diagnosis and Clinical Management of the Most Common Types of Neurologic Failure**

1. **Traumatic brain injury** is the leading cause of death from blunt trauma, and in patients between the age of 5 and 45 years, TBI represents the leading cause of death (Table 56-2). Examination of the pupils can predict neurologic outcome.

a. **Resuscitation.** The goal of resuscitation in traumatic and other types of brain injury is to prevent continuing cerebral insult after a primary injury has occurred. A primary insult is often associated with intracranial hypertension and systemic hypotension, leading to decreased

TABLE 56-2

PREDICTORS OF POOR OUTCOME AFTER TRAUMATIC
BRAIN INJURY

Age >55 years
Poor pupillary reactivity (bilateral dilated and unreactive
  associated with poor neurologic outcome and death as high as
  90%)
Postresuscitation Glasgow Coma Scale score (most widely used
  measure of injury severity; may be unmeasurable initially; injury
  is severe when score is ≤8)
Hypotension
Hypoxia
Unfavorable intracranial diagnosis based on radiologic features
  (CT scan, degree of diffuse injury, and midline shift)
Hyperglycemia (>200 mg/dL)

cerebral perfusion and brain ischemia.
Concomitant hypoxemia aggravates brain
hypoxia, especially in the presence of hyperthermia, which increases the brain's metabolic
demand. The combined effect of these factors
leads to secondary brain injury characterized by
excitotoxicity, oxidative stress, and inflammation. The resulting cerebral ischemia may be the
single most important secondary event affecting
outcome after a cerebral insult.

b. **Prevention of secondary injury** is the main goal
of resuscitative efforts. Traumatized areas of the
brain manifest impaired autoregulation, with
increased dependency of flow on perfusion pressure and disruption of the blood–brain barrier.
The goals of neuroresuscitation are oriented at
restoration of cerebral blood flow by maintenance of adequate CPP, reduction of ICP, evacuation of space-occupying lesions, and initiation of
therapies for cerebral protection and avoidance
of hypoxia (Table 56-3).

c. **Drug-Induced Sedation.** A common practice is to
provide sedation with propofol or benzodiazepines in patients after TBI. These agents have
favorable effects on cerebral oxygen balance.
Despite the induction of systemic hypotension,
propofol decreases cerebral metabolism, resulting

TABLE 56-3

INTENSIVE CARE UNIT MANAGEMENT OF PATIENTS WITH SEVERE TRAUMATIC BRAIN INJURY (ASSUMING INITIAL SURGICAL MANAGEMENT)

Head elevation 30 to 45 degrees*
CPP >70 mm Hg
Euvolemia, vasopressors as needed
ICP <20 mm Hg
  Mannitol, hypertonic saline
  CSF drainage
SaO_2 ≥95%; $PaCO_2$ 35–40 mm Hg
Temperature ≤37°C
Glucose <180 mg/dL
Sedation and analgesia
Early enteral nutrition
Seizure, stress ulcer, and DVT prophylaxis
Refractory intracranial hypertension
  Optimized hyperventilation with SjO2 monitoring, PbrO2
    monitoring, or both
  Barbiturate coma
  Mild therapeutic hypothermia (33°–35°C)
  Decompressive craniectomy

*Unless contraindicated by spine injury or hemodynamic instability.
CPP = cerebral perfusion pressure; DVT = deep vein thrombosis; ICP = intracranial pressure.

in a coupled decline in cerebral blood flow with consequent decrease in ICP. Barbiturates should be considered if ICP is not controlled by moderate doses of propofol. Although neuromuscular blockade may result in a decrease in ICP, the routine use of neuromuscular blockade is discouraged because its use has been associated with longer ICU course, a higher incidence of pneumonia, and a trend toward more frequent sepsis without any improvement in outcome.

d. **Hyperventilation** effectively reduces ICP by reducing CBF, but in small randomized trials, prophylactic hyperventilation has not proven to be beneficial in patients with TBI. Prolonged or prophylactic hyperventilation should be avoided after severe TBI. Hyperventilation may be necessary for brief periods to reduce intracranial hypertension refractory to sedation, osmotic therapy, and cerebrospinal fluid drainage, and should be guided by SjO_2, $PbrO_2$, or both (a decrease in either of these values suggests a harmful effect of hyperventilation).

e. **Hypothermia.** There is insufficient evidence to provide recommendations for the use of moderate hypothermia in patients with TBI.

f. **Corticosteroids** to reduce posttraumatic inflammatory injury should not be administered as therapy for acute TBI.

g. Anticonvulsants may be used to prevent early posttraumatic seizures within 7 days after head trauma. (Evidence does not indicate that prevention of early seizures improves outcome after TBI.)

h. **Albumin** as fluid replacement therapy in patients with TBI may increase mortality when compared with saline.

2. **Subarachnoid hemorrhage** is most commonly caused by the rupture of an intracranial aneurysm with only one third of the patients with SAH being functional survivors. The leading causes of death and disability are the direct effects of the initial bleed—cerebral vasospasm and rebleeding. At the time of aneurysm rupture, a critical reduction in CBF takes place because of an increase in ICP toward arterial diastolic values. The persistence of a no-flow pattern is associated with acute vasospasm. In survivors of the initial bleed, emphasis has been placed on early aneurysm securing with either surgery or interventional neuroradiology (coiling). Early aneurysm occlusion substantially reduces the risk of this rebleeding.

a. **Cerebral vasospasm** after SAH is correlated with the amount and location of subarachnoid blood. A reduction in cerebral blood flow is ultimately responsible for the appearance of delayed ischemic neurologic deficits (DINDS). Oral nimodipine (60 mg every 4 hours for 21 days) as prophylaxis for cerebral vasospasm is recognized as an effective treatment in improving neurologic outcome (reduction of cerebral infarction and poor outcome) and mortality from cerebral vasospasm in patients with SAH. The benefits of nimodipine have been attributed to a cytoprotective effect related to the reduced availability of intracellular calcium and improved microvascular collateral flow.

   b. **Hypervolemic, hypertensive, and hemodilution ("triple-H") therapy** is one of the mainstays of treatment for cerebral ischemia associated with SAH-induced vasospasm despite the lack of evidence for its effectiveness. The rationale for hypertension derives from the concept that a loss of cerebral autoregulation associated with vasospasm results in pressure-dependent blood flow. Hemodilution is a consequence of hypervolemic therapy and is thought to optimize the rheologic properties of the blood and thereby improve microcirculatory flow. Common complications of treatment are pulmonary edema and myocardial ischemia.

   c. **Interventional neuroradiology** with the use of balloon angioplasty (within 6 to 12 hours) can reverse or improve vasospasm-induced neurologic deficits.

   d. **Hyponatremia** usually develops several days after the hemorrhage and is attributed to a syndrome of inappropriate antidiuretic hormone (SIADH) and an excess of free water.

3. **Acute Ischemic Stroke.** More than half of strokes can be attributed to a thrombotic mechanism. Transient ischemic attacks may precede stroke and thus should be considered a warning sign.

   a. **Thrombolysis.** Rapid clot lysis and restoration of circulation using alteplase (rt-PA) should be provided within 3 hours of stroke onset. Patients receiving systemic rt-PA should not receive aspirin, heparin, warfarin, clonidine, or other antithrombotic or antiplatelet aggregating drugs within 24 hours of treatment. Because hyperglycemia is associated with poor outcome in ischemic stroke, tight glucose control is recommended. (The mortality benefit at 90 days has not been demonstrated.)

4. **Anoxic brain injury** most commonly occurs as a result of cardiac arrest. The pathophysiology of anoxic brain injury is multifactorial and includes excitatory neurotransmitter release, accumulation of intracellular calcium, and oxygen free radical generation. A strong experimental literature supports a

role for mild therapeutic hypothermia in anoxic brain injury (temperature. 32°–34°C). Hypothermia is recommended in neonatal hypoxic encephalopathy.

IV. CARDIOVASCULAR AND HEMODYNAMIC ASPECTS OF CRITICAL CARE

A. **Principles of Monitoring and Resuscitation.** Shock states are associated with impairment of adequate oxygen delivery, resulting in decreased tissue perfusion and tissue hypoxia. (Global hemodynamic monitoring may not reflect regional perfusion or the peripheral tissue energy status.) Invasive monitoring in shock states provides insight into the circulatory status, organ perfusion, tissue microcirculation, and cellular metabolic status of the critically ill patient.

B. **Functional Hemodynamic Monitoring**
   1. **Pulmonary Artery Catheter (PAC).** The information provided by the PAC may assist in the differentiation of cardiogenic and noncardiogenic circulatory and respiratory failure and may help guide fluid, inotropic, and vasopressor therapy.
      a. Despite the theoretical benefits of pulmonary artery catheterization, little data support a positive effect of PACs on mortality or other substantive outcome variables. A trial conducted in patients assigned to receive PAC-guided or central venous catheter–guided therapy did not find any survival or organ function differences between the two groups, and there was an equal number of catheter-related complications (dysrhythmias).
      b. Studies do not support the routine use of the PAC for the management of acute lung injury (ALI) or septic shock.
   2. **Arterial Pressure Waveform Analysis.** The variation in systolic blood pressure and pulse pressure during positive pressure ventilation is highly predictive of the response to intravascular fluid administration in both normal subjects and critically ill patients. Cardiac output derived using pulse contour analysis correlates well with thermodilution cardiac output in a variety of conditions and has the advantage of providing continuous measurement without necessitating the

placement of a PAC. The use of pulse contour analysis may potentially obviate the need for pulmonary artery catheterization to measure cardiac output, particularly if combined with the measurement of $ScvO_2$ as an indicator of the balance between oxygen delivery and consumption.

3. **Echocardiography.** Transthoracic and transesophageal echocardiography (TEE) provide accurate noninvasive diagnostic information with regard to right and left ventricular function, valve function, pericardium anatomy, traumatic vascular injury, and pulmonary embolism (direct and indirect signs). TEE can also be used to assess volume status or preload via measurement of left ventricular end-diastolic volume or area.

C. **Definition and Types of Circulatory Failure.** The common denominator of shock is circulatory instability characterized by severe hypotension and inadequate tissue perfusion. Shock states are classified according to the primary cause of circulatory failure. Distributive or vasodilatory shock results from a reduction in systemic vascular resistance (SVR) often associated with an increased cardiac output. On the other hand, cardiogenic (left or right cardiac failure) and hypovolemic shock are low cardiac output states that are usually characterized by increased peripheral resistance. The most common forms of shock encountered in the ICU are cardiogenic, septic, and hypovolemic shock.

1. **Cardiogenic Shock.** The initiating event in cardiogenic shock is a primary pump failure (myocardial infarction, cardiomyopathy, arrhythmias, mechanical complications [mitral regurgitation, ventricular septal defect], tamponade). The onset of pump failure is associated with a compensatory reflex vasoconstriction in systemic vessels that causes an increase in left ventricular workload and myocardial oxygen demand and a redistribution of blood volume toward the heart and the lungs. Consequently, therapy should minimize myocardial oxygen demand and increase oxygen delivery to the ischemic area; this goal is complicated by the fact that many resuscitative approaches to correct hypotension (preload augmentation, inotropes, and vasopressors) increase myocardial oxygen

consumption. In patients without hypotension, pharmacologic vasodilatation using nitrates or sodium nitroprusside may reduce myocardial oxygen consumption and improve ventricular ejection by reducing left ventricular afterload and possibly produce a shift of blood from the lungs to the periphery by reducing venous tone. When pharmacologic interventions are not sufficient to restore hemodynamic stability, the use of mechanical support with the insertion of intra-aortic balloon pump counterpulsation and ventricular assist devices can help unload the ventricles. In patients with myocardial infarction, coronary reperfusion can be achieved with thrombolysis or, preferably, primary percutaneous coronary intervention.

2. **Septic shock** is a form of distributive shock associated with the activation of the systemic inflammatory response, and it is usually characterized by a high cardiac output, low SVR, hypotension, and regional blood flow redistribution, resulting in tissue hypoperfusion. In patients with systemic infections, the physiologic response may be staged on a continuum from a systemic inflammatory response syndrome (SIRS) to sepsis, severe sepsis, and septic shock (Table 56-4). Multiple organ dysfunction syndrome (MODS) refers to the presence of altered organ function in an acutely ill patient such that homeostasis cannot be maintained without intervention. MODS accounts for most deaths in the ICU.

D. **Clinical Management of Shock or Circulatory Failure Based on Hemodynamic Parameters.** The mainstay of treatment of hemodynamic instability is correction of hypotension and restoration of regional blood flow with intravascular volume expansion and vasopressors, inotropes, or both. Adequacy of regional perfusion is usually assessed by evaluating indices of organ function, including myocardial ischemia, renal dysfunction (urine output and renal function tests), arterial lactate levels as an indicator of anaerobic metabolism, central nervous system dysfunction as indicated by abnormal sensorium, and hepatic parenchymal injury by liver function tests. Additional end points of treatment consist of mean arterial pressure and DO_2 or some surrogate of the latter (SvO_2 or $ScvO_2$).

TABLE 56-4

DEFINITIONS OF SEPSIS AND ORGAN FAILURE

Clinical Evidence of Infection
Infection: Microbial phenomenon characterized by an inflammatory response to the presence of microorganisms or the invasion of normally sterile tissue by those organisms.
Bacteremia: Presence of viable bacteria in the blood.

Systemic Inflammatory Response Syndrome (SIRS): Systemic inflammatory response to a variety of severe clinical insults. The response is manifested by two or more of the following conditions:
Core temperature $<36°C$ or $>38°C$
Tachycardia >90 bpm
Tachypnea >20 breaths/min while breathing spontaneously or $PaCO_2$ <32 mm Hg
White blood count $>12,000$ cells/mm^3, <4000 cells/mm^3, or $>10\%$ immature forms

Sepsis: The systemic response to infection. This systemic response is manifested by three or more of the conditions described above (SIRS) and presented clinical or microbiologic evidence of infection.

Severe Sepsis: Sepsis associated with organ dysfunction, hypoperfusion, or hypotension.
Hypoperfusion and perfusion abnormalities may include, but are not limited to, lactic acidosis, oliguria, or an acute alteration in mental status.

Septic Shock: Sepsis with hypotension despite adequate fluid resuscitation along with the presence of perfusion abnormalities that may include, but are not limited to, lactic acidosis, oliguria, or an acute alteration in mental status. Patients taking inotropic or vasopressor agents may not be hypotensive at the time that perfusion abnormalities are measured.

Sepsis-Induced Hypotension: A systolic blood pressure of <90 mm Hg or a reduction of >40 mm Hg from baseline in the absence of other causes of hypotension.

Multiple Organ Dysfunction Syndrome: Presence of several altered organ function in an acutely ill patient such that homeostasis cannot be maintained without intervention.

1. **Management of Hypotension with Fluid Replacement Therapy.** Intravascular volume expansion is the first line of therapy in all forms of shock. Clinical indicators of the response to a fluid challenge (bolus fluid therapy of 250–1000 mL of crystalloids over 5–15 minutes) are heart rate, blood

pressure, and urine output as well as invasively acquired measures, including CVP, PaOP, systolic and pulse pressure variation, and cardiac output.

2. **Management of Shock with Vasopressors or Inotropes.** If patients remain persistently hypotensive despite volume expansion and markers of adequate preload, the use of vasopressors is indicated.

   a. **Norepinephrine** (NE) increases systemic arterial pressure, with variable effects on cardiac output and heart rate. A concern that NE may compromise renal perfusion has led to some hesitancy to use this drug; however, the majority of available evidence suggests that NE improves renal function in volume-resuscitated, hypotensive patients with septic shock. NE is the drug of first choice in the management of septic shock.

   b. **Dopamine** increases mean arterial pressure by increasing cardiac index and less so SVR. Comparing low dose-dopamine with placebo in critically ill patients shows no differences in renal function tests or survival, and the use of low-dose dopamine is therefore not recommended. In addition, dopamine may have detrimental effects on the splanchnic circulation and gastric mucosal perfusion.

   c. **Dobutamine** demonstrates potent inotropic and chronotropic effects and mild peripheral vasodilatation, with the ultimate effect of increasing oxygen delivery and consumption. Dobutamine is the drug of choice in patients with circulatory failure primarily caused by cardiac pump failure (cardiogenic shock). However, dobutamine should not be used as first-line single therapy when hypotension is present.

   d. **Epinephrine** increases cardiac index by increasing contractility and heart rate, and it also increases SVR. In patients with septic shock, epinephrine may reduce splanchnic perfusion despite an increase in global hemodynamic and oxygen transport. In addition, epinephrine therapy consistently increases plasma lactate levels in septic shock. Epinephrine treatment brings no additional benefit to other catecholamine therapy in the management of patients with septic shock.

    e. Vasopressin is a potent vasoconstrictor when administered in low doses to patients in shock, particularly those with distributive shock caused by sepsis or hepatic failure or with circulatory failure after cardiopulmonary bypass. Vasopressin may also be useful in resuscitation from cardiac arrest, particularly if it is caused by asystole. Vasopressin may be added to norepinephrine with the expectation that the effect on blood pressure will be similar to that produced by norepinephrine. Epinephrine should be the first choice alternative agent in patients with septic shock who are poorly responsive to norepinephrine or dopamine.

3. **Additional Treatment Considerations for Critically Ill Patients with Septic Shock**

    a. Activated Protein C. Clinical or subclinical manifestations of disseminated intravascular coagulation and consumption coagulopathy (increase in D-dimers, decreased protein C, thrombocytopenia, and increased prothrombin time) are present in essentially all patients with septic shock. The activation of protein C is thought to be an important mechanism for modulating sepsis-induced consumption coagulopathy. Activated protein C works as an antithrombotic agent by inactivating factors Va and VIIIa. The rationale for replacing activated protein C relates to its anticoagulant and profibrinolytic properties, which interrupt the consumption coagulopathy and are particularly effective at preventing microvascular thrombosis.

    b. Corticosteroids are of no benefit for the treatment of septic shock, but low doses (hydrocortisone 200–300 mg/day) can reduce the dependency on vasopressors.

    c. Treatment of Infection. Identifying the source of the infection and early initiation of appropriate antibiotic therapy are critical priorities in addition to hemodynamic support. Empiric antibiotic therapy should be started as soon as possible after appropriate culture collection.

V. **ACUTE RESPIRATORY FAILURE** is a generic term that encompasses the need for mechanical ventilation or airway intubation, independent of cause.

A. **Principles of Mechanical Ventilation.** Mechanical ventilation in the ICU is provided through the application of positive pressure to the airway; a preset tidal volume and rate are commonly provided, and any breathing that the patient does above this set minute ventilation is either supported (assist-control [AC]) or not (intermittent mandatory ventilation [IMV]). There is little evidence to suggest that the mode of mechanical ventilation contributes significantly to any major outcome measure. Mechanical ventilation using tidal volumes of 10 to 15 mL/kg may be injurious in certain settings.

1. **Air-trapping** and auto PEEP (positive end-expiratory pressure) lead to significant morbidity and mortality in patients with obstructive lung disease. The ventilatory strategy in these patients should focus on prolongation of expiratory time by limiting minute ventilation by using low tidal volumes (≤6–8 mL/kg) and a low rate (8–12 breaths/min) and by reducing the inspiratory time of the respiratory cycle. To accomplish these goals, deep sedation is often required, and rarely neuromuscular blockade must be used. Separation from mechanical ventilation is expedited when respiratory therapy–driven protocols are used that focus on daily assessment of the ability to breath without assistance, assuming improvement of the inciting process, adequate oxygenation, and hemodynamic stability (grade A recommendation). After the patient can breathe comfortably for 30 to 120 minutes without support, the trachea can be extubated, assuming that there are no other precluding factors such as airway abnormalities or coma.

B. **Acute Lung Injury and Acute Respiratory Distress Syndrome** are characterized by acute hypoxemic respiratory failure and diffuse alveolar damage with resulting increased lung permeability. Diffuse alveolar edema and mortality in patients with ARDS and ALI appear to be similar.

1. The treatment of ALI and ARDS is largely supportive and includes aggressive treatment of inciting events, avoidance of complications, and mechanical ventilation. It is critical that tidal volumes (≤6 mL/kg) and static ventilatory pressures (≤30 cm H_2O) are

minimized to avoid further injury to the remaining relatively uninjured lung.

2. Because ARDS is marked by high intrapulmonary shunt, hypoxemia is relatively unresponsive to oxygen therapy. Thus, strategies to recruit the collapsed lung are necessary. This is most commonly achieved by using PEEP. Long-term outcome benefits of inhaled nitric oxide have not been demonstrated, although inhaled nitric oxide may still be useful as "rescue" therapy in selected patients with severe refractory hypoxemia.

3. It is intuitive that administration of excessive fluids be avoided.

4. Corticosteroids administered early in the course of ARDS are of no benefit but may be beneficial during the fibroproliferative phase.

VI. **ACUTE RENAL FAILURE (ARF)** is reported to occur in as many as 1.5% to 24% of critically ill patients. Mortality associated with ARF requiring dialysis has remained approximately 60% for nearly five decades. In the ICU, ARF occurs from prerenal causes and tubular injury (acute tubular necrosis) in the vast majority of cases. Urine sodium concentration and fractional excretion of sodium can help identify prerenal azotemia (Table 56-5).

A. **Treatment.** In incipient and established ARF, supportive care is the rule, with the focus on maintenance of euvolemia, avoidance of renal toxins, adjustment of medication doses, and monitoring of electrolytes and acid–base status. Pharmacologic approaches to the prevention and treatment of ARF, including low-dose dopamine, have been uniformly disappointing.

1. Diuretics should be administered with caution in early ARF and in response to defined physiologic problems (hypervolemia, hyperkalemia.)

2. Prophylactic administration of N-acetyl cysteine and sodium bicarbonate to patients with preexisting renal disease appears to be beneficial in preventing contrast-induced nephropathy.

3. The weight of evidence supports an increased intensity of dialysis using either daily standard hemodialysis, CRRT, or extended daily hemodialysis ("slow dialysis").

TABLE 56-5

URINALYSIS, URINE CHEMISTRIES, AND OSMOLALITY IN ACUTE RENAL FAILURE

	Hypovolemia	Acute Tubular Necrosis	Acute Interstitial Nephritis	Glomerulonephritis	Obstruction
Sediment	Bland	Broad, brownish granular casts	WBCs, eosinophils, cellular casts	RBCs, RBC casts	Bloody
Protein	None or low	None or low	Minimal but may be increased with NSAIDs	Increased, >100 mg/dL	Low
Urine Na$^+$ (mEq/L)*	<20 <40 (days)	>30	>30	<20	<20
Urine osmolality (mOsm/kg)†	>400	<350	<350	>400	<350
FENa+ (%)†	<1	>1	Varies	<1	<1 (acute) >1 (days)

*The sensitivity and specificity of urine sodium of less than 20 in differentiating prerenal azotemia from acute tubular necrosis are 90% and 82%, respectively.

†FENa+: Fractional excretion of sodium is the urine to plasma (U/P) of sodium divided by U/P of creatinine ×100. The sensitivity and specificity of fractional excretion of sodium of less than 1% in differentiating prerenal azotemia from acute tubular necrosis are 96% and 95%, respectively.

NSAID = nonsteroidal anti-inflammatory drug; RBC = red blood cell; WBC = white blood cell.

PERIOPERATIVE

VII. ENDOCRINE ASPECTS OF CRITICAL CARE MEDICINE

A. **Glucose Management in Critical Illness.** Hyperglycemia is associated with increased risk of postoperative infection (wound and otherwise) and poor outcome in patients with stroke or TBI.

1. Strict glycemic control in critically ill patients has been advocated based on evidence from a single randomized trial in surgical patients in the ICU. A subsequent study by the same investigators in medical patients found no benefit of intensive insulin therapy on mortality.

2. The enthusiasm for intensive insulin therapy with tight glycemic control in the ICU has diminished.

B. **Adrenal Function in Critical Illness.** The stress response to injury includes an increase in serum cortisol levels in most critically ill patients. Adrenal insufficiency may also occur in critically ill patients, reflecting inhibition of adrenal stimulation or corticosteroid synthesis by drugs or cytokines and direct injury to or infection of the pituitary or adrenal glands. Until free cortisol assays are more widely available, the diagnosis of adrenal insufficiency in critical illness must be based on clinical suspicion and total cortisol levels. Adrenal insufficiency should be considered in all critically ill patients with pressor-dependent shock.

C. **Thyroid Function in Critical Illness.** Depression of triiodothyronine (T_3) occurs within hours of injury or illness and can persist for weeks. Low thyroid hormone levels, particularly for T_3, correlate with the severity of illness and are associated with an increased risk of death. Hypothyroidism (elevation of thyroid-stimulating hormone in the presence of a low thyroxine level) may be present in critically ill patients, particularly in the geriatric population, and should be considered in the face of refractory shock; adrenal insufficiency; unexplained coma; and prolonged, unexplained respiratory failure.

D. **Somatotropic Function in Critical Illness.** Growth hormone levels are low in patients with prolonged critical illness.

VIII. ANEMIA AND TRANSFUSION THERAPY IN CRITICAL ILLNESS

The vast majority of patients admitted to the ICU are anemic at some point in their hospital stay, and more than one third of them will receive transfused blood. The cause of anemia in critical illness is multifactorial and is related to blood loss from the primary injury or illness, iatrogenic blood loss caused by daily blood sampling, and nutritional deficiencies (e.g., folate). It is assumed that critically ill patients have less efficient compensatory mechanisms and reduced physiologic reserve and thereby require a higher hemoglobin concentration than unstressed individuals. Data collected from ICUs at multiple centers in the United States suggest that the transfusion trigger is nearer 8.6 g/dL than the previously recommended 7 g/dL. Hemoglobin is an important determinant of oxygen delivery (DO_2), and transfusion is an integral component of goal-directed therapeutic strategies that aim to optimize DO_2 in early shock states.

IX. NUTRITION IN CRITICALLY ILL PATIENTS

Poor nutritional status is associated with increased mortality and morbidity rate among critically ill patients; adequate nutritional support should be considered a standard of care. Enteral nutrition is preferred over parenteral nutrition whenever possible because of its lower cost and less frequent complications.

A. **Complications** associated with enteral feedings include aspiration of gastric feeding, diarrhea, and fluid and electrolyte imbalance. To prevent aspiration with gastric feeding, the head of the patient's bed should be raised 30 to 45 degrees during feeding; jejunal access can be considered in patients with recurrent tube feeding aspiration. To prevent or reduce diarrhea, all potential causes should be considered and corrected.

X. SEDATION OF CRITICALLY ILL PATIENTS

Critically ill patients are often deeply sedated because of the potential benefits afforded by a reduction in the sympathoadrenal response to injury. Additionally, complications associated with undersedation include ventilator

PERIOPERATIVE

dyssynchrony, patient injury, agitation, anxiety, stress disorders, and possibly unplanned extubation.

A. Recent studies have tempered the enthusiasm for deep sedation in the ICU. (Daily interruption of continuous sedative and analgesic drug infusions has been shown to be effective in reducing the length of mechanical ventilation and length of ICU stay.)

1. The depth of sedation may also play a role in long-term outcomes after discharge from the ICU. (The extent of ICU recall, including delusional memories, is a function of the extent of sedation.)

2. It is important to titrate medications according to established therapeutic goals and re-evaluate the sedation requirements frequently (Ramsay sedation scale, Richmond agitation sedation scale).

B. **Confusion and agitation** are common in ICU patients and may have unfavorable consequences on patient outcome. Agitation should be distinguished from delirium, which is relatively common in ICU patients and equally associated with increased length of stay, morbidity, and mortality. The distinguishing characteristics of delirium include acute onset and fluctuating course, inattention, disorganized thinking, and altered level of consciousness.

C. **Nonpharmacologic and pharmacologic** means can be used to provide comfort and safety to ICU patients. The former include communication, frequent reorientation, maintenance of a day–night cycle, noise reduction, and ensuring ventilation synchrony.

Pharmacologic agents include hypnotics–anxiolytics, opioids, and antipsychotics.

1. The most commonly used **hypnotics** are propofol, midazolam, and lorazepam. Continuous infusion of propofol is associated with a shorter length of mechanical ventilation and ICU stay compared with lorazepam administration.

2. **Dexmedetomidine** has been effectively used as a single agent or in combination with other drugs in postsurgical and medical ICU patients.

3. **Opioids.** Morphine and fentanyl are the most commonly used opioids to provide analgesia in the ICU. Morphine should be avoided in patients with renal failure because of active metabolites that accumulate in the presence of impaired renal elimination.

4. **Neuromuscular blockade** may be occasionally indicated in ICU patients with severe TBI or respiratory failure, but routine use is discouraged because of concerns that this practice may predispose patients to critical illness, polyneuropathy, and myopathy and because of an increased risk of nosocomial pneumonia in patients receiving these agents.

XI. COMPLICATIONS IN THE INTENSIVE CARE UNIT: DETECTION, PREVENTION, AND THERAPY

A. **Nosocomial infections** are a major source of morbidity and mortality in critically ill patients. At some level, nosocomial infections are unavoidable and occur because of the nature of intensive care: patients are critically ill with altered host defenses; they require invasive devices (endotracheal tubes, intravascular catheters) for support, monitoring, and therapy that provide portals of entry for infectious organisms; and they receive therapies that increase the risk of infection (glucocorticoids, parenteral nutrition). On the other hand, many nosocomial infections are preventable with relatively simple interventions.

1. **Sinusitis** is common in critically ill patients with indwelling oral and nasal tubes. Prevention of sinusitis should focus on efforts to improve sinus drainage, including semi-recumbent positioning and avoidance of nasal tubes. Bacterial sinusitis should be considered in patients with unexplained fever and leukocytosis in the ICU.

2. **Ventilator-Associated Pneumonia (VAP).** Endotracheal intubation and mechanical ventilation increase the risk of VAP. Interventions that can reduce the incidence of VAP include strict hand washing before and after patient contact and semi-recumbent positioning of the patient (head height at 30 degrees or greater from horizontal) (level II evidence). These practices should be rigorously applied in all ICUs (granted that semi-recumbent positioning is not possible in all patients).

a. Gastric and oropharyngeal colonization with resistant organisms appears to be a risk factor for the development of VAP. Oral decontamination with chlorhexidine (not non-absorbable antimicrobial agents) appears to reduce VAP rates without leading to excess antibiotic resistance.

b. Acid-suppression therapies as prophylaxis against gastrointestinal (GI) bleeding have been associated with an increased risk of VAP because they allow bacterial overgrowth in the stomach. (Sucralfate should be considered as an alternative agent to acid-suppressive regimens despite its potentially reduced effectiveness.)

c. An important approach to reduce the overall mortality from VAP involves refinement of the diagnostic process and limitation of antibiotic therapy to avoid the development of antibiotic resistance. Antibiotics can than be narrowed in spectrum or discontinued depending on the results from quantitative cultures after 48 to 72 hours.

3. **Intravascular catheter-associated bacteremia** is strictly defined as clinical suspicion of catheter-related infection plus positive culture of blood drawn from the catheter or of a segment of catheter and matching positive blood culture drawn from another site.

a. Catheter infection is more likely when placement occurs under emergency conditions and is reduced by the use of strict aseptic technique with full barrier precautions. Catheter-related infection and bacteremia increase with the duration of catheterization, particularly for durations of greater than 2 days. However, routine catheter replacement at 3 or 7 days does not reduce the incidence of infection and results in increased mechanical complications. Thus, routine guidewire change of catheters is not recommended.

b. Based on incidence of infection at the insertion site, the subclavian route should be used when possible if the duration of catheterization is predicted to be longer than 2 days.

c. Catheter-related venous thrombosis occurs commonly and is associated with an increased risk of infection. Routine flushing of catheter ports with heparin reduces the incidence of both thrombosis and infection.

    d. When catheter-related bacteremia is confirmed, the offending catheter should be removed and appropriate antibiotics continued for a minimum of 7 days.

4. **Urinary tract infection (UTI)** is the second most common source of infection in the ICU. Its incidence increases with the duration of bladder catheterization.

5. **Invasive fungal infections** in non-neutropenic patients is caused by *Candida* species in the vast majority of cases. These infections are increasingly common in the ICU population, accounting for 5% to 10% of all bloodstream infections in the ICU. A high level of suspicion for invasive *Candida* infection in critically ill patients is necessary, and "pre-emptive" therapy should be considered in patients with a high likelihood of invasive *Candida* infection while awaiting blood culture results. An ophthalmologic examination is warranted in patients with documented or suspected bloodstream infection because patients with endophthalmitis may require longer courses of therapy. Intravascular catheters that are potential sources of bloodstream infection should be removed. Organisms sensitive to the azole derivative fluconazole cause the majority of invasive *Candida* infections in the ICU, and fluconazole is the first-line treatment given its reasonable efficacy and limited toxicity.

B. **Stress Ulceration and Gastrointestinal Hemorrhage.** Gastric mucosal breakdown with resulting gastritis and ulceration ("stress ulceration") can lead to GI bleeding in ICU patients. The major risk factors for stress-related GI bleeding are mechanical ventilation and coagulopathy; secondary risk factors among mechanically ventilated patients include renal failure, thermal injury, and possibly head injury. Enteral nutrition may protect against significant GI bleeding.

1. **Prevention.** Agents used to prevent stress ulceration and GI bleeding include methods to suppress acid production (H2 blockers and proton pump inhibitors) and cytoprotective agents (sucralfate). The agent of choice—and whether any prophylaxis is beneficial or indicated—is somewhat controversial. It appears that stress ulcer prophylaxis is more widely used than necessary.

Thus, although stress ulcer prophylaxis, predominantly with ranitidine, is commonly used in critically ill patients, the utility of this intervention is unclear.

C. **Venous thromboembolism** (VTE) occurs frequently in critically ill patients, with incidences of deep venous thrombosis (DVT) of 10% to 30% and of pulmonary embolism (PE) of 1.5% to 5%. In addition to classic lower extremity DVT, upper extremity DVT occurs with increased frequency in the ICU population. This is directly associated with the use of central venous catheters in the subclavian and internal jugular sites. Upper extremity DVT can result in pulmonary embolism in up to two thirds of cases, with occasional fatalities.

1. **Prophylaxis.** The risks of VTE prophylaxis, including heparin-induced thrombocytopenia and bleeding, must be weighed when considering prophylaxis in the ICU population. Nonetheless, it is generally agreed that high-risk patients without contraindications should receive prophylaxis with low-molecular-weight heparin (LMWH) and that patients with low to moderate risk should receive low-dose unfractionated heparin (UFH) (Table 56-6). To reduce central venous catheter–associated thrombosis and infection, catheter tips should be positioned in the superior vena cava, and catheters should be flushed with a dilute heparin solution. Heparin bonding of catheters may also reduce local thrombosis.

2. **Diagnosis.** Despite the high incidence of DVT, routine screening studies for DVT do not appear to improve clinical outcomes in the ICU. VTE should be considered in critically ill patients in the face of relatively nonspecific findings, such as unexplained tachycardia, tachypnea, fever, asymmetric extremity edema, and gas exchange abnormalities (including high dead space ventilation). Compression Doppler ultrasonography is the most commonly used test for diagnosis of DVT. Ventilation-perfusion scanning and pulmonary angiography may have utility in specific circumstances, including in the presence of renal insufficiency (concerns about contrast-induced nephrotoxicity) or equivocal results on computed tomography scan. Pulmonary angiography may be

TABLE 56-6

RISK FACTORS FOR VENOUS THROMBOEMBOLISM

Strong Risk Factors
Fracture (hip or leg)
Hip or knee replacement
Major trauma
Spinal cord injury

Moderate Risk Factors
Arthroscopic knee surgery
Central venous lines
Chemotherapy
Congestive heart or respiratory failure
Hormone replacement therapy
Malignancy
Oral contraceptive therapy
Paralytic stroke
Pregnancy or postpartum period
Previous venous thromboembolism
Thrombophilia

Weak Risk Factors
Bed rest >3 days
Immobility caused by sitting (prolonged car or air travel)
Increasing age
Laparoscopic surgery (cholecystectomy)
Obesity
Pregnancy or antepartum period
Varicose veins

PERIOPERATIVE

the test of choice when the likelihood of PE is high
and anticoagulation is contraindicated, necessitating
immediate placement of a vena cava filter.

3. **Treatment.** The mainstay of treatment for VTE is
heparin, which should be started before the results
of confirmatory studies if clinical suspicion is high.
LMWH may be superior to UFH in efficacy with
comparable rates of bleeding. The advantage of
UFH in the ICU population is its titratability and
rapid reversibility, which may be desirable in
patients at high risk for bleeding. For patients who
have contraindications to anticoagulation or who
have recurrent PE despite anticoagulation, vena
cava filters can be placed in the SVC or IVC,
depending on DVT location.

D. **Acquired Neuromuscular Disorders in Critical Illness.**
Neuromuscular abnormalities developing as a

consequence of critical illness can be found in the majority of patients hospitalized in the ICU for 1 week or more. These disorders range from isolated nerve entrapment with focal pain or weakness to disuse muscle atrophy with mild weakness to severe myopathy or neuropathy with associated severe, prolonged weakness. It is likely that there is considerable overlap between the neuropathic and myopathic syndromes in terms of risk factors, presentation, and prognosis.

1. Prospective studies suggest that neuromuscular abnormalities are present in 42% to 72% of patients in the ICU for 7 days or more and in 68% to 100% of patients with sepsis or the systemic inflammatory response syndrome. The ultimate role of corticosteroids and neuromuscular blocking agents in the pathogenesis of this problem is undefined.

2. ICU-acquired neuromuscular abnormalities may result in severe weakness with flaccid quadriplegia that last for weeks or months. (This prolongs the duration of mechanical ventilation and is a significant contributor to mortality.)

3. **Prevention** of acquired neuromuscular disorders in the ICU centers on avoidance or minimization of contributory risk factors, including high-dose steroids, prolonged administration of neuromuscular blockade, and hyperglycemia.

4. **Diagnosis** of ICU-acquired neuromuscular abnormalities should be entertained in all critically ill patients with unexplained weakness; electrodiagnostic studies can help confirm the diagnosis and rule out other potentially treatable causes of weakness such as Guillain-Barré syndrome.

5. **Treatment.** No treatment for ICU-acquired neuromuscular abnormalities has been identified; avoidance of potentially contributing agents and aggressive physical therapy are warranted.

CHAPTER 57 ■ ACUTE PAIN MANAGEMENT

Appropriate management of patients with acute perioperative pain using multimodal or balanced analgesia is crucial (Macres SM, Moore PG, Fishman SM: Perioperative pain management. In *Clinical Anesthesia*. Edited by Barash PG, Cullen BF, Stoelting RK, Cahalan MK, Stock MC. Philadelphia: Lippincott Williams & Wilkins, 2009, pp 1473–1504). Inadequate relief of postoperative pain has adverse physiologic effects that may contribute to significant morbidity and mortality, resulting in the delay of patient recovery and return to daily activities.

I. DEFINITION OF ACUTE PAIN

Acute pain has been defined as the normal, predicted, physiological response to an adverse chemical, thermal, or mechanical stimulus. Generally, acute pain resolves within 1 month. Acute pain-induced change in the central nervous system is known as neuronal plasticity. This can result in sensitization of the nervous system, resulting in allodynia and hyperalgesia.

II. ANATOMY OF ACUTE PAIN (Figs. 57-1 and 57-2 and Table 57-1).

α-δ Fibers transmit "first pain," which is described as sharp or stinging in nature and is well localized. Polymodal C fibers transmit "second pain," which is more diffuse in nature and is associated with the affective and motivational aspects of pain.

III. PAIN PROCESSING

Tissue injury tends to fuel neuroplastic changes within the nervous system, which results in both peripheral and central sensitization. Clinically, this can manifest as

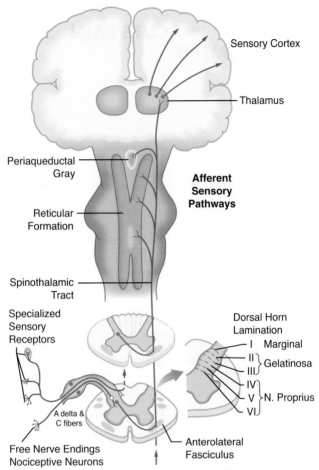

FIGURE 57-1. Afferent pathways involved in nociceptive regulation.

hyperalgesia (exaggerated pain response to a normally painful stimulus) or allodynia (painful response to a typically nonpainful stimulus) (Fig. 57-3).

A. The four elements of pain processing are transduction, transmission, modulation, and perception (Fig. 57-4).

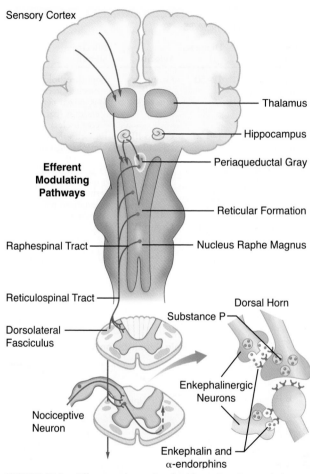

Sensory Cortex

Thalamus

Hippocampus

Efferent Modulating Pathways

Periaqueductal Gray

Reticular Formation

Raphespinal Tract

Nucleus Raphe Magnus

Reticulospinal Tract

Dorsal Horn

Dorsolateral Fasciculus

Substance P

Enkephalinergic Neurons

Nociceptive Neuron

Enkephalin and α-endorphins

FIGURE 57-2. Efferent pathways involved in nociceptive regulation.

1. **Modulation** of pain transmission involves altering afferent neural transmission along the pain pathway. The dorsal horn of the spinal cord is the most common site for modulation of the pain pathway, and modulation can involve either inhibition

PERIOPERATIVE

TABLE 57-1

PRIMARY AFFERENT NERVES

Fiber Class	Diameter (μ)	Velocity	Effective Stimuli
A_{beta} (myelinated)	12–20	Group II (>40–50 m/sec)	Low-threshold mechanoreceptors Specialized nerve endings (pacinian corpuscles)
α-δ (myelinated)	1–4	Group III (<40 m/sec)	Low-threshold mechanical or thermal High-threshold mechanical or thermal Specialized nerve endings
C (unmyelinated)	0.5–1.5	Group IV (<2 msec)	High-threshold thermal, mechanical, and chemical Free nerve endings

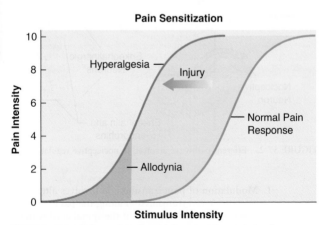

Pain Sensitization

FIGURE 57-3. Pain sensitization. (Adapted with permission from Klemm D: *Am Family Phys* 63(10), 2001.)

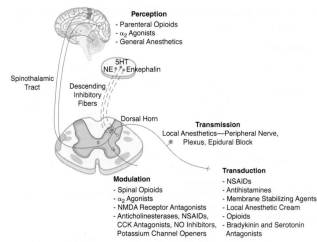

FIGURE 57-4. The four elements of pain processing are transduction, transmission, modulation and perception. 5HT = 5-hydroxytryptamine (serotonin); CCK = cholecystokinin; NE = norepinephrine; NMDA = N-methyl-D-aspartate; NO = nitric oxide; NSAID = nonsteroidal anti-inflammatory drug.

or augmentation of the pain signals. Examples of inhibitory spinal modulation include release of inhibitory neurotransmitters (γ-aminobutyric acid, glycine) and activation of descending efferent neuronal pathways (release of norepinephrine, serotonin, and endorphins in the dorsal horn).

2. Spinal modulation that results in augmentation of pain pathways is a consequence of neuronal plasticity. The phenomenon of "wind-up" is an example of central plasticity that results from repetitive C-fiber stimulation of wide-dynamic range (WDR) neurons in the dorsal horn.

B. A multimodal approach to pain therapy should target all four elements of the pain processing pathway.

IV. **CHEMICAL MEDIATORS OF TRANSDUCTION AND TRANSMISSION** (Table 57-2 and Fig. 57-5)

A. Pain receptors include the NMDA (N-methyl-D-aspartate), AMPA (α-amino-3-hydroxy-5-methylisoxazole-4-

TABLE 57-2

ALGOGENIC SUBSTANCES

Substance	Source	Effect
Bradykinin	Macrophages Plasma kininogen	Activates nociceptors
Serotonin	Platelets	Activates nociceptors
Histamine	Platelets Mast cells	Produces vasodilation, edema, and pruritus Potentiates the response of nociceptors to bradykinin
Prostaglandin	Tissue injury and cyclo-oxygenase pathway	Sensitizes nociceptors
Leukotriene	Tissue injury and lipo-oxygenase pathway	Sensitizes nociceptors
Excess hydrogen ions	Tissue injury and ischemia	Increases pain and hyperalgesia associated with inflammation
Cytokines (interleukins, TNF)	Macrophages	Excite and sensitize nociceptors
Adenosine	Tissue injury	Pain and hyperalgesia
Neurotransmitters (glutamate, substance P)	Antidromic release by peripheral nerve terminals after tissue injury	Substance P activates macrophages and mast cells Glutamate activates nociceptors
Nerve growth factor	Macrophages	Stimulates mast cells to release histamine and serotonin Induces heat hyperalgesia Sensitizes nociceptors

TNF = tissue necrosis factor.

proprionic acid), kainite, and metabotropic receptors (Fig. 57-6).

B. Repetitive C-fiber stimulation of WDR neurons in the dorsal horn at intervals of 0.5 to 1.0 Hz may precipitate the occurrence of "wind-up" and central sensitization and secondary hyperalgesia (Fig. 57-7).

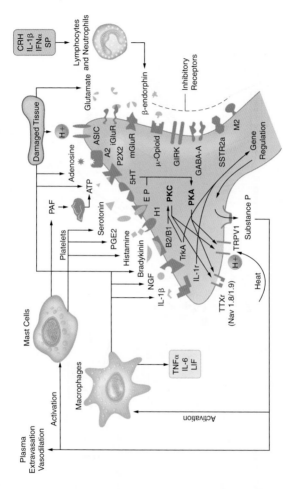

FIGURE 57-5. Substances involved in nociception.

921

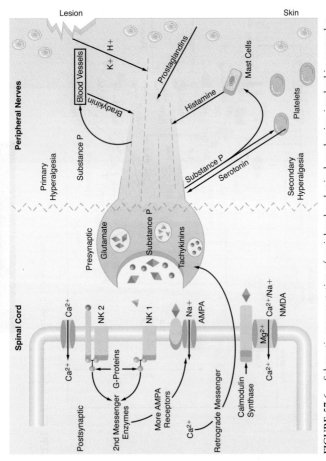

FIGURE 57-6. Schematic representation of peripheral and spinal mechanism involved in neuroplasticity. AAMPA = α-amino-3-hydroxy-5-methylisoxazole-4-proprionic acid; NK = neurokinin; NMDA = N-methyl-D-aspartate.

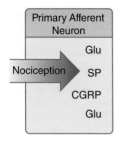

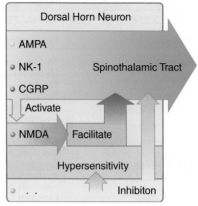

FIGURE 57-7. Primary nociceptive transmission in the spinal cord. NMDA antagonists have an antihyperalgesic rather than an analgesic effect in the spinal cord. AMPA = α-amino-3-hydroxy-5-methylisoxazole-4-proprionic acid; CGRP = calcitonin gene-related peptide; NK = neurokinin; NMDA = N-methyl-D-aspartate.

V. THE SURGICAL STRESS RESPONSE

Although similar, postoperative pain and the surgical stress response are not the same. Surgical stress causes release of cytokines and precipitates adverse neuroendocrine and sympathoadrenal responses (increased secretion of the catabolic hormones [cortisol, glucagon, growth hormone, and catecholamines] and decreased secretion of the anabolic hormones [insulin and testosterone]) (Table 57-3).

VI. PREEMPTIVE ANALGESIA

The goal of preemptive analgesia is to prevent NMDA receptor activation in the dorsal horn which causes "wind-up," facilitation, central sensitization expansion of receptive fields, and long-term potentiation, all of which may lead to a chronic pain state.

VII. STRATEGIES FOR ACUTE PAIN MANAGEMENT

The majority of postoperative pain is nociceptive in character. Evidence suggests that women experience more

PERIOPERATIVE

TABLE 57-3

CONSEQUENCES OF POORLY MANAGED ACUTE PAIN

System	Consequences
Cardiovascular	Tachycardia
	Hypertension
	Increased cardiac workload
Pulmonary	Respiratory muscle spasm (splinting)
	Decreased vital capacity
	Atelectasis
	Arterial hypoxemia
	Increased risk of pulmonary infection
Gastrointestinal	Postoperative ileus
Renal	Increased risk of oliguria and urinary retention
Coagulation	Increased risk of thromboemboli
Immunologic	Impaired immune function
Muscular	Muscle weakness and fatigue
	Limited mobility with increased risk of thromboembolism
Psychological	Anxiety
	Fear and frustration, resulting in poor patient satisfaction

pain after surgery than men and therefore require more morphine to achieve a similar level of pain relief.

VIII. **ASSESSMENT OF ACUTE PAIN** (Fig. 57-8).
Common features of pain are usually reviewed during the assessment for acute pain (Table 57-4).

IX. **OPIOID ANALGESICS** are the mainstay for the treatment of acute postoperative pain, and morphine is the "gold-standard" (Tables 57-5).

A. **Hydromorphone** is a semisynthetic opioid that has four to six times the potency of morphine, making it the ideal drug for long-term subcutaneous administration in opioid-tolerant patients.

B. **Fentanyl** is available for intravenous (IV), subcutaneous, transdermal, transmucosal, and neuraxial administration.

Universal Pain Assessment Tool

This Pain Assessment Tool is Intended to Help Patient Care Providers Assess Pain According to Individual Patient Needs.
Explain and Use 0-10 Scale for Patient Self-assessment. Use the Faces or Behavioral Observations to Interpret Expressed Pain
When Patient Cannot Communicate His/Her Pain Intensity.

	0	1	2	3	4	5	6	7	8	9	10
Verbal Descriptor Scale	No Pain		Mild Pain		Moderate Pain		Moderate Pain		Severe Pain		Worst Pain Possible
Wong-Baker Facial Grimace Scale	Alert Smiling		No Humor Serious Flat		Furrowed brow pursed lips breath holding		Wrinkled nose raised upper lips rapid breathing		Slow Blink Open Mouth		Eyes Closed Moaning Crying
Activity Tolerance Scale	No Pain		Can Be Ignored		Interferes with Tasks		Interferes with Concentration		Interferes with Basic needs		Bedrest Required
Spanish	NADA DE DOLOR		UNPOQUITO DE DOLOR		UN DOLOR LEVE		DOLOR FUERTE		DOLOR DEMASIADO FUERTE		UN DOLOR INSOPORTABLE
Tagalog	Walang Sakit		Konting Sakit		Katamtamang Sakit		Matinding Sakit		Pinaka-Matinding Sakit		Pinaka-Malalang Sakit
Chinese	不痛		輕微		中度		嚴重		非常嚴重		最嚴重
Korean	통증 없음		약한 통증		보통 통증		심한 통증		아주 심한 통증		최악의 통증
Persian (Farsi)	بدون درد		درد ملایم		درد معتدل		درد شدید		درد بسیار شدید		بدترین درد ممکن
Vietnamese	Không Đau		Đau Nhẹ		Đau Vừa Phải		Đau Nặng		Đau Thật Nặng		Đau Đớn Tột Cùng
Japanese	痛みがない		少し痛い		いくらか痛い		かなり痛い		ひどく痛い		ものすごく痛い

FIGURE 57-8. Linear visual analogue scale and faces pain assessment tool.

PERIOPERATIVE

TABLE 57-4

FEATURES OF PAIN COMMONLY ADDRESSED DURING ASSESSMENT

Onset of pain
Temporal pattern of pain
Site of pain
Radiation of pain
Intensity (severity) of pain
Exacerbating features (what makes the pain start or get worse?)
Relieving factors (what prevents the pain or makes it better?)
Response to analgesics (including attitudes and concerns about opioids)
Response to other interventions
Associated physical symptoms
Associated psychological symptoms
Interference with activities of daily living

TABLE 57-5

OPIOID EQUIANALGESIC DOSING

Drug	Intravenous, Intramuscular, or Subcutaneous Dose	Oral Dose
Morphine	10 mg	30 mg
Hydromorphone (Dilaudid)	1.5–2.0 mg	6–8 mg
Hydrocodone (Vicodin)		30–45 mg
Oxymorphone (Opana IR and ER)	1 mg	10 mg
Oxycodone (Percocet, OxyContin)	10–15 mg	20 mg
Levorphanol (Levo-Dromoran)	2 mg	4 mg
Fentanyl	100 μg	
Meperidine (Demerol)	100 mg	300 mg
Codeine	100 mg	200 mg
Methadone	Conversion ratio is variable	

C. **Sufentanil.** The high intrinsic potency of sufentanil makes it an excellent choice for epidural analgesia in opioid-dependent patients.

D. **Methadone** is well absorbed from the gastrointestinal (GI) tract. With repetitive dosing, methadone can accumulate. Opioid rotation is a useful technique to restore analgesic sensitivity in highly tolerant patients, and methadone is a common choice for opioid rotation.

X. **NON-OPIOID ANALGESIC ADJUNCTS** (Table 57-6). Nonsteroidal anti-inflammatory drugs (NSAIDs) have been proven effective in the treatment of postoperative pain. In addition, they are opioid sparing and can significantly decrease the incidence of opioid-related side effects such as postoperative nausea and vomiting and sedation. Platelet dysfunction, GI ulceration, and an increased risk of nephrotoxicity are several reasons why the nonselective NSAIDs may be avoided in the perioperative period.

TABLE 57-6

ADULT DOSING GUIDELINES FOR NON-OPIOID ANALGESICS

Drug	Route	Half-Life (hr)	Dose (mg)
Para-aminophenols			
Acetaminophen	Oral	0.25	500–1000 mg every 4–6 hr Maximum daily dose in healthy adults: 4000 mg
Salicylates			
Acetylsalicylic acid	Oral	0.25	500–1000 mg every 4–6 hr Maximum daily dose in healthy adults: 4000 mg
Diflunisal	Oral	8–12	500 mg every 8–12 hr Loading dose: 1000 mg
Choline magnesium Trisalicylate	Oral	9–17	1000–1500 mg every 12 hr
NSAID's			
Propionic Acids			
Ibuprofen	Oral	2	400 mg every 4–6 hr
Naproxen	Oral	12–15	250 mg every 6–8 hr
Ketoprofen	Oral	2.1	25–50 mg every 6–8 hr
Oxaprozin	Oral	42–50	600 mg every 12–24 hr
Indoleacetic Acids			
Indomethacin	Oral	2	25 mg every 8–12 hr
Sulindac	Oral	7.8	150 mg every 12 h
Etodolac	Oral	7.3	300–400 mg every 12 hr
Pyrrolacetic Acids			
Ketorolac	IV	6	30 mg initially followed by 15–30 mg every 6–8 hr, not to exceed 5 days
Phenylacetic Acids			
Diclofenac potassium	Oral	2	50 mg every 8 hr
Enolic Acids (Oxicams)			
Meloxicam	Oral	15–20	7.5–15.0 mg every 24 hr
Piroxicam	Oral	50	20–40 mg every 24 hr
Naphthylalkalone			
Nabumetone	Oral	22.5	500–750 mg every 8–12 hr
COX-2 Inhibitor			
Celecoxib	Oral	11	100–200 mg every 12 hr

COX = cyclo-oxygenase; IV = intravenous.

PERIOPERATIVE

A. **NMDA receptor antagonists** (ketamine, dextromethorphan) may be analgesic adjuncts.

B. **α2-Adrenergic agonists** (clonidine, dexmedetomidine) may be administered perioperatively to provide analgesia, sedation, and anxiolysis.

C. **Gabapentin** and **pregabalin** are effective analgesics not only for the treatment of neuropathic pain syndromes but also for the treatment of postoperative pain. When these drugs are combined with an NSAID, the combination has been shown to be synergistic in attenuating the hyperalgesia associated with peripheral inflammation.

D. **Lidocaine** has been shown to be analgesic, antihyperalgesic, and anti-inflammatory after IV administration.

E. **Glucocorticoids** possess analgesic, anti-inflammatory, and antiemetic effects.

XI. METHODS OF ANALGESIA

A. **Patient-Controlled Analgesia (PCA)** is any technique of pain management that allows patients to administer their own analgesia on demand.

   1. The five variables associated with all modes of PCA include bolus dose, incremental (demand) dose, lockout interval, background infusion rate, and 1-hour and 4-hour limits (Table 57-7).

   2. **Risk Factors for Use of Opioid Patient-Controlled Analgesia** (Table 57-8)

B. **Neuraxial Analgesia.** Since the discovery of the opioid receptor, the intrathecal administration of opioids and the epidural administration of opioids plus a local anesthetic have produced significant pain control.

TABLE 57-7

UNIVERSAL INTRAVENOUS OPIOID PATIENT-CONTROLLED ANALGESIA REGIMENS FOR OPIOID-NAÏVE ADULT PATIENT

Opioid	Demand Dose	Lockout (min)	Basal Infusion
Morphine	1–2 mg	6–10	0–2 mg/hr
Hydromorphone	0.2–0.4 mg	6–10	0.4 mg/hr
Fentanyl	20–50 µg	5–10	0–60 µg/hr
Sufentanil	4–6 µg	5–10	0–8 µg/hr
Tramadol	10–20 mg	6–10	0–20 mg/hr

TABLE 57-8

RELATIVE RISK FACTORS ASSOCIATED WITH
PATIENT-CONTROLLED ANALGESIA

Pulmonary disease
Obstructive sleep apnea
Renal or hepatic dysfunction
Congestive heart failure
Closed head injury
Altered mental status
Lactating mothers

1. **Epidural analgesia** is a critical component of multi-modal perioperative pain management and improved patient outcome.
   a. The efficacy of an epidural technique is determined by numerous factors, including catheter incision site congruency, choice of analgesic drugs, rates of infusion, duration of epidural analgesia, and type of pain assessment (rest vs dynamic).
   b. Ideally, the epidural catheter is positioned congruent with the surgical incision (Table 57-9).
   c. A local anesthetic plus an opioid in the epidural space is the most common drug combination and is believed to have a synergistic effect.
   d. Epidurally administered opioids have the distinct advantage of producing analgesia without causing significant sympatholytic effect or motor blockade.
   e. Analgesia occurs by way of a spinal mechanism (diffusion of drug into the spinal fluid) and

PERIOPERATIVE

TABLE 57-9

GUIDELINES FOR ADULT EPIDURAL CATHETER DOSING REGIMEN*

Recommended adult dose for epidural bupivacaine (should not exceed 400 mg in 24 hours)
Surgical dermatome: Catheter placement
  Lumbar (total knee, arthroplasty, or lower extremity bypass surgery)
  Low thoracic (exploratory laparotomy, or xiphopubic incision)
  Mid to high thoracic (thoracotomy or sternotomy)

*Rate of infusion, 2–10 mL/hr.

through a supraspinal mechanism after systemic adsorption. Opioids with intermediate lipophilicity (hydromorphone, alfentanil, meperidine) have the ability to easily move between the aqueous and lipid regions of the arachnoid membrane and therefore have high meningeal permeability, which potentially confers higher bioavailability in the spinal cord. Nevertheless, morphine has greater bioavailability in the spinal cord than alfentanil, fentanyl, and sufentanil.

f. In general, epidural administration of hydrophilic opioids tends to have a slow onset, a long duration, and a mechanism of action that is primarily spinal in nature. Epidural administration of lipophilic opioids, on the other hand, has a quick onset, a short duration, and a mechanism of action that is primarily supraspinal and secondary to rapid systemic uptake.

g. Adjuvant medications that may enhance analgesia include clonidine and ketamine.

h. Extended-release epidural morphine (DepoDur) consists of morphine encapsulated within a liposome delivery system, which provides controlled release of morphine for up to 48 hours. DepoDur is only approved for lumbar epidural administration.

2. **Intrathecal analgesia** is provided with a variety of opioid analgesics (morphine, hydromorphone, meperidine, methadone, fentanyl, sufentanil) (Table 57-10).

a. Hydrophilic opioids (morphine) traverse the dura slowly, bind to epidural fat poorly, and slowly enter the plasma. They tend to have a slow onset of action and a long duration and provide a broad band of analgesia. Delayed respiratory depression is more common with hydrophilic opioids secondary to rostral spread.

b. Lipophilic opioids (fentanyl) rapidly cross the dura, are quickly sequestered into epidural fat, and promptly enter the systemic circulation. Lipophilic opioids tend to have a rapid onset of action, a short duration, and a narrow band of analgesia. Delayed respiratory depression is less of a problem with the lipophilic opioids.

TABLE 57-10

INTRATHECAL ANALGESIA

Surgical Procedure	Intrathecal Drug Dose*
Labor analgesia	Sufentanil 2.5–5.0 μg
Cesarean section	Morphine 100 μg
	Addition of clonidine (60 μg) is synergistic and can increase the duration of spinal analgesia after cesarean section but also increases intraoperative sedation
Outpatient knee arthroplasty	Fentanyl (25–50 μg) improves intraoperative analgesia without prolonging postoperative motor blockade
Total knee arthroplasty	Morphine (200–300 μg)
Total hip arthroplasty	Morphine (100–200 μg)
Thoracotomy and major abdominal surgery	Morphine (500 μg)
	Incidence of side effects (nausea and vomiting, urinary retention, pruritus) increases with doses >300 μg

*Intrathecal hydromorphone, 50–100 μg, approximates intrathecal morphine, 100–200 μg.

      c. Other useful analgesic additives include the α2-agonists, NSAIDs, NMDA receptor antagonists, acetylcholinesterase inhibitors, adenosine, epinephrine, and benzodiazepines (Table 57-11).

  C. Peripheral Nerve Blockade. Single injection of peripheral nerve blockade may provide pain control that is superior to opioids with fewer side effects. Single injection techniques are limited in duration, but continuous peripheral nerve block techniques may extend the benefits of peripheral nerve blockade well into the postoperative period (Table 57-12).

    1. The Brachial Plexus

      a. The **interscalene block** is the ideal peripheral nerve block for painful orthopaedic and vascular procedures performed on the shoulder and upper arm but is a poor choice for forearm and hand surgery because the ulnar nerve is commonly spared.

      b. The **supraclavicular approach** to the brachial plexus provides anesthesia to the entire upper

TABLE 57-11

INTRATHECAL ANALGESIA

Intrathecal Drug	Dosing	Comments
Clonidine	15–45 μg improves the quality of spinal blockade in outpatient surgery	Side effects increase significantly at intrathecal doses >150 μg
Epinephrine	0.1–0.6 mg Produces dose-related increase in the return of motor function and micturition	Not recommended for outpatient surgery
Neostigmine	6.25–50 μg Produces dose-related increase in motor blockade, time for resolution of the block, and nausea and vomiting	Further studies of the appropriate intrathecal dose that optimizes analgesia while minimizing side effects are needed

extremity with a single injection of local anesthetic. The safety of this approach has improved dramatically with the use of ultrasonography.

c. The **infraclavicular block** is ideally suited for surgical procedures below the mid-humerus such as the hand, wrist, forearm, or elbow. The block targets the brachial plexus at the level of the cords, where it is in close proximity to the axillary artery. Ultrasound guidance has dramatically improved the safety and success of the infraclavicular approach.

2. **The Lumbar Plexus**

a. **Psoas compartment block** is indicated for major surgeries of the hip and knee. When combined with sciatic nerve blockade, virtually any surgical procedure can be performed on the lower extremity. The incidence of sciatic nerve injury after total knee arthroplasty, unrelated to regional anesthesia technique, is reported to be in the range of 0.2% to 2.4%. Sciatic nerve blockade can mask these complications.

TABLE 57-12

RECOMMENDED DOSING REGIMEN OF LOCAL ANESTHETICS FOR CONTINUOUS PERIPHERAL NERVE BLOCKADE

Catheter	Drug	Rate of Infusion	Patient Controlled Analgesia Bolus (mL)	Lockout (min)
Interscalene	Ropivacaine 0.2%	5–8 mL/hr	2–4	15–20
	Bupivacaine 0.15%–0.2%			
Infraclavicular	Ropivacaine 0.2%	5–8 mL/hr	2–4	15–20
	Bupivacaine 0.15%–0.2%			
Femoral	Ropivacaine 0.2%	5–10 mL/hr	5–10	30–60
	Bupivacaine 0.15%–0.2%			
Popliteal	Ropivacaine 0.2%	5–8 mL/hr	2	15–20
	Bupivacaine 0.15%–0.2%			
Paravertebral	Ropivacaine 0.2%	0.1–0.2 mL/kg/hr		
	Bupivacaine 0.25% with 1:400,000 epinephrine	0.1 mL/kg/hr		

b. **Femoral Nerve Block.** Although the nerve can be visualized with ultrasonography both above and below the inguinal ligament, it is ideally visualized at the level of the inguinal crease; at this level, the nerve is positioned approximately 0.5 cm lateral to the femoral artery. The nerve provides motor innervation to the quadriceps femoris, sartorius, and pectineus muscles as well as sensory innervation to the anterior thigh and knee and the medial aspect of the lower extremity terminating as the saphenous nerve. Femoral nerve blockade is tremendously effective for postoperative pain control after arthroscopic reconstruction of the anterior cruciate ligament with patellar tendon autograft.

    c. **Saphenous nerve blockade** is frequently combined with a lateral popliteal block or sciatic block for procedures involving the lower leg. The saphenous nerve is the only branch of the lumbar plexus below the knee and is the largest sensory terminal branch of the femoral nerve.

3. **Sacral Plexus**

    a. After foot and ankle surgery, sciatic nerve blockade provides safe, effective, and long-lasting postoperative analgesia. Ultrasound guidance provides real-time visualization and high-quality images of the sciatic nerve.

    b. **Paravertebral blockade** may provide segmental analgesia for numerous surgical procedures (thoracotomy, mastectomy, nephrectomy, cholecystectomy, rib fractures, video-assisted thorascopic surgery, inguinal and abdominal procedures).

XII. CONTINUOUS PERIPHERAL NERVE BLOCKADE CAVEATS

Hemorrhagic complications, rather than neurologic deficits, appear to be the predominant risk associated with the performance of peripheral nerve blockade in anticoagulated patients.

XIII. COMPLICATIONS FROM REGIONAL ANESTHESIA

The comparative safety of regional anesthesia compared with general anesthesia cannot be accurately determined. Serious complications associated with the performance of regional anesthesia include cardiac arrest, radiculopathy, cauda equina syndrome, and paraplegia (Table 57-13). The incidences of cardiac arrest and neurologic complications are higher after spinal anesthesia than after all other types of regional procedures.

XIV. PERIOPERATIVE PAIN MANAGEMENT OF OPIOID-DEPENDENT PATIENTS

The onus for the identification of opioid-dependent patients rests with the surgical team, preoperative evaluation staff, and anesthesia team (Table 57-14).

TABLE 57-13

RISK FACTORS FOR NERVE INJURY DURING THE PERFORMANCE
OF REGIONAL ANESTHESIA

Variable	Risk Factors
Patient	Body habitus
	Pre-existing neurologic disorder (diabetes mellitus, past chemotherapy)
	Male gender
	Advanced age
Surgical	Direct surgical trauma or stretch
	Prolonged tourniquet time
	Hematoma
	Infection
	Tightly applied casts or surgical dressings
	Patient positioning
Regional anesthesia	Mechanical injury from the needle or catheter
	Chemical neurotoxicity from the local anesthetic
	Ischemic injury to the nerve

A. **Preoperative management** involves determining the patient's "baseline" opioid requirement and instruction to the patient to take his or her normal opioid dose on the day of surgery.
   1. Patients maintained on methadone should continue their "baseline" dose throughout the perioperative period. Patients receiving greater than 200 mg/day of methadone may develop a prolonged QT interval, which places them at risk for torsades de pointes (a baseline electrocardiogram should be obtained).
   2. Full antagonists (naloxone, naltrexone) and the partial agonists–antagonists (nalbuphine, pentazocine, butorphanol) should be avoided because they precipitate withdrawal symptoms in opioid-dependent patients.
B. **Intraoperative management** of opioid-dependent patients requires the prudent use of fentanyl, morphine, or hydromorphone to provide effective intraoperative anesthesia and postoperative analgesia and to prevent opioid withdrawal. This requires the administration of the patient's "baseline" opioid requirement plus his or her intraoperative requirements secondary to surgical stimulation.

PERIOPERATIVE

TABLE 57-14

SURGICAL GUIDELINES FOR PERIOPERATIVE PAIN MANAGEMENT OF OPIOID-TOLERANT PATIENTS

Preoperative
Evaluation: Early recognition and high index of suspicion.
Identification: Identify factors such as total opioid dose requirement and previous surgery or trauma.
Consultation: Meet with addiction specialists and pain specialists for perioperative planning.
Reassurance: Discuss patient concerns related to pain control, anxiety, and risk of relapse.
Medication: Calculate the opioid dose requirement and modes of administration; provide anxiolytics as needed.

Intraoperative
Maintain baseline opioids (oral, transdermal, intravenous).
Increase the intraoperative and postoperative opioid dose to compensate for tolerance. Provide peripheral neural or plexus blockade (consider neuraxial techniques).
Use non-opioids as analgesic adjuncts.

Postoperative
Plan preoperatively for postoperative analgesia (include an alternative).
Maintain baseline opioids.
Use multimodal analgesic techniques.
Use patient-controlled analgesia (use as primary therapy or as supplementation for neuraxial techniques).
Continue neuraxial opioids.
Continue continuous neural blockade.

After Discharge
If surgery provides complete pain relief, opioids should be tapered rather than abruptly discontinued.
Develop a pain management plan before hospital discharge (provide adequate doses of opioid and non-opioid analgesics).

1. Because of chronic opioid administration, opioid doses may need to be increased 30% to 100% vis-à-vis the opioid-naïve patient.
2. The optimal intraoperative dose of opioid varies considerably from patient to patient; therefore, monitoring intraoperative vital signs such as heart rate, pupil size, and respiratory rate can be useful and allows the clinician to avoid the negative consequences of overdosing or underdosing the patient with opioid.
   a. Titrating fentanyl, morphine, or hydromorphone to a respiratory rate of 12 to 14 breaths/min and a moderately miotic pupil is recommended.

   b. It is also recommend that patients who are receiving chronic methadone therapy may receive an additional intraoperative dose of 0.1 mg/kg IV, which can be titrated to hemodynamic effect and pupillary response.

C. **Postoperative Management**

   1. Upon arrival to the recovery room, IV opioids may be administered on an "as needed" basis; however, initiation of an IV PCA opioid with both a basal and incremental (bolus) dose minimizes the risk of breakthrough pain.
   2. Non-opioid co-analgesics (low-dose ketamine) are opioid sparing and should be part of any multimodal perioperative pain management regimen in opioid-dependent patients.
   3. Regional anesthesia (peripheral nerve blockade, epidural analgesia) is highly recommended in this patient population.
   4. Careful monitoring of the patient for excessive sedation and respiratory depression is mandatory, and caregivers in the recovery room and on the postsurgical units should be alerted to the potential risk for respiratory depression when parenteral and neuraxial opioids are combined.

XV. **ORGANIZATION OF PERIOPERATIVE PAIN MANAGEMENT SERVICES**

The effective management of pain is a crucial component of good perioperative care and recovery from surgery. Unrelieved pain and inadequate pain relief have detrimental physiologic and psychological effects on patients by slowing their recovery. The key components to establishing a successful perioperative pain management service begins with an institutional commitment to support the service. The team must be built around a physician leader with training and experience in pain medicine, and other anesthesiologists must be available to support the service.

XVI. **SPECIAL CONSIDERATIONS IN THE PERIOPERATIVE PAIN MANAGEMENT OF CHILDREN**

Acute pain management in children undergoing surgery and invasive procedures offers several specific and unique challenges for anesthesiologists (Table 57-15).

PERIOPERATIVE

TABLE 57-15

CHALLENGES FOR ACUTE PAIN MANAGEMENT IN CHILDREN

Importance of the child's parents and siblings
Unavoidable preoperative fear and anxiety (adversely impact
  postoperative pain and recovery from surgery)
Developmental and communications issues
Difficulty in evaluating the effectiveness of treatment

A. **Nonparenteral Analgesics**
   1. **Non-opioid analgesics** (oral or suppository
      acetaminophen, ibuprofen, ketorolac) are important
      adjuvant analgesic therapies, often with oral mida-
      zolam.
   2. **Opioid Analgesics.** Codeine in combination with
      acetaminophen is commonly used with good effect
      for the management of moderate postoperative pain
      in ambulatory patients. Intranasal sufentanil can
      also be used to manage preoperative anxiety and
      postoperative analgesia in children.
B. **Patient-Controlled Analgesia.** There are safety
   concerns with use of PCA in children that mandate a
   high level of surveillance with respect to the functioning of the equipment and careful patient monitoring
   that may be a limitation to its use in infants. PCA by
   proxy is a safety risk because there is no complete
   assurance that parents will be competent in assessing
   the intensity of their child's pain or be able to regulate
   bolus doses to avoid opioid overdosage.
C. **Epidural neuraxial analgesia** (single-shot technique or
   continuous catheter technique) has become a key component of the perioperative pain management plan for
   infants and young children undergoing abdominal,
   urologic, and orthopaedic procedures.
D. **Nerve Blocks in Children.** The introduction of small
   stimulating needles and ultrasound imaging along with
   long-acting local anesthetics and continuous catheter
   techniques in selected patients has resulted in an
   increase in the use of peripheral nerve blocks in
   children undergoing orthopaedic extremity procedures.
   Combined ilioinguinal and iliohypogastric nerve
   blocks performed under ultrasound guidance to reduce
   the volume of the injection have gained increasing
   interest for effective pain management in children
   undergoing inguinal herniorrhaphy.

CHAPTER 58 ■ CHRONIC PAIN MANAGEMENT

I. ANATOMY, PHYSIOLOGY, AND NEUROCHEMISTRY OF SOMATOSENSORY PAIN PROCESSING (Fig. 58-1)

A. **Primary Afferents and Peripheral Stimulation.** A variety of mechanical, thermal, and chemical stimuli may result in the sensation and perception of pain (Benzon HT, Hurley R, Deer T: Chronic pain management. In *Clinical Anesthesia*. Edited by Barash PG, Cullen BF, Stoelting RK, Cahalan MK, Stock MC. Philadelphia: Lippincott Williams & Wilkins, 2009, pp 1505–1531). Information about these painful or noxious stimuli is carried to higher brain centers by receptors and neurons that are distinct from those that carry innocuous somatic sensory information (Table 58-1).

B. **Neurochemistry of Peripheral Nerve and the Dorsal Root Ganglion.** The nociceptive primary afferents (the A and C fibers) represent the principal target of pharmacologic manipulation by physicians treating pain. Glutamate receptors, as well as opioid, substance P, somatostatin, and vanilloid receptors, have been identified on the peripheral endings of these nerve fibers.

1. The cell bodies of primary afferents, regardless of the structure they innervate, make up the dorsal root ganglia located just outside the spinal cord within the bony foramen.

2. Primary afferent activation results in a postsynaptic excitatory event in the spinal cord. Glutamate is the primary neurotransmitter serving this function.

C. **Neurobiology of the Spinal Cord and Spinal Trigeminal Nucleus.** Primary afferent fibers enter the gray matter of the spinal cord through the dorsal root entry zone and innervate the spinal cord.

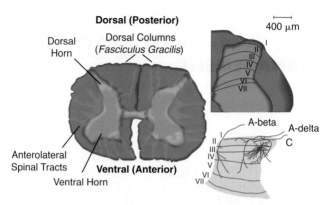

FIGURE 58-1. Anatomy and physiology of somatosensory and pain processing.

1. The gray matter of the spinal cord is made up of synaptic terminations of primary afferents and the second-order neurons, which form the first stage of processing and integration of sensory information.
2. The gray matter of the spinal cord is divided into 10 laminae based on histologic appearance.
   a. The dorsal horn includes laminae I–VI and represents the primary sensory component of the spinal cord.
   b. The ventral horn, including laminae VII–IX and X, is involved in somatic motor and autonomic function, respectively.
   c. Somatic C-fiber nociceptive afferents endings primarily terminate in the laminae I and II of the same or one or two adjacent spinal segments from which they entered from the periphery. The visceral C-fiber nociceptive afferents terminate in the dorsal horn more than five segments rostrally or caudally.
   d. The substantia gelatinosa or lamina II also contains excitatory and inhibitory interneurons but fewer projection neurons.
D. **Neurobiology of Ascending Pathways**
   1. **Dorsal Column Tracts.** The dorsal column contains the axons of second-order spinal cord projection

TABLE 58-1

PRIMARY AFFERENT FIBERS AND THEIR CHARACTERISTICS

Modality	Receptor	Fiber Type	Conduction Velocity (m/s)	Diameter (μ)	Rate of Adaptation	Function
Proprioceptive	Golgi and Ruffini endings, muscle spindle afferents	Aα	70–120	15–20	Slow and rapid	Muscle tension, length, and velocity
Mechanosensitive	Meissner, Ruffini, Pacinian corpuscles and Merkel disc	Aβ	40–70	5–15	Rapid (slow-Merkel)	Touch, flutter, motion, pressure, vibration
Thermoreceptive	Free nerve endings	Aδ	10–35	1–5	Slow	Innocuous cold
	Free nerve endings	C	0.5–1.0	<1	Slow	Innocuous warmth
Nociceptive	Free nerve endings	Aδ	10–35	<1	Slow	Sharp pain
	Free nerve endings	C	0.5–1.0		Slow	Burning pain

neurons in addition to the ascending axons of primary afferent neurons relaying touch, pressure, and vibratory sensation.

2. **Spinothalamic tract** (STT) neurons are the primary relay cells that provide nociceptive input from the spinal cord to supraspinal levels. The axons of STT cells cross the midline of the spinal cord through the anterior white commissure and ascend primarily in the contralateral lateral and anterolateral tracts.

3. **Spinobulbar Pathways.** Major ascending lateral axonal projections relaying information about noxious stimuli terminate in the reticular formation of the ventrolateral medulla.

E. **Neurobiology of Supraspinal Structures Involved in Higher Cortical Processing.** Higher cortical centers play a role in the perception of painful stimuli as well as the integration of the sensory-discriminative and affective components of the noxious stimulation.

F. **Transition from Acute to Persistent Nociception**

1. Pain sensation is unique in that it does not rapidly adapt to prolonged stimulation as do the other sensory modalities, such as fine touch (allodynia, hyperalgesia).

2. Persistent C fiber (but not Aβ fiber) primary afferent activation of lamina I and V, as occurs with tissue injury and inflammation, has been shown to enhance the response to subsequent stimulation and augment the size of the receptive field of the respective dorsal horn neuron. This general phenomenon has come to be termed *wind-up* or *central sensitization.*

3. Although acute noxious stimuli are transmitted to the spinal cord via Aβ and C fibers, the presence of allodynia is thought to be mediated by the activation of large-diameter Aβ fibers through what has been termed a "phenotypic" switch.

II. MANAGEMENT OF COMMON PAIN SYNDROMES

A. **Low Back Pain: Radicular Pain Syndromes** (Table 58-2)

1. Low back and radicular pain secondary to a herniated vertebral disc are caused by mechanical nerve root compression and the subsequent inflammatory process.

TABLE 58-2

COMMON CAUSES OF LOW BACK PAIN

Radiculitis or radiculopathy from a herniated disc or spinal or
  foraminal stenosis
Facet syndrome
Internal disc disruption
Myofascial pain
Sacroiliac joint syndrome and pyriformis syndrome (mostly
  buttock pain)
Vertebral body fractures
Infections
Abdominal aortic aneurysm
Chronic pancreatic lesions

    a. The presence of a herniated disc does not neces-
       sarily result in pain.
    b. Patients with a herniated disc may show sponta-
       neous regression without treatment; absence of
       symptoms in the presence of more abnormali-
       ties; and partial or complete resolution with
       treatment that includes medications, bed rest,
       physical therapy, traction, or epidural steroids.

2. If symptomatic, the patient usually presents with
   low back pain and radicular symptoms that include
   paresthesias and numbness and weakness in the
   distribution of the involved nerve root. Radicular
   pain typically travels along a narrow band and has
   a sharp, shooting, and lancinating quality. Gait
   disturbances, loss of sensation, reduced muscle
   strength, and diminished reflexes involve the appropriate affected dermatomal distribution.

3. Inflammation in the spinal canal secondary to a herniated disc plays an important role in the causation
   of back and radicular pain. A herniated nucleus
   pulposus results in local release of cytokines and
   other inflammatory mediators that cause a chemical
   radiculitis.

4. Epidural steroid injections (ESIs) may be useful to
   treat some forms of low back pain because of their
   anti-inflammatory, local anesthetic, and antinociceptive effect. At best, ESIs may provide transient relief
   (no longer than 3 months) from the injections
   (Table 58-3).

TABLE 58-3

COMPLICATIONS OF EPIDURAL STEROID INJECTIONS

Needle trauma
Vasospasm
Infection
Glucocorticoids reduce the hypoglycemic effect of insulin
Insulin sensitivity may be impaired
Suppress plasma cortisol levels and the ability to secrete cortisol in
   response to synthetic ACTH for up to 3 weeks

ACTH = adrenocorticotrophic hormone.

      a. The transient relief provided by ESIs may minimize the need for potent anti-inflammatory medications or opioids and may reduce the incidence of drug-related side effects.

      b. ESIs should be a component, not the sole modality, of the conservative management of radicular pain.

      c. It is advisable that fluoroscopy be used in ESIs to ensure insertion of the needle at the affected vertebral level and document and follow the flow of the contrast medium (and the drug).

      d. If there is no response to an initial injection, it can be repeated once because some patients require a second injection before they respond. If there is partial response, up to three injections can be performed.

   5. It appears that surgery for a herniated disc produces only short-term relief. The long-term results are comparable to those seen with conservative management. For spinal stenosis, surgery is associated with greater improvements in most outcome measures.

B. Facet Syndrome

   1. Patients with low back pain secondary to facet problems have pain in the low back that radiate to the ipsilateral posterior thigh and usually ends at the knee. On physical examination, paraspinal tenderness and reproduction of pain occur with extension–rotation maneuvers of the back.

   2. The diagnosis of facet syndrome is arrived at by a combination of the patient's history, physical examination findings, and a positive response to diagnostic medial branch blocks or facet joint injections.

C. **Buttock Pain: Sacroiliac Joint (SIJ) Syndrome and Piriformis Syndrome**
   1. The pain of SIJ syndrome is located in the region of the affected SIJ and medial buttock.
   2. Physical examination usually reveals tenderness over the sacroiliac sulcus, reduction in the joint mobility, and reproduction of the pain when the affected SIJ is stressed.
   3. The treatments for SIJ syndrome include physical therapy, manipulation, intra-articular steroid injections, radiofrequency denervation, and surgical fusion of the joint.
D. **Piriformis syndrome** is another pain syndrome that originates in the buttock and affects 5% to 6% of patients referred for the treatment of back and leg pain. The pain is aggravated by hip flexion, adduction, and internal rotation. Neurologic examination findings are usually negative. There may be leg numbness when the sciatic nerve is irritated; the straight leg test result may be normal or limited.
   1. The diagnosis of piriformis syndrome is made on clinical grounds.
   2. Treatment for piriformis syndrome includes physical therapy combined with medications including muscle relaxants, anti-inflammatory drugs, and analgesics to reduce the spasm, inflammation, and pain. Local anesthetic and steroid injections into the piriformis may break the pain/muscle spasm cycle.
E. **Myofascial pain syndrome and fibromyalgia (MFPS)** is a painful regional syndrome characterized by the presence of an active trigger point in a skeletal muscle (Table 58-4).
   1. The management of MFPS includes repeated applications of a cold spray over the trigger point in line with the involved muscle fibers followed by gentle massage of the trigger point and stretching of the affected muscle.
   2. Another treatment is local anesthetic injection or dry needling of the trigger point.
F. **Fibromyalgia.** The American College of Rheumatology criteria for classification of fibromyalgia requires only a history of widespread pain for at least 3 months and allodynia to digital pressure at 11 or more of 18 anatomically defined tender points.

TABLE 58-4

CRITERIA FOR THE DIAGNOSIS OF MYOFASCIAL PAIN
SYNDROME AND FIBROMYALGIA

Palpable taut band
Exquisite spot tenderness of a nodule in the taut band
Pressure on the tender nodule that induces pain
Painful limitation to full passive range of motion for the affected
   muscle
Visual or tactile identification of local twitch response induced
   by needle penetration of a tender nodule
Electromyographic demonstration of spontaneous electrical activity
   characteristic of active loci in the tender nodule of a taut band

III. NEUROPATHIC PAIN SYNDROMES

A. Herpes Zoster and Postherpetic Neuralgia

1. The pain of acute herpes zoster is usually moderate
   in severity and can be managed with analgesics. The
   pain usually subsides with healing of the rash. Ten
   percent to 15% of the patients develop postherpetic
   neuralgia (PHN), or pain that persists more than
   3 months after resolution of the rash; the incidence
   increases to 30% to 50% in elderly individuals.
2. The risk factors for the development of PHN
   include increased pain during the acute stage,
   greater severity of the skin lesion, older age, and the
   presence of a prodrome.
3. The use of antiviral drugs acyclovir, famciclovir, or
   valacyclovir has been shown to hasten the healing
   of the rash, reduce the duration of viral shedding,
   and decrease the increase of PHN.
4. Studies on the efficacy of neuraxial and peripheral
   nerve blocks provide conflicting results. To be effective in preventing PHN, the blocks are preferably
   done within 2 to 4 weeks of the onset of rash.
5. The mainstay of treatment for postherpetic neuralgia is pharmacologic management that includes
   anticonvulsants, opioids, and antidepressants.
   a. Based on efficacy (numbers needed to treat), anti-
      depressants are the first choice for neuropathic
      pain syndromes, followed by opioids, tramadol,
      and gabapentin or pregabalin.
   b. If quality of life, side effects, prevention of addic-
      tion, and regulatory issues are to be considered

TABLE 58-5

SYMPTOMS OF SENSORIMOTOR DISTAL POLYNEUROPATHY

Burning pain
Deep aching pain
Electrical or stabbing sensations
Paresthesias and hyperesthesias (usually worse at night)
Peripheral autonomic dysfunction

along with pain relief, then gabapentin and pregabalin are the first drugs of choice.

c. For allodynia accompanying PHN, the lidocaine patch is recommended.

B. **Diabetic Painful Neuropathy (DPN).** Neuropathies secondary to diabetes can be classified into generalized neuropathies and focal or multifocal neuropathies. Peripheral neuropathy may be present in approximately 65% of patients with insulin-dependent diabetes mellitus (IDDM), most commonly distal symmetric polyneuropathy followed by median nerve mononeuropathy at the wrist and visceral autonomic neuropathy.

1. Chronic sensorimotor distal polyneuropathy is the most common type of diabetic neuropathy (Table 58-5). The lower limbs are usually involved with loss of sensation to vibration, pressure, pain, and temperature along with absent ankle reflexes.

2. The management of DPN includes tight control of the patient's blood glucose and pharmacologic therapy.

a. The anticonvulsants gabapentin and pregabalin appear to be effective in the management of DPN, with the efficacy of gabapentin enhanced by the addition of controlled-release morphine.

b. The tricyclic antidepressants (TCAs) are also effective in patients with DPN; the selective serotonin reuptake inhibitors are not as effective.

c. Opioids and tramadol are also effective in the treatment of DPN.

C. **Chronic Regional Pain Syndrome (CRPS)**

1. There are two types of CRPS. CRPS type I was originally called reflex sympathetic dystrophy, and CRPS type II represents causalgia (Table 58-6). A discrepancy is typically seen between the severity of the symptoms and severity of the inciting injury.

PERIOPERATIVE

TABLE 58-6

SIGNS AND SYMPTOMS OF CHRONIC REGIONAL
PAIN SYNDROME

Spontaneous pain
Hyperalgesia
Allodynia
Trophic, sudomotor, or vasomotor abnormalities
Active and passive movement disorders

The clinical features of CRPS type II are the same as in CRPS type I except there is a preceding nerve injury in CRPS II.

2. The primary treatment for CRPS includes sympathetic blocks, physical therapy, and oral medications.

   a. Intravenous (IV) regional anesthesia with bretylium and lidocaine or ketorolac may also be used.

   b. Pharmacologic therapy for CRPS includes gabapentin and memantine, a neuromuscular blocking drug.

   c. If the patient does not respond to the above treatments, then spinal cord stimulation can be entertained.

D. **Human Immunodeficiency Virus (HIV) Neuropathy.** Symptomatic neuropathy occurs in 10% to 35% of patients who are seropositive for HIV, and pathologic abnormalities exist in almost all patients with end-stage AIDS.

   1. The sensory neuropathies associated with HIV include distal sensory polyneuropathy, the more common neuropathy related to the viral infection, and antiretroviral toxic neuropathy secondary to treatment.

   2. The clinical features of HIV sensory neuropathy typically include painful allodynia and hyperalgesia. The onset is gradual and most commonly involves the lower extremities.

   3. The treatment of HIV sensory neuropathy is symptomatic and includes optimization of the patient's metabolic and nutritional status.

E. **Phantom Pain.** Nearly all patients with amputated extremities experience nonpainful phantom sensations, and phantom pain, or painful sensation referred to the phantom limb, occurs in as many as 80% of amputees. The onset of pain may be immediate but commonly occurs within the first few days after amputation. Approximately 50% of patients experience a decrease of their pain with time; the other 50% report no change or an increase in pain over time.

1. Phantom pain is caused by both peripheral and central factors. Peripheral mechanisms include neuromas, an increase in C-fiber activity, and sodium channel activation. Central mechanisms include abnormal firing of spinal internuncial neurons and supraspinal involvement secondary to the development of new synaptic connections in the cerebral cortex.

2. The treatment of phantom limb pain includes pharmacologic and nonpharmacologic measures. Pharmacologic treatments include the use of opioids and gabapentin and the empirical use of antidepressants. The nonpharmacologic measures include transcutaneous electrical nerve stimulation, spinal cord stimulators, and biofeedback.

IV. CANCER PAIN

Significant pain is present in up to 25% of patients with cancer who are in active treatment and in up to 90% of patients with advanced cancer.

A. Cancer pain can be somatic, visceral, or neuropathic (Table 58-7)
B. Management of cancer pain should be multifaceted.
   1. Pharmacologic therapies include opioids, antidepressants, anticonvulsants, nonsteroidal anti-inflammatory drugs (NSAIDs), corticosteroids, oral local anesthetics, and topical analgesics. Continuous

PERIOPERATIVE

TABLE 58-7

CAUSES AND CHARACTERISTICS OF CANCER PAIN

Somatic pain (responsive to opioids, NSAIDs, COX-2 inhibitors, neural blocks)
Visceral pain (sympathetic blocks)
Neuropathic pain (anticonvulsants, opioids, TCAs)

COX = cyclo-oxygenase; NSAID = nonsteroidal anti-inflammatory drug; TCA = tricyclic antidepressant.

TABLE 58-8

NEUROLYTIC BLOCKS FOR VISCERAL PAIN FROM CANCER

Celiac Plexus Block
Local anesthetics, alcohol, phenol
Complications may include orthostatic hypotension and paralysis

Superior Hypogastric Plexus Block
Indicated for pelvic pain secondary to cancer and chronic
  nonmalignant conditions

Ganglion Impar Block
Pain in the perineal area associated with malignancies can be
  treated with neurolysis of the ganglion impar (Walther's
  ganglion)

IV opioid infusions can be infused during the later
stages of life.

2. Interventional treatments include neurolytic sympathetic blocks and intrathecal opioids.
3. Opioids are the mainstay of treatment for cancer
   pain because approximately 70% to 95% of
   patients are responsive when appropriate guidelines
   are followed. Neurolytic blocks and intrathecal opioids should be considered when pharmacologic
   agents are not completely effective at maximum
   tolerated dosages.

C. **Neurolytic Blocks for Visceral Pain from Cancer**
   (Table 58-8)

D. **Pharmacologic Management**
   1. Morphine is the standard for opioid therapy of can-
      cer pain.
   2. Hydromorphone, a *mu*-receptor agonist, is three to
      five times more potent than morphine when given
      orally and five to seven times more potent when
      given parenterally.
   3. Methadone has a 60% to 95% bioavailability, a
      high potency, and a long duration of action. It is
      ideal in patients with renal failure because it does
      not accumulate in these patients. In 2006, the Food
      and Drug Administration issued an alert advisory
      regarding the hazards of death, opioid overdose,
      and cardiac dysrhythmias associated with
      methadone. The cardiac rhythm abnormalities
      include QT prolongation and torsades de pointes.

4. Oxycodone is mainly a prodrug that acts primarily by being converted by to oxymorphone. The controlled-release preparation (OxyContin) has good analgesic characteristics but has become a popular drug for abuse.
5. The weak opioids include codeine, hydrocodone, propoxyphene, and tramadol.
   a. Codeine is transformed to morphine via the enzyme cytochrome P450 2D6 (approximately 9% of white people do not have the enzyme and do not experience analgesia from codeine). Children younger than 12 years of age lack maturity of the enzyme and cannot convert the drug to morphine, so they experience the drug's side effects with minimal analgesia.
   b. Propoxyphene is a synthetic opioid structurally related to methadone.
   c. Tramadol is an opioid agonist and a monoaminergic drug.
6. There is considerable public concern regarding the effect of opioids on driving performance. Patients taking stable doses of opioids can probably drive, but those who are starting to take opioids and those who have had a recent dose increase should be warned about the hazards of driving.
7. Opioids are mostly used for cancer pain, with long-acting opioids supplemented by short-acting ones for breakthrough pain.
   a. Because of controversial issues associated with the use of opioids, such as addiction, aberrant behaviors, and regulatory issues, opioids are often second-line drugs for neuropathic pain.
   b. The combination of gabapentin and an opioid has been shown to result in better analgesia, fewer side effects, and the need for lower doses of each drug. Combination therapy is now commonly practiced in the treatment of patients with neuropathic pain.
   c. When considering the use of opioids for treatment of low back pain, it should be noted that although individual studies show the efficacy of opioids in low back pain, a meta-analysis did not show reduced pain compared with a placebo or a non-opioid control group. In addition to NSAIDs and muscle relaxants, opioids may be efficacious for short-term relief of acute low back pain, but

the long-term efficacy of opioids (≥16 weeks) is unclear. Antidepressants are preferred for treatment of chronic low back pain.

E. **Antidepressants**

1. The TCAs exert analgesic effects via multiple mechanisms (serotonergic, noradrenergic, opioidergic, and anti-inflammatory effects).

2. The side effects of antidepressants include cholinergic effects such as dry mouth, sedation, and urinary retention. Accidental or intentional overdose may lead to fatal dysrhythmias. TCAs impair driving ability during the first week of treatment and during dose escalation, but driving performance returns to baseline shortly thereafter.

F. **Anticonvulsants**

1. Anticonvulsants block sodium channels, explaining their efficacy in patients with neuropathic pain syndromes.

2. Randomized, controlled studies demonstrate the efficacy of the anticonvulsants in patients with neuropathic pain syndromes, including trigeminal neuralgia, postherpetic neuralgia, DPN, phantom limb pain, spinal cord injury pain, and Guillain-Barré syndrome.

3. Gabapentin is an effective drug in patients with neuropathic pain and has few side effects.

4. Lamotrigine has been shown to be effective in HIV polyneuropathy, pain from spinal cord injury, and central poststroke pain.

G. **Lidocaine Patch, Mexiletine, and Intravenous Lidocaine**

1. The 5% lidocaine patch delivers drug locally at the site of neuropathic pain generation, limiting its systemic effects and reducing its interactions with other concomitantly administered medications. Analgesia is provided through local sodium channel blockade rather than through its systemic effects.

2. Mexiletine is oral lidocaine. Its efficacy is similar to IV lidocaine, although a favorable response to IV lidocaine does not necessarily mean a similar response to mexiletine.

3. A meta-analysis has shown IV lidocaine to be superior to placebo and equal to morphine, gabapentin, and amitriptyline for treatment of patients with neuropathic pain.

V. INTERVENTIONAL PROCEDURES

Anesthesiologists who have completed a pain management fellowship are well suited to perform invasive procedures for the treatment of chronic pain. Complications from some of these invasive procedures can be serious (discitis, worsening neuropathy, paraplegia).

A. Discography

1. The symptoms of discogenic pain are nonspecific and include nonradicular back pain that is worse in the sitting position. The pain is provoked by bending and may involve the buttock, hip, groin, and thighs. The neurologic examination results, including results for the straight leg raise, are usually normal. Magnetic resonance imaging may show a high-intensity zone on the T2 sagittal images, indicating an annular tear.

2. Treatments include stabilization, exercise training, education, activity modification, and ESIs.

3. Functional discography involves the insertion of a catheter and injection of a local anesthetic followed by observation of the patient's response.

4. Discitis is the most feared complication of discography. The incidence of discitis is considerably decreased with prophylactic antibiotic use.

   a. The diagnosis of discitis includes worsening back pain the week after discography and elevated erythrocyte sedimentation rate and C-reactive protein that usually peak 3 weeks after the procedure.

   b. The most common causative organism in discitis is *Staphylococcus aureus*.

B. Intradiscal electrothermal therapy (IDET) is a procedure in which a thermal resistance catheter is placed percutaneously in the posterolateral portion of the disc. Heat causes the collagen of the annulus fibrosis to contract.

1. The complications of IDET may include catheter kinking or breakage, nerve root injury, nondermatomal leg pain, dural puncture, infection, bleeding, cauda equina syndrome, and spinal cord damage.

2. A review comparing IDET with surgical fusion in patients with intractable discogenic low back pain showed similar improvements in both groups.

C. In percutaneous disc decompression (nucleoplasty), a portion of the nucleus pulposus is removed or coagulated using radiofrequency energy.

TABLE 58-9

CONTRAINDICATIONS TO PERCUTANEOUS DISC DECOMPRESSION

Large, noncontained disc herniation
Free fragments
Herniation greater than one third the sagittal diameter of the
   spinal canal
Equivocal results from discography
Tumor, infection, or fracture
Spinal stenosis
Cauda equina syndrome or newly developed signs of neurologic
   deficit
Uncontrolled coagulopathy and bleeding disorders

    1. Discography may be performed before nucleoplasty
       to help determine which disc is involved.
    2. Contraindications to Percutaneous Disc Decompres-
       sion (Table 58-9)
  D. **Vertebroplasty and kyphoplasty** are percutaneous inter-
    ventional modalities to treat vertebral compression
    fractures, a condition that is usually secondary to
    osteoporosis in elderly patients.
    1. Vertebroplasty involves the injection of polymethyl-
       methacrylate into the affected vertebral body;
       kyphoplasty involves the insertion of a balloon
       before injection of the cement.
    2. Vertebroplasty is usually performed under
       fluoroscopic guidance, although a combination of
       fluoroscopy and computed tomography guidance
       has been described.
    3. Pulmonary embolism may result from leakage of
       cement into the paravertebral veins and bone mar-
       row or embolism of fat particles. Neurologic com-
       plications may include radiculopathy, spinal claudi-
       cation, and paraplegia.
    4. Kyphoplasty is associated with a greater restoration
       of vertebral height compared with vertebroplasty.
  E. **Spinal Cord Stimulation**
    1. The analgesic effect of spinal cord stimulation (SCS)
       involves the **gate control theory.** It has been hypoth-
       esized that SCS increases the input of the large nerve
       fibers, thus closing the "gate" at the substantia
       gelatinosa of the dorsal horn of the spinal cord
       (Table 58-10).

TABLE 58-10

INDICATIONS FOR SPINAL CORD STIMULATOR IMPLANTATION

Failed back surgery syndrome or neuropathic pain syndromes
Failed conservative therapy
Trial demonstrating pain relief
Significant psychological issues ruled out

---

    2. Placement of the permanent stimulator is preceded by a trial period of 5 to 7 days to confirm its efficacy (Fig. 58-2).
    3. Complications may include nerve and spinal cord injury, infection, hematoma, and lead breakage or migration.
  F. **Intrathecal Pumps**
    1. Intrathecal drug delivery systems (IDDS) are a valuable option in patients in whom oral or transdermal opioids are ineffective at reasonable doses or cause unacceptable side effects.
    2. The main indications for IDDS is cancer pain followed by pain of spinal origin, with the majority of pumps placed in the United States for failed back surgery syndrome.
    3. Several factors should be considered before instituting IDDS (Table 58-11).

TABLE 58-11

QUESTIONS TO CONSIDER BEFORE INTRATHECAL PUMP PLACEMENT

Are the pain complaints related to an objective physiological diagnosis?
Have less invasive therapies been tried or considered?
Is the patient's life expectancy 3 months or longer?
Is the patient's function limited by the pain symptoms?
Is the patient psychologically stable? Does the patient have uncontrolled psychosis, severe depression, intractable anxiety, or a significant personality disorder?
Is the patient compliant with other treatment recommendations?
Does the patient have any contraindications to pump placement such as bacteremia, bleeding disorders, or localized infection?
Has an acceptable trial been performed to document adequate pain response and controllable side effects?
Is the patient aware of the expectations of the procedure?
Is the patient agreeable to permanent pump placement despite the risks of the procedure and the long-term risks of the drugs to be infused?

PERIOPERATIVE

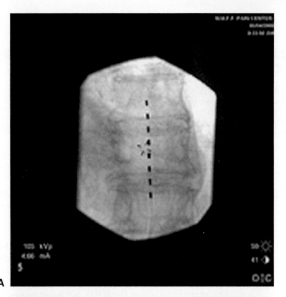

A

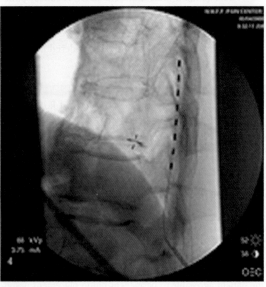

B

FIGURE 58-2. Anteroposterior (**A**) and lateral (**B**) views of a spinal cord stimulator placed over the T11–T12 vertebral levels. The stimulator was placed for peripheral ischemia.

2007 POLYANALGESIC ALGORITHM FOR INTRATHECAL THERAPIES

	(a)	(b)	(c)
Line #1:	Morphine ↔	Hydromorphone ↔	Ziconotide

	(d)	(e)	(f)
Line #2:	Fentanyl ↔	Morphine/Hydromorphone + Ziconotide ↔	Morphine/Hydromorphone + Bupivacaine/Clonidine ↕

	(g)	(h)	
Line #3:	Clonidine ↔	Morphine/Hydromorphone/Fentanyl Bupivacaine +/Clonidine + Ziconotide	

	(i)	(j)	
Line #4:	Sufentanil ↔	Sufentanil + Bupivacaine +/Clonidine + Ziconotide	

	(k)		
Line #5:	Ropivacaine, Buprenophine, Midazolam Meperidine, Ketorolac		

Line #6:	*Experimental Drugs* Gabapentin, Octreotide, Conepetide, Neostigmine, Adenosine, XEN2174, AM336, XEN, ZGX 160		

FIGURE 58-3. Recommendations for the management of pain by intrathecal drug delivery.

TABLE 58-12

COMPLICATIONS OF INTRATHECAL DRUG DELIVERY SYSTEMS

Infection
Bleeding
Respiratory depression
Pump malfunction
Catheter failure
Hormonal dysfunction (decreased testosterone levels)
Peripheral edema
Formation of an inflammatory mass (morphine concentrations
  >20 mg/mL or hydromorphone >10 mg/mL)

4. A treatment algorithm recommends morphine and hydromorphone as acceptable first-line agents. If either morphine or hydromorphone does not produce relief or causes side effects, then one drug is switched to the other first-line drug if the patient has primary nociceptive pain, or clonidine or bupivacaine is added for patients with primary neuropathic or mixed pain syndromes.
   a. In 2007, a panel of experts included ziconotide as a first-line drug (Fig. 58-3).
   b. Fentanyl was moved to a second-line agent because the more hydrophilic agents cause intractable side effects.
5. **Complications of Intrathecal Drug Delivery Systems** (Table 58-12)

CHAPTER 59 ■
CARDIOPULMONARY RESUSCITATION

The cardiopulmonary physiology, and pharmacology that form the basis of anesthesia practice are applicable to treating the victims of cardiac arrest (Otto CW: Cardiopulmonary resuscitation. In *Clinical Anesthesia*. Edited by Barash PG, Cullen BF, Stoelting RK, Cahalan MK, Stock MC. Philadelphia: Lippincott Williams & Wilkins, 2009, pp 1532–1558).

I. HISTORY (Table 59-1)

II. SCOPE OF THE PROBLEM

A. Cardiopulmonary resuscitation (CPR) is systematic therapy that is aimed at sustaining vital organ function until natural cardiac function can be restored.

B. In clinical practice, the severity of underlying cardiac disease is the major determining factor in the success or failure of CPR.

C. Brain adenosine triphosphate is depleted in 4 to 6 minutes of no blood flow. It returns nearly to normal within 6 minutes of starting effective CPR.

D. Factors associated with poor outcomes are long arrest time before CPR is begun, prolonged ventricular fibrillation without definitive therapy, and inadequate coronary and cerebral perfusion during cardiac massage.

1. Optimum outcome from ventricular fibrillation is obtained only if basic life support is begun within 4 minutes of arrest and defibrillation is applied within 8 minutes.

2. Blood flow decreases rapidly with interruptions of chest compressions (checking the pulse, intubation, defibrillation attempts, starting intravenous [IV] lines) and resumes slowly with reinstitution of com-

TABLE 59-1

HISTORY OF CARDIOPULMONARY RESUSCITATION

Bible story of Elisha breathing life back into the son of a Shunammite woman

Andreas Versalius described tracheostomy and artificial ventilation in 1543

Teaching of resuscitation by the Society for the Recovery of Persons Apparently Drowned founded in London in 1774

Establishment of mouth-to-mouth ventilation as the only effective means of artificial ventilation in the 1950s by Elam, Safar, and Gordon

Successful use of the internal defibrillator in 1947

External defibrillation introduced in the late 1950s

Description by Kouwenhoven, Jude, and Knickerbocker of closed chest compression

Description by Redding and Pearson of the value of epinephrine

pressions, emphasizing the importance of continued chest compressions in overall outcome.

III. ETHICAL ISSUES: "DO NOT RESUSCITATE" ORDERS IN THE OPERATING ROOM

A. The patient's right to limit medical treatment, including refusing CPR (with a "do not resuscitate" order) is firmly established in modern medical practice based on the ethical principle of respect for patient autonomy.

B. There are ethically sound arguments on both sides of the issue of whether DNR orders should be upheld in the operating room.

1. A desire by the anesthesiologist or surgeon to suspend DNR orders during surgery is often based on the knowledge that nearly 75% of cardiac arrests in the operating room are related to surgical or anesthetic complications and that resuscitation attempts are highly successful.

2. A mutual decision to suspend or limit a DNR order in the perioperative period may be achieved by communication among the patient, family, and caregivers.

   a. Many interventions used commonly in the operating room (mechanical ventilation, vasopressors, cardiac antidysrhythmics, blood products) may be considered forms of resuscitation in other situations. The only modalities that are not routine anesthetic care are cardiac massage and defibrillation.

    b. Specific interventions included in a DNR status must be clarified with allowance made for methods necessary to perform anesthesia and surgery.

IV. COMPONENTS OF RESUSCITATION

The major components of resuscitation from cardiac arrest are airway, breathing, circulation, drugs, and electrical therapy (ABCDE). Traditionally, these have been divided into basic life support (BLS) and advanced cardiac life support (ACLS) (Fig. 59-1). Recent advances in resuscitation (public access to automatic external defibrillators [AEDs]) have tended to blur the lines between BLS and ACLS.

A. Airway Management. The techniques used for airway maintenance during anesthesia are also applicable to cardiac arrest victims (Table 59-2).

1. **Foreign body airway obstruction** must be considered in any person who suddenly stops breathing and becomes cyanotic and unconscious. (This occurs most commonly during eating and is usually caused by food, especially meat, impacting in the laryngeal inlet, at the epiglottis, or in the vallecula.)

2. The signs of total airway obstruction are the lack of air movement despite respiratory efforts and the inability of the victim to speak or cough.

3. Treatment is the abdominal thrust maneuver (chest thrusts are an alternative for parturients and massively obese individuals) and the finger sweep.

4. In an awake victim, the rescuer reaches around the victim from behind, placing the fist of one hand in the epigastrium between the xiphoid and umbilicus. The fist is grasped with the other hand and pressed into the victim's epigastrium with a quick upward thrust. If the first attempt is unsuccessful, repeated attempts should be made because hypoxia-related muscular relaxation may eventually allow success.

B. Ventilation (see Fig. 59-1). When ventilation is provided in the rescue setting, mouth-to-mouth or mouth-to-nose ventilation is the most effective immediately available method. Although inspired gas with this method contains only about 17% oxygen and nearly 4% carbon dioxide (composition of exhaled air), it is sufficient to maintain viability.

PERIOPERATIVE

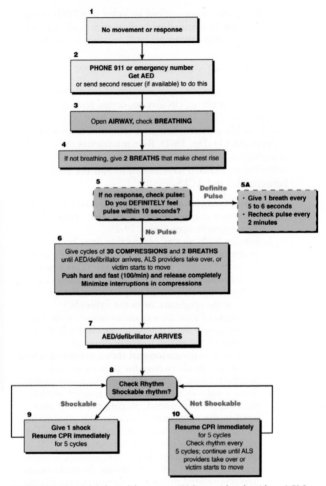

FIGURE 59-1. Adult basic life support (BLS) provider algorithm. ACLS = advanced cardiac life support; AED = automatic external defibrillator; CPR = cardiopulmonary resuscitation.

TABLE 59-2

TECHNIQUES USED FOR AIRWAY MAINTENANCE DURING
CARDIOPULMONARY RESUSCITATION

Head tilt and chin lift (the head is extended by pressure applied to
the brow while the mandible is pulled forward by pressure on
the front of the jaw, lifting the tongue away from the posterior
pharynx)
Jaw thrust (applying pressure behind the rami of the mandible)
Oropharyngeal or nasopharyngeal airway (danger of inducing
vomiting or laryngospasm in a semiconscious victim)
Tracheal intubation (should not be performed until adequate
ventilation and chest compression have been established)
Alternatives to tracheal intubation
    Laryngotracheal mask airway
    Airway Combitube
    Translaryngeal ventilation
    Tracheostomy

1. **Physiology of Ventilation During Cardiopulmonary
Resuscitation**
   a. Avoiding gastric insufflation requires that peak
   inspiratory airway pressures remain below
   esophageal opening pressure ($\sim$20 cm H_2O).
   Partial airway obstruction by the tongue and
   pharyngeal tissues is a major cause of increased
   airway pressure contributing to gastric insufflation during CPR. Properly applied pressure to
   the anterior arch of the cricoid (Sellick maneuver) causes the cricoid lamina to seal the esophagus and can prevent air from entering the stomach at airway pressures up to 100 cm H_2O.
   b. Achievement of an acceptable tidal volume during low inspiratory pressures characteristic of
   rescue breathing requires a slow inspiratory flow
   rate and long inspiratory time (breaths over
   1.5–2.0 seconds during a pause in chest compressions).
2. **Techniques of Rescue Breathing** (Table 59-3)
C. **Circulation**
   1. **Physiology of Circulation During Closed Chest
   Compression.** Two theories of the mechanism of
   blood flow during closed chest compression have

PERIOPERATIVE

TABLE 59-3

TECHNIQUES OF RESCUE BREATHING

Mouth-to-mouth ventilation (the rescuer delivers exhaled air to victim, and exhalation by the victim is passive)

Mouth-to-nose ventilation

Oropharyngeal airway with an external extension mouthpiece (it is often difficult to obtain a good mouth seal)

Mouth-to-mask ventilation (the mask may include one-way valve to direct the victim's exhaled gases away from the rescuer and a side port for delivery of supplemental oxygen)

Self-inflating resuscitation bag

Tracheal intubation (after placement of the tracheal tube, no pause should be made for ventilation because blood flow during CPR decreases rapidly when chest compressions are stopped)

CPR = cardiopulmonary resuscitation.

been suggested. The mechanism that predominates varies from victim to victim and even during the resuscitation of the same victim.

  a. The **cardiac pump mechanism** proposes that pressure on the chest compresses the heart between the sternum and spine. Compressions increase the pressure in the ventricular chambers (closing the atrioventricular valves) and eject blood into the lungs and aorta. During the relaxation phase of closed chest compression, expansion of the thoracic cage causes a subatmospheric intrathoracic pressure, facilitating blood return.

  b. The **thoracic pump mechanism** proposes that the increase in intrathoracic pressure caused by sternal compressions forces blood out of the chest (backward flow into veins is prevented by valves) with the heart acting as a passive conduit.

2. **Distribution of Blood Flow During Cardiopulmonary Resuscitation.** Cardiac output is decreased between 10% to 33% of normal during CPR, and nearly all the blood flow is directed to organs above the diaphragm (abdominal viscera and lower extremity blood flow are decreased to <5% of normal).

  a. Myocardial perfusion is 20% to 50% of normal, and cerebral perfusion is maintained at 50% to 90% of normal.

  b. Total flow tends to decrease with time during CPR, but the relative distribution is not altered.

Epinephrine may help sustain cardiac output over time during CPR.

3. **Gas Transport During Cardiopulmonary Resuscitation**
   a. During the low-flow state of CPR, excretion of carbon dioxide is decreased to the same extent that cardiac output is reduced.
   b. Exhaled carbon dioxide concentrations reflect only the metabolism of the part of the body that is being perfused.
   c. When normal circulation is restored, carbon dioxide that has accumulated in nonperfused tissues is washed out, and a temporary increase in carbon dioxide excretion is seen.
   d. Although carbon dioxide excretion is decreased during CPR, measurement of blood gases reveals an arterial respiratory alkalosis and a venous respiratory acidosis, reflecting the severely reduced cardiac output.

4. **Technique of Closed Chest Compression**
   a. Some circulation may be present in a "pulseless" patient (systolic blood pressure of about 50 mm Hg is necessary to palpate a peripheral pulse) with primary respiratory arrest. In such a patient, opening the airway and ventilation of the lungs may be sufficient for resuscitation. For this reason, a further search for a pulse should be made after artificial ventilation before beginning sternal compressions.
   b. Important considerations in performing closed chest compressions are the position of the rescuer relative to the victim, the position of the rescuer's hands, and the rate and force of compression (Table 59-4).

5. **Alternative Methods of Circulatory Support.** Standard CPR can sustain most patients for only 15 to 30 minutes. If return of spontaneous circulation has not been achieved in that time, the outcome is dismal.
   a. Alternatives to standard techniques for CPR are based on the thoracic pump mechanism with the goal of improving hemodynamics. Unfortunately, none of these alternatives has proven reliably superior to the standard technique.
   b. **Invasive Techniques.** Open chest cardiac massage or cardiopulmonary bypass must be instituted

PERIOPERATIVE

TABLE 59-4

TECHNIQUES OF CLOSED CHEST COMPRESSION

The rescuer should stand or kneel next to the victim's side.

The heel of one hand is placed on the lower sternum, and the other hand is placed on top of the hand on the victim. Pressing on the xiphoid, which can lead to liver laceration, should be avoided. Even with proper technique, costochondral separation and rib fractures are common.

Pressure is applied only with the heel of the hand (with the fingers free of contact with the chest) straight down on the sternum with the arms straight and the elbows locked into position so the entire weight of the upper body is used to apply force.

During relaxation, all pressure is removed, but the hands should not lose contact with the chest wall.

The sternum must be depressed 3.5 to 5.0 cm in the average adult (palpable pulse when systolic pressure >50 mm Hg).

The duration of compression should equal that of relaxation.

The compression rate should be 80 to 100/min.

early to improve survival. If open chest massage is begun after 30 minutes of ineffective closed chest compressions, there is no better survival even though hemodynamics are improved.

6. **Assessing the Adequacy of Circulation During Cardiopulmonary Resuscitation** (Table 59-5).

   a. The adequacy of closed chest compressions is usually judged by palpation of a pulse in the carotid or femoral artery (palpable pulse primarily reflects systolic blood pressure).

   b. The return of spontaneous circulation is greatly dependent on restoring oxygenated blood flow to the myocardium. Obtaining such flow depends on closed chest compressions developing adequate cardiac output and coronary perfusion

TABLE 59-5

CRITICAL VARIABLES ASSOCIATED WITH SUCCESSFUL RESUSCITATION

Myocardial blood flow	>15–20 mL/min/100 g
Aortic diastolic pressure	>40 mm Hg
Coronary perfusion pressure	>15–25 mm Hg
End-tidal carbon dioxide	>10 mm Hg

pressure (diastolic blood pressure minus central venous pressure). Damage to the myocardium from underlying disease may preclude survival no matter how effective the CPR efforts.

c. During CPR with a tracheal tube in place, exhalation of carbon dioxide is dependent on pulmonary blood flow (cardiac output) rather than alveolar ventilation. End-tidal carbon dioxide concentrations can be used to judge the effectiveness of chest compressions. Attempts should be made to maximize the end-tidal carbon dioxide concentration by alterations in technique or drug therapy (epinephrine). It should be remembered that sodium bicarbonate produces a transient (3–5 minutes) increase in end-tidal carbon dioxide concentration.

V. PHARMACOLOGIC THERAPY (Table 59-6).

Establishing IV access and pharmacologic therapy should come after other interventions have been instituted. Of the drugs given during CPR, only epinephrine is acknowledged as being useful in helping restore spontaneous circulation. Asystole and pulseless electrical

TABLE 59-6
ADULT ADVANCED CARDIAC LIFE SUPPORT DRUGS AND DOSES

	Dose (IV)	Dosing Interval	Maximum Dose
Epinephrine	1 mg	3–5 min	None
	3–7 mg*	3–5 min	
Vasopressin	40 U	May replace first or second dose of epinephrine	
Amiodarone	300 mg	Repeat 150 mg in 5 min	2 g
Lidocaine	1.0–1.5 mg/kg	Repeat 0.5–0.75 mg/kg in 5 min	3 mg/kg
Atropine	1 mg	3–5 min	0.04 mg/kg
Sodium bicarbonate	1 mEq/kg	As needed	Check pH

*Consider if there is no response to lower doses of epinephrine.

activity (electromechanical dissociation) are circumstances in which drugs are most frequently given.

A. **Routes of Administration**

1. The preferred route of administration of all drugs during CPR is IV. (Central injection produces a higher drug level and more rapid onset than peripheral injection.) Because of poor blood flow below the diaphragm during CPR, drugs administered into the lower extremity may not reach sites of action.

2. If venous access cannot be established, the endotracheal tube is an alternative route of administration for epinephrine, lidocaine, and atropine (not sodium bicarbonate). Doses 2 to 2.5 times the established IV dose administered in 5- to 10-mL volumes are recommended when the tracheal route of administration is used.

B. **Catecholamines and Vasopressors**

1. **Mechanism of Action.** The efficacy of **epinephrine** lies entirely in its α-adrenergic actions. (Peripheral vasoconstriction leads to an increase in aortic diastolic pressure, causing an increase in coronary perfusion pressure and myocardial blood flow.)

   a. It is commonly believed that the ability of epinephrine to increase the amplitude of ventricular fibrillation (α-adrenergic effect) makes defibrillation easier. There is no proof, however, that epinephrine improves the success or decreases the energy necessary for successful defibrillation.

   b. When added to chest compressions, epinephrine helps develop the critical coronary perfusion pressure necessary to provide myocardial blood flow for restoration of spontaneous circulation.

2. **Epinephrine** is given 1 mg IV every 3 to 5 minutes in adults. If this dose remains ineffective, higher doses (3–7 mg IV) should be considered.

3. **Vasopressin** is recommended as an alternative to epinephrine in a dose of 40 U IV as a one-time injection. If additional vasopressor doses are need, epinephrine should be administered.

C. **Amiodarone and Lidocaine**

1. These drugs are used during cardiac arrest to aid in defibrillation when ventricular fibrillation is refractory to electrical countershock or when ventricular fibrillation recurs. Amiodarone may be considered

the first drug for treatment of ventricular fibrillation that is resistant to electrical countershock.

   a. Lidocaine has few hemodynamic effects when given IV.

   b. Amiodarone can cause hypotension and tachycardia, especially with rapid IV administration.

2. Ventricular fibrillation threshold is decreased by acute myocardial ischemia or infarction, and this effect is partially reversed by lidocaine and amiodarone.

3. To rapidly achieve and maintain therapeutic blood levels during CPR, relatively large doses of lidocaine or amiodarone are necessary (see Table 59-6).

D. Atropine

1. Atropine (1 mg IV repeated every 3 to 5 minutes to a total dose of 0.04 mg/kg, which is totally vagolytic) is commonly administered during cardiac arrest associated with a pattern of asystole or slow, pulseless electrical activity on the electrocardiogram (ECG). Atropine enhances sinus node automaticity and atrioventricular conduction via its vagolytic effects.

   a. Excessive parasympathetic tone probably contributes little to asystole or pulseless electrical activity in adults (most often caused by myocardial ischemia).

   b. Even in children, it is doubtful that parasympathetic tone plays a significant role during most cardiac arrests.

2. Full vagolytic doses of atropine may be associated with fixed mydriasis after successful resuscitation confounding neurologic evaluation.

E. Sodium Bicarbonate

1. The use of sodium bicarbonate during CPR is based on theoretical considerations that acidosis lowers ventricular fibrillation threshold and respiratory acidosis impairs the physiologic response to catecholamines.

2. Little to no evidence supports the efficacy of sodium bicarbonate treatment during CPR. The lack of effect of buffer therapy may be explained by the slow onset of metabolic acidosis during cardiac arrest. (Acidosis as measured by blood lactate concentrations does not become severe for 15–20 minutes of cardiac arrest.)

3. In contrast to the lack of evidence that buffer therapy during CPR improves survival, the adverse effects of excessive sodium bicarbonate administration are well documented and include metabolic alkalosis, hypernatremia, and hyperosmolarity.

   a. IV sodium bicarbonate combines with hydrogen ions to produce carbonic acid that dissociates into carbon dioxide and water. ($PaCO_2$ is temporarily increased until ventilation eliminates the excess carbon dioxide.)

   b. Tissue acidosis during CPR is caused primarily by low tissue blood flow and accumulation of carbon dioxide in the tissues. (Theoretically, there is concern that carbon dioxide liberated from sodium bicarbonate could worsen existing tissue acidosis.)

4. Current practice restricts the use of sodium bicarbonate (1 mEq/kg IV initially with additional doses of 0.5 mEq/kg every 10 minutes [better if guided by blood gas determinations]) primarily to cardiac arrests that are associated with hyperkalemia, severe pre-existing metabolic acidosis, and tricyclic antidepressant overdose.

F. **Calcium**

1. The only indications for administration of calcium during CPR are hyperkalemia, hypocalcemia, or calcium blocker toxicity.

2. When calcium is administered, the chloride salt (2–4 mg/kg of the 10% solution IV) is recommended because it produces higher and more consistent levels of ionized calcium than other salts. (Calcium gluconate contains one third as much molecular calcium as the chloride salt.)

VI. ELECTRICAL THERAPY (see Fig. 59-1)

A. **Electrical Pattern and Duration of Ventricular Fibrillation.** Ventricular fibrillation is the most common ECG pattern found during cardiac arrest in adults, and the only effective treatment is electrical defibrillation. *Defibrillation should be performed as soon as the ventricular fibrillation is diagnosed and equipment is available.* Immediate defibrillation is only effective when applied within 4 to 5 minutes of collapse. Otherwise, a brief period of 2 to 3 minutes of chest compressions before defibrillation is necessary.

1. The most important controllable determinant of failure to resuscitate a patient with ventricular fibrillation is the duration of fibrillation. (The fibrillating heart has a high oxygen consumption.)
2. If defibrillation occurs within 1 minute of fibrillation, CPR is not necessary.
3. Defibrillation should not be delayed for epinephrine administration. (There is no evidence that epinephrine improves the success of defibrillation or decreases the energy setting needed for defibrillation.)
4. Fibrillation amplitude on an ECG lead varies with the orientation of that lead to the vector of the fibrillatory wave. (A flat line can be present if lead is oriented at right angles to the fibrillatory wave.)
5. A nonfibrillatory rhythm will not respond to defibrillation.

B. **Defibrillators: Energy, Current, and Voltage**
1. The typical defibrillator consists of a variable transformer that allows selection of a variable voltage potential, an AC to DC converter to provide a direct current that is stored in a capacitor, a switch to charge the capacitor, and discharge switches to complete the circuit from the capacitor to the paddle electrodes.
2. Defibrillation is accomplished by direct current passing through a critical mass of myocardium, resulting in simultaneous depolarization of the myofibrils.
3. Even at a constant delivered energy, the delivered current (critical determinant of defibrillation) is decreased as impedance (resistance) increases.

C. **Transthoracic Impedance** (Table 59-7)

TABLE 59-7

DETERMINANTS OF TRANSTHORACIC IMPEDANCE

Diameter of electrode paddles (most common diameter, 8–10 cm)
Impedance between metal electrode and skin (decreased with gel designed to conduct electricity in the defibrillation setting)
Successive shocks (may decrease impedance and partially explain why an additional shock of the same energy can cause defibrillation when previous shocks have failed)
Lung volume (air is a poor electrical conductor, so impedance is slightly higher during inspiration)
Paddle pressure (pressure of at least 11 kg decreases resistance by improving contact between the paddle and the skin and by expelling air from the lungs)

PERIOPERATIVE

D. **Adverse Effects and Energy Requirements**
  1. Repeated defibrillation with high-energy shocks, especially if repeated at short intervals, may result in myocardial damage.
  2. Current recommendations for adults are to use 200 J for the initial shock followed by a second shock at 200 to 300 J if the first is unsuccessful. If both fail to defibrillate the patient's heart, additional shocks should be given at 300 to 360 J.

VII. PUTTING IT ALL TOGETHER

Specific guidelines for the teaching and practice of CPR are published periodically (Figs. 59-1 and 59-2). The two levels of CPR care are referred to as BLS for ventilation and chest compressions without additional equipment and ACLS for using all modalities available for resuscitation. Medical personnel need to be well versed in both levels of care.

A. **Cardiocerebral Resuscitation.** An approach to victims of sudden cardiac death has been called cardiocerebral resuscitation or minimally interrupted cardiac resuscitation.
  1. **Time-Sensitive Model of Ventricular Fibrillation.** Untreated ventricular fibrillation has been described as a time-sensitive model consisting of the electrical (first 4–5 minutes), hemodynamic (next 10–15 minutes when perfusing the brain and heart with oxygenated blood is critical), and metabolic (not clear what intervention will be successful) phases.
     a. Prompt defibrillation during the **electrical phase** is when CPR has had the most dramatic effect and why public access AED has proven beneficial. The longer ventricular fibrillation continues, the more difficult it is to defibrillate and the less likely successful resuscitation is.
     b. If an arrest is witnessed and a defibrillator or AED is immediately available, then defibrillation should be the first priority in resuscitation.
  2. The most important intervention during the **hemodynamic phase** of cardiac arrest is producing coronary perfusion with chest compressions before any attempt to defibrillate.
  3. In the absence of prompt defibrillation, the most important intervention for neurologically normal survival from cardiac arrest is restoration and

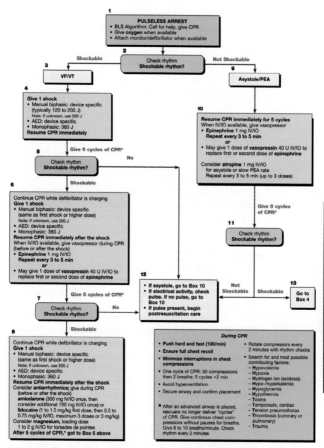

FIGURE 59-2. Adult advanced cardiac life support pulseless arrest algorithm. AED = automatic external defibrillator; CPR = cardiopulmonary resuscitation; IV = intravenous; PEA = pulseless electrical activity; VF = ventricular fibrillation; VT = ventricular tachycardia.

maintenance of cerebral and myocardial blood flow. This is the main principle behind the concept of **cardiocerebral resuscitation**.

B. **Bystander Cardiopulmonary Resuscitation.** Restoration of cerebral and myocardial blood flow must begin at the scene of the cardiac arrest. Much of the reluctance

PERIOPERATIVE

to initiate CPR as a bystander is the concern of applying mouth-to-mouth ventilation on a stranger.

1. If the airway remains patent during CPR, chest compressions cause substantial air exchange. Some data suggest that eliminating mouth-to-mouth ventilation early in the resuscitation of witnessed fibrillatory cardiac arrest is not detrimental to outcome and may improve survival.

2. Recognizing the deleterious effects of prolonged pauses in chest compressions for ventilation, the 2005 American Heart Association's guidelines change the compression-to-ventilation ratio from 15:2 to 30:2, recommending that ventilation be done in 2 to 4 seconds.

3. A public education program stresses an immediate call to 911 and prompt institution of continuous chest compressions without ventilation in the case of witnessed unexpected sudden collapse in adults.

C. **Cardiocerebral Resuscitation During Advanced Life Support**

1. The principle of not interrupting chest compressions to maintain cerebral and myocardial perfusion applies to resuscitation attempts by health care providers as well as lay bystanders.

2. The adverse hemodynamic consequences of interrupting chest compressions have been well documented. Blood flow stops almost immediately with cessation of chest compressions and returns slowly when they are resumed. Consequently, in cardiocerebral resuscitation, the emphasis is that chest compressions are to be paused only when absolutely necessary and then for the shortest time possible.

3. Positive pressure ventilation increases intrathoracic pressure, reducing venous return, cardiac output, and coronary perfusion pressure and adversely affecting survival.

D. **Rhythm Analysis and Defibrillation**

1. Defibrillation during the hemodynamic phase is counterproductive, usually producing either asystole or pulseless electrical activity.

2. The success rate of a single shock is between 70% and 85%, with most monophasic waveform defibrillators and more than 90% with the newer biphasic waveform units.

3. In prolonged ventricular fibrillation, successful defibrillation almost always results in asystole or pulseless electrical activity. Immediately restarting chest compressions (without waiting to check a pulse or reanalyze the ECG rhythm) after defibrillation to provide coronary perfusion nearly always results in reversion to a perfusing rhythm.

VIII. PEDIATRIC CARDIOPULMONARY RESUSCITATION

A. The basic approach to pediatric cardiac arrest victims is the same as in adults (see Fig. 59-1).
   1. Cardiac arrest is less likely to be a sudden event and more likely related to progressive deterioration of ventilation and cardiac function in the pediatric age group.
   2. Effective ventilation of the lungs is critical because ventilatory problems are frequently the cause of cardiac arrest in this age group.
B. Cardiac compression in infants is provided with two fingers on the midsternum or by encircling the chest with the hands and using the thumbs to provide compression.
C. Defibrillation is less frequently necessary in children, but the same principles apply as in adults. (The recommended starting energy is 2 J/kg, which is doubled if defibrillation is unsuccessful.)
D. Drug therapy is similar to that in adults but plays a larger role because electrical therapy is less often needed.

IX. POSTRESUSCITATION CARE

A. The major factors contributing to mortality after successful resuscitation are progression of the primary disease and cerebral damage experienced as a result of the cardiac arrest. Furthermore, even brief cardiac arrest causes generalized decreases in myocardial function (global myocardial stunning) and may require treatment with inotropic drugs.
   1. When cerebral blood flow is restored after a period of global cerebral ischemia, there are initially multifocal areas of the brain with no reflow (this may reflect the effects of epinephrine administered during

PERIOPERATIVE

CPR) followed within 1 hour by global hyperemia, which is followed quickly by global hypoperfusion.

2. Support after resuscitation is focused on providing stable oxygenation (PaO_2 >100 mm Hg), ventilation ($PaCO_2$ 25–35 mm Hg), neuromuscular blockers to prevent coughing or restlessness, and optimal hemodynamics (hematocrit, 30%–35%).

   a. A brief (5 min) period of hypertension (mean arterial pressure, 120–140 mm Hg) may help overcome the initial cerebral no reflow.

   b. Hyperglycemia during cerebral ischemia results in increased neurologic damage. Although it is unknown if hyperglycemia in the postresuscitation period influences outcome, it seems prudent to maintain the blood glucose level between 100 and 250 mg/dL.

   c. Increased intracranial pressure (ICP) is unusual after resuscitation from cardiac arrest. (Ischemic injury may lead to cerebral edema and increased ICP in the ensuing days.)

   d. In contrast to general supportive care, specific pharmacologic therapy directed at brain preservation has not been shown to have further benefit.

3. Most severely damaged victims die of multisystem organ failure within 1 to 2 weeks.

4. It is recommended that unconscious patients with spontaneous circulation after out-of-hospital cardiac arrest should be cooled to 32° to 34°C for 12 to 24 hours when the initial rhythm was ventricular fibrillation. Such cooling may also be beneficial for other rhythms or in-hospital cardiac arrest.

B. **Prognosis.** Most patients who completely recover show rapid improvement in the first 48 hours.

CHAPTER 60 ■ DISASTER PREPAREDNESS

Hurricane Katrina, 9/11, the Sago mine, and severe acute respiratory syndrome (SARS) have entered our national consciousness and connote vivid images of tragic circumstances (Murray MJ: Disaster preparedness and weapons of mass destruction. In *Clinical Anesthesia*. Edited by Barash PG, Cullen BF, Stoelting RK, Cahalan MK, Stock MC. Philadelphia: Lippincott Williams & Wilkins, 2009, pp 1559–1578). The term *mass casualty* refers to a large number of injuries or deaths that occur in a short period of time and have the potential to exceed the capabilities of local facilities. Mass casualty incidents include naturally occurring as well as intentional or unintentional events (Table 60-1).

I. THE JOINT COMMISSION

After the events of September 11, 2001, and the subsequent anthrax attacks, The Joint Commission (previously the Joint Commission on Accreditation of Healthcare Organizations) published a "white paper" to help hospitals develop systems to create and sustain community-wide emergency preparedness (Table 60-2). Ever-increasing demands on an underfunded health care system may limit the surge capacity to handle major emergencies (Fig. 60-1).

II. DISASTER PREPAREDNESS

Although the critical importance of planning and preparing to deal with the use of weapons of mass destruction is recognized, the reality is that we are far more likely to have to manage patients and health care facilities that are victims of natural and unintentional disasters (see Table 60-1).

TABLE 60-1
DISASTERS THAT MAY RESULT IN MASS CASUALTIES

Natural
Hurricanes
Tornados
Floods
Earthquakes
Forest fires

Unintentional
Airplane, train, or bus crash
Boat sinking

Fire
Nuclear accident
Industrial accident
Building collapse or sports stadium disaster

Intentional
Bombing
Nuclear
Biologic
Chemical

TABLE 60-2
DISASTER PREPAREDNESS AND RESPONSE

Enlisting the Community to Develop the Local Response
The initial response needs to be a coordinated local response.
There has traditionally been poor communication between law enforcement agencies, fire and rescue services, and emergency medical services.
Community planning needs to occur, and the plans must be widely disseminated.

Focusing on the Key Aspects of the System That Prepares Community Health Care Resources to Mobilize to Care for Patients, Protect Their Staff Members, and Serve the Public
To respond to a mass casualty event, an emergency medical system must be able to assess and expand its surge capacity.
To maintain surge capacity, it is imperative that every health care provider recognize the importance of protecting her- or himself.
After having established the basics, the most important aspect of managing a mass casualty event is having a command and control structure with which everyone is familiar.

Establishing the Accountabilities, Oversight, Leadership, and Sustainment of a Community Preparedness System
Responsibility for preparedness is with local, state, and federal governments and with hospitals and hospital organizations.

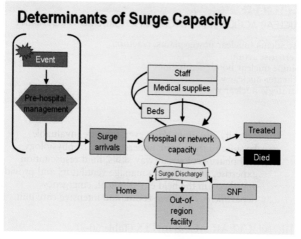

FIGURE 60-1. SNF: Skilled Nursing Facility. Published with permission: Nathaniel Hupert, MD, MPH, "Addressing Surge Capacity in a Mass Casualty Event" Web Conference, broadcast on October 26, 2004. Agency for Healthcare Research and Quality, Rockville, MD. Available at http://www.ahrq.gov/news/ulp/btsurgemass/

A. **Role of Government**
1. The initial response to any disaster, whether natural, unintended, or terrorist initiated, begins at the local level and would involve law enforcement agencies (especially if criminal activity is suspected), firefighters, and paramedics.
2. If the event supersedes the state's ability to respond, the federal government would become involved. The Federal Emergency Management Agency is the lead agency for assistance to state and local governments.
3. Physicians who wish to volunteer can become members of the National Disaster Medical System.
4. The Centers for Disease Control and Prevention has established a National Pharmaceutical Stockpile program as a national repository of antibiotics, chemical antidotes, life support medications, intravenous administration and airway maintenance supplies, and medical and surgical items.
B. **Role of Anesthesiologists in Managing Mass Casualties.** It is difficult to anticipate every measure in which anesthesiologists could be asked to assist in managing mass

TABLE 60-3

NUCLEAR ACCIDENTS IN DECREASING ORDER OF PROBABILITY

Accidents (nuclear power plants, reactors)
Terrorist action
Single nuclear bomb detonation
Theater nuclear war
Strategic nuclear war

casualty situations. However, they are invaluable because of their basic understanding of physiology and pharmacology, airway skills, fluid resuscitation expertise, and ability to manage ventilators and provide anesthesia in the field environment, emergency department, operating room, and intensive care unit.

III. NUCLEAR ACCIDENTS (Table 60-3)

A. **Radiation Injury.** The experience from Chernobyl indicates the kind of injuries and results that anesthesiologists can anticipate from nuclear accidents, including radiation burns, bone marrow suppression, the destruction of the lining of the gastrointestinal (GI) tract, GI bleeding with translocation of bacteria, infection, sepsis, septic shock, and death.

   1. Potassium iodide is indicated to protect the thyroid gland from taking up ^{131}I, and other drugs, such as 5-androstenediol, are being considered.
   2. Because of the possibility of exposure to ionizing radiation (such as from nuclear power plants), the American Academy of Pediatrics has recommended that at least two tablets of potassium iodide be available for all inhabitants within 16 km of any nuclear power plant.

B. **Potential Sources of Ionizing Radiation Exposure**

   1. The greatest concern is the exposure to ionizing radiation that is unintentional as occurred at the Chernobyl nuclear power plants or exposure that is intentional.
   2. Exposure to ionizing radiation may be the result of terrorism. (A radiologic dispersion device remains the most likely cause of the event.)
   3. Individuals should be familiar with the types of ionizing radiation (Table 60-4).

TABLE 60-4

TYPES OF RADIATION

Ionizing radiation (a high-frequency, low-amplitude form of radiation that interacts significantly with biologic systems)

α Particles (poor penetration and pose little hazard after external exposure but can produce tissue injury when inhaled or ingested)

β Particles (high-speed particles identical to electrons that are emitted from the nucleus of an atom)

Neutrons (emitted only after a nuclear detonation, neutrons are highly destructive, producing 10 times more tissue damage than gamma rays)

Gamma rays (significant penetrance; these are the most important external radiation hazard after a radiation disaster)

X-rays (energy is emitted from electrons)

4. The most likely injury from ionizing radiation is to the tissues that have the greatest turnover rate (greatest for lymphoid tissue).
   a. Thrombocytopenia, granulocytopenia, and GI injury lead to bleeding and bacterial translocation across the GI epithelium. The net results are sepsis and bleeding—the hallmarks of acute radiation syndrome—which lead to death.
   b. Because ionizing radiation is invisible, individuals may appear normal or may present with nausea, vomiting, diarrhea, fever, hypotension, erythema, and central nervous system (CNS) dysfunction.
   c. Patients who present with nausea, vomiting, diarrhea, and fever are likely to have severe acute radiation syndrome. Hypotension, erythema, and CNS dysfunction manifest later.
   d. Long-term effects include thyroid cancer and psychologic injury as have been documented many times in the past.
C. **Management**
   1. Depending on the type of radiation event, the first step is immediate evacuation of the area.
   2. The principle of disaster management always involves containment (bringing patients with material emitting ionizing radiation to the hospital should be avoided). To the extent possible, patients should be decontaminated at the site.

PERIOPERATIVE

3. Potassium iodide can prevent radiation-induced thyroid effects. (It should be given with 24 hours.)
4. Acute radiation syndrome manifests as bleeding and sepsis.

IV. BIOLOGIC DISASTERS

Anesthesiologists need to be familiar with contagious diseases that are not initiated by terrorist groups (influenza, SARS, West Nile virus). Influenza has killed more people in the 20th century than has any other infectious disease.

A. **Epidemics**
   1. **Influenza.** Only subtypes of influenza A virus normally infect people (and birds, who are natural hosts). A new pathogenic virus is usually detected several months in advance of major outbreaks, but vaccines remain in short supply principally because of manufacturing liability issues. Antiviral drugs have some benefit in treating patients with flu, but development of resistance is a concern. Isolation and quarantine practices are effective, low-cost methods.
   2. **Severe acute respiratory syndrome** is caused by coronavirus, and health care workers are at risk because they often manage these patients. (The virus is airborne, and protective masks are indicated.) Strict quarantine prevents the spread of SARS.

V. BIOLOGIC TERRORISM

The ideal biologic agent is one that has the greatest potential for adverse public health impact, generating mass casualties and with the potential for easy large-scale dissemination that could cause mass hysteria and civil disruption. There are three categories of biologic weapons (Table 60-5). Category A includes weapons that are highly contagious and fit all the characteristics of a relatively ideal biologic agent.

A. **Smallpox** (Table 60-6). Routine vaccination for smallpox was discontinued in the United States in 1972. It is precisely because of this that we are at most risk for terrorists using smallpox as a biologic weapon.
B. **Anthrax** has appeal as a bioterrorism agent because it can be "weaponized" (aerosolized). The three primary

TABLE 60-5

BIOLOGIC AGENTS USED FOR WARFARE

Category A	Category B	Category C
Anthrax	Q fever	Various equine encephalitic viruses
Smallpox	Cholera	
Plague	Glanders	
Botulism	Enteric pathogens (salmonella, shigella)	
Tularemia	Cholera	
Viral hemorrhagic fever (Ebola, Lassa, Marburg, Argentine)	Various encephalitic viruses Various biologic toxins	

types of anthrax infection are cutaneous, inhalation, and GI. Ninety-five percent of cases are cutaneous. Inhalation anthrax is hard to detect and manifests as an influenza-like disease with fever, myalgias, malaise, and a nonproductive cough with or without chest pain.

1. The most notable finding on physical examination and laboratory and imaging testing is a widened mediastinum. When a patient develops profound dyspnea, death usually ensues within 1 to 2 days.
2. In the past, penicillin G was the treatment of choice, but because weaponized anthrax has been engineered to be resistant to penicillin G, ciprofloxacin or doxycycline is more commonly used.

C. **Plague** (bubonic and pneumonic). The virus has a 2- to 6-day incubation period at which time there is a sudden onset of fever, chills, weakness, and headache. Without treatment, patients become septic and develop septic shock with cyanosis and gangrene

TABLE 60-6

COMPARISON OF SMALLPOX AND CHICKENPOX

Sign	Chickenpox	Smallpox
Fever	Simultaneous with rash	Precedes rash by 2–4 days
Rash	Lesions at various stages (papules, pustules, scabs)	Lesions are all in the same stage of development

PERIOPERATIVE

in peripheral tissues, leading to the "black death" descriptor that was used during the epidemics in Europe.

1. The treatment of choice is streptomycin, but chloramphenicol and tetracycline are acceptable alternatives.
2. Because the respiratory secretions are highly infectious, patients with pneumonic plague should be managed as one would manage patients with drug resistance to tuberculosis.

D. **Tularemia.** Normally, humans acquire tularemia from direct contact with an infected animal or from the bite of an infected tick or deerfly. The virus has a 3- to 5-day incubation period, and then the onset of disease is marked by fever, pharyngitis, bronchitis, pneumonia, pleuritis, and hilar lymphadenopathy. Prophylaxis with streptomycin, ciprofloxacin, or doxycycline has been recommended.

E. **Botulism** is a neuroparalytic disease caused by the toxin *Botulinum*, the most potent poison known. Victims develop progressive weakness and a flaccid paralysis that begins in the extremities and progresses until the respiratory muscles are paralyzed. Patients with profound respiratory impairment should have their tracheas protected and mechanical ventilation initiated.

F. **Hemorrhagic Fevers.** At least 18 viruses cause human hemorrhagic fevers, which form a special group of viruses characterized by viral replication in lymphoid cells. Infected individuals develop fever and myalgia, evidence of capillary leak (peripheral or pulmonary edema), disseminated intravascular coagulation, and thrombocytopenia. There are no specific antiviral therapies for this class of viruses.

G. **Role of Anesthesiologists in Bioterrorism.** Airway management and ventilator management may be critical, as are the establishment of intravascular access and volume resuscitation. Anesthesiologists must protect themselves by using 100% effective respiratory protection, going so far as to consider an oxygen-rebreathing system.

VI. CHEMICAL (Table 60-7)

A. Nerve agents are chemicals that affect nerve transmission by inhibiting acetylcholinesterase so that acetylcholine accumulates at the muscarinic and nicotinic acetylcholine receptor and within the CNS.

TABLE 60-7

TYPES OF CHEMICAL AGENTS

Nerve (tabun, sarin, soman)
Pulmonary (chlorine, phosgene)
Blood (hydrogen cyanide, cyanogen chloride)
Vesicants (sulfur mustard, nitrogen mustard)

1. Nicotinic stimulation leads to tachycardia and hypertension at the preganglionic site and at the nicotinic acetylcholine receptor on the neuromuscular junction. Signs and symptoms include fasciculations, twitching, fatigue, and flaccid paralysis.
2. Excess parasympathetic activity leads to miosis and loss of accommodation, so patients complain of blurred vision.
   a. Within the respiratory system, the increased parasympathetic activity leads to bronchospasm, dyspnea, and rhinorrhea.
   b. Within the cardiovascular system, activity within the muscarinic system leads to bradycardia. Activity within the nicotinic site leads to preganglionic nodes and increases in heart rate.
3. Treatment for nerve agent poisoning is with atropine, pralidoxime chloride (2-PAM-Cl) (a continuous infusion may be used), or both.
   a. The US military travels with automatic injectors containing 2 mg of atropine and 600 mg of 2-PAM-Cl.
   b. For situations in which one is anticipating nerve agent exposure, pyridostigmine may be used. It is a long-acting agent that binds with acetylcholinesterase, allowing the enzyme to spontaneously regenerate. It does not cross the blood–brain barrier and must be taken more than 30 minutes before exposure.
   c. Patients are decontaminated by removing their clothing and washing with copious amounts of water in 5% hypochlorite (household bleach).
B. **Pulmonary agents** include chloropicrin (PS), chlorine (CL), phosgene (CG), diphosgene (DP), and Ricin.
   1. Phosgene is a prototypical agent because it is deadlier than any of the other compounds. It is a colorless gas and has an odor of recently cut hay at 22° to 28°C and normal pressure conditions.

PERIOPERATIVE

      a. Phosgene is highly soluble in lipids, so it can easily penetrate the pulmonary epithelium and the cells lining the alveoli.

      b. Although it is very lipid soluble, phosgene reacts rapidly with water, forming hydrochloric acid (it is extremely toxic to tissues, causing acute respiratory distress syndrome) and carbon dioxide.

      c. For individuals who are exposed, gas masks provide the best protection.

C. Blood agents (cyanogens) are inhaled and release hydrogen cyanide, which impairs cytochrome oxidase and aerobic metabolism at the level of the mitochondria (metabolic acidosis).

    1. The blood agents are hydrogen cyanide (AC), hydrocyanic acid (HCN), cyanogen chloride (CK), and arsine (SA).

    2. Hydrogen cyanide is a colorless liquid that can be taken up through the skin as a liquid or inhaled.

    3. Treatment for cyanide toxicity involves the administration of sodium thiosulfate with supportive care in terms of tracheal intubation, ventilation, 100% oxygen, and cardiac support with inotropes and vasopressors. (Nitroprusside is a medical cause of cyanide toxicity.)

D. Vesicants

    1. Sodium mustard and related compounds, such as nitrogen mustard, phosgene oxime, and lewisite, also known as "blister agents," get their names by the fact that with contact with skin, these compounds produce burns and blisters. Although these are the most readily apparently manifestations, these compounds are also inhaled and can inflict severe damage to the respiratory system and eyes and can also produce multiple organ dysfunction syndrome.

    2. Blister agents are colorless and almost odorless. If the temperature is high enough, odor is present, which smells like rotten onions or mustard.

      a. Individuals loose their sight, and nausea, vomiting, and diarrhea develop along with severe respiratory difficulty. (The effects seen on the skin can also happen in the pulmonary epithelium.)

      b. A nuclear–biologic–chemical protective suit and gas mask provide the best protection.

APPENDIX A ■ **FORMULAS**

HEMODYNAMIC FORMULAS

HEMODYNAMIC VARIABLES: CALCULATIONS AND NORMAL VALUES

Variable	Calculation	Normal Values
Cardiac index (CI)	CO/BSA	$2.5–4.0$ L/min/m^2
Stroke volume (SV)	CO $\times$ 1000/HR	$60–90$ mL/beat
Stroke index (SI)	SV/BSA	$40–60$ mL/beat/m^2
Mean arterial pressure (MAP)	Diastolic pressure $+ \frac{1}{3}$ pulse pressure	$80–120$ mm Hg
Systemic vascular resistance (SVR)	$\dfrac{\text{MAP} - \overline{\text{CVP}}}{\text{CO}} \times 79.9$	$1200–1500$ dyne-cm-sec^{-5}
Pulmonary vascular resistance (PVR)	$\dfrac{\overline{\text{PAP}} - \text{PCWP}}{\text{CO}} \times 79.9$	$100–300$ dyne-cm-sec^{-5}
Right ventricular stroke work index (RVSWI)	0.0136 (PAP − CVP) $\times$ SI	$5–9$ g-m/beat/m^2
Left ventricular stroke work index (LVSWI)	0.0136 (MAP − PCWP) $\times$ SI	$45–60$ g-m/beat/m^2

HR = heart rate; $\overline{\text{CVP}}$ = mean central venous pressure; BSA = body surface area; CO = cardiac output; $\overline{\text{PAP}}$ = mean pulmonary artery pressure; PCWP = pulmonary capillary wedge pressure; MAP = mean arterial blood pressure.

RESPIRATORY FORMULAS

	Normal Values (70 kg)
Alveolar oxygen tension $P_{AO_2} = (P_B - 47)\, F_{IO_2} - P_{ACO_2}$	110 mm Hg ($F_{IO_2} = 0.21$)
Alveolar-arterial oxygen gradient $A_{aO_2} = P_{AO_2} - P_{aO_2}$	<10 mm Hg ($F_{IO_2} = 0.21$)
Arterial-to-alveolar oxygen ratio, a/A ratio	>0.75
Arterial oxygen content $C_{aO_2} = (S_{aO_2})(Hb \times 1.34) + P_{aO_2}\,(0.0031)$	21 mL/100 mL
Mixed venous oxygen content $C\bar{v}_{O_2} = (S\bar{v}_{O_2})(Hb \times 1.34) + P\bar{v}_{O_2}\,(0.0031)$	15 mL/100 mL
Arterial-venous oxygen content difference $a{-}v\,O_2 = C_{aO_2} - C\bar{v}_{O_2}$	4–6 mL/100 mL
Intrapulmonary shunt $\dot{Q}_S/\dot{Q}_T = (C_{CO_2} - C_{aO_2})/(C_{CO_2} - C\bar{v}_{O_2})$ $C_{CO_2} = (Hb \times 1.34) + (P_{AO_2} \times 0.0031)$	<5%
Physiologic dead space $\dot{V}_D/\dot{V}_T = (P_{aCO_2} - P_{ECO_2})/P_{aCO_2}$	0.33
Oxygen consumption $\dot{V}_{O_2} = CO\,(C_{aO_2} - C\bar{v}_{O_2})$	240 mL/min
Oxygen transport $O_2T = CO\,(C_{aO_2})$	1000 mL/min

C_{aO_2} = arterial oxygen content; $C\bar{v}_{O_2}$ = mixed venous oxygen content; C_{CO_2} = pulmonary capillary oxygen content; CO = cardiac output; F_{IO_2} = fraction inspired oxygen; O_2T = oxygen transport; P_B = barometric pressure; $\dot{Q}_S/\dot{Q}_T$ = intrapulmonary shunt; P_{aCO_2} = alveolar carbon dioxide tension; P_{aCO_2} = arterial carbon dioxide tension; P_{AO_2} = alveolar oxygen tension; P_{aO_2} = arterial oxygen tension; P_{ECO_2} = expired carbon dioxide tension; V_D = dead space gas volume; V_T = tidal volume; $\dot{V}_{O_2}$ = oxygen consumption (minute).

LUNG VOLUMES AND CAPACITIES

	Lung Volume (% TLC)
IRV	45–50%
TV	10–15%
ERV	15–20%
RV	20–25%

		Normal Values (70 kg)
Vital capacity	VC	4,800 mL
Inspiratory capacity	IC	3,800 mL
Functional residual capacity	FRC	2,400 mL
Inspiratory reserve volume	IRV	3,500 mL
Tidal volume	TV	1,500 mL
Expiratory reserve volume	ERV	1,200 mL
Residual volume	RV	1,200 mL
Total lung capacity	TLC	6,000 mL

ELECTROCARDIOGRAPHY ATLAS

ELECTROCARDIOGRAM

LEAD PLACEMENT

	Electrode	
	Positive	Negative
BIPOLAR LEADS		
I	LA	RA
II	LL	RA
III	LL	LA
AUGMENTED UNIPOLAR		
aVR	RA	LA, LL
aVL	LA	RA, LL
aVF	LL	RA, LA
	Position	
PRECORDIAL		
V_1	4 ICS–RSB	
V_2	4 ICS–LSB	
V_3	Midway between V_2 and V_4	
V_4	5 ICS–MCL	
V_5	5 ICS–AAL	
V_6	5 ICS–MAL	

We wish to thank Dr. Malcom S. Thaler for graciously permitting reproduction of electrocardiographic tracings from his book. *The Only EKG Book You'll Ever Need* (Philadelphia, JB Lippincott, 1988).

THREE-LEAD SYSTEMS

Bipolar Lead System	Electrode Placement	ECG Lead[a]	Advantage
II	RA R–clavicle LA L–10th rib (midclavicular line) LL Ground	II (II)	Dysrhythmias
MCL 1	RA Ground LA L-clavicle LL V_1	III (V_1)	Dysrhythmias and conduction defects
CS 5	RA R-clavicle LA V_5 LL Ground	I (V_5)	Precordial ischemia
CB 5	RA R-scapula LA V_5 LA Ground	I (V_5)	Precordial ischemia and dysrhythmias

MCL = modified central lead; CB = central back; CS = central subclavian.
[a]Selected lead on monitor; () = simulated ECG lead.

THE NORMAL ELECTROCARDIOGRAM—CARDIAC CYCLE

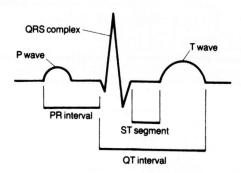

In this section the ECG complex is divided into the atrial (PR interval) and ventricular (QT interval) components.

ASHMAN BEATS

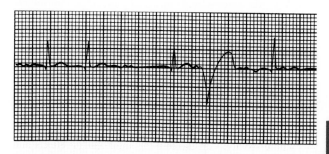

Rate: Variable.

Rhythm: Irregular.

PR interval: P wave may be present if supraventricular premature beat.

QT interval: QRS prolonged (>0.12 s) and altered, revealing bundle-branch pattern, most commonly right bundle. ST segment abnormal.

Note: Ashman beats are often confused with ventricular premature contractions. Ashman beats, usually seen with atrial fibrillation, have no compensatory pause and are a benign ECG finding requiring no treatment.

ATRIAL FIBRILLATION

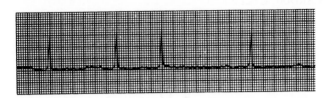

Rate: Variable (~150–200 beats/min).
Rhythm: Irregular.
PR interval: No P wave, and PR interval not discernible.
QT interval: QRS normal.

Note: Must be differentiated from atrial flutter: (1) absence of flutter waves and presence of fibrillatory line; (2) flutter usually associated with higher ventricular rates (>150 beats/min). Loss of atrial contraction reduces cardiac output (10–20%). Mural atrial thrombi may develop. Considered controlled if ventricular rate <100 beats/min.

ATRIAL FLUTTER

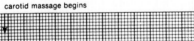

carotid massage begins

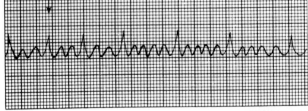

Rate: Rapid, atrial usually regular (250–350 beats/min); ventricular usually regular (<100 beats/min).
Rhythm: Atrial and ventricular regular.
PR interval: Flutter (F) waves are saw-toothed. PR interval cannot be measured.
QT interval: QRS usually normal; ST segment and T waves are not identifiable.

Note: Carotid massage will slow ventricular response, simplifying recognition of the F waves.

ATRIOVENTRICULAR BLOCK
(First Degree)

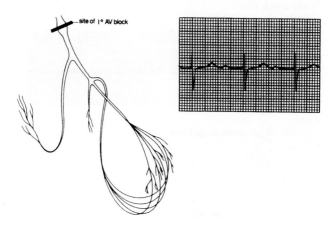

Rate: 60–100 beats/min.
Rhythm: Regular.
PR interval: Prolonged (>0.20 s) and constant.
QT interval: Normal.

Note: Usually clinically insignificant; may be early harbinger of drug toxicity.

ATRIOVENTRICULAR BLOCK
(Second Degree), Mobitz Type I/
Wenckebach Block

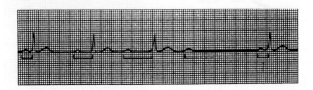

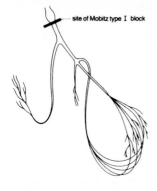

site of Mobitz type I block

Rate: 60–100 beats/min.

Rhythm: Atrial regular; ventricular irregular.

PR interval: P wave normal; PR interval progressively lengthens with each cycle until QRS complex is dropped (dropped beat). PR interval following dropped beat is shorter than normal.

QT interval: QRS complex normal but dropped periodically.

Note: Commonly seen (1) in trained athletes and (2) with drug toxicity.

ATRIOVENTRICULAR BLOCK
(Second Degree), Mobitz Type II

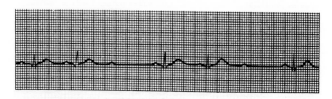

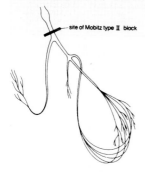

site of Mobitz type II block

Rate: <100 beats/min.

Rhythm: Atrial regular; ventricular regular or irregular.

PR interval: P waves normal, but some are not followed by QRS complex.

QT interval: Normal but may have widened QRS complex if block is at level of bundle branch. ST segment and T wave may be abnormal, depending on location of block.

Note: In contrast to Mobitz type I block, the PR and RR intervals are constant and the dropped QRS occurs without warning. The wider the QRS complex (block lower in the conduction system), the greater the amount of myocardial damage.

ATRIOVENTRICULAR BLOCK
(Third Degree), Complete Heart Block

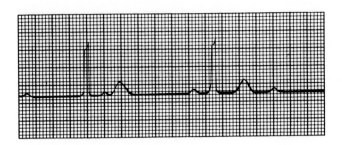

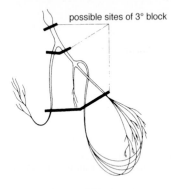

possible sites of 3° block

Rate: <45 beats/min.

Rhythm: Atrial regular; ventricular regular; no relationship between P wave and QRS complex.

PR interval: Variable because atria and ventricles beat independently.

QT interval: QRS morphology variable, depending on the origin of the ventricular beat in the intrinsic pacemaker system (atrioventricular junctional versus ventricular pacemaker). ST segment and T wave normal.

Note: Immediate treatment with atropine or isoproterenol is required if cardiac output is reduced. Consideration should be given to insertion of a pacemaker. Seen as a complication of mitral valve replacement.

ATRIOVENTRICULAR DISSOCIATION

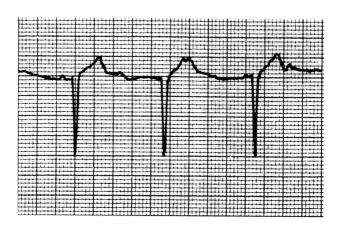

Rate: Variable.

Rhythm: Atrial regular; ventricular regular; ventricular rate faster than atrial rate; no relationship between P wave and QRS complex.

PR interval: Variable because atria and ventricles beat independently.

QT interval: QRS morphology depends on location of ventricular pacemaker. ST segment and T wave abnormal.

Note: Digitalis toxicity can present as atrioventricular dissociation.

BUNDLE-BRANCH BLOCK—LEFT (LBBB)

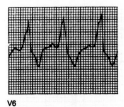

V6

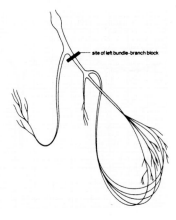

site of left bundle-branch block

Rate: <100 beats/min.
Rhythm: Regular.
PR interval: Normal.
QT interval: Complete LBBB (QRS >0.12 s); incomplete LBBB (QRS = 0.10–0.12 s). Lead V_1 negative rS complex; I, aVL, V_6 wide R wave without Q or S component. ST segment and T wave defection opposite direction of the R wave.

Note: LBBB does not occur in healthy patients and usually indicates serious heart disease with a poorer prognosis. In patients with LBBB, insertion of a pulmonary artery catheter may lead to complete heart block.

BUNDLE-BRANCH BLOCK—RIGHT (RBBB)

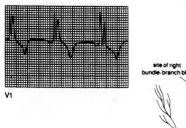

V1

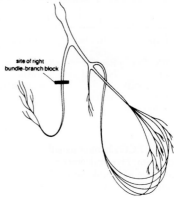

site of right
bundle-branch block

Rate: <100 beats/min.
Rhythm: Regular.
PR interval: Normal.
QT interval: Complete RBBB (QRS >0.12 s); incomplete RBBB
　(QRS = 0.10–0.12 s). Varying patterns of QRS complex; rSR
　(V₁); RS, wide R with M pattern. ST segment and T wave
　opposite direction of the R wave.

Note: In the presence of RBBB, Q waves may be seen with a
myocardial infarction.

ELECTROLYTE DISTURBANCES

	$\downarrow Ca^{2+}$	$\uparrow Ca^{2+}$	$\downarrow K^+$	$\uparrow K^+$
Rate	<100 beats/min	<100 beats/min	<100 beats/min	<100 beats/min
Rhythm	Regular	Regular	Regular	Regular
PR interval	Normal	Normal/increased	Normal	Normal
QT interval	Increased	Decreased	T flat U wave	T peaked QT decreased

Note: ECG changes usually do not correlate with serum calcium. Hypocalcemia rarely causes dysrhythmias in the absence of hypokalemia. In contrast, abnormalities in serum potassium concentration can be diagnosed by ECG.

DIGITALIS EFFECT

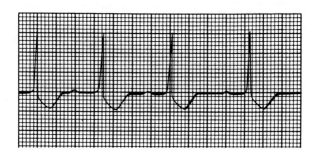

Rate: <100 beats/min.
Rhythm: Regular.
PR interval: Normal or prolonged.
QT interval: ST segment sloping ("digitalis effect").

Note: Digitalis toxicity can be the cause of many common dysrhythmias (e.g., premature ventricular contractions, second-degree heart block). Verapamil, quinidine, and amiodarone cause an increase in serum digitalis concentration.

CORONARY ARTERY DISEASE—Ischemia

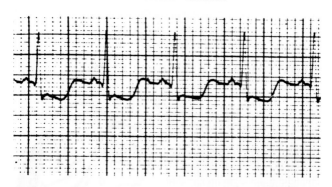

Rate: Variable.
Rhythm: Usually regular, but may show atrial and/or ventricular dysrhythmias.
PR interval: Normal.
QT interval: ST segment depressed; J point depression; T-wave inversion: conduction disturbances. Coronary vasospasm (Prinzmetal) ST segment elevation.

Note: Intraoperative ischemia is usually seen in the presence of "normal" vital signs (e.g., ± 20% of preinduction values).

CORONARY ARTERY DISEASE—
Myocardial Infarction

Anatomic Site	Leads	ECG Changes	Coronary Artery
Inferior	II, III, aVF	Q, ST, T	Right
Lateral	I, aVL, V_5–V_6	Q, ST, T	Left circumflex
Anterior	I, aVL, V_1–V_4	Q, ST, T	Left
Anteroseptal	V_1–V_4	Q, ST, T	Left anterior descending

SUBENDOCARDIAL MYOCARDIAL INFARCTION (SEMI)

Persistent ST segment depression and/or T-wave inversion in the absence of Q wave. Usually requires additional laboratory data (e.g., isoenzymes) to confirm diagnosis.

TRANSMURAL MYOCARDIAL INFARCTION (TMI)

Q waves seen on ECG useful in confirming diagnosis. Associated with poorer prognosis and more significant hemodynamic impairment; dysrhythmias frequently complicate course.

PAROXYSMAL ATRIAL TACHYCARDIA (PAT)

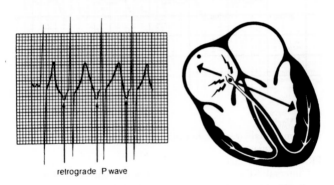

retrograde P wave

Rate: 150–250 beats/min.
Rhythm: Regular.
PR interval: Difficult to distinguish because of tachycardia obscuring P wave. P wave may precede, be included in, or follow QRS complex.
QT interval: Normal, but ST segment and T wave may be difficult to distinguish.

Note: Therapy depends on degree of hemodynamic compromise. In contrast to management of PAT in awake patients, synchronized cardoversion rather than pharmacologic treatment is preferred in hemodynamically unstable anesthetized patients.

PREMATURE ATRIAL CONTRACTION (PAC)

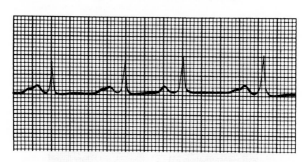

Rate: <100 beats/min.

Rhythm: Irregular.

PR interval: P waves may be lost in preceding T waves. PR interval is variable.

QT interval: QRS normal configuration; ST segment and T wave normal.

Note: Nonconducted PAC appears similar to that of sinus arrest; T waves with PAC may be distorted by inclusion of P wave in the T wave.

PREMATURE VENTRICULAR CONTRACTION (PVC)

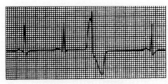

A

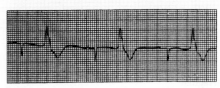

B

Rate: Usually <100 beats/min.

Rhythm: Irregular.

PR interval: P wave and PR interval absent; retrograde conduction of P wave can be seen.

QT interval: Wide QRS (>0.12 s); ST segment cannot be evaluated (e.g., ischemia); T wave opposite direction of QRS with compensatory pause (*A*). Bigeminy: every other beat a PVC (*B*); trigeminy: every third beat a PVC. R-on-T occurs when PVC falls in the T wave and can lead to ventricular tachycardia or fibrillation.

Note: If compensatory pause is not seen following an ectopic beat, the complex is most likely supraventricular in origin.

SINUS TACHYCARDIA

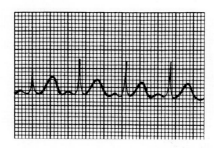

Rate: 100–160 beats/min.
Rhythm: Regular.
PR interval: Normal; P wave may be difficult to see.
QT interval: Normal.

Note: Should be differentiated from paroxysmal atrial tachycardia (PAT). With PAT, carotid massage terminates dysrhythmia. Sinus tachycardia may respond to vagal maneuvers but reappears as soon as vagal stimulus is removed.

TORSADES DE POINTES

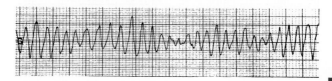

Rate: 150–250 beats/min.
Rhythm: No atrial component seen; ventricular rhythm regular or irregular.
PR interval: P wave buried in QRS complex.
QT interval: QRS complexes usually wide and with phasic variation twisting around a central axis (a few complexes point upward, then a few point downward). ST segments and T waves difficult to discern.

Note: Type of ventricular tachycardia associated with prolonged QT interval. Seen with electrolyte disturbances (e.g., hypokalemia, hypocalcemia, and hypomagnesemia) and bradycardia. Administering standard antidysrhythmics (lidocaine, procainamide, etc.) may worsen Torsades de Pointes. Treatment includes increasing heart rate pharmacologically or by pacing.

VENTRICULAR FIBRILLATION

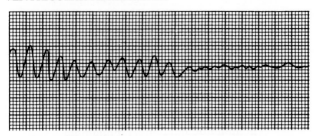

Rate: Absent.
Rhythm: None.
PR interval: Absent.
QT interval: Absent.

Note: "Pseudoventricular fibrillation" may be the result of a monitor malfunction (e.g., ECG lead disconnect). Always check for carotid pulse before instituting therapy.

VENTRICULAR TACHYCARDIA

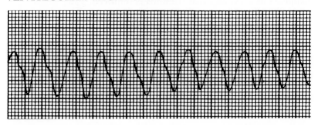

Rate: 100–250 beats/min.
Rhythm: No atrial component seen; ventricular rhythm irregular or regular.
PR interval: Absent; retrograde P wave may be seen in QRS complex.
QT interval: Wide, bizarre QRS complex. ST segment and T wave difficult to determine.

Note: In the presence of hemodynamic compromise, immediate DC synchronized cardioversion is required. If the patient is stable, with short bursts of ventricular tachycardia, pharmacologic management is preferred. Should be differentiated from supraventricular tachycardia with aberrancy (SVT-A). Compensatory pause and atrioventricular dissociation suggest a PVC. P waves and SR' (V_1) and slowing to vagal stimulus suggest SVT-A.

WOLFF-PARKINSON-WHITE SYNDROME (WPW)

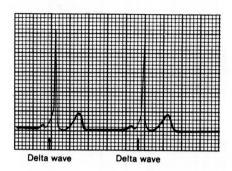

Delta wave   Delta wave

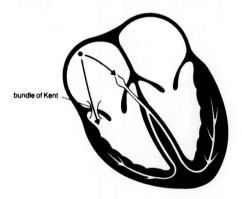

bundle of Kent

Rate: <100 beats/min.
Rhythm: Regular.
PR interval: P wave normal; PR interval short (<0.12 s).
QT interval: Duration (>0.10 s) with slurred QRS complex.
Type A has delta wave, RBBB, with upright QRS complex V_1.
Type B has delta wave and downward QRS-V_1. ST segment
and T wave usually normal.

Note: Digoxin should be avoided in the presence of WPW
because it increases conduction through the accessory bypass
tract (bundle of Kent) and decreases atrioventricular node conduction; consequently, ventricular fibrillation can occur.

PACEMAKER

GENERIC PACEMAKER CODE (NBG*): NASPE/BPEG REVISED (2002)

Position I, Pacing Chamber(s)	Position II, Sensing Chamber(s)	Position III, Response(s) to Sensing	Position IV, Programmability	Position V, Multisite Pacing
O = none	O = none	O = none	O = none	O = none
A = atrium	A = atrium	I = Inhibited	R = rate modulation	A = atrium
V = ventricle	V = ventricle	T = triggered		V = ventricle
D = dual (A + V)	D = dual (A + V)	D = dual (T + I)		D = dual (A + V)

ICD, implanted cardioverter defibrillator.

*NBG: N refers to North American Society of Pacing and Electrophysiology (NASPE), now called the Heart Rhythm Society (HRS), B refers to British Pacing and Electrophysiology Group (BPEG), and G refers to generic.

From Practice Advisory for Perioperative Management of Patients with Cadiac Rhythm Management Devices: Pacemakers and Implantable Cardioverter Defibrillators. Anesthesiology, 103:186, 2005.

GENERIC DEFIBRILLATOR CODE (NBD): NASPE/BPEG

Position I, Shock Chamber(s)	Position II, Antitachycardia Pacing Chamber(s)	Position III, Tachycardia Detection	Position IV,* Antibradycardia Pacing Chamber(s)
O = none	O = none	E = electrogram	O = none
A = atrium	A = atrium	H = hemodynamic	A = atrium
V = ventricle	V = ventricle		V = ventricle
D = dual (A + V)	D = dual (A + V)		D = dual (A + V)

*For robust identification position IV is expanded into its complete NBD code. For example, a biventricular pacing–defibrillator with ventricular shock and antitachycardia pacing functionality would be identified as VVE-DDDRV, assuming that the pacing section was programmed DDDRV. Currently, no hemodynamic sensors have been approved for tachycardia detection (position III).

From Practice Advisory for Perioperative Management of Patients with Cardiac Rhythm Management Devices: Pacemakers and Implantable Cardioverter Defibrillators. Anesthesiology, 103:186, 2005.

EXAMPLE OF A STEPWISE APPROACH TO THE PERIOPERATIVE TREATMENT OF THE PATIENT WITH A CARDIAC RHYTHM MANAGEMENT DEVICE (CRMD)

Preoperative Period	Patient/CRMD Condition	Intervention
Preoperative evaluation	Patient has CRMD	• Focused history • Focused physical examination • Manufacture's CRMD identification card • Chest x-ray studies (no data available) • Supplemental resources*
	Determine CRMD type (pacemaker, ICD, CRT)	• Verbal history
	Determine whether patient is CRMD-dependent for pacing function	• Bradyarrhythmia symptoms • Atrioventricular node ablation • No spontaneous ventricular activity†
	Determine CRMD function	• Comprehensive CRMD evaluation‡ • Determine whether pacing pulses are present and create paced beats
Preoperative preparation	EMI unlikely during procedure	• If EMI unlikely, special precautions are not needed
	EMI likely: CRMD is pacemaker	• Reprogram to asynchronous mode when indicated • Suspend rate-adaptive functions§
	EMI likely: CRMD is ICD	• Suspend antitachyarrhythmia functions • If patient is dependent on pacing function, alter pacing functions as above
	EMI likely: all CRMD	• Use bipolar cautery; ultrasonic scalpel • Temporary pacing and external cardioversion–defibrillation available
	Intraoperative physiologic changes likely (e.g., bradycardia, ischemia)	• Plan for possible adverse CRMD-patient interaction

(Continued)

EXAMPLE OF A STEPWISE APPROACH TO THE PERIOPERATIVE TREATMENT OF THE PATIENT WITH A CRMD (*Continued*)

Perioperative Period	Patient/CRMD Condition	Intervention
Intraoperative management	Monitoring	• Electrocardiographic monitoring per ASA standard • Peripheral pulse monitoring
	Electrocautery interference	• CT/CRP—no current through PG/leads • Avoid proximity of CT to PG/leads • Short bursts at lowest possible energy • Use bipolar cautery; ultrasonic scalpel
	Radiofrequency catheter ablation	• Avoid contact of radiofrequency catheter with PG/leads • Radiofrequency current path far away from PG/leads • Discuss these concerns with operator
	Lithotripsy	• Do not focus lithotripsy beam near PG • R wave triggers lithotripsy? Disable atrial pacing[∥]
	MRI	• Generally contraindicated • If required, consult ordering physician, cardiologist, radiologists, and manufacturer
	RT	• PG/leads must be outside of RT field • Possible surgical relocation of PG • Verify PG function during/after RT course
	ECT	• Consult with ordering physician, patient's cardiologist, a CRMD service, or CRMD manufacturer

1014

Emergency defibrillation–cardioversion	ICD: magnet disabled	• Terminate all EMI sources • Remove magnet to reenable therapies • Observe for appropriate therapies
	ICD: programming disabled	• Programming to reenable therapies or proceed directly with external cardioversion–defibrillation
	ICD: either of above	• Minimize current flow through PG/leads • PP as far as possible from PG • PP perpendicular to major axis PG/leads • To extent possible, PP in anterior–posterior location • Use clinically appropriate cardioversion/defibrillation energy
	Regardless of CRMD type	• Monitor cardiac R&R continuously • Backup pacing and cardioversion/defibrillation capability
Postoperative management	Immediate postoperative period	• Interrogation to assess function • Setting appropriate?# • Is CRMD an ICD?**
	Postoperative interrogation and restoration of CRMD function	• Use cardiology/pacemaker–ICD service if needed

*Manufacturer's databases, pacemaker clinic records, cardiology consultation. †With cardiac rhythm management device (CRMD) programmed WI at lowest programmable rate. ‡Ideally CRMD function assessed by interrogation, with function altered by reprogramming if required. §Most times this will be necessary; when in doubt, assume so. ‖Atrial pacing spikes may be interpreted by the lithotriptor as R waves, possibly inciting the lithotriptor to deliver a shock during a vulnerable period in the heart. #If necessary, reprogram appropriate setting. **Restore all antitachycardia therapies.

CRP, current return pad; CRT, cardiac resynchronization therapy; CT, cautery tool; ECT, electroconvulsive therapy; EMI, electromagnetic interference; ICD, internal cardioverter–defibrillator; MRI, magnetic resonance imaging; PG, pulse generator; PP, external cardioversion–defibrillation pads or paddles; R&R, rhythm and rate; RT, radiation therapy.

From Practice Advisory for Perioperative Management of Patients with Cardiac Rhythm Management Devices: Pacemakers and Implantable Cardioverter Defibrillators. Anesthesiology, 103:186, 2005.

TREATMENT OF PACEMAKER FAILURE

Rate	Possible Treatment
Adequate to maintain blood pressure	1. Observe, oxygen
	2. Atropine
	3. Try magnet
Severe bradycardia hypotension	1. Oxygen, airway control
	2. Atropine
	3. Isoproterenol
	4. Try magnet
	5. Transcutaneous pacing
No escape rhythm	1. CPR
	2. Isoproterenol
	3. Try magnet
	4. Transcutaneous pacing

Reprinted with permission from Zaldan JR: Pacemakers. In Youngberg JA, Lake CL, Roizeu MF, Wilson KS (eds): Cardiac, Vascular and Thoracic Anesthesia. New York, Churchill Livingston, 2000.

ATRIAL PACING

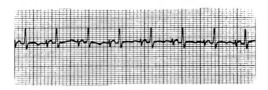

Atrial pacing as demonstrated in this figure is used when the atrial impulse can proceed through the AV node. Examples are sinus bradycardia and junctional rhythms associated with clinically significant decreases in blood pressure.

VENTRICULAR PACING

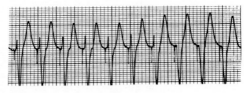

In this tracing ventricular pacing is evident by absence of atrial wave (*P wave*) and pacemaker spike preceding QRS complex. Ventricular pacing is used in the presence of bradycardia secondary to AV block or atrial fibrillation.

DDD PACING

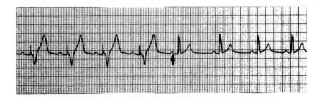

The DDD pacemaker (generator), one of the most commonly used, paces and senses both atrium and ventricle. In the first four beats, the P waves were not followed by a QRS complex within the programmed PR interval. Therefore, a ventricular pacing spike and a ventricular paced beat occurred. In the last four beats (*after the arrow*), atrial activity proceeded through the AV node in the allotted amount of time; therefore, ventricular pacing was inhibited.

ATRIAL ELECTROGRAM (AEG)

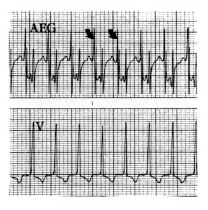

The AEG is useful in differentiating various atrial dysrhythmias. The AEG is obtained from an intracardiac or esophageal lead, if P waves are not clearly seen on the surface ECG. In this trace the V lead does not have obvious P waves; however, the AEG reveals large P waves (*arrows*) that precede each QRS complex. Locate the QRS on the AEG by matching the R wave on the surface ECG to the AEG. The surface and AEG must be simultaneously recorded.

GUIDELINES FOR USING THE ELECTROCAUTERY

1. Electromagnet interference created by an electrocautery can cause a number of problems with pacemaker or ICD function including, but not limited to, reprogramming, inhibition, noise reversion mode, electrical reset, myocardial burns, increase in threshold, rate increment changes in rate adaptive pacemakers, and inappropriate sensing and charging in ICDs.[2,3]
2. When positioning the return plate of the electrocautery,
   a. Ensure it is located so the pacemaker or ICD is not between this return plate and the active electrode.
   b. Ensure the plane described by the return plate and the active electrode of the electrocautery is perpendicular to a plane described by the pacemaker or ICD and the pacemaker's electrodes.
3. Use the smallest current required to cut or coagulate.
4. Use the electrocautery in short bursts.
5. Avoid using the electrocautery within 6 in. of the device or leads.
6. Consider using the bipolar electrocautery or the ultrasonic scalpel[4,5] to minimize interference with pacemaker or ICD function.
7. Activating the electrocautery in the area of the pacemaker or ICD, even if the active electrode is not touching the patient, will cause interference.
8. Do not use the electrocautery when an ICD is programmed to sense and deliver therapy.
9. Convert the ICD to no response either by programming or by using the magnet, depending on the manufacturer of the ICD so the device will not deliver therapy secondary to misinterpretation of signals from the electrocautery as a dysrhythmia. These maneuvers will not change the program of a pacemaker that is incorporated into an ICD.
10. If desired, convert a pacemaker that does not have an ICD to the asynchronous mode so it is not inhibited by the electrocautery.
11. A magnet will not change bradycardia-related pacing parameters in the ICD.
12. ICDs must be programmed to respond to a magent.

ICD, implanted cardioverter defibrillator.

ADDITIONAL ISSUES FOR PATIENTS WITH IMPLANTED CARDIOVERTER DEFIBRILLATORS

1. All ICDs have pacemakers incorporated into the circuitry.
2. Preoperative assessments should include those procedures that are standard for patients with heart disease.
3. Obtain a cardiology consult to help assess the patient, interrogate the ICD, program the device to no response, and program the device to respond to the magnet.
4. There is no particular anesthetic technique that is clearly right or wrong for a patient who has an ICD.
5. Apply patches for external defibrillation when the ICD is programmed to no response. Ensure these external patches are as far away as possible from the device and, if possible, not in the same plane as the device and electrodes.
6. Monitor as required for patient care. If monitoring with a pulmonary arterial catheter, discuss the issues of dislodgment of the ICD's electrodes with the patient and cardiologist. Document in the chart your discussions and the logic supporting the necessity for a pulmonary arterial catheter. Maintain sterile technique, and consider administering antibiotics just before inserting central lines.
7. Continue antidysrhythmic agents until the time of surgery. Discuss with the cardiologist the necessity of administering an additional dose of an antidysrhythmic agent if the patient experiences an intraoperative dysrhythmia.
8. Intraoperative dysrhythmias:
   a. If the patient has a dysrhythmia, rule out and treat the usual intraoperative causes to prevent a recurrence.
   b. If the dysrhythmia continues and a magnet has been used to create the no response mode, remove the magnet from the ICD and allow the ICD to charge and deliver a response.
   c. If the ICD has been programmed to the no response mode, then either quickly reprogram the ICD to deliver a response or proceed directly to external defibrillation.
   d. If external defibrillation or cardioversion is required, apply the defibrillator paddles in an anterior-posterior position if possible and deliver the shock at a level sufficient to terminate the dysrhythmia.
   e. External pacing might be required if the pacemaker/ICD is damaged with the shock.
9. Monitor the patient's ECG and be prepared to deliver an external defibrillation when transporting the patient to and from the operating room.
10. Interrogate and reprogram the ICD when the patient has entered the postoperative care unit.

ECG, electrocardiogram; ICD, implanted cardioverter defibrillator.

APPENDICES

References

1. Practice advisory for perioperative management of patients with cardiac rhythm management devices: Pacemakers and implantable cardioverter-defibrillators. A Report by the American Society of Anesthesiologists Task Force on Perioperative Management of Patients with Cardiac Rhythm Management Devices. Anesthesiology, 103:186, 2005

2. Hayes DL, Strathmore NF: Electromagnetic interference with implantable devices. In Ellenbogen KA, Kay GN, Wilkoff BL (eds): Clinical Cardiac Pacing and Defibrillation, 2nd ed, p 939. Philadelphia, WB Saunders, 2000

3. Atlee JL, Bernstein AD: Cardiac rhythm management devices (part II): Perioperative management. Anesthesiology 95:1492, 2001

4. Epstein MR, Mayer JE Jr, Duncan BW: Use of an ultrasonic scalpel as an alternative to electrocautery in patients with pacemakers. Ann Thorac Surg 65:1802, 1998

5. Ozeren M, Dogan OV, Duzgun C, Yucel E: Use of an ultrasonic scalpel in the open-heart reoperation of a patient with a pacemaker. Eur J Cardiothorac Surg 21:761, 2002

APPENDIX C ■ **AMERICAN HEART ASSOCIATION (AHA) RESUSCITATION PROTOCOLS**

Adult
Pediatric
Neonatal

For more detailed information, the reader is referred to the American Heart Association: Guidelines 2000 for Cardiopulmonary Resuscitation and Emergency Cardiovascular Care: International Concensus on Science. Circulation 102(8), 2000.

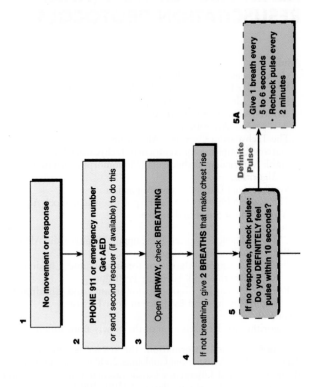

1 No movement or response

2 PHONE 911 or emergency number
Get AED
or send second rescuer (if available) to do this

3 Open AIRWAY, check **BREATHING**

4 If not breathing, give **2 BREATHS** that make chest rise

5 If no response, check pulse:
Do you DEFINITELY feel pulse within 10 seconds?

Definite Pulse

5A
- Give 1 breath every 5 to 6 seconds
- Recheck pulse every 2 minutes

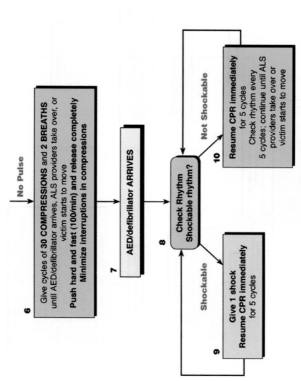

No Pulse

6
Give cycles of **30 COMPRESSIONS and 2 BREATHS**
until AED/defibrillator arrives, ALS providers take over, or
victim starts to move
Push hard and fast (100/min) and release completely
Minimize interruptions in compressions

7
AED/defibrillator **ARRIVES**

8
Check Rhythm
Shockable rhythm?

Shockable

9
Give 1 shock
Resume CPR immediately
for 5 cycles

Not Shockable

10
Resume CPR immediately
for 5 cycles
Check rhythm every
5 cycles; continue until ALS
providers take over or
victim starts to move

FIGURE 1. Adult basic life support (BLS) healthcare provider algorithm.

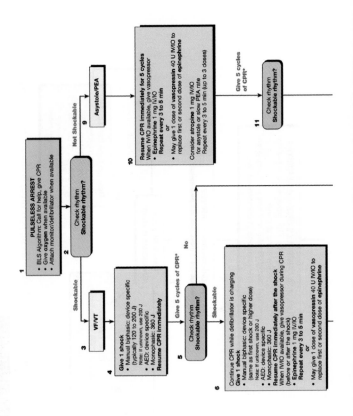

PULSELESS ARREST
- BLS Algorithm: Call for help, give CPR
- Give oxygen when available
- Attach monitor/defibrillator when available

2 Check rhythm
Shockable rhythm?

Shockable → **VF/VT** **3**

Not Shockable → **Asystole/PEA** **9**

4
Give 1 shock
- Manual biphasic: device specific
  (typically 120 to 200 J)
  Note: If unknown, use 200 J
- AED: device specific
- Monophasic: 360 J
Resume CPR immediately

Give 5 cycles of CPR*

5 Check rhythm
Shockable rhythm?

Shockable →

6
Continue CPR while defibrillator is charging
Give 1 shock
- Manual biphasic: device specific
  (same as first shock or higher dose)
  Note: If unknown, use 200 J
- AED: device specific
- Monophasic: 360 J
Resume CPR immediately after the shock
When IV/IO available, give vasopressor during CPR
(before or after the shock)
- **Epinephrine** 1 mg IV/IO
  Repeat every 3 to 5 min
  or
- May give 1 dose of vasopressin 40 U IV/IO to
  replace first or second dose of **epinephrine**

No →

9 Asystole/PEA

10
Resume CPR immediately for 5 cycles
When IV/IO available, give vasopressor
- **Epinephrine** 1 mg IV/IO
  Repeat every 3 to 5 min
  or
- May give 1 dose of vasopressin 40 U IV/IO to
  replace first or second dose of **epinephrine**

- Consider atropine 1 mg IV/IO
  for asystole or slow PEA rate
  Repeat every 3 to 5 min (up to 3 doses)

Give 5 cycles
of CPR*

11 Check rhythm
Shockable rhythm?

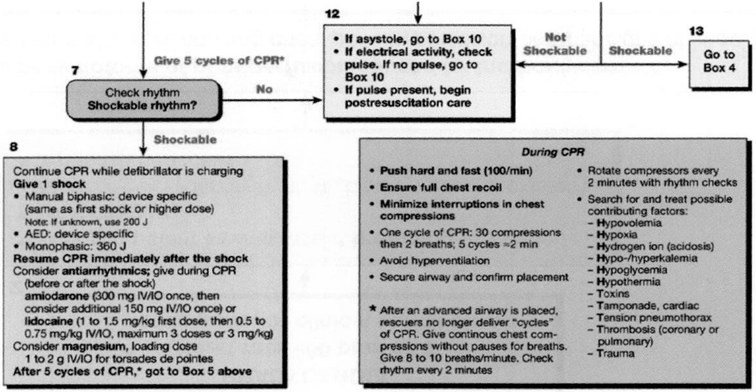
Give 5 cycles of CPR*
7
Check rhythm
Shockable rhythm?
No
Shockable
12
• If asystole, go to Box 10
• If electrical activity, check pulse. If no pulse, go to Box 10
• If pulse present, begin postresuscitation care
Not Shockable
Shockable
13
Go to Box 4
8
Continue CPR while defibrillator is charging
Give 1 shock
• Manual biphasic: device specific (same as first shock or higher dose)
Note: If unknown, use 200 J
• AED: device specific
• Monophasic: 360 J
Resume CPR immediately after the shock
Consider antiarrhythmics; give during CPR (before or after the shock)
amiodarone (300 mg IV/IO once, then consider additional 150 mg IV/IO once) or
lidocaine (1 to 1.5 mg/kg first dose, then 0.5 to 0.75 mg/kg IV/IO, maximum 3 doses or 3 mg/kg)
Consider magnesium, loading dose
1 to 2 g IV/IO for torsades de pointes
After 5 cycles of CPR,* got to Box 5 above
During CPR
• Push hard and fast (100/min)
• Ensure full chest recoil
• Minimize interruptions in chest compressions
• One cycle of CPR: 30 compressions then 2 breaths; 5 cycles ≈2 min
• Avoid hyperventilation
• Secure airway and confirm placement
* After an advanced airway is placed, rescuers no longer deliver "cycles" of CPR. Give continous chest compressions without pauses for breaths. Give 8 to 10 breaths/minute. Check rhythm every 2 minutes
• Rotate compressors every 2 minutes with rhythm checks
• Search for and treat possible contributing factors:
- Hypovolemia
- Hypoxia
- Hydrogen ion (acidosis)
- Hypo-/hyperkalemia
- Hypoglycemia
- Hypothermia
- Toxins
- Tamponade, cardiac
- Tension pneumothorax
- Thrombosis (coronary or pulmonary)
- Trauma

FIGURE 2. Adult advanced cardiac life support pulseless arrest algorithm.

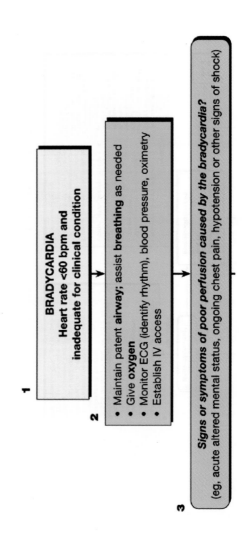

1

BRADYCARDIA
Heart rate <60 bpm and
inadequate for clinical condition

2
- Maintain patent airway; assist **breathing** as needed
- Give **oxygen**
- Monitor ECG (identify rhythm), blood pressure, oximetry
- Establish IV access

3
Signs or symptoms of poor perfusion caused by the bradycardia?
(eg, acute altered mental status, ongoing chest pain, hypotension or other signs of shock)

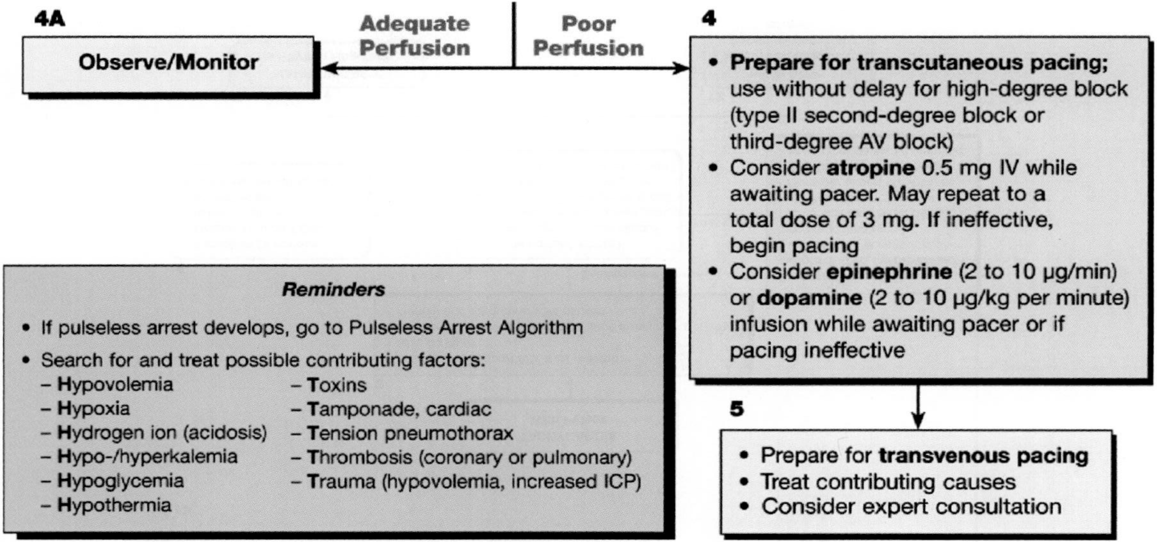

FIGURE 3. Bradycardia algorithm.

4A
- Observe/Monitor

Adequate Perfusion | **Poor Perfusion**

4
- **Prepare for transcutaneous pacing;** use without delay for high-degree block (type II second-degree block or third-degree AV block)
- Consider **atropine** 0.5 mg IV while awaiting pacer. May repeat to a total dose of 3 mg. If ineffective, begin pacing
- Consider **epinephrine** (2 to 10 μg/min) or **dopamine** (2 to 10 μg/kg per minute) infusion while awaiting pacer or if pacing ineffective

5
- **Prepare for transvenous pacing**
- Treat contributing causes
- Consider expert consultation

Reminders
- If pulseless arrest develops, go to Pulseless Arrest Algorithm
- Search for and treat possible contributing factors:
  - Hypovolemia
  - Hypoxia
  - Hydrogen ion (acidosis)
  - Hypo-/hyperkalemia
  - Hypoglycemia
  - Hypothermia
  - Toxins
  - Tamponade, cardiac
  - Tension pneumothorax
  - Thrombosis (coronary or pulmonary)
  - Trauma (hypovolemia, increased ICP)

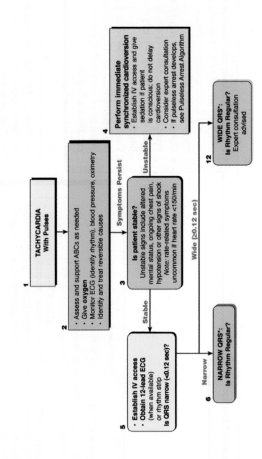

TACHYCARDIA
With Pulses

1

2
- Assess and support ABCs as needed
- Give **oxygen**
- Monitor ECG (identify rhythm), blood pressure, oximetry
- Identify and treat reversible causes

Symptoms Persist

3
Is patient stable?
Unstable signs include altered mental status, ongoing chest pain, hypotension or other signs of shock.
Note: rate-related symptoms uncommon if heart rate <150/min

Unstable

Stable

4
Perform immediate synchronized cardioversion
- Establish IV access and give sedation if patient is conscious; do not delay cardioversion
- Consider expert consultation
- If pulseless arrest develops, see Pulseless Arrest Algorithm

---

5
- Establish IV access
- Obtain 12-lead ECG (when available) or rhythm strip
Is QRS narrow (<0.12 sec)?

Wide (≥0.12 sec)

Narrow

6
NARROW QRS*:
Is Rhythm Regular?

12
WIDE QRS*:
Is Rhythm Regular?
Expert consultation advised

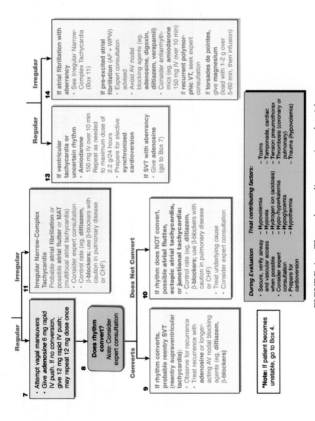

FIGURE 4. The tachycardia overview algorithm.

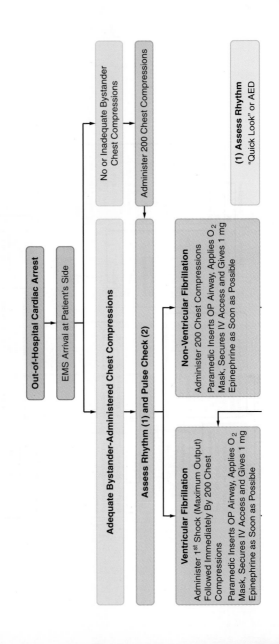

Out-of-Hospital Cardiac Arrest

EMS Arrival at Patient's Side

Adequate Bystander-Administered Chest Compressions

No or Inadequate Bystander Chest Compressions

Administer 200 Chest Compressions

Assess Rhythm (1) and Pulse Check (2)

(1) Assess Rhythm
"Quick Look" or AED

Non-Ventricular Fibrillation
Administer 200 Chest Compressions
Paramedic Inserts OP Airway, Applies O_2 Mask, Secures IV Access and Gives 1 mg Epinephrine as Soon as Possible

Ventricular Fibrillation
Administer 1st Shock (Maximum Output) Followed Immediately By 200 Chest Compressions
Paramedic Inserts OP Airway, Applies O_2 Mask, Secures IV Access and Gives 1 mg Epinephrine as Soon as Possible

1030

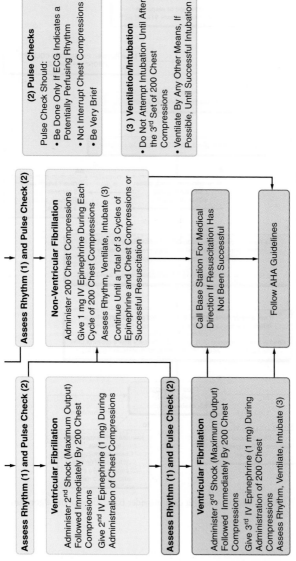

(2) Pulse Checks

Pulse Check Should:
- Be Done Only If ECG Indicates a Potentially Perfusing Rhythm
- Not Interrupt Chest Compressions
- Be Very Brief

(3) Ventilation/Intubation

- Do Not Attempt Intubation Until After the 3rd Set of 200 Chest Compressions
- Ventilate By Any Other Means, If Possible, Until Successful Intubation

Assess Rhythm (1) and Pulse Check (2)

Non-Ventricular Fibrillation

Administer 200 Chest Compressions
Give 1 mg IV Epinephrine During Each Cycle of 200 Chest Compressions
Assess Rhythm, Ventilate, Intubate (3)
Continue Until a Total of 3 Cycles of Epinephrine and Chest Compressions or Successful Resuscitation

Assess Rhythm (1) and Pulse Check (2)

Ventricular Fibrillation

Administer 2nd Shock (Maximum Output) Followed Immediately By 200 Chest Compressions
Give 2nd IV Epinephrine (1 mg) During Administration of Chest Compressions

Assess Rhythm (1) and Pulse Check (2)

Ventricular Fibrillation

Administer 3rd Shock (Maximum Output) Followed Immediately By 200 Chest Compressions
Give 3rd IV Epinephrine (1 mg) During Administration of 200 Chest Compressions
Assess Rhythm, Ventilate, Intubate (3)

Call Base Station For Medical Direction If Resuscitation Has Not Been Successful

Follow AHA Guidelines

FIGURE 5. Cardiocerebral resuscitation algorithm.

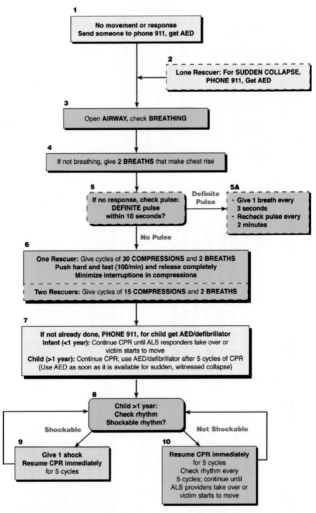

FIGURE 6. Pediatric health care provider basic life support algorithm.

TABLE App-C1

PEDIATRIC ADVANCED LIFE SUPPORT MEDICATION FOR CARDIAC ARREST AND
SYMPTOMATIC ARRHYTHMIAS

■ DRUG	■ DOSAGE (PEDIATRIC)	■ REMARKS
Adenosine	0.1 mg/kg (maximum, 6 mg) Repeat: 0.2 mg/kg (maximum, 12 mg)	Monitor ECG during dose Rapid IV/IO bolus
Amiodarone	5 mg/kg IV/IO Repeat up to 15 mg/kg Maximum: 300 mg	Monitor ECG and blood pressure Adjust administration rate to urgency Use caution when administering with other drugs that prolong QT
Atropine	0.02 mg/kg IV/IO 0.03 mg/kg ET^d Repeat once if needed Minimum dose: 0.1 mg Maximum single dose: Child, 0.5 mg Adolescent, 1.0 mg	Higher doses may be given with organophosphate poisoning
Calcium chloride (10%)	20 mg/kg IV/IO (0.2 mL/kg)	Give slow IV push for hypocalcemia, hypermagnesemia, calcium channel blocker toxicity
Epinephrine	0.01 mg/kg (0.1 mL/kg 1: 10,000) IV/IO 0.1 mg/kg (0.1 mL/kg 1: 1,000) ET$^\alpha$ Maximum dose: 1 mg IV/IO; 10 mg ET	May repeat every 3–5 min
Glucose	0.5–1.0 g/kg IV/IO	D$_{10}$W: 5–10 mL/kg D$_{25}$W: 2–4 mL/kg D$_{50}$W: 1–2 mL/kg
Lidocaine	Bolus: 1 mg/kg IV/IO Maximum dose: 100 mg Infusion: 20–50 μg/kg per minute ET$^\alpha$: 2–3 mg/kg	—
Magnesium sulfate	25–50 mg/kg IV/IO over 10–20 min; faster in torsades Maximum dose: 2 g	—
Naloxone	≤5 years or ≤20 kg: 0.1 mg/kg IV/IO/ET$^\alpha$ ≥5 y or >20 kg: 2 mg IV/IO/ET$^\alpha$	Use lower doses to reverse respiratory depression associated with therapeutic opioid use (1–15 μg/kg)
Procainamide	15 mg/kg IV/IO over 30 to 60 min Adult dose: 20 mg/min IV infusion up to total maximum dose of 17 mg/kg	Monitor ECG and blood pressure Use caution when administering with other drugs that prolong QT
Sodium bicarbonate	1 mEq/kg IV/IO slowly	After adequate ventilation

ECG, electrocardiogram; IV, intravenous; IO, intraosseous; ET, endotracheal.
^{d}Flush with 5 mL of normal saline and follow with five ventilations.
Adapted from 2005 American Heart Association Guidelines for cardiopulmonary resuscitation and
emergency cardiovascular care. Circulation 2005; 112(Suppl IV): IV.

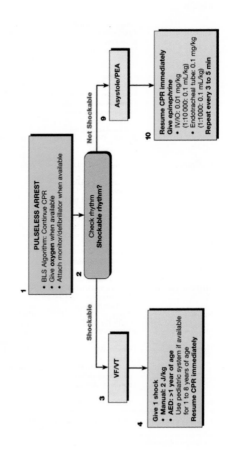

PULSELESS ARREST
- BLS Algorithm: Continue CPR
- Give **oxygen** when available
- Attach monitor/defibrillator when available

1

Check rhythm
Shockable rhythm?

2

Shockable

VF/VT

3

Give 1 shock
- Manual: 2 J/kg
- AED: >1 year of age
  Use pediatric system if available
  for 1 to 8 years of age
Resume CPR immediately

4

Not Shockable

Asystole/PEA

9

Resume CPR immediately
Give **epinephrine**
- IV/IO: 0.01 mg/kg
  (1:10 000: 0.1 mL/kg)
- Endotracheal tube: 0.1 mg/kg
  (1:1000: 0.1 mL/kg)
Repeat every 3 to 5 min

10

1034

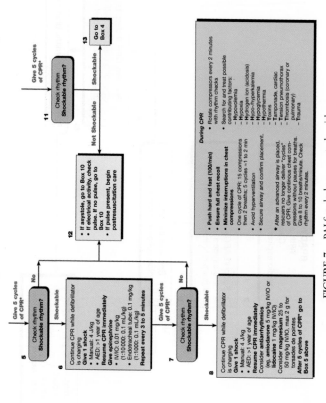

FIGURE 7.   PALS pulseless arrest algorithm.

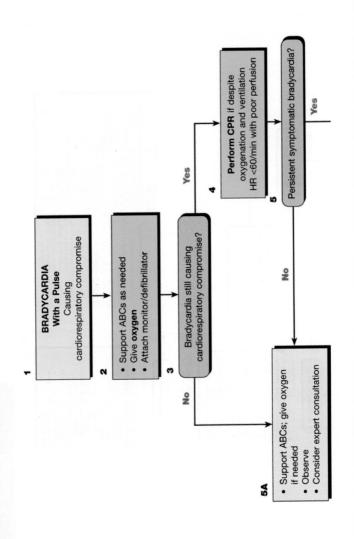

1

**BRADYCARDIA
With a Pulse**
Causing
cardiorespiratory compromise

2

- Support ABCs as needed
- Give **oxygen**
- Attach monitor/defibrillator

3

Bradycardia still causing
cardiorespiratory compromise?

No

Yes

4

Perform CPR if despite
oxygenation and ventilation
HR <60/min with poor perfusion

5

Persistent symptomatic bradycardia?

Yes

No

5A

- Support ABCs; give oxygen
  if needed
- Observe
- Consider expert consultation

6

- Give epinephrine
  - IV/IO: 0.01 mg/kg
    (1:10 000: 0.1 mL/kg)
  - Endotracheal tube:
    0.1 mg/kg
    (1:1000: 0.1 mL/kg)
  Repeat every 3 to
  5 minutes

- If increased vagal tone
  or primary AV block:
  Give atropine, first dose:
  0.02 mg/kg, may repeat.
  (Minimum dose: 0.1 mg;
  maximum total dose for
  child: 1 mg.)

- Consider cardiac pacing

7

If pulseless arrest develops,
go to Pulseless Arrest
Algorithm

Reminders

- During CPR, push hard and fast
  (100/min)

  Ensure full chest recoil
  Minimize interruptions in chest
  compressions
- Support ABCs
- Secure airway if needed; confirm
  placement

- Search for and treat possible
  contributing factors:
  - Hypovolemia
  - Hypoxia or ventilation problems
  - Hydrogen ion (acidosis)
  - Hypo-/hyperkalemia
  - Hypoglycemia
  - Hypothermia
  - Toxins
  - Tamponade, cardiac
  - Tension pneumothorax
  - Thrombosis (coronary or pulmonary)
  - Trauma (hypovolemia, increased ICP)

FIGURE 8. PALS (Pediatric Advanced Life Support) bradycardia algorithm.

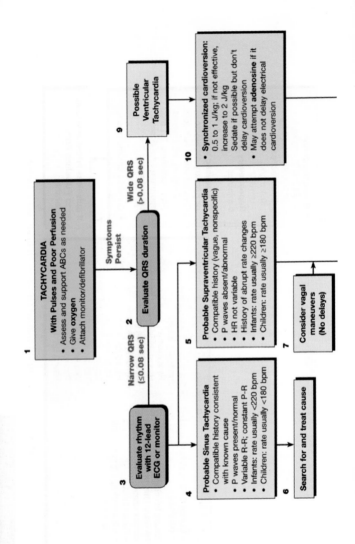

1

TACHYCARDIA
With Pulses and Poor Perfusion
• Assess and support ABCs as needed
• Give oxygen
• Attach monitor/defibrillator

Symptoms Persist

2

Evaluate QRS duration

Narrow QRS (≤0.08 sec)

Wide QRS (>0.08 sec)

3

Evaluate rhythm with 12-lead ECG or monitor

4

Probable Sinus Tachycardia
• Compatible history consistent with known cause
• P waves present/normal
• Variable R-R; constant P-R
• Infants: rate usually <220 bpm
• Children: rate usually <180 bpm

5

Probable Supraventricular Tachycardia
• Compatible history (vague, nonspecific)
• P waves absent/abnormal
• HR not variable
• History of abrupt rate changes
• Infants: rate usually ≥220 bpm
• Children: rate usually ≥180 bpm

6

Search for and treat cause

7

Consider vagal maneuvers
(No delays)

9

Possible Ventricular Tachycardia

10

• Synchronized cardioversion: 0.5 to 1 J/kg; if not effective, increase to 2 J/kg
  Sedate if possible but don't delay cardioversion
• May attempt **adenosine** if it does not delay electrical cardioversion

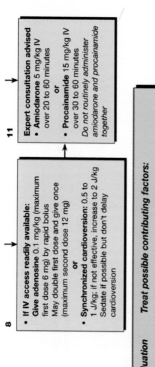

8

- If IV access readily available:
  - Give adenosine 0.1 mg/kg (maximum first dose 6 mg) by rapid bolus
    May double first dose and give once (maximum second dose 12 mg)

  or

  - Synchronized cardioversion: 0.5 to 1 J/kg; if not effective, increase to 2 J/kg
    Sedate if possible but don't delay cardioversion

11

Expert consultation advised
- **Amiodarone** 5 mg/kg IV over 20 to 60 minutes

  or

- **Procainamide** 15 mg/kg IV over 30 to 60 minutes
  Do not routinely administer amiodarone and procainamide together

During Evaluation

- Secure, verify airway and vascular access when possible
- Consider expert consultation
- Prepare for cardioversion

Treat possible contributing factors:

- Hypovolemia
- Hypoxia
- Hydrogen ion (acidosis)
- Hypo-/hyperkalemia
- Hypoglycemia
- Hypothermia
- Toxins
- Tamponade, cardiac
- Tension pneumothorax
- Thrombosis (coronary or pulmonary)
- Trauma (hypovolemia)

FIGURE 9. PALS tachycardia algorithm for infants and children with rapid rhythm and evidence of poor perfusion.

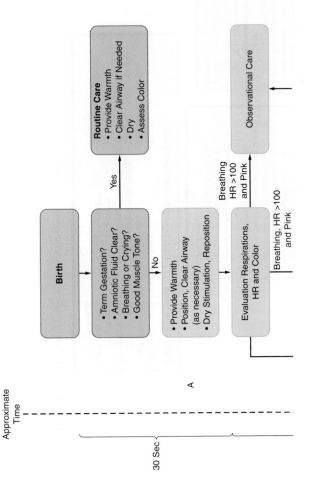

Approximate
Time

Birth

- Term Gestation?
- Amniotic Fluid Clear?
- Breathing or Crying?
- Good Muscle Tone?

Yes

Routine Care
- Provide Warmth
- Clear Airway if Needed
- Dry
- Assess Color

No

- Provide Warmth
- Position, Clear Airway (as necessary)
- Dry Stimulation, Reposition

Evaluation Respirations, HR and Color

Breathing, HR >100 and Pink

Breathing HR >100 and Pink

Observational Care

30 Sec

A

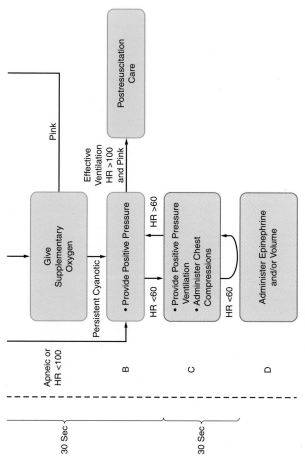

FIGURE 10. Algorithm for resuscitation of the newly born infant.

NOTES

APPENDIX D ■ AMERICAN SOCIETY OF ANESTHESIOLOGISTS STANDARDS, GUIDELINES, AND PRACTICE PARAMETERS

STANDARDS FOR BASIC ANESTHETIC MONITORING

(Approved by the ASA House of Delegates on October 21, 1986, and last amended on October 25, 2005)

These standards apply to all anesthesia care although, in emergency circumstances, appropriate life support measures take precedence. These standards may be exceeded at any time based on the judgment of the responsible anesthesiologist. They are intended to encourage quality patient care, but observing them cannot guarantee any specific patient outcome. They are subject to revision from time to time, as warranted by the evolution of technology and practice. They apply to all general anesthetics, regional anesthetics and monitored anesthesia care. This set of standards addresses only the issue of basic anesthetic monitoring, which is one component of anesthesia care. In certain rare or unusual circumstances, 1) some of these methods of monitoring may be clinically impractical, and 2) appropriate use of the described monitoring methods may fail to detect untoward clinical developments. Brief interruptions of continual[†] monitoring may be unavoidable. *Under extenuating circumstances, the responsible anesthesiologist may waive the requirements marked with an asterisk (*); it is recommended that when this is done, it should be so stated (including the reasons) in a note in the patient's medical record.* These standards are not intended for application to the care of the obstetrical patient in labor or in the conduct of pain management.

Standard I
Qualified anesthesia personnel shall be present in the room throughout the conduct of all general anesthetics, regional anesthetics and monitored anesthesia care.

Objective
Because of the rapid changes in patient status during anesthesia, qualified anesthesia personnel shall be continuously present to monitor the patient and provide anesthesia care. In the event there is a direct known hazard, e.g., radiation, to the anesthesia personnel which might require intermittent remote observation of the patient, some provision for monitoring the patient must be made. In the event that an emergency requires the temporary absence of the person primarily responsible for the anesthetic, the best judgment of the

---

[†]Note that "continual" is defined as "repeated regularly and frequently in steady rapid succession" whereas "continuous" means "prolonged without any interruption at any time."

anesthesiologist will be exercised in comparing the emergency with the anesthetized patient's condition and in the selection of the person left responsible for the anesthetic during the temporary absence.

Standard II
During all anesthetics, the patient's oxygenation, ventilation, circulation and temperature shall be continually evaluated.

Oxygenation
Objective
To ensure adequate oxygen concentration in the inspired gas and the blood during all anesthetics.

Methods
1. Inspired gas: During every administration of general anesthesia using an anesthesia machine, the concentration of oxygen in the patient breathing system shall be measured by an oxygen analyzer with a low oxygen concentration limit alarm in use.*
2. Blood oxygenation: During all anesthetics, a quantitative method of assessing oxygenation such as pulse oximetry shall be employed.* When the pulse oximeter is utilized, the variable pitch pulse tone and the low threshold alarm shall be audible to the anesthesiologist or the anesthesia care team personnel.* Adequate illumination and exposure of the patient are necessary to assess color.*

Ventilation
Objective
To ensure adequate ventilation of the patient during all anesthetics.

Methods
1. Every patient receiving general anesthesia shall have the adequacy of ventilation continually evaluated. Qualitative clinical signs such as chest excursion, observation of the reservoir breathing bag and auscultation of breath sounds are useful. Continual monitoring for the presence of expired carbon dioxide shall be performed unless invalidated by the nature of the patient, procedure or equipment. Quantitative monitoring of the volume of expired gas is strongly encouraged.*
2. When an endotracheal tube or laryngeal mask is inserted, its correct positioning must be verified by clinical assessment and by identification of carbon dioxide in the expired gas. Continual end-tidal carbon dioxide analysis, in use from the time of endotracheal tube/laryngeal mask placement, until extubation/removal or initiating transfer to a postoperative care location, shall be performed using a quantitative method

such as capnography, capnometry or mass spectroscopy.*
When capnography or capnometry is utilized, the end tidal
CO_2 alarm shall be audible to the anesthesiologist or the
anesthesia care team personnel.*

3. When ventilation is controlled by a mechanical ventilator,
   there shall be in continuous use a device that is capable of
   detecting disconnection of components of the breathing system. The device must give an audible signal when its alarm
   threshold is exceeded.
4. During regional anesthesia and monitored anesthesia care,
   the adequacy of ventilation shall be evaluated by continual
   observation of qualitative clinical signs and/or monitoring for
   the presence of exhaled carbon dioxide.

Circulation
Objective
To ensure the adequacy of the patient's circulatory function dur-
ing all anesthetics.

Methods
1. Every patient receiving anesthesia shall have the electrocardiogram continuously displayed from the beginning of anesthesia
   until preparing to leave the anesthetizing location.*
2. Every patient receiving anesthesia shall have arterial blood
   pressure and heart rate determined and evaluated at least
   every five minutes.*
3. Every patient receiving general anesthesia shall have, in addition to the above, circulatory function continually evaluated
   by at least one of the following: palpation of a pulse, auscultation of heart sounds, monitoring of a tracing of intra-arterial pressure, ultrasound peripheral pulse monitoring, or
   pulse plethysmography or oximetry.

Body Temperature
Objective
To aid in the maintenance of appropriate body temperature dur-
ing all anesthetics.

Methods
Every patient receiving anesthesia shall have temperature monitored when clinically significant changes in body temperature are
intended, anticipated or suspected.

---

[1]To become effective July 1, 1999.

CONTINUUM OF DEPTH OF SEDATION DEFINITION OF GENERAL ANESTHESIA AND LEVELS OF SEDATION/ANALGESIA*

(Approved by ASA House of Delegates on October 13, 1999, and amended on October 27, 2004)

	Minimal Sedation (Anxiolysis)	Moderate Sedation/ Analgesia ("Conscious Sedation")	Deep Sedation/ Analgesia	General Anesthesia
Responsiveness	Normal response to verbal stimulation	Purposeful** response to verbal or tactile stimulation	Purposeful** response following repeated or painful stimulation	Unarousable even with painful stimulus
Airway	Unaffected	No intervention required	Intervention may be required	Intervention often required
Spontaneous Ventilation	Unaffected	Adequate	May be inadequate	Frequently inadequate
Cardiovascular Function	Unaffected	Usually maintained	Usually maintained	May be impaired

Minimal Sedation (Anxiolysis) is a drug-induced state during which patients respond normally to verbal commands. Although cognitive function and coordination may be impaired, ventilatory and cardiovascular functions are unaffected.

Moderate Sedation/Analgesia ("Conscious Sedation") is a drug-induced depression of consciousness during which patients respond purposefully** to verbal commands, either alone or accompanied by light tactile stimulation. No interventions are required to maintain a patent airway, and spontaneous ventilation is adequate. Cardiovascular function is usually maintained.

Deep Sedation/Analgesia is a drug-induced depression of consciousness during which patients cannot be easily aroused but respond purposefully** following repeated or painful stimulation. The ability to independently maintain ventilatory function

---

*Monitored Anesthesia Care does not describe the continuum of depth of sedation, rather it describes "a specific anesthesia service in which an anesthesiologist has been requested to participate in the care of a patient undergoing a diagnostic or therapeutic procedure."

**Reflex withdrawal from a painful stimulus is NOT considered a purposeful response.

may be impaired. Patients may require assistance in maintaining a patent airway, and spontaneous ventilation may be inadequate. Cardiovascular function is usually maintained.

General Anesthesia is a drug-induced loss of consciousness during which patients are not arousable, even by painful stimulation. The ability to independently maintain ventilatory function is often impaired. Patients often require assistance in maintaining a patent airway, and positive pressure ventilation may be required because of depressed spontaneous ventilation or drug-induced depression of neuromuscular function. Cardiovascular function may be impaired.

Because sedation is a continuum, it is not always possible to predict how an individual patient will respond. Hence, practitioners intending to produce a given level of sedation should be able to rescue*** patients whose level of sedation becomes deeper than initially intended. Individuals administering Moderate Sedation/Analgesia ("Conscious Sedation") should be able to rescue*** patients who enter a state of Deep Sedation/Analgesia, while those administering Deep Sedation/Analgesia should be able to rescue*** patients who enter a state of General Anesthesia.

***Rescue of a patient from a deeper level of sedation than intended is an intervention by a practitioner proficient in airway management and advanced life support. The qualified practitioner corrects adverse physiologic consequences of the deeper-than-intended level of sedation (such as hypoventilation, hypoxia and hypotension) and returns the patient to the originally intended level of sedation.

BASIC STANDARDS FOR PREANESTHESIA CARE

(Approved by the House of Delegates on October 14, 1987, and amended October 25, 2005)

These standards apply to all patients who receive anesthesia care. Under exceptional circumstances, these standards may be modified. When this is the case, the circumstances shall be documented in the patient's record.

An anesthesiologist shall be responsible for determining the medical status of the patient and developing a plan of anesthesia care.

The anesthesiologist, before the delivery of anesthesia care, is responsible for:

1. Reviewing the available medical record.
2. Interviewing and performing a focused examination of the patient to:
   a. Discuss the medical history, including previous anesthetic experiences and medical therapy.
   b. Assess those aspects of the patient's physical condition that might affect decisions regarding perioperative risk and management.
3. Ordering and reviewing pertinent available tests and consultations as necessary for the delivery of anesthesia care.
4. Ordering appropriate preoperative medications.
5. Ensuring that consent has been obtained for the anesthesia care.
6. Documenting in the chart that the above has been performed.

STANDARDS FOR POSTANESTHESIA CARE

*(Approved by House of Delegates on October 12, 1988
and last amended on October 27, 2004)*

These standards apply to postanesthesia care in all locations. These standards may be exceeded based on the judgment of the responsible anesthesiologist. They are intended to encourage quality patient care, but cannot guarantee any specific patient outcome. They are subject to revision from time to time as warranted by the evolution of technology and practice. *Under extenuating circumstances, the responsible anesthesiologist may waive the requirements marked with an asterisk (*); it is recommended that when this is done, it should be so stated (including the reasons) in a note in the patient's medical record.*

Standard I

All patients who have received general anesthesia, regional anesthesia or monitored anesthesia care shall receive appropriate postanesthesia management.[1]

1. A Postanesthesia Care Unit (PACU) or an area which provides equivalent postanesthesia care (for example, a Surgical Intensive Care Unit) shall be available to receive patients after anesthesia care. All patients who receive anesthesia care shall be admitted to the PACU or its equivalent **except** by specific order of the anesthesiologist responsible for the patient's care.
2. The medical aspects of care in the PACU (or equivalent area) shall be governed by policies and procedures that have been reviewed and approved by the Department of Anesthesiology.
3. The design, equipment and staffing of the PACU shall meet requirements of the facility's accrediting and licensing bodies.

Standard II

A patient transported to the PACU shall be accompanied by a member of the anesthesia care team who is knowledgeable about the patient's condition. The patient shall be continually evaluated and treated during transport with monitoring and support appropriate to the patient's condition.

Standard III

Upon arrival in the PACU, the patient shall be re-evaluated and a verbal report provided to the responsible PACU nurse by the member of the anesthesia care team who accompanies the patient.

---

[1]Refer to *Standards of Post Anesthesia Nursing Practice 1992* published by ASPAN, for issues of nursing care.

1. The patient's status on arrival in the PACU shall be documented.
2. Information concerning the preoperative condition and the surgical/anesthetic course shall be transmitted to the PACU nurse.
3. The member of the Anesthesia Care Team shall remain in the PACU until the PACU nurse accepts responsibility for the nursing care of the patient.

Standard IV
The patient's condition shall be evaluated continually in the PACU.

1. The patient shall be observed and monitored by methods appropriate to the patient's medical condition. Particular attention should be given to monitoring oxygenation, ventilation, circulation, level of consciousness and temperature. During recovery from all anesthetics, a quantitative method of assessing oxygenation such as pulse oximetry shall be employed in the initial phase of recovery.* This is not intended for application during the recovery of the obstetrical patient in whom regional anesthesia was used for labor and vaginal delivery.
2. An accurate written report of the PACU period shall be maintained. Use of an appropriate PACU scoring system is encouraged for each patient on admission, at appropriate intervals prior to discharge and at the time of discharge.
3. General medical supervision and coordination of patient care in the PACU should be the responsibility of an anesthesiologist.
4. There shall be a policy to assure the availability in the facility of a physician capable of managing complications and providing cardiopulmonary resuscitation for patients in the PACU.

Standard V
A physician is responsible for the discharge of the patient from the postanesthesia care unit.

1. When discharge criteria are used, they must be approved by the Department of Anesthesiology and the medical staff. They may vary depending upon whether the patient is discharged to a hospital room, to the Intensive Care Unit, or to a short stay unit or home.
2. In the absence of the physician responsible for the discharge, the PACU nurse shall determine that the patient meets the discharge criteria. The name of the physician accepting responsibility for discharge shall be noted on the record.

APPENDICES

PRACTICE ADVISORY FOR THE PREVENTION AND MANAGEMENT OF OPERATING ROOM FIRES

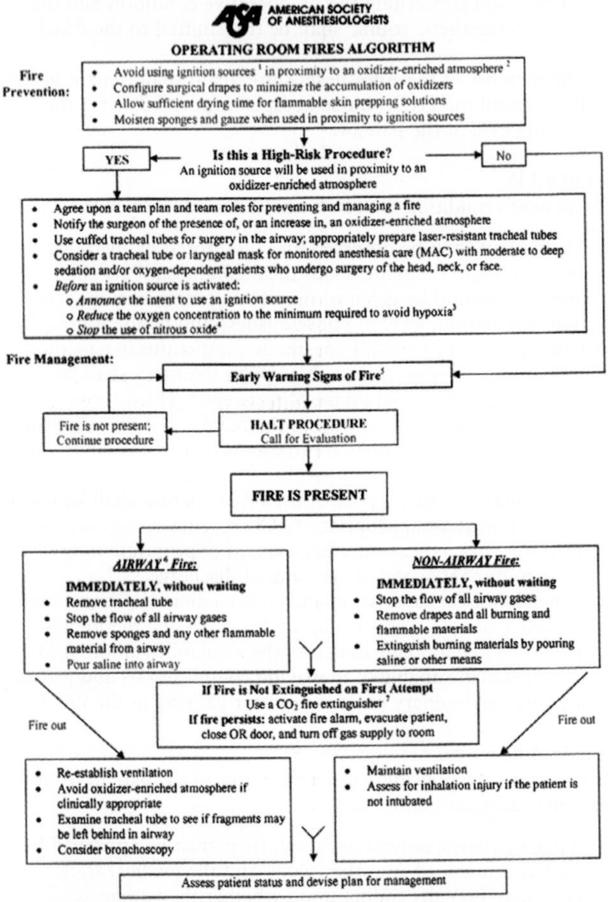

AMERICAN SOCIETY OF ANESTHESIOLOGISTS

OPERATING ROOM FIRES ALGORITHM

Fire Prevention:
- Avoid using ignition sources [1] in proximity to an oxidizer-enriched atmosphere [2]
- Configure surgical drapes to minimize the accumulation of oxidizers
- Allow sufficient drying time for flammable skin prepping solutions
- Moisten sponges and gauze when used in proximity to ignition sources

Is this a High-Risk Procedure?
An ignition source will be used in proximity to an oxidizer-enriched atmosphere

YES → | No →

- Agree upon a team plan and team roles for preventing and managing a fire
- Notify the surgeon of the presence of, or an increase in, an oxidizer-enriched atmosphere
- Use cuffed tracheal tubes for surgery in the airway; appropriately prepare laser-resistant tracheal tubes
- Consider a tracheal tube or laryngeal mask for monitored anesthesia care (MAC) with moderate to deep sedation and/or oxygen-dependent patients who undergo surgery of the head, neck, or face.
- *Before* an ignition source is activated:
  o *Announce* the intent to use an ignition source
  o *Reduce* the oxygen concentration to the minimum required to avoid hypoxia [3]
  o *Stop* the use of nitrous oxide [4]

Fire Management:

Early Warning Signs of Fire [5]

Fire is not present; Continue procedure ← **HALT PROCEDURE** Call for Evaluation

FIRE IS PRESENT

AIRWAY [6] *Fire:*

IMMEDIATELY, without waiting
- Remove tracheal tube
- Stop the flow of all airway gases
- Remove sponges and any other flammable material from airway
- Pour saline into airway

NON-AIRWAY Fire:

IMMEDIATELY, without waiting
- Stop the flow of all airway gases
- Remove drapes and all burning and flammable materials
- Extinguish burning materials by pouring saline or other means

If Fire Is Not Extinguished on First Attempt
Use a CO₂ fire extinguisher [7]
If fire persists: activate fire alarm, evacuate patient, close OR door, and turn off gas supply to room

Fire out

- Re-establish ventilation
- Avoid oxidizer-enriched atmosphere if clinically appropriate
- Examine tracheal tube to see if fragments may be left behind in airway
- Consider bronchoscopy

Fire out

- Maintain ventilation
- Assess for inhalation injury if the patient is not intubated

Assess patient status and devise plan for management

[1] Ignition sources include but are not limited to electrosurgery or electrocautery units and lasers.
[2] An oxidizer-enriched atmosphere occurs when there is any increase in oxygen concentration above room air level, and/or the presence of any concentration of nitrous oxide.
[3] After minimizing delivered oxygen, wait a period of time (*e.g.*, 1-3 min) before using an ignition source. For oxygen dependent patients, *reduce* supplemental oxygen delivery to the minimum required to avoid hypoxia. Monitor oxygenation with pulse oximetry, and if feasible, inspired, exhaled, and/or delivered oxygen concentration.
[4] After stopping the delivery of nitrous oxide, wait a period of time (*e.g.*, 1-3 min) before using an ignition source.
[5] Unexpected flash, flame, smoke or heat, unusual sounds (*e.g.*, a "pop," snap or "foomp") or odors, unexpected movement of drapes, discoloration of drapes or breathing circuit, unexpected patient movement or complaint.
[6] In this algorithm, airway fire refers to a fire in the airway or breathing circuit.
[7] A CO₂ fire extinguisher may be used on the patient if necessary.

FIGURE 1. Operating room fires algorithm. CO_2 = carbon dioxide; OR = operating room.

DISTINGUISHING MONITORED ANESTHESIA CARE ("MAC") FROM MODERATE SEDATION/ANALGESIA (CONSCIOUS SEDATION)

Approved by the ASA House of Delegates on October 27, 2004)

Moderate Sedation/Analgesia (Conscious Sedation; hereinafter known as Moderate Sedation) is a physician service recognized in the CPT procedural coding system. During Moderate Sedation, a physician supervises or personally administers sedative and/or analgesic medications that can allay patient anxiety and control pain during a diagnostic or therapeutic procedure. Such drug-induced depression of a patient's level of consciousness to a "moderate" level of sedation, as defined in JCAHO standards, is intended to facilitate the successful performance of the diagnostic or therapeutic procedure while providing patient comfort and cooperation. Physicians providing moderate sedation must be qualified to recognize "deep" sedation, manage its consequences and adjust the level of sedation to a "moderate" or lesser level. The continual assessment of the effects of sedative or analgesic medications on the level of consciousness and on cardiac and respiratory function is an integral element of this service.

The American Society of Anesthesiologists has defined Monitored Anesthesia Care (*see Position on Monitored Anesthesia Care, last amended October 15, 2003*). This physician service can be distinguished from Moderate Sedation in several ways. An essential component of MAC is the anesthesia assessment and management of a patient's actual or anticipated physiological derangements or medical problems that may occur during a diagnostic or therapeutic procedure. While Monitored Anesthesia Care may include the administration of sedatives and/or analgesics often used for Moderate Sedation, the provider of MAC must be prepared and qualified to convert to general anesthesia when necessary. Additionally, a provider's ability to intervene to rescue a patient's airway from any sedation induced compromise is a prerequisite to the qualifications to provide Monitored Anesthesia Care. By contrast, Moderate Sedation is not expected to induce depths of sedation that would impair the patient's own ability to maintain the integrity of his or her airway. These components of Monitored Anesthesia Care are unique aspects of an anesthesia service that are not part of Moderate Sedation.

The administration of sedatives, hypnotics, analgesics, as well as anesthetic drugs commonly used for the induction and maintenance of general anesthesia is often, but not always, a part of Monitored Anesthesia Care. In some patients who may require only minimal sedation, MAC is often indicated because even small doses of these medications could precipitate adverse physiologic responses that would necessitate acute clinical interventions and resuscitation. If a patient's condition and/or a procedural require-ment is likely to require sedation to a "deep" level or even to a transient period of general anesthesia, only a practitioner privi-leged to provide anesthesia services should be allowed to manage the sedation. Due to the strong likelihood that "deep" sedation may, with or without intention, transition to general anesthesia, the skills of an anesthesia provider are necessary to manage the effects of general anesthesia on the patient as well as to return the patient quickly to a state of "deep" or lesser sedation.

Like all anesthesia services, Monitored Anesthesia Care includes an array of post-procedure responsibilities beyond the expectations of practitioners providing Moderate Sedation, including assuring a return to full consciousness, relief of pain, management of adverse physiological responses or side effects from medications administered during the procedure, as well as the diagnosis and treatment of co-existing medical problems.

Monitored Anesthesia Care allows for the safe administration of a maximal depth of sedation in excess of that provided during Moderate Sedation. The ability to adjust the sedation level from full consciousness to general anesthesia during the course of a procedure provides maximal flexibility in matching sedation level to patient needs and procedural requirements. In situations where the procedure is more invasive or when the patient is especially fragile, optimizing sedation level is necessary to achieve ideal pro-cedural conditions.

In summary, Monitored Anesthesia Care is a physician service which is clearly distinct from Moderate Sedation due to the expec-tations and qualifications of the provider who must be able to uti-lize all anesthesia resources to support life and to provide patient comfort and safety during a diagnostic or therapeutic procedure.

POSITION ON MONITORED ANESTHESIA CARE

(Approved by the House of Delegates on October 21, 1986, and last amended on October 25, 2005)

Monitored anesthesia care is a specific anesthesia service for a diagnostic or therapeutic procedure. Indications for monitored anesthesia care include the nature of the procedure, the patient's clinical condition and/or the potential need to convert to a general or regional anesthetic.

Monitored anesthesia care includes all aspects of anesthesia care—a preprocedure visit, intraprocedure care and postprocedure anesthesia management. During monitored anesthesia care, the anesthesiologist provides or medically directs a number of specific services, including but not limited to:

- Diagnosis and treatment of clinical problems that occur during the procedure
- Support of vital functions
- Administration of sedatives, analgesics, hypnotics, anesthetic agents or other medications as necessary for patient safety
- Psychological support and physical comfort
- Provision of other medical services as needed to complete the procedure safely.

Monitored anesthesia care may include varying levels of sedation, analgesia, and anxiolysis as necessary. The provider of monitored anesthesia care must be prepared and qualified to convert to general anesthesia when necessary. If the patient loses consciousness and the ability to respond purposefully, the anesthesia care is a general anesthetic, irrespective of whether airway instrumentation is required.

Monitored anesthesia care is a physician service provided to an individual patient. It should be subject to the same level of payment as general or regional anesthesia. Accordingly, the ASA Relative Value Guide provides for the use of proper base procedural units, time units and modifier units as the basis for determining reimbursement.

ETHICAL GUIDELINES FOR THE ANESTHESIA CARE OF PATIENTS WITH DO-NOT-RESUSCITATE ORDERS

*(Approved by House of Delegates on October 13, 1993
and last amended on October 17, 2001)*

These guidelines apply to competent patients and also to incompetent patients who have previously expressed their preferences.

I. Given the diversity of published opinions and cultures within our society, an essential element of preoperative preparation and perioperative care for patients with Do-Not Resuscitate (DNR) orders or other directives that limit treatment is communication among involved parties. It is necessary to document relevant aspects of this communication.

II. Policies automatically suspending DNR orders or other directives that limit treatment prior to procedures involving anesthetic care may not sufficiently address a patient's rights to self-determination in a responsible and ethical manner. Such policies, if they exist, should be reviewed and revised, as necessary, to reflect the content of these guidelines.

III. The administration of anesthesia necessarily involves some practices and procedures that might be viewed as "resuscitation" in other settings. Prior to procedures requiring anesthetic care, any existing directives to limit the use of resuscitation procedures (that is, do-not-resuscitate orders and/or advance directives) should, when possible, be reviewed with the patient or designated surrogate. As a result of this review, the status of these directives should be clarified or modified based on the preferences of the patient. One of the three following alternatives may provide for a satisfactory outcome in many cases.

    A. Full Attempt at Resuscitation: The patient or designated surrogate may request the full suspension of existing directives during the anesthetic and immediate postoperative period, thereby consenting to the use of any resuscitation procedures that may be appropriate to treat clinical events that occur during this time.

    B. Limited Attempt at Resuscitation Defined With Regard to Specific Procedures: The patient or designated surrogate may elect to continue to refuse certain specific resuscitation procedures (for example, chest compressions, defibrillation or tracheal intubation). The anesthesiologist should inform the patient or designated surrogate about which procedures are 1) essential to the success of the anesthesia and the proposed procedure, and 2) which procedures are not essential and may be refused.

C. Limited Attempt at Resuscitation Defined With Regard to the Patient's Goals and Values: The patient or designated surrogate may allow the anesthesiologist and surgical team to use clinical judgment in determining which resuscitation procedures are appropriate in the context of the situation and the patient's stated goals and values. For example, some patients may want full resuscitation procedures to be used to manage adverse clinical events that are believed to be quickly and easily reversible, but to refrain from treatment for conditions that are likely to result in permanent sequelae, such as neurologic impairment or unwanted dependence upon life-sustaining technology.

IV. Any clarifications or modifications made to the patient's directive should be documented in the medical record. In cases where the patient or designated surrogate requests that the anesthesiologist use clinical judgment in determining which resuscitation procedures are appropriate, the anesthesiologist should document the discussion with particular attention to the stated goals and values of the patient.

V. Plans for postoperative care should indicate if or when the original, pre-existent directive to limit the use of resuscitation procedures will be reinstated. This occurs when the patient leaves the postanesthesia care unit or when the patient has recovered from the acute effects of anesthesia and surgery. Consideration should be given to whether continuing to provide the patient with a time-limited or event-limited postoperative trial of therapy would help the patient or surrogate better evaluate whether continued therapy would be consistent with the patient's goals.

VI. It is important to discuss and document whether there are to be any exceptions to the injunction(s) against intervention should there occur a specific recognized complication of the surgery or anesthesia.

VII. Concurrence on these issues by the primary physician (if not the surgeon of record), the surgeon and the anesthesiologist is desirable. If possible, these physicians should meet together with the patient (or the patient's legal representative) when these issues are discussed. This duty of the patient's physicians is deemed to be of such importance that it should not be delegated. Other members of the health care team who are (or will be) directly involved with the patient's care during the planned procedure should, if feasible, be included in this process.

VIII. Should conflicts arise, the following resolution processes are recommended:
   A. When an anesthesiologist finds the patient's or surgeon's limitations of intervention decisions to be irreconcilable with one's own moral views, then the anesthesiologist should withdraw in a nonjudgmental fashion, providing an alternative for care in a timely fashion.
   B. When an anesthesiologist finds the patient's or surgeon's limitation of intervention decisions to be in conflict with generally accepted standards of care, ethical practice or institutional policies, then the anesthesiologist should voice such concerns and present the situation to the appropriate institutional body.
   C. If these alternatives are not feasible within the time frame necessary to prevent further morbidity or suffering, then in accordance with the American Medical Association's Principles of Medical Ethics, care should proceed with reasonable adherence to the patient's directives, being mindful of the patient's goals and values.

IX. A representative from the hospital's anesthesiology service should establish a liaison with surgical and nursing services for presentation, discussion and procedural application of these guidelines. Hospital staff should be made aware of the proceedings of these discussions and the motivations for them.

X. Modification of these guidelines may be appropriate when they conflict with local standards or policies, and in those emergency situations involving incompetent patients whose intentions have been previously expressed.

APPENDIX E ■ THE AIRWAY APPROACH ALGORITHM AND DIFFICULT AIRWAY ALGORITHM

AIRWAY APPROACH ALGORITHM

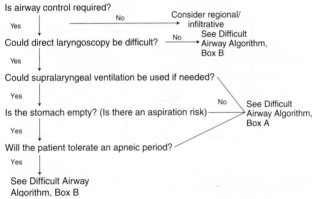

FIGURE 1. Airway Approach Algorithm. From: Rosenblatt W: The airway approach algorithm. J Clin Anes 16:312, 2004.

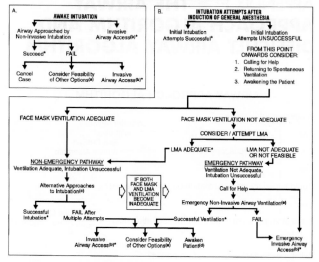

FIGURE 2. Difficult Airway Algorithm. From: Practice guidelines for the management of the difficult airway: An updated report by the American Society of Anesthesiologists Task Force on Management of the Difficult Airway. Anesthesiology 98(5): 1273, 2003.

APPENDIX F ■ **MALIGNANT HYPERTHERMIA PROTOCOL**

DIAGNOSIS
Signs of Malignant Hyperthermia (MH)
    A. Increased $ETCO_2$
    B. Trunk or limb rigidity
    C. Masseter spasm or trismus
    D. Tachycardia/tachypnea
    E. Acidosis
    E Increased temperature (late sign)
Sudden/Unexpected Cardiac Arrest in Young Patients
    A. Presume hyperkalemia and initiate treatment (see #6).
    B. Measure CK, myoglobin, ABGs, until normalized.
    C. Consider dantrolene.
    D. Realize it is usually secondary to occult myopathy (e.g., muscular dystrophy).
    E. Understand resuscitation may be difficult and prolonged
Trismus or Masseter Spasm with Succinylcholine
    A. Early sign of MH in many patients.
    B. If limb muscle rigidity, begin treatment with dantrolene.
    C. For emergent procedures, continue with nontriggering agents, consider dantrolene.
    D. Follow CK and urine myoglobin for 36 hours at least.
    E. Observe in ICU for at least 12 hours.

ACUTE PHASE TREATMENT

1. **GET HELP. GET DANTROLENE—Notify surgeon.**
    A. Discontinue volatile agents and succinylcholine (SCh).
    B. Hyperventilate with 100% oxygen at flows of 10 L/min or more.
    C. Halt the procedure as soon as possible; if emergent, use nontriggers.
2. **Dantrolene 2.5 mg/kg rapidly iv**
    A. Repeat until there is control of the signs of MH.
    B. Sometimes more than 10 mg/kg is necessary.
    C. Dissolve the 20 mg in each vial with at least 60 mL sterile **distilled water** for injection.
    D. The crystals also contain NaOH for a pH of 9, mannitol 3 g.

3. **Bicarbonate for metabolic acidosis**
   A. 1 to 2 mEq/kg if blood gas values are not yet available.
4. **Cool** the patient with core temperature >39°C, via cold saline iv, surface, open body cavities, stomach, bladder, or rectum. Stop cooling if temp <38°C and falling. Avoid excess cooling to prevent drift <36°.
5. **Dysrhythmias** usually respond to treatment of acidosis and hyperkalemia.
   A. Use standard drug therapy except calcium channel blockers, which may cause hyperkalemia or cardiac arrest in the presence of dantrolene sodium.
6. **Hyperkalemia**—Treat with hyperventilation, bicarbonate, glucose/insulin, calcium
   A. 10 units regular insulin and 50 mL 50% glucose (adult) OR
   B. 0.15 units insulin/kg and 1 mL/kg 50% glucose (pediatric)
   C. Calcium chloride 10 mg/kg or calcium gluconate 10 to 50 mg/kg for life-threatening hyperkalemia
7. **Follow** ETCO$_2$, electrolytes, blood gases, CK, core temperature, urine output and color, coagulation factors.
   A. Venous blood gas (e.g., femoral vein) values may document hypermetabolism better than arterial values.
   B. Central venous or PA monitoring as needed.

POST ACUTE PHASE

A. Observe the patient in an ICU for a minimum of 36 hours.
B. Dantrolene 1 mg/kg q4 to 6 hours for 24 to 48 hours, depending on recovery phase.
C. Follow vitals and labs as above (see #7)
   ▪ Frequent ABG
   ▪ CK every 6 to 8 hours
D. Counsel the patient and family regarding MH and further precautions. Refer them to MHAUS, fill and send in the Adverse Metabolic Reaction to Anesthesia (AMRA) form, and send a letter to the patient and his or her physician.
E. Refer patient to the nearest biopsy center for follow up.

CAUTION: This protocol may not apply to every patient and may require alteration according to specific patient needs.

APPENDIX G ■ **DRUG LIST**

The authors and publisher have exerted every effort to ensure that the drug selection and dosage set forth in this appendix are in accord with current recommendations and practice at the time of publication. However, in view of ongoing research, changes in government regulations, and the constant flow of information relating to drug therapy and drug reactions, the reader is urged to check the package insert for each drug for any change in indications and dosage and for added warnings and precautions. This is particularly important when the recommended agent is a new or infrequently used drug. Unless specified otherwise, all doses are for adults.

The editors acknowledge the contribution of Stella A. Haddadin, BSc, PharmD, Yale–New Haven Hospital, Department of Pharmacy Services, in the preparation of this appendix.

ABBREVIATIONS

BBW:	black box warning **BBW**
CrCl:	creatinine clearance
ESRD:	end-stage renal disease
HTN:	hypertension
IV:	intravenous
IM:	intramuscular
MR:	may repeat
N/A:	not available
NTE:	not to exceed
PO:	orally
SC:	subcutaneous
t½:	half-life

ACETAMINOPHEN (VARIOUS)

- **Uses:** analgesic, antipyretic
- **Dose:** Adults: (PO) 325–650 mg q4h, max daily dose 4 g. Children >12 yr: (PO) 10–15 mg/kg q4h, NTE 5 doses. Children 6–12 yr: (rectal) 325 mg q4–6h, max daily dose 2.6 g. Children 3–6 yr: (rectal) 120 mg q4h, max daily dose 720 mg. Children 1–3 yr: (rectal) 80 mg q4–6h.
- **Site of clearance:** hepatic
- **t½:** 1–3 h

■ **Interaction/toxicity:** Has no significant anti-inflammatory effect. Causes severe liver toxicity when combined with alcohol. Use with caution in patients with alcoholic-related liver disease. Therapeutic doses can cause liver failure in alcoholics. Potentiates toxicity of barbiturates, carbamazepine, and hydantoins. Beta-blockers and anticholinergics intensify effect.

ACETAZOLAMIDE (VARIOUS)

■ **Uses:** reduce intraocular pressure, acute altitude sickness, diuretic

■ **Dose:** *Glaucoma:* Adults: (IV) 250 mg q6h; (PO) 250–1,000 mg/day qid, max 1 g/24 h. Children: (IV, IM) 5–10 mg/kg q6h; (PO) 10–15 mg/kg/day q6–8h.

   Acute altitude sickness: (PO) 250 mg q8–12h; begin Rx 24–48 h before and continue for 24–48 h after arrival at altitude.

■ **Site of clearance:** renal

■ **t½:** 2.4–5.8 h

■ **Interaction/toxicity:** Contraindicated in sulfonamide allergy, hepatic disease, decreased serum sodium or potassium levels, adrenocortical insufficiency, hyperchloremic acidosis, renal disease, long-term use in glaucoma. Use with caution in respiratory acidosis, diabetes mellitus (may cause significant blood glucose increase). Paresthesias and myalgias may be experienced. Decreased effects of lithium. Increases toxicity of cyclosporine and digitalis toxicity (hypokalemia present). Salicylates may cause accumulation.

ADENOSINE (ADENOCARD)

■ **Uses:** antidysrhythmic (paroxysmal supraventricular tachycardia)

■ **Dose:** Adults: (IV) 6 mg, if not effective within 1–2 min give 12 mg, MR 12 mg bolus prn, max single dose 12 mg. Infants and children: (IV) 0.1 mg/kg, if not effective give 0.2 mg/kg, medium dose 0.15 mg/kg, max single dose 12 mg.

■ **Site of clearance:** enzymatic

■ **t½:** <10 sec

■ **Interaction/toxicity:** Transient dysrhythmias seen before conversion to sinus rhythm. Excessive doses may cause significant hypotension, shortness of breath, and flushing. Adenosine does not convert atrial flutter/atrial fibrillation/ventricular tachycardia to sinus rhythm but may be used to distinguish paroxysmal supraventricular tachycardia and other tachycardias.

ALBUTEROL (VARIOUS)

- ▓ **Uses:** bronchodilator
- ▓ **Dose:** Adults: (PO) regular release 2–4 mg/dose tid-qid NTE 32 mg/day (divided doses); (inhalation) 90 mcg/spray, 1–2 inhalations q4–6h, NTE 12 inhalations/day. Children 6–12 yr: (PO) 4 mg bid, NTE 24 mg/day; (inhalation) 90 mcg/spray, 1–2 inhalations q6–8h, NTE 12 inhalations/day.
- ▓ **Site of clearance:** hepatic
- ▓ **t½:** 1.5–2.5 h
- ▓ **Interaction/toxicity:** Use with spacer for inhalations. Use with caution in patients with hypothyroidism, diabetes mellitus, CAD, and HTN, and those using MAOIs, tricyclic antidepressants. Decreased effect with beta-blockers. Enhanced effect with sympathomimetics. Excessive use leads to tolerance. May contain sulfites.

ALFENTANIL (ALFENTA)

- ▓ **Uses:** analgesia
- ▓ **Dose:** (IV) induction 130–245 mcg/kg, maintenance 0.5–1.5 mcg/kg/min.
- ▓ **Site of clearance:** hepatic
- ▓ **t½:** 83–97 min
- ▓ **Interaction/toxicity:** Diazepam potentiates hypotensive action; truncal muscle rigidity may be seen during induction and emergence. Erythromycin delays clearance.

AMINOCAPROIC ACID (VARIOUS)

- ▓ **Uses:** antifibrinolytic
- ▓ **Dose:** (IV, PO) loading 5 g, then 1.25 g/h, max daily dose 30 g.
- ▓ **Site of clearance:** renal
- ▓ **t½:** 1–2 h
- ▓ **Interaction/toxicity:** Adjust dose in renal dysfunction. Rapid IV administration may cause hypotension, bradycardia, or dysrhythmias. Do not administer if DIC is present. Use with caution in presence of upper urinary tract bleeding (may cause intrarenal thrombosis).

AMIODARONE (CORDARONE)

- ▓ **Uses:** antidysrhythmic
- ▓ **Dose:** *Cardiac arrest:* Pulseless VF or VT: (IV) Initial: 300 mg in 20–30 ml NS or D$_5$W; if VF or VT recurs, supplemental dose

of 150 mg followed by infusion of 1 mg/min for 6 h, then 0.5 mg/min × 18 hr (max daily dose 2.2 gm)

Break through VF or VT: (IV) 150 mg supplemental dose in 100 ml D$_5$W over 10 min (PO) loading 800–1,000 mg divided bid–tid, then 400 mg/day.

- ■ **Site of clearance:** hepatic
- ■ **t½:** 13–37 days
- ■ **Interaction/toxicity:** Contraindicated in cardiogenic shock, severe sinus node dysfunction, second- and third-degree heart arteriovenous block and bradycardia-induced syncope in absence of pacemaker. Pulmonary toxicity (hypersensitivity pneumonitis) and optic neuropathy can occur. Inhibits peripheral conversion of T$_4$ to T$_3$. Potentiates anticoagulants, beta-blockers, calcium channel blockers, digoxin, fentanyl, hydantoins, lidocaine, procainamide, quinidine, and theophylline.

AMINOPHYLLINE (VARIOUS)

- ■ **Uses:** bronchodilator
- ■ **Dose:** *Acute bronchospasm:* Adults and children >1 yr: (IV) loading 6 mg/kg (diluted in 100 mL D$_5$W or NS), NTE 25 mg/min use ideal body weight for obese patients (each 0.6 mg/kg increases serum theophylline level 1 mcg/mL); maintenance 0.5–1 mg/kg/h (adjust dose based on serum level).
- ■ **Site of clearance:** hepatic
- ■ **t½:** infants (4–52 wk) 4–30 h, children/adolescents 2–16 h, adults 4–16 h
- ■ **Interaction/toxicity:** Increases effects on sympathomimetics, digitalis, oral anticoagulants; decreases effects of phenytoin, lithium, nondepolarizing muscle relaxants. Phenobarbital increases aminophylline metabolism. Antagonizes beta-blockers; toxicity with halothane (dysrhythmias) and ketamine (seizures).

AMITRIPTYLINE (VARIOUS)

- ■ **Uses:** antidepressant, chronic pain, migraine headaches
- ■ **Dose:** *Antidepressant:* (IM) 20–30 mg qid; (PO) 10–25 mg tid.
  Pain management: (PO) initial 25 mg qhs, may increase to 100 mg/day.
- ■ **Site of clearance:** hepatic
- ■ **t½:** 16–26 h
- ■ **Interaction/toxicity:** Contraindicated in patients with narrow-angle glaucoma, Rx with MAOIs within previous 14 days. Use with caution in patients receiving electroshock Rx, and those

with cardiac dysrhythmias, hyperthyroidism, renal or hepatic dysfunction. Blocks antihypertensive effect of guanethidine. Barbiturates increase metabolism. Increases amount of inhalation anesthesia required. Potentiates sympathomimetics, CNS depressants, and anticoagulants. Cimetidine decreases metabolism. Do not discontinue abruptly. Cardiovascular toxicity leading cause of death.

AMOBARBITAL (VARIOUS)

- Uses: hypnotic, sedative, anticonvulsant, premedicant
- Dose: (IV, IM) 60–500 mg; (PO) 30–50 mg tid, 60–200 mg qhs.
- Site of clearance: hepatic
- t½: 8–42 h
- Interaction/toxicity: Contraindicated in patients with severe liver dysfunction or porphyria. Potentiates sedatives, hypnotics tranquilizers, and other CNS depressants. Decreases effects of beta-blockers, theophylline, and corticosteroids. MAOIs increase actions. Increases metabolism of methadone and can result in withdrawal. Tolerance can develop.

AMOXICILLIN (VARIOUS)

- Uses: antibiotic
- Dose: Adults: (PO) 250–500 mg q8h. Children: (PO) 20–40 mg/kg q8h.
  Prophylaxis for bacterial endocarditis (dental, respiratory, oral procedures): Adults: (PO) 2 g 1 h before procedure. Children: (PO) 50 mg/kg 1 h before procedure.
- Site of clearance: renal
- t½: infants and children 1–2 h, adults 0.7–1.4 h
- Interaction/toxicity: Adjust dose with renal dysfunction. Potentiates anticoagulants.

AMPICILLIN (VARIOUS)

- Uses: antibiotic
- Dose: Adults: (IV) 500 mg to 2 g q4–6h, max daily dose 12 g; (IM) 0.5–1.5 g q4–6h; (PO) 250–500 mg q6h. Children: (IV, IM) 100–400 mg/kg/day divided q4–6h; (PO) 50–100 mg/kg/day divided q6h, max daily dose 2–3 g.
  Sepsis/meningitis: Adults: (IV) 150–250 mg/kg/day divided q4h, max 2 g q4h. Children: (IV) 200 mg/kg/day divided q4–6h, max daily dose 12 g.
- Site of clearance: renal
- t½: 1–1.8 h

▪ **Interaction/toxicity:** Adjust dose with renal dysfunction. Potentiates anticoagulants. Rapid infusion >100 mg/min may cause rigors.

ANTITHROMBIN III (THROMBATE III)

▪ **Uses:** antithrombin III replacement
▪ **Dose:** (IV) International units required = [(desired − baseline AT III level)/(1.4)](weight in kg); administer over 10–20 min.
▪ **Site of clearance:** N/A
▪ **t½:** 2.6–3.8 days
▪ **Interaction/toxicity:** Derived from human plasma; risk of HIV and infectious viruses. Potentiates action of heparin.

ARGATROBAN (ARGATROBAN)

▪ **Uses:** anticoagulant, thrombin inhibitor
▪ **Dose:** *Prophylaxis of thrombosis (heparin-induced thrombocytopenia):* (IV) initial 2 mcg/kg/min, NTE 10 mcg/kg/min.
  Myocardial infarction: 100 mcg/kg bolus followed by 1–3 mcg/kg/min for 6–72 h. *Percutaneous coronary interventions:* 350 mcg/kg IV over 3–5 min and 25 mcg/kg/min IV continuous infusion. Check ACT 5–10 min after bolus.
▪ **Site of clearance:** liver
▪ **t½:** 30–51 min
▪ **Interaction/toxicity:** Use with caution in patients with increased risk of hemorrhage: severe HTN, lumbar puncture, spinal anesthesia, major surgery, bleeding disorders, GI ulcers hepatic impairment.

ATENOLOL (TENORMIN) **BBW**

▪ **Uses:** antianginal, antihypertensive, antidysrhythmic
▪ **Dose:** Adults: (IV) 5 mg over 5 min, MR after 10 min; (PO) 25–50 mg/day.
▪ **Site of clearance:** renal
▪ **t½:** 6–9 h, ESRD 15–35 h
▪ **Interaction/toxicity:** Adjust dose in renal dysfunction. Administer with caution to patients with diabetes mellitus, bronchospastic disorders, CHF, second- and third-degree heart block, and myasthenia gravis. Increases effects of calcium channel blockers, H_2 antagonists, MAOIs, IV anesthetic agents, and local anesthetics. Avoid abrupt withdrawal. Clonidine may cause life-threatening HTN.

ATRACURIUM (TRACRIUM) BBW

▨ **Uses:** nondepolarizing neuromuscular blocker
▨ **Dose:** Dose to effect; doses will vary due to interpatient variability; use ideal body weight for obese patients. Adults and children >2 yr: (IV) 0.4–0.5 mg/kg, then 0.08–0.1 mg/kg 20–45 min after initial dose to maintain neuromuscular block, followed by repeat doses of 0.08–0.1 mg/kg at 15–25 min intervals.

Initial dose after succinylcholine for intubation: Adults and Children >2 yr: 0.2–0.4 mg/kg.

Neuromuscular blockade: Children 1 mo to 2 yr: (IV) 0.3–0.5 mg/kg followed by 0.25 mg/kg maintenance doses.

Continuous infusion: Adults and Children >2 yr: surgery initial 9–10 mcg/kg/min at initial signs of recovery from bolus dose, block usually maintained by a rate of 5–9 mcg/kg/min under balanced anesthesia.

ICU: Adults and Children >2 yr: neuromuscular blockade usually maintained by rate of 11–13 mcg/kg/min.

▨ **Site of clearance:** plasma (Hofmann elimination) and ester hydrolysis; hepatic
▨ **t½:** 16–20 min
▨ **Interaction/toxicity:** Potentiated by volatile anesthetics, hypokalemia, antibiotics (aminoglycosides), lithium, verapamil, trimethaphan, and procainamide. Antagonized by theophylline and phenytoin (decrease action). Releases histamine at high doses.

ATROPINE (VARIOUS)

▨ **Uses:** antisialagogue; vagolysis
▨ **Dose:** *Paradoxical bradycardia has been associated with the following doses:* Adults: <0.5 mg. Neonates, infants, and children: <0.1 mg.

Asystole or pulseless electrical activity: (IV) 1 mg, MR in 3–5 min if asystole persists to a total dose of 0.04 mg/kg; (intratracheal) 2–2.5 times the IV dose in 10 mL NS.

Pre-anesthetic: Adults: (IV, IM, SC) 0.4–0.6 mg 30–60 min preop then q4–6h prn. Children >5 kg: (IV, IM, SC, PO) 0.01–0.02 mg/kg to a max 0.4 mg/dose 30–60 min preop, min dose 0.1 mg. Children <5 kg: (IV, IM, SC, PO) 0.02 mg/kg 30–60 min preop then q4–6h prn. Use of a minimum dosage of 0.1 mg in neonates <5 kg will result in dosages >0.02 mg/kg. There is no documented minimum dosage in this age group.

Bradycardia: Adults: (IV) 0.5–1 mg q5min, NTE total 3 mg or 0.04 mg/kg; may give intratracheally in 10 mL NS.

Children: (IV, intratracheal) 0.02 mg/kg, min dose 0.1 mg, max single dose 0.5 mg in children and 1 mg in adolescents; MR in 5-min intervals to max total dose 1 mg in children and 2 mg in adolescents (for intratracheal administration, dilute in NS to total volume of 1–2 mL). When treating bradycardia in neonates, reserve use for patients unresponsive to improved oxygenation and epinephrine.

Neuromuscular blockade reversal: (IV) 25–30 mcg/kg 60 sec before neostigmine or 7–10 mcg/kg in combination with edrophonium.
- **Site of clearance:** renal
- **t½:** 2–3 h
- **Interaction/toxicity:** Potentiated by antihistamines, procainamide, tricyclic antidepressants, and monoamine oxidase inhibitors. Antagonizes effects of cholinesterase inhibitors and metoclopramide.

BENZOCAINE (AMERICAINE, HURRICAINE)

- **Uses:** topical anesthesia
- **Dose:** (topical) Spray applied for ≤1 sec. A spray >2 sec is contraindicated. The average expulsion rate of residue from the spray is 200 mg/sec.
- **Site of clearance:** plasma cholinesterase
- **t½:** N/A
- **Interaction/toxicity:** methemoglobinemia

BISOPROLOL (ZEBETA)

- **Uses:** antianginal, antihypertensive, antidysrhythmic
- **Dose:** Adults: (PO) 5 mg/day, may be increased to 10 mg and then up to 20 mg/day if necessary. Elderly: (PO) initial 2.5 mg/day, may be increased by 2.5–5 mg/day, max daily dose 20 mg.
- **Site of clearance:** renal
- **t½:** 9–12 h
- **Interaction/toxicity:** Adjust dose in renal dysfunction. Administer with caution to patients with diabetes mellitus, bronchospastic disorders, CHF, second- and third-degree heart block, and myasthenia gravis. Increases effects of calcium channel blockers, H_2 antagonists, MAOIs, IV anesthetic agents, and local anesthetics. Avoid abrupt withdrawal. Clonidine may cause life-threatening HTN.

BIVALRUDIN (ANGIOMAX)

- **Uses:** anticoagulant, thrombin inhibitor

- **Dose:** PTCA/PCI or PCI with HIT: (IV): 0.75 mg/kg bolus followed by 1.75 mg/kg/hr for duration of proceedure up to 4 hrs post proceedure if needed. Check ACT 5 min after bolus.

  Renal impairment: for CrCl 30–59 mL/min reduce dose by 20%; for CrCl 10–29 mL/min reduce dose by 60%; for CrCl <10 mL/min reduce dose by 90%.
- **Site of clearance:** renal and proteolysis
- **t½:** 25 min
- **Interaction/toxicity:** Contraindicated in patients with active bleeding. Use with caution in patients for brachytherapy procedures (increased risk of thrombus formation with possible fatal outcomes), cerebral aneurysm, renal impairment, gastrointestinal ulceration (risk of hemorrhage). There is limited data to support use in patients with heparin induced thrombocytopenia-thrombosis syndromes (HIT/HITTS) undergoing PTCA. However, in vitro studies exhibited no platelet aggregation response against serum from patients with a history of HIT/HITTS.

  Cardiac Surgery: Off pump: (IV) 0.75 mg/kg followed by 1.75 mg/kg/hr to maintain ACT>300 sec. On pump: (IV) 1 mg/kg followed by 2.5 mg/kg/hr; 50 mg bolus added to priming solution of CPB circuit.

BUPIVACAINE (MARCAINE, SENSORCAINE) `BBW`

- **Uses:** local/regional anesthesia
- **Dose:** Doses vary; max daily dose 3 mg/kg.

  Local anesthesia: infiltration 0.25% infiltrated locally, max dose 175 mg.

  Caudal block (with or without epinephrine, preservative free): Adults: 15–30 mL of 0.25% or 0.5%. Children: 1–3.7 mg/kg.

  Epidural block (other than caudal block with or without epinephrine, preservative free): Adults: 10–20 mL of 0.25% or 0.5%. Children: 1.25 mg/kg/dose. Always administer in 3–5 mL increments, allowing sufficient time to detect toxic manifestations of inadvertent IV or IT administration.

  Surgical procedures requiring a high degree of muscle relaxation and prolonged effects only: 10–20 mL of 0.75% (do not use in obstetrical cases).

  Maxillary and mandibular infiltration and nerve block: 9 mg (1.8 mL) of 0.5% (with epinephrine) per injection site, MR after 10 min to produce adequate anesthesia, max 90 mg per dental appointment.

APPENDICES

Obstetrical anesthesia: incremental 3–5 mL of 0.5%, NTE 50–100 mg in any dosing interval; allow sufficient time to detect toxic manifestations or inadvertent IV or IT injection.

Peripheral nerve block: 5 mL of 0.25 or 0.5%, max daily dose 400 mg

Sympathetic nerve block: 20–50 mL of 0.25%

Retrobulbar anesthesia: 2–4 mL of 0.75%

Spinal anesthesia: solution of 0.75% bupivacaine in 8.25% dextrose (a hyperbaric solution); lower extremity and perineal procedures 1 mL, lower abdominal procedures 1.6 mL.

Obstetrical: normal vaginal delivery 0.8 mL (higher doses may be required); C section 1–1.4 mL

- **Site of clearance:** hepatic
- **t½:** 3–5 h
- **Interaction/toxicity:** Bupivacaine 0.75% not recommended for obstetrics or IV regional anesthesia. Diazepam increases bioavailability. Acute CV collapse following accidental injection; cardiac toxicity greater than CNS toxicity.

BUPRENORPHINE (BUPRENEX)

- **Uses:** analgesia, opioid agonist-antagonist
- **Dose:** *Acute pain (moderate to severe):* Adults and children ≥13 yr: (IM, slow IV) opiate-naïve initial 0.3 mg q6–8h prn, MR once 30–60 min after initial dose, usual range 0.15–0.6 mg q4–6h prn. Children 2–12 yr: 2–6 mcg/kg q4–6h. Elderly: 0.15 mg q6h. Doses should be titrated to pain relief and control.
- **Site of clearance:** hepatic
- **t½:** 2.2–3 h
- **Interaction/toxicity:** Potentiates barbiturates and CNS depressants. Potentiated in patients with hepatic disease. May precipitate withdrawal in opioid-dependent patient. Increases intracholedochal pressure.

BUTORPHANOL (STADOL)

- **Uses:** analgesia; opioid agonist-antagonist
- **Dose:** *Acute pain (moderate to severe):* Adults: (IM) initial 2 mg, MR q3–4h prn, usual range 1–4 mg q3–4h prn; (IV) initial 1 mg, MR q3–4h prn, usual range 0.5–2 mg q3–4h prn.

Preoperative medication: (IM) 2 mg 60–90 min before surgery.

Supplement to balanced anesthesia: (IV) 2 mg shortly before induction and/or incremental dose of 0.5–1 mg (up to 0.06 mg/kg).

Pain during labor (fetus >37 wk gestation and no signs of fetal distress): (IM, IV) 1–2 mg, MR in 4 h.

■ **Site of clearance:** hepatic, renal
■ **t½:** 3–6 h
■ **Interaction/toxicity:** May precipitate withdrawal in opioid-dependent patients.

CALCIUM CHLORIDE (VARIOUS)

■ **Uses:** electrolyte replacement; inotropic
■ **Dose:** 1 g = 13.6 mEq calcium. Calcium chloride is 3 times as potent as calcium gluconate.

Cardiac arrest in the presence of hyperkalemia or hypocalcemia, magnesium toxicity, or calcium antagonist toxicity: Adults: (IV) 2–4 mg/kg (10% solution), MR q10min if necessary. Infants and children: (IV) 20 mg/kg, MR in 10 min.

Hypocalcemia: Children: (IV) 2.7–5 mg/kg q4–6h. Alternate dosing for infants and children: (IV) 10–20 mg/kg (infants <1 mEq, children 1–7.0 mEq), repeat q4–6h prn.

Hypocalcemic tetany: Adults: (IV) 1 g over 10–30 min, MR after 6 h. Infants and children: (IV) 10 mg/kg (0.5–0.7 mEq/kg) over 5–10 min, MR after 6–8 h or follow with an infusion, max daily dose 200 mg/kg.

Hypocalcemia secondary to citrated blood transfusion: Adults: (IV) 1.35 mEq calcium for each 100 mL of citrated blood infused. Neonates, infants, and children: (IV) 0.45 mEq elemental calcium for each 100 mL citrated blood infused.

■ **Site of clearance:** GI, renal
■ **t½:** N/A
■ **Interaction/toxicity:** Increases risk of dysrhythmias in digitalized patients; antagonizes verapamil; skin slough (necrosis) seen with extravasation.

CALCIUM GLUCONATE (VARIOUS)

■ **Uses:** electrolyte replacement; inotropic
■ **Dose:** (IV) 500–2,000 mg (1 g = 4.5 mEq calcium).
■ **Site of clearance:** GI, renal
■ **t½:** N/A

■ **Interaction/toxicity:** Increases risk of dysrhythmias in digitalized patients; antagonizes verapamil; risk of skin slough (necrosis) seen with extravasation.

CAPSAICIN (VARIOUS)

■ **Uses:** chronic pain Rx
■ **Dose:** (topical) apply tid–qid.
■ **Site of clearance:** N/A
■ **t½:** N/A
■ **Interaction/toxicity:** Burning diminishes with repeated use. Do not bandage area tightly.

CAPTOPRIL (CAPOTEN) `BBW`

■ **Uses:** antihypertensive; CHF
■ **Dose:** *Acute HTN (urgency/emergency):* (PO) 12.5–25 mg, MR prn.

HTN: (PO) initial 12.5–25 mg bid–tid, may increase by 12.5–25 mg/dose at 1–2-wk intervals up to 50 mg tid, add diuretic before further dosage increase, max dose 150 mg tid.

CHF: (PO) initial 6.25–12.5 mg tid, max dose 150 mg tid.

LVD after MI: (PO) initial 6.25 mg followed by 12.5 mg tid, increase to 25 mg tid during next several days to weeks to target dose 50 mg tid.

Diabetic nephropathy: Adults: (PO) 25 mg tid; other antihypertensives given concurrently. Adolescents: (PO) initial 12.5–25 mg given q8–12h, increase by 25 mg/dose to max daily dose 450 mg. Older children: (PO) initial 6.25–12.5 mg q12–24h, titrate up to max daily dose 6 mg/kg. Children: (PO) initial 0.5 mg/kg, titrate up to max 6 daily dose mg/kg in 2–4 divided doses. Infants: (PO) initial 0.15–0.3 mg/kg, titrate up to max daily dose 6 mg/kg in 1–4 divided doses; usual dose 2.5–6 mg/kg/day.

Renal dosing: (PO) for CrCl 10–50 mL/min reduce to 75% of normal dose; for CrCl <10 mL/min reduce to 50% of normal dose.
■ **Site of clearance:** renal
■ **t½:** adults 1.9 h, CHF 2 h, anuria 20–40 h; renal and cardiac function dependent
■ **Interaction/toxicity:** Potentiates hypotensive effects of anesthetics; elevates serum digoxin level; enhances hemodynamic effects of vasodilators, calcium channel blockers, and beta-blockers.

CARBAMAZEPINE (VARIOUS) `BBW`

- **Uses:** anticonvulsant, chronic pain
- **Dose:** *Anticonvulsant:* Adults and children >12 yr: (PO) initial 200 mg bid, increase by 200 mg/day at weekly intervals until therapeutic levels achieved, usual dose 400–1,200 mg/day divided bid–qid, max daily dose 12–15 yr 1,000 mg. Children >15 yr: (PO) 1,200 mg; some patients require up to 1.6 to 2 g/day. Children 6–12 yr: (PO) initial 100 mg bid or 10 mg/kg/day divided bid; increase by 100 mg/day at weekly intervals depending on response, usual maintenance 20–30 mg/kg/day divided bid–qid, max daily dose 1,000 mg. Children <6 yr: (PO) initial 5 mg/kg/day; may be increased q5–7days to 10 mg/kg/day, up to 20 mg/kg/day if necessary divided bid to qid.

  Trigeminal or glossopharyngeal neuralgia: Adults: (PO) initial 100 mg q12h, gradually increase in increments of 100 mg bid prn, maintenance 400–600 mg bid, max daily dose 1,200 mg. Elderly: (PO) 100 mg qd–bid, increase in increments of 100 mg/day at weekly intervals until therapeutic levels are achieved, usual dose 400–1,000 mg/day.

  Renal impairment: for CrCl <10 mL/min reduce dose to 75%.
- **Site of clearance:** hepatic
- **t½:** 10–20 h
- **Interaction/toxicity:** Contraindicated in patients with bone-marrow suppression and liver dysfunction, and those using MAOIs. Discontinue MAOIs for 14 days before starting carbamazepine Rx. Induces its own metabolism as well as that of other drugs (e.g., benzodiazepines, corticosteroids, tricyclic antidepressants). Potentiated by cimetidine, verapamil, and barbiturates. Enhances the toxicity of acetaminophen. Risk of aplastic anemia.

CEFAZOLIN (VARIOUS)

- **Uses:** antibiotic
- **Dose:** Adults: (IV, IM) 250 mg to 2 g q6–12h (usually q8h) depending on severity of infection, max daily dose 12 g. Children and infants >1 mo: (IV, IM) 25–100 mg/kg/day divided q6–8h, max daily dose 6 g.

  Prophylaxis against bacterial endocarditis: Adults: (IV) 1 g 30 min before procedure. Infants/children: 25 mg/kg 30 min before procedure, max 1 g.

Renal adjustment: for CrCl 10–30 mL/min dose q12h, for CrCl <10 mL/min dose q24h.
- **Site of clearance:** renal
- **t½:** 1.5–2.5 h
- **Interaction/toxicity:** Adjust dose with renal dysfunction. May increase toxicity of nephrotoxic drugs such as aminoglycosides. Large doses in patients with renal failure may cause seizures. Potentiates anticoagulants. Ingestion of alcohol may cause a disulfiram-like reaction.

CEFOTAXIME (CLAFORAN)

- **Uses:** antibiotic
- **Dose:** *Bacterial infections:* Adults and children >12 yr: (IV, IM) 1–2 g q6–8h. Infants and children 1 mo to 12 yr <50 kg: (IV, IM) 50–180 mg/kg/day divided q4–6h. *Meningitis/other serious infections:* Adults and children >12 yr: 2 g q4–6h, max daily dose 12 g. Infants and children 1 mo to 12 yr <50 kg: 200 mg/kg/day divided q6h.

  Preoperative: (IM, IV) 1 g 30–90 min before surgery.

  C section: 1 g when umbilical cord clamped, then 1 g q6–12h.

  Renal adjustment: for CrCl 10–50 mL/min dose q8–12 h, for CrCl <10 mL/min dose q24h.
- **Site of clearance:** renal
- **t½:** adults 1–1.5 h; prolonged with renal or hepatic impairment
- **Interaction/toxicity:** Adjust dose in renal dysfunction. Potentiates aminoglycoside nephrotoxicity. Alcohol ingestion causes disulfiram-like reaction. Potentiates anticoagulants.

CEFOTETAN (CEFOTAN)

- **Uses:** antibiotic
- **Dose:** Adults: (IV, IM) 1–2 g q12h, max daily dose 6 g. Children: (IV, IM) 20–40 mg/kg q12h.

  Perioperative prophylaxis: Adults: (IV) 1–2 g 30–60 min before procedure. Children: (IV) 20–40 mg/kg 30–60 min before procedure.

  Renal adjustment: for CrCl 10–30 mL/min dose q24h, for CrCl <10 mL/min dose q48h.
- **Site of clearance:** renal
- **t½:** 3–5 h

▓ **Interaction/toxicity:** Adjust dose in renal dysfunction. Potentiates aminoglycoside nephrotoxicity. Alcohol ingestion causes disulfiram-like reaction. Potentiates anticoagulants.

CELECOXIB (CELEBREX) BBW

▓ **Uses:** nonsteroidal analgesic (selective COX-2 inhibitor)
▓ **Dose:** (PO) 100–200 mg/day
▓ **Site of clearance:** hepatic
▓ **t½:** 11 h
▓ **Interaction/toxicity:** GI bleeding (including ulceration and perforation), liver dysfunction, renal impairment, and worsening of aspirin-sensitive asthma have been reported. Aspirin potentiates GI ulceration. Reduces natriuretic effect of furosemide. Diminish antihypertensive effect of ACE inhibitors. Increased INR and PTT in patients receiving warfarin. Fluconazole and lithium increase plasma levels. Contraindicated in patients with sulfa allergy. Use increases the risk of cardiovascular events such as heart attack and stroke.

CHLORAL HYDRATE (VARIOUS)

▓ **Uses:** sedative
▓ **Dose:** Adults: (PO) 250 mg tid, 500–1,000 mg qhs, max daily dose 2 g. Children: (PO/rectal) 25 mg/kg.
   Preoperative: Adults: (PO) 500–1,000 mg 30–60 min before procedure, NTE 2 g in 24 h. Children (PO/rectal): 50–75 mg/kg 30–60 min before procedure, NTE 1 g in single dose.
▓ **Site of clearance:** renal
▓ **t½:** 8–11 h
▓ **Interaction/toxicity:** Contraindicated in patients with severe hepatic or renal dysfunction. Use with caution in patients with porphyria. Potentiates CNS depressants and warfarin.

CHLORAMPHENICOL (VARIOUS) BBW

▓ **Uses:** antibiotic
▓ **Dose:** Adults: (IV) 50 mg/kg/day q6h, max daily dose 4 g. Children: (IV) 50–75 mg/kg/day q6h. Neonates: (IV) 25 mg/kg/day.
▓ **Site of clearance:** renal
▓ **t½:** 1.6–3.3 h
▓ **Interaction/toxicity:** Adjust dose with renal or hepatic dysfunction. Use with caution in patients with porphyria or G6PD deficiency. Barbiturates antagonize effect. Potentiates barbitu-

rates, anticoagulants, hydantoins. Severe blood dyscrasias seen. Causes gray syndrome in neonates.

CHLORDIAZEPOXIDE (LIBRIUM)

- **Uses:** antianxiety
- **Dose:** *Anxiety:* Adults: (IM, IV) initial 50–100 mg followed by 25–50 mg tid–qid prn; up to 300 mg may be given IM or IV during a 6-h period but not more than this in any 24-h period; (PO) 15–100 mg divided tid–qid. Children >6 yr: (PO, IM) 0.5 mg/kg/24 h divided q6–8h. Children <6 yr: not recommended.

   Preoperative anxiety: (IM) 50–100 mg.

   Ethanol withdrawal symptoms: (PO, IV) initial 50–100 mg, MR in 2–4 h prn to max 300 mg/24 h.

   Renal adjustment: for CrCl <10 mL/min reduce dose to 50%.

   Hepatic impairment: avoid use
- **Site of clearance:** hepatic
- **t½:** 10–48 h
- **Interaction/toxicity:** Cimetidine, metoprolol, propranolol decrease elimination. Increases effect of digoxin.

CHLOROPROCAINE (NESACAINE)

- **Uses:** regional anesthesia
- **Dose:** Dosage varies with anesthetic procedure; range 1.5–25 mL of 2–3% solution, max 800 mg.

   Infiltration and peripheral nerve block: 1–2%.

   Infiltration, peripheral and central nerve block, including caudal and epidural block: 2–3%, without preservative.
- **Site of clearance:** plasma cholinesterase
- **t½:** 1.5–4.7 min
- **Interaction/toxicity:** Rapid inadvertent IT injection of low pH and bisulfite-containing solution may be associated with residual motor/sensory deficit.

CHLORPROMAZINE (THORAZINE)

- **Uses:** psychiatric disorders; premedication; vasodilator
- **Dose:** *Nausea/vomiting:* Adults: (IV, IM) 25–50 mg q4–6h; (PO) 10–25 mg q4–6h; (rectal) 50–100 mg q6–8h. Children: (IV, IM) 0.5–1 mg/kg q6–8h, max daily dose 40 mg for ≤5 yr (22.7 kg), max daily dose 75 mg for 5–12 yr (22.7–45.5 kg). Infants >6 mo: (PO) 0.5–1 mg/kg q6h prn; (rectal) 1 mg/kg q6–8h prn.

   Hepatic impairment: avoid use if severe.
- **Site of clearance:** hepatic

■ t½: 2 h
■ **Interaction/toxicity:** Potentiates sedative–hypnotics. Lithium reduces bioavailability. Mephentermine and epinephrine potentiate chlorpromazine-induced hypotension.

CIMETIDINE (TAGAMET)

■ **Uses:** histamine antagonist (H$_2$)
■ **Dose:** *Premedication:* (IV) 300 mg (dilute in 20–100 mL NS); (PO) 300 mg.
   Children: (PO, IM, IV) 20–40 mg/kg/day divided q4h
   Adults: Short-term treatment of active ulcers: (PO) 300 mg qid or 800 mg at bedtime or 400 mg bid for up to 8 weeks
   (IM, IV) 300 mg q6h or 37.5 mg/hr by continuous infusion; IV dosage should be adjusted to maintain intragastric pH ≥5.
   Renal adjustment: for CrCl 20–40 mL/min dose q8h or reduce dose to 75%, for CrCl 0–20 mL/min dose q12h or reduce dose to 50%.
   Hepatic impairment: caution and reduce dose in severe liver disease; increased risk of CNS toxicity in cirrhosis.
■ **Site of clearance:** renal
■ **t½:** children 1.4 h, adults 2 h
■ **Interaction/toxicity:** Rapid IV administration may cause hypotension and dysrhythmias. Potentiates respiratory depressant effects of morphine. High serum level associated with confusional states in the elderly. Reduces hepatic metabolism of drugs requiring cytochrome P-450 (beta-blockers, calcium channel blockers, theophylline, tranquilizers).

CIPROFLOXACIN (CIPRO)

■ **Uses:** antibiotic
■ **Dose:** (IV) 200–400 mg q12h; (PO) 250–500 mg q12h.
■ **Site of clearance:** renal and hepatic
■ **t½:** 3–5 h
■ **Interaction/toxicity:** Adjust dose in renal or hepatic failure. May cause CNS stimulation (e.g., tremor, confusion, and seizures). Potentiates anticoagulants and theophylline. Cimetidine potentiates. Antagonizes hydantoins. Not recommended in children <18 yr.

CISATRACURIUM BESYLATE (NIMBEX)

■ **Uses:** nondepolarizing neuromuscular blocker
■ **Dose:** Children 2–12 yr: (IV) intubating 0.1 mg over 5–15 sec.

Adults: (IV) intubating 0.15–0.2 mg/kg; maintenance 0.03 mg/kg 40–60 min after initial dose, then at ~20-min intervals based on clinical criteria.

Continuous infusion: Adults and children ≥2 yr: (IV) initial rate of 3 mcg/kg/min may be required to rapidly counteract spontaneous recovery of neuromuscular function; thereafter a rate of 1–2 mcg/kg/min should be adequate to maintain continuous neuromuscular block in the 89 to 99% range in most pediatric and adult patients. Consider reduction of infusion rate by 30–40% when administering during stable level of anesthesia.

▪ **Site of clearance:** plasma (Hofmann elimination)
▪ **t½:** 22–29 min
▪ **Interaction/toxicity:** Potentiated by volatile anesthetics, hypokalemia, antibiotics (aminoglycosides), lithium, magnesium, verapamil, local anesthetics, quinidine, and procainamide. Antagonized by phenytoin and carbamazepine. Does not release histamine at high doses.

CLINDAMYCIN (VARIOUS) `BBW`

▪ **Uses:** antibiotic
▪ **Dose:** Adults: (IM, IV) 1.2–1.8 g/day q6–12h, max daily dose 4,800 mg; (PO) 150–450 mg q6–8h. Children >1 mo: (IM, IV) 20–40 mg/kg/day q6–8h; (PO) 8–16 mg/kg/day q6–8h.
▪ **Site of clearance:** hepatic
▪ **t½:** 1.6–5.3 h
▪ **Interaction/toxicity:** Adjust dose in renal or hepatic dysfunction. Rapid injection may cause cardiac arrest. Potentiates effects of nondepolarizing neuromuscular blockers and digoxin. Theophylline antagonizes effects. May cause fatal colitis.

CLONAZEPAM (VARIOUS)

▪ **Uses:** anticonvulsant, chronic pain
▪ **Dose:** *Seizure disorders:* Adults: (PO) initial NTE 1.5 mg in 3 divided doses, may increase by 0.5–1 mg every third day until seizures are controlled or adverse effects seen, maintenance 0.05–0.2 mg/kg, max daily dose 20 mg. Children: (PO) initial 0.01–0.03 mg/kg/day in 2–3 divided doses (max 0.05 mg/kg/day), increase by no more than 0.5 mg every third day until seizures controlled or adverse effects seen, maintenance 0.1–0.2 mg/kg/day divided TID, NTE 0.2 mg/kg/day.

Panic disorder: (PO) 0.25 mg bid; increase in increments of 0.125–0.25 mg bid q3days; target dose 1 mg/day, max daily dose 4 mg.

▪ **Site of clearance:** renal

- t½: children 22–33 h, adults 19–50 h
- **Interaction/toxicity:** Use with caution in patients with chronic respiratory or renal dysfunction. Abrupt withdrawal may cause seizures. Potentiated by general anesthetics, cimetidine, CNS depressants, and verapamil.

CLONIDINE (CATAPRES) BBW

- **Uses:** antihypertensive
- **Dose:** *HTN:* Adults: (PO) initial 0.1 mg bid, usual maintenance 0.2–1.2 mg/day in 2–4 divided doses, max daily dose 2.4 mg; (transdermal) apply once q7days; for initial therapy start with 0.1 mg and increase by 0.1 mg at 1–2 week intervals; dosages >0.6 mg do not improve efficacy. Children: (PO) initial 5–10 mcg/kg/day divided q8–12h, increase gradually at 5–7 day intervals to 25 mcg/kg/day divided q6h, max daily dose 0.9 mg.

  Acute HTN (urgency): (PO) initial 0.1–0.2 mg, may be followed by additional doses of 0.1 mg q1h prn to max total 0.6 mg.

  Pain management: Adults: (epidural infusion) initial 30 mcg/h, titrate for relief of pain or presence of side effects. Minimal experience with doses >40 mcg/h; should be considered an adjunct to intraspinal opiate therapy. Children (reserved for patients with severe intractable pain, unresponsive to other analgesics or epidural or spinal opiates): (epidural infusion) initial 0.5 mcg/kg/h; adjust with caution, based on clinical effect.
- **Site of clearance:** renal, hepatic
- t½: adults 6–20 h, renal impairment 18–41 h
- **Interaction/toxicity:** Rebound HTN follows abrupt withdrawal. Enhances effects of anesthetics, tranquilizers, sedatives, and hypnotics. Tolazoline and tricyclic antidepressants can block antihypertensive effects.

COCAINE (VARIOUS)

- **Uses:** topical anesthesia
- **Dose:** (topical) 1–4% solution to mucous membranes, max 1–3 mg/kg (or 400 mg); generally 1 mg/kg sufficient
  Doses reduced for children, elderly or debilitated patients.
- **Site of clearance:** plasma cholinesterase
- t½: 75 min
- **Interaction/toxicity:** Potentiates vasopressors; cardiac dysrhythmias and seizures at high doses.

CODEINE (VARIOUS)

- **Uses:** analgesic
- **Dose:** Adults: (IV, IM, SC, PO) 15–60 mg q4–6h, max daily dose 360 mg. Children: (IV, IM, SC, PO) 0.5–1 mg/kg q4–6h, max dose 60 mg.
- **Site of clearance:** hepatic
- **t½:** 2.5–3.5 h
- **Interaction/toxicity:** Use with caution with other CNS depressants and MAOIs, and in patients with respiratory diseases. May contain sulfites.

DALTEPARIN (FRAGMIN) **BBW**

- **Uses:** anticoagulant (LMW heparin)
- **Dose:** *Abdominal surgery:* (DVT prophylaxis) Low to moderate risk: (SQ) 2,500 IU 1–2 h before surgery, then 2,500 IU, then once daily 5–10 days postoperatively. High-risk: (SQ) 5,000 IU 1–2 h before surgery, then 5,000 IU qd for 5–10 days.

  Hip replacement surgery: (DVT prophylaxis) (SQ) 2,500 IU 1–2 h before surgery, then 2,500 IU on evening of surgery (>6 h after last dose), then 5,000 IU qd for 5–10 days.

  Unstable angina: 120 IU/kg (max 10,000 IU) q12h concurrently with aspirin.
- **Site of clearance:** renal
- **t½:** 2–5 h
- **Interaction/toxicity:** Adjust dose with renal dysfunction. Administer as deep SQ (not IM) injection. Contraindicated in patients with pork allergy, active hemorrhage, severe HTN, and thrombocytopenia (ardeparin induced antiplatelet antibodies). Use with caution in patients with HIT. Concomitant use with other anticoagulants, antiplatelet drugs, aspirin, or NSAIDs may cause bleeding. May cause epidural or spinal hematoma in presence of spinal or epidural anesthetic. Single-dose spinal anesthetic may be safest technique. Needle placement should occur 10–12 h after last dose of LMW heparin; 24-h delay is required with higher doses of LMW heparin. For neuraxial catheter techniques, do not administer LMW heparin for 24 h postoperatively. Remove catheters before initiating LMW heparin Rx. Delay catheter removal 10–12 h after last dose of LMW heparin. Subsequent dosing should not occur for <2 h after catheter removal. Presence of blood during spinal, epidural needle, or catheter placement should delay administration of LMW heparin for 24 h. Overdose treated with protamine.

DANTROLENE (DANTRIUM) `BBW`

- Uses: malignant hyperthermia
- Dose: *Preoperative prophylaxis:* Adults and children: (IV) 2.5 mg/kg about 75 min prior to anesthesia and infused over 1 h with additional doses prn (dilute 20 g in 60 mL sterile distilled H_2O); (PO) 4–8 mg/kg/day in 4 divided doses 1–2 days prior to surgery with last dose 3–4 h before surgery.

  Crisis: Adults and children: (IV) 2.5 mg/kg, MR to cumulative dose of 10 mg/kg; if physiologic and metabolic abnormalities reappear, repeat regimen.

  Postcrisis follow-up: Adults and children: (PO) 4–8 mg/kg/day in 4 divided doses for 1–3 days. IV used when PO not practical. Individualize dosage beginning with 1 mg/kg, then switch to PO dosage.
- Site of clearance: hepatic
- t½: 8.7 h
- Interaction/toxicity: Skeletal muscle weakness.

DESIPRAMINE (VARIOUS) `BBW`

- Uses: antidepressant, chronic pain
- Dose: (PO) 100–200 mg/day tid.
- Site of clearance: hepatic
- t½: 7–60 h
- Interaction/toxicity: Contraindicated in patients with narrow-angle glaucoma, Rx with MAOIs within previous 14 days. Use with caution in patients with cardiac dysrhythmias and conduction defects, seizure disorders, hyperthyroidism, renal or hepatic dysfunction. Phenobarbital increases metabolism. Increases amount of inhalation anesthesia required. Potentiates sympathomimetics, CNS depressants, and anticoagulants. Cimetidine decreases metabolism. Do not discontinue abruptly. Cardiovascular toxicity leading cause of death.

DESMOPRESSIN ACETATE (DDAVP, STIMATE)

- Uses: antidiuretic hormone, coagulation (von Willebrand disease type I)
- Dose: *Diabetes insipidus:* Adults and children >12 yr: (IV, SC) 2–4 mcg/day (0.5–1 mL) in 2 divided doses; (intranasal) 100 mcg/mL nasal solution at 10–40 mcg/day (0.1–0.4 mL) divided 1–3 times/day; adjust morning and evening doses for an adequate diurnal rhythm of water turnover; (PO) initial 0.05 mg bid, total daily dose increased or decreased prn to obtain adequate antidiuresis, range 0.1–1.2 mg divided 2–3 times/day.

Hemophilia A and mild to moderate von Willebrand disease (type 1): Adults and children >12 yr: (IV) 0.3 mcg/kg by slow infusion begun 30 min before procedure (dilute in 50–100 mL NS).
- **Site of clearance:** renal
- **t½:** IV 75 min, PO 1.5–2.5 h.
- **Interaction/toxicity:** Chlorpropamide, clofibrate, and carbamazepine potentiate antidiuretic effects.

DEXMEDETOMIDINE (PRECEDEX)

- **Uses:** sedative
- **Dose:** (IV) loading 1 mcg/kg over 10 min, infusion 0.2–0.7 mcg/kg/h, not indicated for infusions >24 h; (IM) 0.5–1.5 mcg/kg.
- **Site of clearance:** hepatic
- **t½:** 6 min
- **Interaction/toxicity:** HTN and bradycardia following rapid IV injection. Hypotension and bradycardia can be seen with sedation. Potentiates sedative, hypnotics, and inhalation anesthetics. May impair recognition of signs of light anesthesia (tearing, movement, or sweating). Renal and hepatic impairment prolong actions.

DEXAMETHASONE (HEXADROL, DECADRON)

- **Uses:** cerebral edema; allergic reactions; replacement Rx
- **Dose:** *Cerebral edema:* Adults: (IV) 10 mg, then 4 mg IV or IM q6h. Children: (IV) loading 1–2 mg/kg as single dose, maintenance 1–1.5 mg/kg/day to max daily dose 16 mg, divided q4–6h for 5 days then taper for 5 days.
  Extubation or airway edema: Children: (IV, IM, PO) 0.5–2 mg/kg/day divided q6h beginning 24 h before extubation and continuing for 4–6 doses afterward.
  Physiologic replacement: Adults and children: (IV, IM, PO) 0.03–0.15 mg/kg/day divided q6–12h.
- **Site of clearance:** hepatic
- **t½:** 1.8–3.5 h
- **Interaction/toxicity:** Increases insulin requirements; phenytoin, phenobarbital, and ephedrine may increase metabolic clearance of steroid.

DIAZEPAM (VALIUM)

- **Uses:** antianxiety
- **Dose:** *Anxiety/sedation/skeletal muscle relaxant:* Adults: (IV, IM) 2–10 mg, MR in 3–4 h prn; (PO) 2–10 mg tid–qid. Children:

(PO) 0.12–0.8 mg/kg/day divided q6–8h; (IM, IV): 0.04–0.3 mg/kg q2–4h to max 0.6 mg/kg in 8-h period.

Sedation in the ICU: (IV) 0.03–0.1 mg/kg q30min to q6h.

Conscious sedation for procedures: Children: (PO) 0.2–0.3 mg/kg to max 10 mg 45–60 min prior to procedure.

- ▪ **Site of clearance:** hepatic, renal
- ▪ **t½:** 20–50 h
- ▪ **Interaction/toxicity:** Elimination reduced by cimetidine, metoprolol, propranolol. Increases effect of digoxin.

DICLOFENAC (VARIOUS) **BBW**

- ▪ **Uses:** anti-inflammatory, analgesic, antipyretic
- ▪ **Dose:** *Analgesia:* (PO) initial 50 mg tid.

Rheumatoid arthritis: 150–200 mg/day in 2–4 divided doses (100 mg/day of sustained-release product).

Osteoarthritis: 100–150 mg/day in 2–3 divided doses (100–200 mg/day of sustained-release product).

- ▪ **Site of clearance:** hepatic
- ▪ **t½:** 2 h
- ▪ **Interaction/toxicity:** Adjust dose in renal failure. Use with caution in patients with CHF, hepatic or renal dysfunction, HTN, history of GI bleed. Higher doses are associated with adverse CNS effects, especially in the elderly (agitation, confusion, and hallucination). Aspirin decreases effect. Potentiates digoxin, lithium, and anticoagulants. Inhibits loop diuretics, ACE inhibitors, and beta-blockers.

DIGOXIN (LANOXIN)

- ▪ **Uses:** heart failure; antidysrhythmic
- ▪ **Dose:** Loading (IV) 0.5–1 mg, (PO) 0.75–1.5 mg; give half total digitalizing dose initially, then one-fourth in two subsequent doses at 8–12-h intervals; maintenance (IV, PO) 0.125–0.5 mg once daily.
- ▪ **Site of clearance:** renal, hepatic
- ▪ **t½:** 38–48 h
- ▪ **Interaction/toxicity:** Potentiated by hypokalemia; synergistic with catecholamines, calcium.

DILTIAZEM (CARDIZEM)

- ▪ **Uses:** antidysrhythmic (atrial fibrillation/flutter paroxysmal supraventricular tachycardia), HTN

▓ **Dose:** *Antidysrhythmic:* (IV) 0.25 mg/kg (bolus over 2 min), wait 15 min; if inadequate response 0.35 mg/kg (bolus over 2 min); infusion 2 mcg/kg/min or 10 mg/h.

HTN: (PO) usual starting dose 30 mg tid; sustained release 120–180 mg/day; increase gradually at 14 day intervals until optimal dose obtained.

▓ **Site of clearance:** hepatic, renal
▓ **t½:** 4–6 h
▓ **Interaction/toxicity:** Potentiated by hepatic and renal disease. Potentiates theophylline and CV depressant effects of volatile anesthetics. Cimetidine and ranitidine may increase bioavailability. Intensifies sick sinus syndrome, second- and third-degree arteriovenous block, hypotension, and cardiogenic shock. Should not be used in patients with Wolf-Parkinson-White syndrome or short PR interval.

DIPHENHYDRAMINE (BENADRYL)

▓ **Uses:** histamine blocker (H_1); allergic reaction
▓ **Dose:** Adults: (IV, IM) 25–50 mg; (PO) 25–50 mg q6–8h. Children >10 kg: (IV) 5 mg/kg/day divided q6–8h; (PO)12.5–25 mg tid–qid.
▓ **Site of clearance:** hepatic
▓ **t½:** 2–8 h, elderly 13.5 h
▓ **Interaction/toxicity:** MAOIs intensify effects; may antagonize effect of heparin.

DIPYRIDAMOLE (VARIOUS)

▓ **Uses:** antiplatelet agent, coronary vasodilator
▓ **Dose:** Adults: (PO) 75–400 mg divided tid–qid. Children: (PO) 3–6 mg/kg/day divided tid–qid.
▓ **Site of clearance:** hepatic
▓ **t½:** 10 h
▓ **Interaction/toxicity:** Use with caution in patients receiving other anticoagulants, aspirin, and NSAIDs. May cause hypotension and "coronary steal." Theophylline inhibits effects.

DOBUTAMINE (DOBUTREX)

▓ **Uses:** inotropic support
▓ **Dose:** Adults and children: (IV) 2.5–20 mcg/kg/min, max 20 mcg/kg/min; titrate to desired response
▓ **Site of clearance:** hepatic
▓ **t½:** 2 min

■ **Interaction/toxicity:** Halogenated anesthetics (especially halothane) sensitize myocardium to sympathomimetic effects (dysrhythmias).

DOPAMINE (INTROPIN)

■ **Uses:** inotropic support
■ **Dose:** (IV) 2–20 mcg/kg/min (dilute 200 mg in 250 mL D$_5$W or NS).
■ **Site of clearance:** enzymatic transformation (COMT and MAOI)
■ **t½:** 2 min
■ **Interaction/toxicity:** Reduce dose in patients receiving MAOIs; combined with phenytoin, causes seizures, hypotension, and bradycardia; halogenated anesthetics (especially halothane) sensitize myocardium to sympathomimetic effects (dysrhythmias).

DOXAPRAM (DOPRAM)

■ **Uses:** respiratory and CNS stimulant
■ **Dose:** (IV) 0.5–1 mg/kg, repeat q5min prn, max 2 mg/kg; infusion 5 mg/min then 1–3 mg/min then taper, max daily dose 300 mg.
■ **Site of clearance:** hepatic
■ **t½:** 2.4–9.9 h
■ **Interaction/toxicity:** Contraindicated in patients with epilepsy, cerebral edema, cerebral vascular accident, severe cardiopulmonary disease, HTN, mechanical obstruction to ventilation, pheochromocytoma, and hyperthyroidism. Associated with cholestatic hepatitis. Continuous infusion in neonates can deliver large amounts of benzyl alcohol.

DROPERIDOL (INAPSINE) **BBW**

■ **Uses:** antianxiety; antiemetic
■ **Dose:** *Nausea and vomiting:* Adults: (IV, IM) 0.625–2.5 mg. Children 2–12 yr: (IV, IM) 0.05–0.06 mg/kg, max initial dose 0.1 mg/kg.
■ **Site of clearance:** hepatic
■ **t½:** 2.3 h
■ **Interaction/toxicity:** Intensifies hypotension of vasodilators; produces extrapyramidal signs. Contraindicated in patients with known or suspected QT-interval prolongation (QTc

APPENDICES

interval above 440 msec for males and above 450 msec for females) and congenital long QT syndrome.

DROTRECOGIN ALFA (XIGRIS)

■ Uses: anti-inflammatory, blood modifier, coagulation inhibitor, profibrinolytic
■ Dose: *Severe sepsis:* (IV) 24 mcg/kg/h for 96 h.
■ Site of clearance: endogenous plasma protease inhibitors
■ t½: 13 min
■ Interaction/toxicity: Hypersensitivity to drotrecogin alfa, active internal bleeding, recent hemorrhagic stroke (within 3 months), recent intracranial, intraspinal surgery; severe head trauma (within 2 months), intracranial neoplasm or mass lesion or evidence of cerebral herniation, existing epidural catheter, trauma with an increased risk of life-threatening bleeding. May prolong activated partial thromboplastin time (aPTT) but has minimal effect of the prothrombin time (PT); the PT should be used to monitor the status of the coagulopathy in these patients, should be discontinued 2 hours prior to procedures with an inherent risk of bleeding.

EDROPHONIUM (TENSILON)

■ Uses: anticholinesterase; antidysrhythmic
■ Dose: *Titration of oral anticholinesterase therapy:* Adults: (IV) 1–2 mg given 1 h after oral dose of anticholinesterase. If strength improves an increase in neostigmine or pyridostigmine dose is indicated. Children: (IV) 0.04 mg/kg given 1 h after oral intake of the drug being used in treatment.
■ Site of clearance: hepatic, renal
■ t½: 1.8 h
■ Interaction/toxicity: Bradycardia, salivation. Overdosage can cause cholinergic crisis which may be fatal. IV atropine should be readily available for treatment of cholinergic reactions.

ENOXAPARIN (LOVENOX) BBW

■ Uses: anticoagulant (LMW heparin)
■ Dose: *Abdominal surgery:* DVT prophylaxis (SQ) 40 mg 2 h before surgery, then 40 mg qd for 7–10 days.
   Hip or knee replacement: DVT prophylaxis (SQ) 40 mg 9–15 h before surgery and 40 mg qd for 3 wk; alternatively 30 mg q12h with first dose given 12–24 h postoperatively in presence of adequate hemostasis; continue for 7–14 days.

Treatment of DVT with or without PE: 1 mg/kg q12h or 1.5 mg/kg qd.

Anticoagulant prophylaxis: Infants >2 mo and children ≤18 yr: (SQ) 0.5 mg/kg q12h.

Anticoagulant treatment: Infants >2 mo and children ≤18 yr: (SQ) 1 mg/kg q12h.

- **Site of clearance:** renal
- **t½:** 4.5–7 h
- **Interaction/toxicity:** Adjust dose with renal dysfunction. Administer as deep SQ (not IM) injection. Contraindicated in patients with pork allergy, active hemorrhage, severe HTN, and thrombocytopenia (ardeparin induced antiplatelet antibodies). Contraindicated in patients with heparin induced thrombocytopenia. Concomitant use with other anticoagulants, antiplatelet drugs, aspirin, or NSAIDs may cause bleeding. May cause epidural or spinal hematoma in presence of spinal or epidural anesthetic. Single-dose spinal anesthetic may be safest technique. Needle placement should occur 10–12 h after last dose of LMW heparin; 24-h delay is required with higher doses of LMWH. For neuraxial catheter techniques, do not administer LMW heparin for 24 h postoperatively. Remove catheters before initiating of LMW heparin Rx. Delay catheter for 10–12 h after last dose of LMW heparin. Subsequent dosing should not occur for <2 h after catheter removal. Presence of blood during spinal, epidural needle, or catheter placement should delay administration of LMW heparin for 24 h. In elderly there is increased incidence of bleeding with therapeutic doses. Careful attention should be paid to elderly patients <45 kg. Overdose treated with protamine.

EPHEDRINE (VARIOUS)

- **Uses:** sympathomimetic
- **Dose:** (IV) 5–10 mg.
- **Site of clearance:** hepatic
- **t½:** 3–6 h
- **Interaction/toxicity:** Potentiated by tricyclic antidepressants and MAOIs; halogenated anesthetics sensitize myocardium to sympathomimetic effects (dysrhythmias).

EPINEPHRINE (VARIOUS)

- **Uses:** sympathomimetic; allergic reaction
- **Dose:** (IV) 2–8 mcg; infusion 0.01–0.02 mcg/kg/min.

- **Site of clearance:** enzymatic transformation (COMT and MAOI)
- **t½:** 2 min
- **Interaction/toxicity:** Halogenated anesthetics (especially halothane) sensitize myocardium to sympathomimetic effects (dysrhythmias); potentiated by tricyclic antidepressants, MAOIs, and antihistamines.

EPINEPHRINE, RACEMIC (VAPONEFRIN, MICRONEFRIN)

- **Uses:** bronchodilator, croup (laryngotracheobronchitis)
- **Dose:** (inhalation) q4h (dilute 1:6 with NS).
- **Site of clearance:** enzymatic transformation (COMT and MAOI)
- **t½:** 2 min
- **Interaction/toxicity:** Halogenated anesthetics (especially halothane) sensitize myocardium to sympathomimetic effects (dysrhythmias).

ERGONOVINE (ERGOTRATE)

- **Uses:** increases uterine contractions
- **Dose:** (IM) 0.2 mg q2–4h for uterine bleeding.
- **Site of clearance:** hepatic
- **t½:** 0.5–3.5 h
- **Interaction/toxicity:** Can induce coronary artery spasm.

ERYTHROMYCIN (VARIOUS)

- **Uses:** antibiotic
- **Dose:** Adults: (IV) 15–20 mg/kg/day q4–6h, max daily dose 4 g; (PO) base 250–500 mg q6h; preop bowel prep 1 g erythromycin base at 1:00, 2:00, and 11:00 PM on the day before surgery combined with mechanical cleansing of the large intestine and oral neomycin. Children: (IV) lactobionate 20–40 mg/kg/day q6h; (PO) 30–50 mg/kg/day q6–8h, max daily dose 1–2 g; preop bowel prep 20 mg/kg erythromycin base at 1:00, 2:00, and 11:00 PM on the day before surgery combined with mechanical cleansing of the large intestine and oral neomycin.
- **Site of clearance:** hepatic
- **t½:** 1.5–2 h, ESRD 5–6 h
- **Interaction/toxicity:** Modify dose in hepatic dysfunction. Ventricular dysrhythmias including ventricular tachycardia and

abnormal prolongation of the QT interval (Torsades de Pointes) have been reported. Potentiates effects of warfarin, benzodiazepines, alfentanil, carbamazepine, corticosteroids, cyclosporine, digoxin, ergot alkaloids, and theophylline. May potentiate effects of myasthenia gravis.

ESMOLOL (BREVIBLOC)

- ▪ **Uses:** supraventricular tachycardia, HTN
- ▪ **Dose:** (IV) bolus 0.25–0.5 mg/kg,; continuous infusion loading dose 500 mcg/kg/min over 1–2 min; maintenance 50–200 mcg/kg/min (dilute 5 g in 500 mL D_5W or NS).
- ▪ **Site of clearance:** red blood cell esterase
- ▪ **t½:** 9 min
- ▪ **Interaction/toxicity:** Increases digoxin and serum morphine levels.

ETHACRYNIC ACID (EDECRIN)

- ▪ **Uses:** diuretic
- ▪ **Dose:** Adults: (IV) 0.5–1 mg/kg, max 100 mg/dose; repeat doses not routinely recommended but if indicated repeat doses q8–12h; (PO) 50–200 mg/day in 1–2 divided doses, may increase up to max 200 mg bid. Children: (PO) 1 mg/kg/dose qd, increase to max of 3 mg/kg/day.
- ▪ **Site of clearance:** renal
- ▪ **t½:** 2–4 h
- ▪ **Interaction/toxicity:** Administration with aminoglycoside antibiotics can cause ototoxicity. Reduces renal clearance of lithium. Reduce warfarin dose.

ETIDOCAINE (DURANEST)

- ▪ **Uses:** regional anesthesia
- ▪ **Dose:** *Neural blockade:* 300 mg (with epinephrine 1:200,000).
- ▪ **Site of clearance:** hepatic
- ▪ **t½:** 2.5 h
- ▪ **Interaction/toxicity:** Not recommended for obstetric anesthesia because of profound motor blockade.

ETOMIDATE (AMIDATE)

- ▪ **Uses:** induction agent
- ▪ **Dose:** Adults and children >10 yr: (IV) initial 0.2–0.6 mg/kg over 30–60 sec, maintenance 5–20 mcg/kg/min.

■ **Site of clearance:** hepatic
■ **t½:** 2.6–3.5 h
■ **Interaction/toxicity:** Interferes with adrenal function (reduced release of cortisol). Myoclonus and pain with rapid IV injection.

FACTOR VIIa RECOMBINANT (NOVOSEVEN)

■ **Uses:** factor replacement for hemophiliacs
■ **Dose:** (IV) 90 mcg/kg q2h until adequate coagulation occurs.
■ **Site of clearance:** N/A
■ **t½:** 2.3 h
■ **Interaction/toxicity:** Contraindicated in patients with known allergies to mouse, hamster, or bovine proteins. Increase in thrombotic events in DIC, advanced arteriosclerotic disease, and crush injury.

FACTOR VIII (ANTIHEMOPHILIAC FACTOR [AHF]; VARIOUS)

■ **Uses:** factor VIII replacement
■ **Dose:** (IV) 10–25 AHF IU/kg q12–24h to increase level to 80%–100% of normal.
■ **Site of clearance:** N/A
■ **t½:** 12–17 h
■ **Interaction/toxicity:** Ineffective for von Willebrand's disease. Risk of HIV and infectious viral agents (hepatitis). Patients with factor VIII inhibitor may not respond appropriately. Hemolysis may occur due to AHF solution containing anti-A and anti-B isoagglutinins.

FACTOR IX CONCENTRATE (VARIOUS)

■ **Uses:** factor IX deficiency (hemophilia B, Christmas disease)
■ **Dose:** (IV) IU (recombinant) = (1.2 IU/kg)(kg)(desired increase % of normal); IU (human derived factor) = (1 IU/kg)(kg)(desired increase % of normal) (titrate to >20% normal). 1 IU/kg will increase level by 1%.
■ **Site of clearance:** N/A
■ **t½:** 18–36 h
■ **Interaction/toxicity:** Contraindicated in patients with known allergy to mouse protein. Risk of HIV, infectious viruses (human-derived factor). May cause thromboembolic complications including MI, pulmonary embolism, venous throm-

bosis, and DIC. Rapid infusion can cause hemodynamic instability.

FAMOTIDINE (PEPCID)

■ **Uses:** histamine blocker (H_2)
■ **Dose:** Adults: (PO, IV) 20 mg q12h (dilute in 10 mg D_5W or NS). Children 1–16 yr: (PO) 0.5 mg/kg/day qhs or divided q12h; (IV) 0.25 mg/kg q12h.
■ **Site of clearance:** renal
■ **t½:** 2.5–3.5 h
■ **Interaction/toxicity:** Antacids decrease oral absorption.

FENOLDOPAM (CORLOPAM)

■ **Uses:** HTN
■ **Dose:** (IV) infusion 0.1 mcg/kg/min, increase 0.05–0.2 mcg/kg/min until target blood pressure is achieved; average rate 0.25–0.5 mcg/kg/min; usual length of treatment 1–6 h with tapering of 12% q15–30 min.
■ **Site of clearance:** hepatic
■ **t½:** 9.8 min
■ **Interaction/toxicity:** Use with caution in patients with cirrhosis, glaucoma, unstable angina. Causes dose-related tachycardia. Hypokalemia may occur. Contains sulfites.

FENTANYL (SUBLIMAZE)

■ **Uses:** analgesia
■ **Dose:** *Sedation for minor procedures/analgesia:* Adults and children >12 yr: (IM, IV) 0.5–1 mcg/kg/dose; higher doses are used for major procedures. Children 1–12 yr: (IM, IV): 1–2 mcg/kg/dose, MR at 30–60 min intervals. Note: Children 18–38 mo may require 2–3 mcg/kg/dose.

General anesthesia without additional anesthetic agents: Adults and children >12 yr: (slow IV) 50–100 mcg/kg.

Mechanically ventilated adults and children >12 yr: (IV) 0.35–1.5 mcg/kg every 30–60 min prn, infusion 0.7–10 mcg/kg/h.

Continuous sedation: Children 1–12 yr: (IV) initial bolus 1–2 mcg/kg then 1 mcg/kg/h, titrate upward, usual 1–3 mcg/kg/h.
■ **Site of clearance:** hepatic
■ **t½:** 2–4 h

■ **Interaction/toxicity:** Diazepam potentiates hypotensive action; truncal muscle rigidity may be seen during induction and emergence.

FENTANYL (DURAGESIC) **BBW**

■ **Uses:** analgesia
■ **Dose:** (transdermal) 2.5 mg patch (therapeutically equivalent to 15 mg morphine IM or 90 mg morphine PO).
■ **Site of clearance:** hepatic
■ **t½:** 17 h
■ **Interaction/toxicity:** Potentiates opioid analgesics, tranquilizers, and sedatives.

FENTANYL ORALET (ACTIQ) **BBW**

■ **Uses:** analgesia
■ **Dose:** 5 mcg/kg, suck on lozenge vigorously for approximately 20–40 min before start of procedure; drug effect begins in 10 min. Available in 200 mcg, 300 mcg, 400 mcg.
■ **Site of clearance:** hepatic
■ **t½:** 6.6 h
■ **Interaction/toxicity:** Potentiates opioid analgesics, tranquilizers, and sedatives.

FLUMAZENIL (MAZICON) **BBW**

■ **Uses:** benzodiazepine receptor antagonist
■ **Dose:** *Reversal of conscious sedation:* Adults: (IV) 0.1–0.2 mg over 30 sec, MR 0.2 mg at 1 min intervals if desired level of consciousness not obtained, max cumulative dose 3 mg. Children: (IV) initial 0.01 mg/kg (max 0.2 mg) over 15 sec, MR 0.005–0.01 mg/kg (max 0.2 mg) at 1 min intervals, max cumulative dose 1 mg.
■ **Site of clearance:** hepatic
■ **t½:** 7–15 min
■ **Interaction/toxicity:** Benzodiazepine reversal may be associated with seizures in high-risk populations: major hypnotic drug withdrawal, previous seizure activity, and cyclic antidepressant poisoning. May precipitate withdrawal syndrome in benzodiazepine dependent patients.

FLURAZEPAM (DALMANE)

■ **Uses:** antianxiety
■ **Dose:** (PO) 15–30 mg

■ **Site of clearance:** hepatic
■ **t½:** single dose 74–90 h, multiple doses 111–113 h; elderly (61–85 yr) single dose 120–160 h, multiple doses 126–158 h
■ **Interaction/toxicity:** Significantly longer elimination half-time in the elderly. Caution in patients with chronic pulmonary insufficiency.

FUROSEMIDE (LASIX)

■ **Uses:** diuretic
■ **Dose:** Adults: (IM, IV) 20–40 mg, MR in 1–2 h prn and increase by 20 mg/dose until desired effect; (PO) 20–80 mg initially increased in increments of 20–40 mg/dose at intervals of 6–8 h; usual maintenance dosing interval is q12h or q24h. Infants and children: (IM, IV) initial 1 mg/kg, increasing each succeeding dose by 1 mg/kg at intervals of 6–12 h up to 6 mg/kg/dose; (PO) initial 1–2 mg/kg, increasing by 1 mg/kg/dose no more frequently than q6h until desired effect up to 6 mg/kg/dose.
■ **Site of clearance:** renal
■ **t½:** 0.5–1.1 h, ESRD 9 h
■ **Interaction/toxicity:** Stimulates release of renal prostaglandin E_2 (increases incidence of patent ductus arteriosus in premature infants). Administration with aminoglycoside antibiotics can cause ototoxicity.

GABAPENTIN (NEURONTIN)

■ **Uses:** epilepsy
■ **Dose:** Adults and children >12 yr: (PO) 300–600 mg tid.
■ **Site of clearance:** renal
■ **t½:** 5–6 h
■ **Interaction/toxicity:** Antacids reduce bioavailability; cimetidine and oral contraceptives increase bioavailability.

GALLAMINE (FLAXEDIL)

■ **Uses:** nondepolarizing neuromuscular blocker
■ **Dose:** (IV): initial 1 mg/kg up to 100 mg, maintenance 0.5 to 1 mg/kg q30–40min prn, max 100 mg.
■ **Site of clearance:** renal
■ **t½:** 134 minutes
■ **Interaction/toxicity:** Tachycardia. Do not administer to patients with iodide allergy.

GENTAMICIN (VARIOUS) `BBW`

- ▓ **Uses:** antibiotic
- ▓ **Dose:** Adults: (IV, IM) (use ideal body weight) 1–1.7 mg/kg q8h. Children >5 yr: (IV, IM): 1.5–2.5 mg/kg q8h. Infants and children <5 yr: (IV, IM) 2.5 mg/kg q8h.
  Renal impairment: extend dosing interval.
- ▓ **Site of clearance:** renal
- ▓ **t½:** 1.5–4 h
- ▓ **Interaction/toxicity:** Adjust dose with renal dysfunction. Associated with significant nephrotoxicity and ototoxicity. In burn patients, reduced serum concentration of gentamicin may be observed. Potentiates nondepolarizing neuromuscular blockers and effects of myasthenia gravis. Antibiotics, loop diuretics, cyclosporine, and enflurane increase risk of nephrotoxicity and/or ototoxicity.

GLUCAGON (GLUCAGON)

- ▓ **Uses:** treatment of hypoglycemia; relaxes sphincter of Oddi
- ▓ **Dose:** *Hypoglycemia or insulin shock therapy:* Adults: (IV, IM, SQ) 0.5–1 mg, MR in 20 min prn. Children: (IV, IM, SQ) 0.025–0.1 mg/kg, NTE 1 g/dose, MR in 20 min prn.
- ▓ **Site of clearance:** renal
- ▓ **t½:** 3–10 min
- ▓ **Interaction/toxicity:** Intensifies action of anticoagulants; causes significant increase in BP.

GLYCOPYRROLATE (ROBINUL)

- ▓ **Uses:** anticholinergic
- ▓ **Dose:** *Preoperative:* Adult: (IM) 0.004 mg/kg 30–60 min before procedure. Children <2 yr: (IM) 0.004–0.008 mg/kg 30–60 in before procedure. Children >2 yr: (IM) 0.004 mg/kg 30–60 min before procedure.
  Intraoperative: Adult: (IV) 0.1 mg repeated prn at 2–3-min intervals. Children: (IV) 0.004 mg/kg, NTE 0.1 mg, MR at 2–3-min intervals prn.
  Control of secretions: Children: (PO) 0.04–0.1 mg/kg q3–4h; (IM, IV) 0.004–0.01 mg/kg q3–4h, max 0.2 mg/dose or 0.8 mg/24 h.
- ▓ **Site of clearance:** renal
- ▓ **t½:** 20–40 min

■ **Interaction/toxicity:** Contraindicated in patients with myasthenia gravis; paralytic ileus, obstructive diseases of GI tract; obstructive uropathy; tachycardia; acute hemorrhage; ulcerative colitis; narrow-angle glaucoma. Incompatible with secobarbital, sodium bicarbonate, thiopental.

GRANISETRON (KYTRIL)

■ **Uses:** antiemetic
■ **Dose:** *PONV prevention:* 1 mg undiluted over 30 sec, administered before induction of anesthesia or before reversal of anesthesia.
   PONV treatment: 1 mg undiluted over 30 sec.
   Chemotherapy-related emesis: Adults and children >2 yr: (IV) 10 mcg/kg or 1 mg/dose infused over 5 min; (PO) 1 mg bid.
■ **Site of clearance:** hepatic
■ **t½:** 9 h
■ **Interaction/toxicity:** Use with caution in patients with liver disease. Has minimal sedative properties.

HALOPERIDOL (HALDOL)

■ **Uses:** tranquilizer
■ **Dose:** *Psychosis:* (IM) (as lactate) 2–5 mg q4–8h prn; (PO) 0.5–5 mg bid–tid, max daily dose 30 mg.
   ICU delirium: (IV, IM): 2–10 mg; MR bolus doses q20–30 min until calm achieved then administer 25% of max dose q6h; monitor ECG and QT_c interval.
   Sedation/psychotic disorders: Children 6–12 yr: (IM, as lactate) 1–3 mg q4–8h to max daily dose 0.15 mg/kg; change to PO as soon as possible. Children 3–12 yr (15–40 kg): (PO) initial 0.05 mg/kg/day or 0.25–0.5 mg/day in 2–3 divided doses; increase by 0.25–0.5 mg q5–7days, max daily dose 0.15 mg/kg.
■ **Site of clearance:** hepatic
■ **t½:** 20 h
■ **Interaction/toxicity:** Coadministration with lithium may produce neurotoxicity.

HEPARIN (VARIOUS) **BBW**

■ **Uses:** anticoagulant
■ **Dose:** *Cardiopulmonary bypass:* (IV) 350–400 units/kg, using ACT as therapeutic guide.

Deep vein thrombosis and pulmonary embolism: (IV) 80 units/kg IV bolus then 18 units/kg/h.

Low-dose prophylaxis: (SC) 5,000 units q8–12h.

- ■ **Site of clearance:** hepatic
- ■ **t½:** 1.5 h
- ■ **Interaction/toxicity:** Increases diazepam plasma levels; digitalis and antihistamines interfere with anticoagulant properties; nitroglycerin may antagonize heparin.

HETASTARCH (HESPAN)

- ■ **Uses:** volume expander
- ■ **Dose:** (IV) 500–1,000 mL with total dosage NTE 1,500 mL/day (or ~20 mL/kg/day).
- ■ **Site of clearance:** enzymatic
- ■ **t½:** 12 h
- ■ **Interaction/toxicity:** Anaphylactoid reaction. Large volumes may cause coagulopathy.

HYDRALAZINE (APRESOLINE)

- ■ **Uses:** antihypertensive
- ■ **Dose:** *HTN:* Adults: (IM, IV) 5–10 mg q4–6h prn, may increase to 40 mg/dose; change to PO as soon as possible. Children: (IM, IV) 0.1–0.2 mg/kg (max 20 mg) q4–6h prn, up to 1.7–3.5 mg/kg/day in 4–6 divided doses.

Pre-eclampsia/eclampsia: 5 mg then 5–10 mg q20–30 min prn.

- ■ **Site of clearance:** hepatic
- ■ **t½:** 3–5 h
- ■ **Interaction/toxicity:** Increases bioavailability of beta-blockers; may require coadministration of beta-blockers to blunt cardiac stimulation.

HYDROCORTISONE (SOLU-CORTEF)

- ■ **Uses:** anti-inflammatory; steroid replacement; allergic reaction
- ■ **Dose:** *Acute adrenal insufficiency:* Adults: (IV, IM) 100 mg q8h. Older children: (IV, IM) 1–2 mg/kg bolus then 150–250 mg/day divided q6–8h. Infants and young children: (IV, IM) 1–2 mg/kg bolus, then 25–150 mg/day divided q6–8h.
- ■ **Site of clearance:** hepatic
- ■ **t½:** 8–12 h
- ■ **Interaction/toxicity:** Increases insulin requirements; phenytoin, phenobarbital, and ephedrine may increase metabolic clearance.

HYDROMORPHONE (DILAUDID) **BBW**

▪ **Uses:** analgesia
▪ **Dose:** Adults and older children >50 kg: (PO) start at 2–4 mg q3–4h in opiate-naïve patients, usual range 2–8 mg q3–4h; (IV) start at 0.2–0.6 mg q2–3h or (IM, SC) 0.8–1 mg q4–6h in opiate-naïve patients, usual range 1–4 mg (IV, IM, SC) q4–6h; (epidural) bolus 0.5–1 mg, continuous infusion 0.10–0.15 mg/h. Young children ≥6 mo and <50 kg: (PO) 0.03–0.08 mg/kg q3–4h prn; (IV) 0.015 mg/kg q3–6h prn.
▪ **Site of clearance:** liver
▪ **t½:** 1–3 h
▪ **Interaction/toxicity:** Hypotension, respiratory depression, nausea, and pruritus. Potentiated by sedatives, hypnotics, tranquilizers; decreases effects of diuretics in CHF.

IBUPROFEN (VARIOUS) **BBW**

▪ **Uses:** analgesia, antipyretic, anti-inflammatory drug
▪ **Dose:** Adults: (PO) 200–800 mg q4–8h, max daily dose 3.2 g. Children: (PO) 30–70 mg/kg/day divided q6–8h.
▪ **Site of clearance:** hepatic
▪ **t½:** 2–4 h
▪ **Interaction/toxicity:** Use with caution in patients with CHF, hepatic or renal dysfunction, HTN, history of GI bleed. May inhibit platelet aggregation. Higher doses are associated with adverse CNS effects, especially in the elderly (agitation, confusion, and hallucination). Aspirin decreases effect. Potentiates digoxin, lithium, and warfarin. Inhibits loop diuretics, beta-blockers, ACE inhibitors, anticoagulants, lithium, and dipyridamole.

IMIPENEM AND CILASTIN (PRIMAXIN)

▪ **Uses:** antibiotic
▪ **Dose:** Adults: (IV) 125–500 mg over 30 min q6–8h. Children: (IV) 15–25 mg/kg q6h, max daily dose 2 g.
▪ **Site of clearance:** renal
▪ **t½:** 60 min
▪ **Interaction/toxicity:** Adjust dose in renal dysfunction. May cause allergic reaction in patients with penicillin allergy. Benzyl alcohol preservative associated with toxicity in neonates.

IMIPRAMINE (VARIOUS) `BBW`

- **Uses:** antidepressant, chronic pain management
- **Dose:** Adults: (PO) 25 mg q6–8h, max daily dose 300 mg. Children: (PO) 25 mg/day, max daily dose 2.5 mg/kg.
- **Site of clearance:** hepatic
- **t½:** 6–18 h
- **Interaction/toxicity:** Contraindicated in patients with narrow-angle glaucoma, Rx with MAOIs within previous 14 days. Use with caution in patients with cardiac dysrhythmias, hyperthyroidism, renal or hepatic dysfunction. Barbiturates increase metabolism. Increases amount of inhalation anesthesia required. Potentiates sympathomimetics, CNS depressants, and anticoagulants. Cimetidine decreases metabolism. Do not abruptly discontinue. Intermediate metabolite has tricyclic activity. May contain sulfites. Cardiovascular toxicity leading cause of death.

INAMRINONE (INOCOR)

- **Uses:** inotropic support
- **Dose:** (IV) loading 0.75 mg/kg, maintenance 5–10 mcg/kg/min.
- **Site of clearance:** renal
- **t½:** 3.6 h; CHF 5.8 h
- **Interaction/toxicity:** Marked vasodilator action seen in hypovolemic patients. Thrombocytopenia following long-term therapy. Should not be diluted with D_5W or given in same IV tubing with furosemide. Contains sodium metabisulfate, which may cause allergic and/or anaphylactic reactions in patients allergic to sulfites.

INDOMETHACIN (VARIOUS) `BBW`

- **Uses:** analgesia, antipyretic, anti-inflammatory drug, closure PDA in neonates
- **Dose:** (PO) 25–50 mg q8–12h, max daily dose 200 mg.
  Closure of PDA: Neonates: (IV) initial 0.2 mg/kg, followed by 2 doses depending on postnatal age. (Withhold with anuria or oliguria.)
- **Site of clearance:** hepatic
- **t½:** 4.5 h
- **Interaction/toxicity:** Contraindicated in patients with active GI bleed, neonates with necrotizing enterocolitis, and active bleeding. Use with caution in patients with CHF, hepatic or renal dysfunction, HTN, history of GI bleed. Higher doses are

associated with adverse CNS effects, especially in the elderly (agitation, confusion, and hallucination). Aspirin decreases effect. Potentiates digoxin, lithium, and anticoagulants. Inhibits loop diuretics. Inhibits effect of antihypertensives, beta-blockers, and furosemide.

ISOPROTERENOL (ISUPREL)

- **Uses:** inotropic/chronotropic; bronchodilator
- **Dose:** Adults: (IV) initial 2 mcg/min, titrate to patient response, usual effective dose 2–10 mcg/min (dilute 2–4 mg/500 mL D_5W). Children: (IV) initial 0.1 mcg/kg/min, usual effective dose 0.2–2 mcg/kg/min.
- **Site of clearance:** hepatic
- **t½:** 2.5–5 min
- **Interaction/toxicity:** Halogenated anesthetics (especially halothane) sensitize myocardium to sympathomimetic effects (dysrhythmias); effects of MAOIs and tricyclic antidepressants are potentiated.

KANAMYCIN (KANTREX)   **BBW**

- **Uses:** antibiotic
- **Dose:** *Infection:* Adults: (IV, IM) 5–7.5 mg/kg q8–12h, max daily dose 1.5 g. Children: (IV, IM) 15 mg/kg/day divided q8–12h.
    Preoperative intestinal antisepsis: (PO) 1 g q1h for 4 h, then q4–6h for 36–72 h.
    Intraperitoneal irrigation: (PO) 500 mg diluted in 20 mL distilled water.
- **Site of clearance:** renal
- **t½:** 2.2–2.4 h
- **Interaction/toxicity:** Use with caution in patients with renal dysfunction, otologic impairment, and myasthenia gravis. Potentiates nondepolarizing neuromuscular blockers. Antibiotics, loop diuretics, cyclosporins, and enflurane increase risk of nephrotoxicity and ototoxicity. Antagonizes digoxin.

KETAMINE (KETALAR)   **BBW**

- **Uses:** induction agent; anesthesia
- **Dose:** Adults: (IV) 1–2 mg/kg; (IM) 5–10 mg/kg. Children: (IM) 3–7 mg/kg. (IV) 0.5–2 mg/kg, with smaller doses (0.5–1 mg/kg) for sedation for minor procedures; usual induction dosage 1–2 mg/kg.
- **Site of clearance:** hepatic

- **t½:** 11–17 min
- **Interaction/toxicity:** Potentiates action of sedatives, hypnotics, and opioids; dysphoric reactions; increases cerebral blood flow and IOP. Increases upper airway secretions and heightens laryngeal reflexes.

KETOROLAC (TORADOL) **BBW**

- **Uses:** analgesic
- **Dose:** (IV, IM) 60 mg as single dose or 30 mg q6h.
- **Site of clearance:** renal
- **t½:** 2–8 h, prolonged in elderly
- **Interaction/toxicity:** Potentiates NSAIDs. Reversibly inhibits platelet aggregation and is contraindicated before major surgery or intraoperatively where hemostasis is critical. May cause renal toxicity and is potentiated by acute renal failure; contraindicated in patients with advanced renal impairment or those at risk for renal failure due to hypovolemia. May cause peptic ulcers, GI bleeding, and/or perforation. Anaphylactic allergic reaction may be seen with first dose. Contraindicated in patients with previously demonstrated hypersensitivity to ketorolac, aspirin, or other NSAIDs. Contraindicated for spinal or epidural anesthesia. Contraindicated in labor and delivery due to adverse effects on fetal circulation and inhibition of fetal contractions. Contraindicated for patients receiving other NSAIDs or aspirin (cumulative risk of serious adverse effects). Duration of oral Ketorolac not to be >5 days, and oral dose is significantly lower than IV or IM routes. For patients aged >65, those who weigh <110 lbs, and those with elevated serum creatinine, IV/IM dose is not to be >60 mg/day.

LABETALOL (NORMODYNE, TRANDATE)

- **Uses:** Alpha- and beta-adrenergic blockade; antihypertensive
- **Dose:** (IV) 5–20 mg (0.25 mg/kg for an 80 kg patient) over 2 min, may administer 40–80 mg at 10 min intervals, up to 300 mg total; infusion 2 mg/min, titrate to response up to 300 mg total dose prn.
- **Site of clearance:** hepatic
- **t½:** 2.5–8 h
- **Interaction/toxicity:** Cimetidine increases bioavailability; halothane or diazepam prolongs effects.

LEPIRUDIN (REFLUDAN)

▨ **Uses:** anticoagulant for heparin-induced thrombocytopenia
▨ **Dose:** (IV) bolus 0.4 mg/kg over 15–20 sec, continuous infusion 0.15 mg/kg/h. Bolus and infusion must be reduced in renal insufficiency.
▨ **Site of clearance:** renal
▨ **t½:** 0.8–2 h
▨ **Interaction/toxicity:** Adjust dose in renal dysfunction. Contraindicated in patient with renal failure, intracranial bleeding, concomitant thrombolytic Rx, active bleeding, recent puncture of large blood vessels, recent surgery, neuraxial anesthesia, and bacterial endocarditis. Should not be administered to patients receiving other anticoagulant drugs.

LEVOBUPIVACAINE (CHIROCAINE)

▨ **Uses:** local anesthetic
▨ **Dose:** infiltration 5–200 mg; epidural 50–150 mg; peripheral nerve block 75–150 mg.
▨ **Site of clearance:** renal
▨ **t½:** 1.3 h
▨ **Interaction/toxicity:** CV toxicity less than that of bupivacaine, otherwise similar.

LIDOCAINE (XYLOCAINE)

▨ **Uses:** local anesthetic; antidysrhythmic
▨ **Dose:** *Antidysrhythmic:* (IV) 1 mg/kg over 2–3 min, then infusion 2–4 mg/min (20–50 mcg/kg/min).
  Anesthetic: (topical) <4 mg/kg, do not repeat within 2 h; (infiltration) 4 mg/kg, with epinephrine (1:200,000), max dose 7 mg/kg.
▨ **Site of clearance:** hepatic
▨ **t½:** 1.5–2 h
▨ **Interaction/toxicity:** Beta-blockers decrease hepatic clearance; cimetidine increases serum level. Plasma concentration >8 mcg/mL may cause seizures, respiratory/cardiac depression.

LIDOCAINE/PRILOCAINE (EMLA)

▨ **Uses:** anesthetic, local, topical
▨ **Dose:** *Anesthesia for major dermal procedure:* Adult: (topical) apply 2 g of cream per 10 cm² of skin, allow to remain

in contact with skin for at least 2 h. Children 0–3 mo or <5 kg: (topical) max dose 1 g, max application area 10 cm^2, max application time 1 h. Children 3–12 mo or >5 kg: (topical) max dose 2 g, max application area 20 cm^2, max application time 4 h. Children 1–6 yr or >10 kg: (topical) max dose 10 g, max application area 100 cm^2, max application time 4 h. Children 7–12 yr or >20 kg: (topical) max dose 20 g, max application area 200 cm^2, max application time 4 h.

- **Site of clearance:** hepatic
- **t½:** lidocaine 65–150 min; prilocaine 10–150 min
- **Interactions/toxicity:** Neonates and infants up to 3 months of age should be monitored for Met-hemoglobin levels before, during, and after the application of EMLA, provided the test results can be obtained quickly. Patients taking drugs associated with drug-induced methemoglobinemia such as sulfonamides, acetaminophen, acetanilid, aniline dyes, benzocaine, chloroquine, dapsone, naphthalene, nitrates and nitrites, nitrofurantoin, nitroglycerin, nitroprusside, pamaquine, para-aminosalicylic acid, phenacetin, phenobarbital, phenytoin, primaquine, quinine, are also at greater risk for developing methemoglobinemia. EMLA should be used with caution in patients receiving Class I antiarrhythmic drugs (such as tocainide and mexiletine) since the toxic effects are additive and potentially synergistic.

  Repeated doses of EMLA may increase blood levels of lidocaine and prilocaine. EMLA should be used with caution in patients who may be more sensitive to the systemic effects of lidocaine and prilocaine including acutely ill, debilitated, or elderly patients.

  Lidocaine and prilocaine have been shown to inhibit viral and bacterial growth. The effect of EMLA on intradermal injections of live vaccines has not been determined.

LORAZEPAM (ATIVAN)

- **Uses:** antianxiety agent
- **Dose:** *Preoperative:* (IM) 0.05 mg/kg administered 2 h before surgery, max 4 mg/dose; (IV) 0.44 mg/kg 15–20 min before surgery, max 2 mg/dose.

  Operative amnesia: (IV) up to 0.05 mg/kg, max 4 mg/dose.

  Agitation in ICU: (IV) 0.02–0.06 mg/kg q2–6h; infusion 0.01–0.1 mg/kg/h.

  Sedation/anxiety: Adults: (PO) usual 2–6 mg/day in 2–3 divided doses. Infants and children: (PO, IM, IV) 0.05 mg/kg (range 0.02–0.09 mg/kg) q4–6h prn.

- **Site of clearance:** hepatic, renal

- t½: 12 h
- **Interaction/toxicity:** Cimetidine, metoprolol, propranolol decrease elimination. Increases effect of digoxin.

MAGNESIUM (VARIOUS)

- **Uses:** toxemia, preeclampsia, hypomagnesemia
- **Dose:** *Hypomagnesemia:* Adults: (IV) 1–4 g; infusion <2 mL/min (4 g in 250 mL). Children: (IM, IV) 25–50 mg/kg q4–6h for 3–4 doses, max single dose 2g. Neonates: (IV) 25–50 mg/kg q4–6h for 2–3 doses.
- **Site of clearance:** renal
- **t½:** N/A
- **Interaction/toxicity:** Potentiates neuromuscular blockade (nondepolarizing/depolarizing), potentiates CNS effects of anesthetics, hypnotics, and opioids. Toxicity seen with serum levels >7–10 mEq/L.

MANNITOL (OSMITROL)

- **Uses:** osmotic diuretic
- **Dose:** *Osmotic diuretic:* Adults: Test dose to produce urine flow of at least 30–50 mL/h over next 2–3 h: (IV) 12.5 g (200 mg/kg) over 3–5 min; initial 0.5–1 g/kg, maintenance 0.25–0.5 g/kg q4–6h, usual dose 20–200 g/24h. Children: Test dose to produce urine flow of at least 1 mL/kg for 1–3 h: (IV) 200 mg/kg over 3–5 min; initial 0.5–1 g/kg, maintenance 0.25–0.5 g/kg q4–6h.
    Neurosurgery: Adults (IV) 0.5–2 g/kg (10–20% solution over 30–60 min) 1–1.5 h before surgery.
- **Site of clearance:** renal
- **t½:** 1–2 h
- **Interaction/toxicity:** Abrupt increases in intravascular volume.

MEPERIDINE (DEMEROL)

- **Uses:** analgesia, antishivering
- **Dose:** Adults: (IM, SC) 50–75 mg q3–4h prn. Children: (IV, IM, SC) 1–1.5 mg/kg q3–4h prn.
    Preoperative: Adults: (IM, SC) 50–100 mg 30–90 min before beginning of anesthesia; (slow IV) initial 5–10 mg q5min prn. Children: (IV, IM, SC) 1–2 mg/kg as single dose, max 100 mg/dose.
- **Site of clearance:** hepatic

- t½: adults 2.5–4 h, liver disease 7–11 h; normeperidine (active metabolite) 15–30 h; accumulates with high doses or decreased renal function.
- **Interaction/toxicity:** Combined with MAOIs can cause hyperthermia and death. High doses may cause seizures.

MEPHENTERMINE (WYAMINE)

- **Uses:** sympathomimetic
- **Dose:** (IV) 15–30 mg.
- **Site of clearance:** hepatic
- t½: 17–18 h
- **Interaction/toxicity:** Pressor effect exaggerated in patients treated with MAOIs; halogenated anesthetics (especially halothane) sensitize myocardium to sympathomimetic effects (dysrhythmias).

MEPIVACAINE (CARBOCAINE)

- **Uses:** regional; local anesthesia
- **Dose:** nerve blockade 400 mg; epidural 400 mg, with epinephrine (1:200,000), max dose 500 mg.
- **Site of clearance:** hepatic
- t½: 1.9 h
- **Interaction/toxicity:** Beta-blockers decrease hepatic clearance; cimetidine increases serum level. High plasma concentration causes seizures, respiratory/cardiac depression.

MEROPENEM (MERREM)

- **Uses:** antibiotic
- **Dose:** Adults and children >50 kg: (IV) 1 g q8h infused over 5–30 min. Children >3 mo and <50 kg: (IV) 20–40 mg/kg q8h, max dose 2g q8h.
- **Site of clearance:** renal
- t½: 1–1.5 h
- **Interaction/toxicity:** Adjust dose in renal dysfunction. Use with caution in seizure disorders. May cause allergic reaction in patients with penicillin allergy.

METAPROTERENOL (VARIOUS)

- **Uses:** bronchodilator
- **Dose:** Adults: (PO) 20 mg q6–8h. Children >9 yr: (PO) 10 mg q6–8h. Children 6–9 yr: (PO) 10 mg q6h. Children 2–6 yr: (PO) 1.3–2.6 mg/kg/day q6h. Children <2 yr: (PO) 0.4 mg/kg tid–qid. Infants: (PO) 0.4 mg/kg q8–12h. Adults and children: (inhalation) 2–3 inhalations q3–4h, not >12 inhalations/day.

- ■ **Site of clearance:** N/A
- ■ **t½:** N/A
- ■ **Interaction/toxicity:** Use with spacer for inhalations. Use with caution in patients with hypothyroidism, diabetes mellitus, CAD, and HTN, and those using MAOIs, tricyclic antidepressants. Decreased effect with beta-blockers. Enhanced effect with sympathomimetics. Excessive use leads to tolerance.

METARAMINOL BITARTRATE (ARAMINE)

- ■ **Uses:** vasoconstrictor
- ■ **Dose:** Adult: (IV, IM, SC) bolus 0.5–10 mg. Children: (IV) bolus 0.01 mg/kg; infusion 5 mcg/kg/min. May be given via ETT.
- ■ **Site of clearance:** N/A
- ■ **t½:** N/A
- ■ **Interaction/toxicity:** Contraindicated in patients receiving MAOIs. May sensitize myocardium to halogenated anesthetics. Use with caution in patients with hyperthyroidism. Extravasation may cause sloughing of skin. Prolonged action associated with cumulative effect. May contain sulfites.

METHADONE (DOLOPHINE) `BBW`

- ■ **Uses:** analgesia, opioid addiction
- ■ **Dose:** *Analgesia:* Adults: (IM, IV, SQ) 2.5–10 mg q6–8h; (PO) 2.5–5 mg q6–8h prn; patients with prior opiate exposure may require higher initial doses. Children: (PO, IM, SC) 0.7 mg/kg/day divided q4–6h prn or 0.1–0.2 mg/kg q4–12h prn, max 10 mg/dose; (IV) 0.1 mg/kg q4h initially for 2–3 doses, then q6–12h prn, max 10 mg/dose.
- ■ **Site of clearance:** hepatic
- ■ **t½:** 15–29 h; prolonged with alkaline pH
- ■ **Interaction/toxicity:** Phenytoin reduces bioavailability by increasing hepatic clearance.

METHOHEXITAL (BREVITAL) `BBW`

- ■ **Uses:** induction agent; cardioversion; electroconvulsive shock Rx
- ■ **Dose:** Adults: (IV) induction 50–120 mg to start, 20–40 mg q4–7min. Children and infants ≥1 mo: (IM) induction 6.6–10 mg/kg of a 5% solution; (rectal) induction usually 25 mg/kg of a 1% solution.
- ■ **Site of clearance:** hepatic
- ■ **t½:** 3.9 h
- ■ **Interaction/toxicity:** Infrequent allergic reactions; myoclonus, hiccups, and seizures.

METHOXAMINE (VASOXYL)

- ■ **Uses:** vasoconstrictor
- ■ **Dose:** (IV) 3–5 mg administered slowly; (IM, SQ) 10–15 mg may be used to supplement IV administration to provide more prolonged effect. May be given via ETT.
- ■ **Site of clearance:** N/A
- ■ **t½:** N/A
- ■ **Interaction/toxicity:** Potentiated by bretylium, guanethidine, oxytocics, and tricyclic anti-depressants. May contain sulfites. Sloughing may be seen with extravasation.

METHYLDOPA (ALDOMET, METHYLDOPATE) `BBW`

- ■ **Uses:** antihypertensive
- ■ **Dose:** Adults: (IV) 250–500 mg q6–8h, max dose 1 g q6h. Children (IV): 5–10 mg/kg q6–8h up to total dose of 65 mg/kg/24 h or 3 g/24 h.
- ■ **Site of clearance:** hepatic, renal
- ■ **t½:** 75–80 min, ESRD 6–16 h
- ■ **Interaction/toxicity:** Reduces anesthetic requirements, potentiates sympathomimetics and levodopa. Concomitant Rx with propranolol may cause paradoxical HTN.

METHYLENE BLUE (VARIOUS)

- ■ **Uses:** antidote cyanide poisoning, methemoglobinemia.
- ■ **Dose:** *Methemoglobinemia:* Adults and children: (IV) 1–2 mg/kg over several minutes, MR in 1 h prn.
  Genitourinary antiseptic: Adults: (PO) 65–130 mg TID with full glass of water.
- ■ **Site of clearance:** renal
- ■ **t½:** 5–6.5 h
- ■ **Interaction/toxicity:** Contraindicated in patients with renal insufficiency. May cause hemolysis in patients with G6PD deficiency. Rapid injection may cause increased levels of methemoglobinemia. Turns urine and stool blue-green.

METHYLERGONOVINE (METHERGINE)

- ■ **Uses:** increases uterine contractions
- ■ **Dose:** (IM) 0.2 mg after delivery of anterior shoulder or placenta or during puerperium, MR q2–4h; (PO) 0.2 mg 3–4 times/day for 2–7 days.
- ■ **Site of clearance:** hepatic
- ■ **t½:** 1–5 min

■ **Interaction/toxicity:** Acute HTN; additive effects with sympathomimetics.

METHYLPREDNISOLONE (SOLU-MEDROL)

■ **Uses:** anti-inflammatory, allergic reaction, steroid replacement
■ **Dose:** *Anti-inflammatory or immunosuppressive:* Adults: (PO) 2–60 mg/day in 1–4 divided doses, followed by gradual reduction to the lowest possible level to maintain adequate clinical response; (IM) 10–80 mg/day; (IV) 10–40 mg over several minutes and repeated IV or IM depending on clinical response; when high dosages needed, give 30 mg/kg over ≥30 min and MR q4–6h for 48 h. Children: (PO, IM, IV) 0.5–1.7 mg/kg/day in divided q6–12h; "pulse" therapy 15–30 mg/kg/dose over ≥30 min given once daily for 3 days.

  Status asthmaticus: Adults and children: (IV) loading 2 mg/kg, then 0.5–1 mg/kg q6h for up to 5 days.

  Acute spinal cord injury: Adults and children: (IV) 30 mg/kg over 15 min, followed in 45 min by continuous infusion of 5.4 mg/kg/h for 23 h.
■ **Site of clearance:** hepatic
■ **t½:** 3–3.5 h
■ **Interaction/toxicity:** Increases insulin requirements; phenytoin, phenobarbital, and ephedrine may increase metabolic clearance of steroid.

METOCLOPRAMIDE (REGLAN)

■ **Uses:** stimulates gastric emptying; antiemetic
■ **Dose:** *Reduce risk of aspiration:* Adults: (IV) 10 mg. Children <6 yr: (IV) 0.1 mg/kg. Children 6–14 yr: (IV) 2.5–5 mg.

  Postoperative nausea and vomiting: (IM) 10 mg near end of surgery.

  Gastroesophageal reflux: Adults: (PO) 10–15 mg qid. Children: (PO): 0.1–0.2 mg/kg qid.
■ **Site of clearance:** renal
■ **t½:** 4–7 h
■ **Interaction/toxicity:** Antagonized by anticholinergics and opioids; potentiated by sedatives, hypnotics, opioids, and tranquilizers. Potentiates extrapyramidal effects of phenothiazines.

METOCURINE (METUBINE)

■ **Uses:** nondepolarizing neuromuscular blocker
■ **Dose:** (IV) 0.2–0.4 mg/kg.

▨ **Site of clearance:** renal
▨ **t½:** 6 h
▨ **Interaction/toxicity:** Histamine release. Cross-sensitivity in patients allergic to other muscle relaxants. Do not administer to patients with iodide allergy.

METOPROLOL (LOPRESSOR) `BBW`

▨ **Uses:** cardioselective beta-blocker; antidysrhythmic
▨ **Dose:** Adults: *HTN/ventricular rate control:* (IV) initial 1.25–5 mg q6–12h.
    Myocardial infarction: (IV) 2–5 mg q2min for 3 doses then 50 mg PO q6h starting 15 min after last IV dose and continuing for 48 h; maintenance max 100 mg q12h.
    Children: (PO) 1–5 mg/kg/24 h divided q12h.
▨ **Site of clearance:** hepatic
▨ **t½:** 3–4 h
▨ **Interaction/toxicity:** Increases digoxin and morphine serum levels.

METRONIDAZOLE (VARIOUS) `BBW`

▨ **Uses:** amebicide and antibiotic
▨ **Dose:** *Anaerobic infections:* Adults: (PO, IV) 250–500 mg q6–8h. Infants and children: (PO) 15–35 mg/kg/day divided q8h for 10 days; (IV) 30 mg/kg/day divided q6h.
▨ **Site of clearance:** hepatic
▨ **t½:** 6–8 h
▨ **Interaction/toxicity:** Reduce dose in hepatic or renal dysfunction. High sodium content. Disulfiram-like reaction seen with alcohol ingestion. Potentiates anticoagulants, lithium, phenytoin. Cimetidine potentiates effect. Antagonizes barbiturates. Barbiturates interfere with therapeutic effects.

MIDAZOLAM (VERSED) `BBW`

▨ **Uses:** premedicant, induction agent
▨ **Dose:** Depends on patient physical status and/or concomitant administration of opioids or other CNS depressants.
    Adults: Preoperative sedation: (IM): 0.07–0.08 mg/kg 30–60 min prior to surgery/procedure; usual dose: 5 mg; (IV): 1–2 mg MR q5min prn to desired effect (max dose <5 mg).
    Conscious sedation: (IV): 0.5–1 mg over at least 2 min; usual dose 2–4 mg

Anesthesia Induction: Unpremedicated patients: (IV) 0.3–0.35 mg/kg (in resistant cases total dose <0.6 mg/kg)

Premedicated patients: (IV): 0.15–0.35 mg/kg

Continuous infusion: Loading dose: (IV) 0.01–0.05 mg/kg, MR at 10–15 min intervals until sedation achieved. Maintenance: (IV): 0.02–0.1 mg/kg/hr

Infants and Children: Conscious sedation for procedures or preoperative sedation: (PO): 0.25–1 mg/kg as a single dose preprocedural dose or anxiolysis (max <20 mg); Children <6 years, or less cooperative patients may require as much as 1 mg/kg as a single dose; 0.25 mg/kg may suffice for children 6–16 yrs of age. (IM): 0.01–0.15 mg/kg; range 0.05–0.15 mg/kg; doses up to 0.5 mg/kg have been used in more anxious patients; max dose <10 mg.

(IV): Infants <6 months: Limited information is available therefore dosing recommendations unclear.

Infants 6 mos to Children 5 yrs: Initial: 0.05–0.1 mg/kg; total dose <0.6 mg/kg may be required; max dose <6 mg.

Children 6–12 yrs: Initial: 0.025–0.05 mg/kg; total doses of 0.4 mg/kg may be required; max <10 mg.

Children 12–16 yrs: Dose as adults; max dose <10 mg

- **Site of clearance:** renal
- **$t^{1/2}$:** 1–4 h; prolonged with cirrhosis, CHF, obesity, and in elderly
- **Interaction/toxicity:** Intensifies effects of CNS depressants, sedatives, hypnotics, opioids, and tranquilizers. Potentiated by antimycotics and erythromycin.

MILRINONE (PRIMACOR)

- **Uses:** inotropic support
- **Dose:** (IV) loading 50 mcg/kg over 10 min; infusion rate 0.375–0.75 mcg/kg/min (dilute in sodium chloride or D_5W). Adjust for renal insufficiency.
- **Site of clearance:** renal
- **$t^{1/2}$:** 1–3 h
- **Interaction/toxicity:** Marked vasodilator effect seen in hypovolemic patients. Use with caution in patients with atrial fibrillation/flutter (milrinone may decrease AV nodal conduction and increase ventricular rate), electrolyte abnormalities, hypotension, recent myocardial infarction, renal disease, severe aortic or pulmonic valvular disease (may aggravate outflow tract obstruction in hypertrophic subaortic stenosis).

MIVACURIUM (MIVACRON)

■ **Uses:** nondepolarizing neuromuscular blocker
■ **Dose:** Adults: (IV) initial 0.15–0.25 mg/kg bolus, then 0.1 mg/kg at 15 min intervals; for prolonged neuromuscular block, initial infusion 9–10 mcg/kg/min used on evidence of spontaneous recovery from initial dose, usual infusion rate 6–7 mcg/kg/min (1–15 mcg/kg/min) under balanced anesthesia. Children 2–12 yr: (IV) (duration of action is shorter and disease requirements are higher) 0.2 mg/kg bolus, then 14 mcg/kg/min (5–31 mcg/kg/min) on evidence of spontaneous recovery from initial dose.
■ **Site of clearance:** plasma cholinesterase
■ **t½:** 2 min
■ **Interaction/toxicity:** Potentiated by volatile anesthetics, hypokalemia, antibiotics (aminoglycosides), lithium, magnesium local anesthetics, procainamide, quinidine. Chronic administration of oral contraceptives, glucocorticoids, MAOIs, or echothiophate enhances neuromuscular block by decreasing plasma cholinesterase activity. Releases histamine at high doses.

MORPHINE (VARIOUS) BBW

■ **Uses:** analgesia
■ **Dose:** *Acute pain:* Adults: (PO) initial for opiate naïve 10 mg q3–4h prn; initial for prior opiate exposure 10–30 mg q3–4h prn; (IV) opiate naïve 2.5–5 mg q3–4h; patients with prior opiate exposure may require higher initial doses; (IM, SC) initial for opiate naïve 5–10 mg q3–4h prn; initial for prior opiate exposure 5–20 mg q3–4h prn. Children >6 mo and <50 kg: (PO) 0.15–0.3 mg/kg q3–4h prn; (IM):0.1 mg/kg q3–4h prn; (IV) 0.05–0.1 mg/kg q3–4h prn.
Patient-controlled analgesia (PCA): usual concentration 1 mg/mL, usual demand dose 1 mg (range 0.5–2.5 mg), lockout interval 5–10 min.
Epidural: bolus 1–6 mg, infusion rate 0.1–1 mg/h, max dose 10 mg/24 h.
Intrathecal: opiate naïve 0.2 mg/dose.
■ **Site of clearance:** hepatic
■ **t½:** 2–4 h
■ **Interaction/toxicity:** Hypotension and respiratory depression. Potentiates cimetidine; increases anticoagulation with warfarin. Releases histamine in high doses.

MORPHINE, CONTROLLED RELEASE (MS CONTIN) **BBW**

- ■ **Uses:** opioid analgesic
- ■ **Dose:** (PO) 15 mg q12h.
- ■ **Site of clearance:** hepatic
- ■ **t½:** 15 h
- ■ **Interaction/toxicity:** Hypotension and respiratory depression. Potentiates sedatives, hypnotics, general anesthetics, and cimetidine (increases anticoagulation with warfarin). Causes nausea and pruritus and can release histamine in high doses. Higher plasma concentrations seen in hepatic and renal failure.

NAFCILLIN (VARIOUS)

- ■ **Uses:** antibiotic
- ■ **Dose:** Adults: (IV, IM) 500 mg q4–6h, max daily dose 18 g; (PO) 250–500 mg q4–6h.
   Children: (IV) 25 mg/kg bid; (PO) 25–50 mg/kg/day q6h.
- ■ **Site of clearance:** renal
- ■ **t½:** Children (3 mo to 14 yr) 0.75–2 h, adults 30 min to 2 h
- ■ **Interaction/toxicity:** Antagonizes effect of warfarin ("warfarin resistance").

NALBUPHINE (NUBAIN)

- ■ **Uses:** analgesia, opioid agonist-antagonist
- ■ **Dose:** Adults: (IV) 10 mg/70 kg q3–6h, max single dose 20 mg, max daily dose 160 mg.
   Premedication: Children 10 mo to 14 yr: (IV) 0.2 mg/kg; max 20 mg/dose.
- ■ **Site of clearance:** hepatic
- ■ **t½:** 3–3.5 h
- ■ **Interaction/toxicity:** Does not antagonize effects of opioids in nondependent patient.

NALMEFENE HYDROCHLORIDE (REVEX)

- ■ **Uses:** opioid antagonist
- ■ **Dose:** (IV) 0.25 mcg/kg, cumulative total dose NTE 1 mcg/kg.
- ■ **Site of clearance:** hepatic
- ■ **t½:** 11 h
- ■ **Interaction/toxicity:** Can cause abrupt CV stimulation and pulmonary edema; withdrawal in opioid-dependent patients.

NALOXONE (NARCAN)

- ▦ **Uses:** opioid antagonist
- ▦ **Dose:** Adults: (IV) 40–100 mcg prn. Children: (IV) 10 mcg/kg.
- ▦ **Site of clearance:** hepatic
- ▦ **t½:** 1–1.5 h
- ▦ **Interaction/toxicity:** Can cause abrupt CV stimulation and pulmonary edema; causes withdrawal in opioid-dependent patients.

NAPROXEN (VARIOUS) `BBW`

- ▦ **Uses:** analgesia, antipyretic, anti-inflammatory
- ▦ **Dose:** Adults: (PO) 250–500 mg bid, max daily dose 1.25 g. Children: (PO) 5–10 mg/kg/day divided bid.
- ▦ **Site of clearance:** hepatic
- ▦ **t½:** 12–15 h
- ▦ **Interaction/toxicity:** Use with caution in patients with CHF, hepatic or renal dysfunction, HTN, history of GI bleed. Higher doses are associated with adverse CNS effects, especially in the elderly (agitation, confusion, and hallucination). Aspirin decreases effect. Potentiates digoxin, lithium, and anticoagulant. Inhibits loop diuretics. Antagonizes ACE inhibitors and beta-blockers.

NEOSTIGMINE (PROSTIGMIN)

- ▦ **Uses:** anticholinesterase
- ▦ **Dose:** Adults: (IV) 0.5–2.5 mg, total dose NTE 5 mg. Children: (IV) 0.025–0.08 mg/kg. Infants: (IV) 0.025–0.1 mg/kg.
- ▦ **Site of clearance:** hepatic
- ▦ **t½:** 0.5–2 h, prolonged in ESRD
- ▦ **Interaction/toxicity:** Bradycardia, salivation.

NESIRITIDE (NATRECOR)

- ▦ **Uses:** natriuretic peptide, B-type, human, vasodilator
- ▦ **Dose:** *Congestive heart failure:* (IV) loading 2 mcg/kg IV bolus over 60 sec, followed by 0.01 mcg/kg/min continuous IV infusion; titration may increase by 0.005 mcg/kg/min (after a bolus of 1 mcg/kg IV) no more frequently than q3h up to a max dose of 0.03 mcg/kg/min. If hypotension occurs, discontinue drug; restart at 70% of dose (without bolus).
- ▦ **Site of clearance:** renal
- ▦ **t½:** 18 min, biologic effects persist longer than expected half-life.

- **Interaction/toxicity:** cardiogenic shock (not as primary therapy), hypersensitivity to nesiritide or any of its components, systolic blood pressure less than 90 mm Hg.

NICARDIPINE (CARDENE IV)

- **Uses:** antihypertensive, antidysrhythmic, and antianginal
- **Dose:** (IV) 1–2 mcg/kg/min or 5 mg/h (dilute in 250 mL NS or D_5W; incompatible with LR solution). Increase by 2.5 mg/hr q 15 min to max of 15 mg/hr. Titrate to lowest dose necessary to maintain blood pressure.
- **Site of clearance:** hepatic
- **t½:** 2–4 h
- **Interaction/toxicity:** Cimetidine and ranitidine may increase bioavailability. Potentiated in patient with liver disease may increase hepatic portal pressure in cirrhotic patients.

NIFEDIPINE (PROCARDIA, ADALAT)

- **Uses:** coronary vasospasm; angina; antihypertensive
- **Dose:** (PO) 10–20 mg tid.
- **Site of clearance:** hepatic, renal
- **t½:** 2–5 h, cirrhosis 7 h, elderly 6–7 h
- **Interaction/toxicity:** Decreases platelet aggregation. Cimetidine and ranitidine may increase bioavailability. Potentiates theophylline.

NIMODIPINE (NIMOTOP) BBW

- **Uses:** prevent cerebral arterial spasm (subarachnoid hemorrhage)
- **Dose:** (PO) 60 mg q4h for 21 days.
- **Site of clearance:** hepatic
- **t½:** 3 h
- **Interaction/toxicity:** Potentiated in patients with hepatic disease. Potentiates effects of antihypertensive drugs.

NITRIC OXIDE (INOMAX)

- **Uses:** selective pulmonary vasodilator
- **Dose:** (inhalation) 10–20 ppm.
- **Site of clearance:** enzymatic and renal
- **t½:** 3–6 sec
- **Interaction/toxicity:** Abrupt withdrawal can result in hypoxemia and pulmonary HTN. Inspiratory N_2O, NO_2, and blood methemoglobin concentrations should be monitored. May cause thrombocytopenia and decrease in platelet aggregation.

NITROGLYCERIN (TRIDIL, NITROL IV, NITROSTAT IV)

▪ **Uses:** vasodilator, antianginal; controlled hypotension
▪ **Dose:** (IV) 1–3 mcg/kg/min (dilute 50 mg in 250 mL D_5W or NS).
▪ **Site of clearance:** hepatic, renal
▪ **t½:** 1–4 min
▪ **Interaction/toxicity:** Increases bioavailability of dihydroergotamine. Methemoglobinemia seen with high doses, especially in individuals with methemoglobin reductase deficiency. Treat with O_2 and methylene blue (0.2 mL/kg IV). Dose may be increased to 1–2 mg/kg.

NITROPRUSSIDE (NIPRIDE, NITROPRESS) `BBW`

▪ **Uses:** antihypertensive; vasodilator; controlled hypotension
▪ **Dose:** *Antihypertensive, vasodilator, controlled hypotension:*
Adults: (IV) initial 0.3–0.5 mcg/kg/min, increase in increments of 0.5 mcg/kg/min, titrating to the desired hemodynamic effect or the appearance of headache or nausea; usual dose 3 mcg/kg/min, rarely need >4 mcg/kg/min, max 10 mcg/kg/min.
Pulmonary HTN: Children: (IV) initial 0.5–1 mcg/kg/min by continuous IV infusion, increase in increments of 1 mcg/kg/min at intervals of 20–60 min, titrating to the desired response; usual dose 3 mcg/kg/min, rarely need >4 mcg/kg/min, max 5 mcg/kg/min.
▪ **Site of clearance:** hepatic
▪ **t½:** <10 min
▪ **Interaction/toxicity:** Cyanide toxicity may occur at doses >10 mcg/kg/min. Tachyphylaxis, elevated mixed venous O_2 tension (saturation), and acidosis suggest diagnosis of cyanide toxicity. Hydroxocobalamin may reduce risk of cyanide toxicity. Treatment of cyanide toxicity is IV administration of sodium thiosulfate, 150 mg/kg over 15 min. Thiocyanate ion can be removed by hemodialysis.

NOREPINEPHRINE (LEVOPHED)

▪ **Uses:** vasoconstrictor
▪ **Dose:** Adults: (IV) initial 0.5–1 mcg/min and titrate to desired response (dilute 4 mg in 250 mL D_5W). Children: (IV) initial 0.03–0.1 mcg/kg/min, max dose 1–2 mcg/kg/min.
▪ **Site of clearance:** enzymatic
▪ **t½:** 2–3 min
▪ **Interaction/toxicity:** MAOIs and tricyclic antidepressants may cause severe HTN. Halogenated anesthetics (especially

halothane) may sensitize myocardium to sympathomimetic effects (dysrhythmias). Furosemide may decrease arterial vaso-constrictor properties. Extravasation may cause skin slough.

NORTRIPTYLINE (VARIOUS) **BBW**

- ▓ **Uses:** antidepressant, chronic pain management, migraine headaches
- ▓ **Dose:** (PO) 25 mg tid.
- ▓ **Site of clearance:** hepatic
- ▓ **t½:** 28–31 h
- ▓ **Interaction/toxicity:** Contraindicated in patients with narrow-angle glaucoma, Rx treated with MAOIs within previous 14 days. Use with caution in patients with cardiac dysrhythmias, hyperthyroidism, renal or hepatic dysfunction. Phenobarbital increases metabolism. Increases amount of inhalation anesthesia required. Potentiates sympathomimetics, CNS depressants, and anticoagulants. Cimetidine decreases metabolism. Should not be abruptly discontinued. May contain sulfites.

ONDANSETRON (ZOFRAN)

- ▓ **Uses:** antiemetic
- ▓ **Dose:** Postoperative nausea and vomiting: Adults: (IV) 4 mg as a single dose 30 min before the end of anesthesia. Children 2–12 yr and ≤40 kg: (IV) 0.1 mg/kg. Children >40 kg: (IV) 4 mg.
- ▓ **Site of clearance:** hepatic
- ▓ **t½:** children (<15 yr) 2–3 h, adults 3–6 h
- ▓ **Interaction/toxicity:** Potentiated by hepatic disease. ECG abnormalities with rapid injection.

OXACILLIN (VARIOUS)

- ▓ **Uses:** antibiotic
- ▓ **Dose:** Adults: (IV, IM) 250–500 mg q4–6h; (PO) 500 mg q4–6h. Children: (IV) 50 mg/day q6h; (PO) 50 mg/kg/day q6h.
- ▓ **Site of clearance:** hepatic
- ▓ **t½:** Children (1 wk to 2 yr) 1–2 h, adults 23–60 min
- ▓ **Interaction/toxicity:** Potentiates anticoagulants.

OXYCODONE, CONTROLLED RELEASE (OXYCONTIN) **BBW**

- ▓ **Uses:** opioid analgesic
- ▓ **Dose:** Adults: (PO) 10 mg q12h.

- Site of clearance: renal
- t½: 4.5–8 h
- Interaction/toxicity: Hypotension and respiratory depression. Potentiates sedatives, hypnotics, general anesthetics and cimetidine (increases anticoagulation with warfarin). Causes nausea and pruritus and can release histamine in high doses. Higher plasma concentrations in hepatic and renal failure.

OXYTOCIN (PITOCIN) [BBW]

- Uses: increases uterine contraction
- Dose: (IV) 10 units, infusion 0.002 units/min.
- Site of clearance: hepatic
- t½: 1–5 min
- Interaction/toxicity: Potentiates sympathomimetics.

PANCURONIUM (PAVULON) [BBW]

- Uses: nondepolarizing neuromuscular blocker
- Dose: Adults, children, and infants >1 mo: (IV) initial 0.05–0.10 mg/kg prn.
- Site of clearance: renal, hepatic
- t½: 110 min
- Interaction/toxicity: Potentiated by volatile anesthetics, hypokalemia, antibiotics (aminoglycosides), magnesium local anesthetics, procainamide, quinidine. Conditions associated with increased volume of distribution (e.g., slower circulation time, edematous states, and old age) may be associated with delay in onset. Prolongation of neuromuscular blockade may occur in patients with renal and/or hepatic disease. Patients receiving tricyclic antidepressants who are anesthetized with halothane and receive pancuronium may develop dysrhythmias.

PENICILLIN G (VARIOUS)

- Uses: antibiotic
- Dose: Adults: (IV) 10,000,000–20,000,000 units/day divided q4–6h. Children: (IV) 100,000–250,000 units/kg/day divided q6h.
- Site of clearance: renal
- t½: 20–50 min
- Interaction/toxicity: Reduce dose with renal dysfunction. May exacerbate seizure disorders. Large doses may prolong bleeding

time and potentiates anticoagulants. Electrolyte abnormalities (sodium and potassium) may be seen with large IV doses.

PENTAZOCINE (TALWIN)

- **Uses:** analgesia; opioid agonist–antagonist
- **Dose:** Adults: (IV, IM) 30 mg q4h. Adults and children >12 yr: (PO) 50 mg q4h.
- **Site of clearance:** hepatic, renal
- **t½:** 2–3 h
- **Interaction/toxicity:** Potentiates barbiturates and CNS depressants. Potentiated in patients with hepatic and/or renal disease. May precipitate withdrawal in opioid-dependent patients.

PENTOBARBITAL (NEMBUTAL)

- **Uses:** hypnotic; premedication
- **Dose:** *Hypnotic, preoperative sedation:* Adults: (IM) 150–200 mg; (IV) initial 100 mg, MR q1–3min up to 200–500 mg total dose. Children ≥6 mo: (IM) 2–6 mg/kg, max 100 mg/dose; (IV) 1–3 mg/kg to max of 100 mg until asleep.

  Conscious sedation prior to a procedure: Adolescents: (IV) 100 mg before procedure. Children 5–12 yr: (IV) 2 mg/kg 5–10 min before procedure, MR once.

  Barbiturate coma in head injury patients: Adults and children: (IV) loading 5–10 mg/kg over 1–2 h while monitoring blood pressure and respiratory rate; maintenance initial 1 mg/kg/h, may increase to 2–3 mg/kg/h; maintain burst suppression on EEG.
- **Site of clearance:** hepatic, renal
- **t½:** adults 22 h, children 25 h (range 15–50 h)
- **Interaction/toxicity:** Barbiturates decrease effects of theophylline, β-adrenergic blockers, corticosteroids, and tricyclic antidepressants. MAOIs increase action.

PHENOBARBITAL (VARIOUS)

- **Uses:** sedative, hypnotic, anticonvulsant
- **Dose:** *Sedation:* Adults (IV, IM): 30–120 mg in 2–3 divided doses; (PO) 30–120 mg/day q8–12h. Children: 2 mg/kg tid.

  Premedication: Adults: (IM) 100–200 mg. Children: 1–3 mg/kg 1–1.5 h before procedure.

  Anticonvulsant, status epilepticus, loading: Adults (IV): 300–800 mg followed by 120–240 mg/dose at 20 min intervals until seizures controlled or total dose of 1–2 g in 24 h. Infants and children: (IV) loading 10–20 mg/kg in single or divided doses q15–30min until seizures controlled or total dose of 40 mg/kg in 24 h.

Anticonvulsant, maintenance: Adults and children >12 yr: (PO, IV) 1–3 mg/kg/day in divided doses or 50–100 mg 2–3 times/day. Children 5–12 yr: (PO, IV) 4–6 mg/kg/day in 1–2 divided doses. Children 1–5 yr (PO, IV) 6–8 mg/kg/day in 1–2 divided doses. Infants (PO, IV) 5–8 mg/kg/day in 1–2 divided doses.

▪ **Site of clearance:** hepatic
▪ **t½:** adults 53–140 h, children 37–73 h
▪ **Interaction/toxicity:** Contraindicated in patients with severe liver or renal dysfunction or porphyria. Rapid IV injection may laryngospasm, respiratory depression, and hypotension. Potentiates sedatives, hypnotics, tranquilizers, and other CNS depressants. Decreases the effects of beta-adrenergic blockers, theophylline, verapamil, corticosteroids, tricyclic antidepressants. MAOIs increase actions. Increases metabolism of methadone and can result in withdrawal. Tolerance may develop. Avoid abrupt withdrawal.

PHENOXYBENZAMINE (DIBENZYLINE)

▪ **Uses:** antihypertensive, vasodilator, pheochromocytoma
▪ **Dose:** (PO) 10 mg bid, increase by 10 mg every other day, usual range 20–40 mg bid–tid.
▪ **Site of clearance:** renal
▪ **t½:** 24 h
▪ **Interaction/toxicity:** Use with caution in patients with coronary, cerebral, renal dysfunction. Exaggerated response (hypotension and tachycardia) may be seen with catecholamine administration such as epinephrine.

PHENTOLAMINE (REGITINE)

▪ **Uses:** arterial dilator
▪ **Dose:** *Diagnosis of pheochromocytoma:* Adults: (IM, IV) 5 mg. Children: (IM, IV) 0.05–0.1 mg/kg, max single dose 5 mg.
   Surgery for pheochromocytoma, HTN: Adults: (IM, IV) 2.5–5.0 mg 1–2 h before procedure and MR prn q2–4h. Children: (IM, IV) 0.05–0.1 mg/kg given 1–2 h before procedure, MR prn q2–4h until controlled, max single dose of 5 mg.
▪ **Site of clearance:** unknown
▪ **t½:** 19 min
▪ **Interaction/toxicity:** Vasoconstrictor effects of epinephrine and ephedrine are blocked by phentolamine.

PHENYLEPHRINE (NEO-SYNEPHRINE) **BBW**

- ■ **Uses:** vasoconstrictor
- ■ **Dose:** *Hypotension/shock:* Adults: (IV) bolus 50–100 mcg; infusion 0.5–1 mcg/kg/min (dilute 4 mg in 250 mL D_5W or NS). Children: (IV) bolus 5–20 mcg/kg q10–15min prn; infusion 0.1–0.5 mcg/kg/min.
- ■ **Site of clearance:** hepatic
- ■ **t½:** 2.5 h, prolonged after long-term infusion
- ■ **Interaction/toxicity:** Effects potentiated by oxytocic drugs, MAOIs, and tricyclic antidepressants.

PHENYTOIN (DILANTIN)

- ■ **Uses:** anticonvulsant; antidysrhythmic
- ■ **Dose:** *Status epilepticus:* Adults: (IV, PO) loading 10–20 mg/kg in single or divided dose, maintenance 5–6 mg/kg/day in 3 divided doses. Infants and children: (IV, PO) loading 15–20 mg/kg in a single or divided dose, maintenance initial 5 mg/kg/day in 2 divided doses.
- ■ **Site of clearance:** hepatic
- ■ **t½:** 22 h
- ■ **Interaction/toxicity:** Increased effects seen with cimetidine and diazepam; decreased effects seen with barbiturates, theophylline, and antacids. Decreases effectiveness of corticosteroids, dicumarol, haloperidol, quinidine, furosemide, dopamine, and nondepolarizing muscle relaxants. Increases toxicity of lithium.

PHYSOSTIGMINE (ANTILIRIUM)

- ■ **Uses:** anticholinesterase; nonspecific reversal of CNS side effects of benzodiazepines, scopolamine, and ketamine
- ■ **Dose:** Adults: (IV) initial 0.5–1 mg, MR q20min until response or adverse effect occurs. Children (reserve for life-threatening situations): (IV) 0.02 mg/kg/dose (max 0.5 mg/min), MR after 5–10 min to max total dose of 2 mg or until response or adverse cholinergic effects occur.
- ■ **Site of clearance:** cholinesterase enzyme
- ■ **t½:** 15–40 min
- ■ **Interaction/toxicity:** Rapid administration can cause bradycardia, salivation, and seizures.

PHYTONADIONE (AQUAMEPHYTON, KONAKION) **BBW**

- ■ **Uses:** hepatic synthesis of prothrombin (II); proconvertin (VII); plasma thromboplastin (IX); and Stuart factor (X)

■ **Dose:** Adults: (slow IV) 2.5–10.0 mg. Children: (slow IV) 0.5–2.0 mg.
■ **Site of clearance:** hepatic
■ **t½:** 26–193 h
■ **Interaction/toxicity:** Severe reaction resembling anaphylaxis has been seen even with administration of dilute phytonadione.

PIPECURONIUM (ARDUAN) `BBW`

■ **Uses:** nondepolarizing neuromuscular blocker
■ **Dose:** (IV) 0.07 mg/kg.
■ **Site of clearance:** renal
■ **t½:** 137–161 min
■ **Interaction/toxicity:** Potentiated by volatile anesthetics, hypokalemia, antibiotics (aminoglycosides), lithium, magnesium, local anesthetics, procainamide, quinidine. Conditions associated with increased volume of distribution (e.g., slower circulation time, edematous states, and old age) may be associated with delay in onset. Contains benzyl alcohol, which may be associated with increased incidence of neurologic complications in neonates. Due to long duration of action not recommended for patient undergoing cesarean section.

PREDNISOLONE (VARIOUS)

■ **Uses:** anti-inflammatory, steroid replacement, allergic reaction
■ **Dose:** Adults: (PO) 5–60 mg/day. Children: (PO) 0.5–1 mg/kg q12–24h.
■ **Site of clearance:** hepatic
■ **t½:** 3.6 h
■ **Interaction/toxicity:** Contraindicated in patients with serious infections or varicella. Use with caution in patients with hypothyroidism, CHF, peptic ulcer disease. Increases insulin requirements. Hydantoins, barbiturates, and ephedrine increase metabolic clearance of steroid. Withdraw drug gradually if used for chronic Rx. Must be metabolized by liver to active form.

PRILOCAINE (CITANEST)

■ **Uses:** regional anesthesia
■ **Dose:** nerve block 600 mg.
■ **Site of clearance:** hepatic
■ **t½:** 10–150 min

■ **Interaction/toxicity:** Methemoglobinemia may be associated with doses >500 mg; treat with methylene blue (IV), 1–2 mg/kg over 5 min.

PROCAINAMIDE (PRONESTYL) BBW

■ **Uses:** antidysrhythmic
■ **Dose:** Adults: (IV) 100–200 mg, MR q5min prn to a total dose of 1 g, maintenance 1–4 mg/min by continuous infusion (dilute 1,000 mg in 500 mL D_5W). Children: (IV) 3–6 mg/kg/dose over 5 min NTE 100 mg/dose, MR q5–10min to max 15 mg/kg/load, maintenance as continuous infusion 20–80 mcg/kg/min, max 2 g/24 h.
■ **Site of clearance:** hepatic
■ **t½:** children 1.7 h, adults 2.5–4.7 h, anephric 11 h; NAPA (dependent on renal function): children 6 h, adults 6–8 h, anephric 42 h.
■ **Interaction/toxicity:** Enhances anticholinergic drugs and potentiates neuromuscular blockers.

PROCAINE (NOVOCAIN)

■ **Uses:** regional anesthesia
■ **Dose:** nerve block 1,000 mg; epidural 1,000 mg; spinal 50–200 mg.
■ **Site of clearance:** plasma cholinesterase
■ **t½:** 7.7 min
■ **Interaction/toxicity:** Potential for allergic reaction with repeated use.

PROCHLORPERAZINE (COMPAZINE)

■ **Uses:** antiemetic, antipsychotic
■ **Dose:** *Antiemetic:* Adults: (PO) tablet 5–10 mg tid–qid, max 40 mg/day; (rectal) 25 mg bid; (IV, IM) 5–10 mg, max 10 mg/dose and 40 mg/day.
   Surgical nausea and vomiting: Adults: (IV) 5–10 mg 15–30 min before induction. Children >10 kg: (PO, rectal) 0.4 mg/kg/24 h divided tid–qid; (IM) 0.1–0.15 mg/kg/dose.
■ **Site of clearance:** hepatic
■ **t½:** PO 3–5 h, IV ~7 h
■ **Interaction/toxicity:** Hypersensitivity reaction may manifest as jaundice and/or extrapyramidal symptoms.

PROMETHAZINE (PHENERGAN) BBW

■ **Uses:** antiemetic
■ **Dose:** *Allergic conditions (including allergic reactions to blood or plasma):* Adults: (IM, IV, PO, rectal) 12.5–25 mg, MR in

2 h. Children ≥2 yr: (PO, rectal) 0.1 mg/kg q6h max 12.5 mg/dose.

Antiemetic: Adults: (IV, IM, PO, rectal) 12.5–25 mg q4–6h prn. Children: (IV, IM, PO, rectal) 0.25–1 mg/kg 4–6 times/day prn, max 25 mg/dose.

- ■ **Site of clearance:** hepatic
- ■ **t½:** 9–16 h
- ■ **Interaction/toxicity:** Hypersensitivity reaction may manifest as jaundice.

PROPOFOL (DIPRIVAN)

- ■ **Uses:** induction agent
- ■ **Dose:** Adults: (IV) induction 1.5–2.5 mg/kg approximately 40 mg q10sec until induction onset; (IV infusion) maintenance initial 150–200 mcg/kg/min, usual infusion rate 100–200 mcg/kg/min. Children: (IV) induction 2.5–3.5 mg/kg over 20–30 sec; (IV infusion) maintenance initial 200–300 mcg/kg/min, titrate 50–100 mcg/kg/min, usual infusion rate 125–150 mcg/kg/min.
- ■ **Site of clearance:** hepatic
- ■ **t½:** 40 min
- ■ **Interaction/toxicity:** Hypotension, respiratory depression, and pain with injection. Prepared in lipid emulsion; infection potential, allergic reaction.

PROPRANOLOL (INDERAL) ▮BBW▮

- ■ **Uses:** Beta blockade, antidysrhythmic, antihypertensive
- ■ **Dose:** *Tachyarrhythmias:* Adults: (IV) 0.5–1 mg, repeat q5min up to total of 5 mg, titrate initial dose to desired response. Children and infants: (IV) 0.01–0.1 mg/kg over 10 min; max 1 mg for infants, 3 mg for children.
- ■ **Site of clearance:** hepatic
- ■ **t½:** children 3.9–6.4 h, adults 4–6 h
- ■ **Interaction/toxicity:** Increases digoxin, local anesthetic, and morphine serum levels. Bradycardia, hypotension, and bronchospasm can be seen.

PROSTAGLANDIN E₁, ALPROSTADIL (PROSTIN VR)

- ■ **Uses:** maintain patency of ductus arteriosus; vasodilator
- ■ **Dose:** (IV) continuous infusion into large vein, or alternatively through umbilical artery catheter placed at ductal opening at 0.05–0.1 mcg/kg/min with therapeutic response, rate reduced to lowest effective dosage; with unsatisfactory response, rate is

increased gradually; maintenance 0.01–0.4 mcg/kg/min (dilute 500 mcg in 250 mL D_5W or sodium chloride).
- **Site of clearance:** lungs
- $t^{1/2}$: 5–10 min
- **Interaction/toxicity:** In premature newborns produces apnea; inhibits platelet aggregation.

PROTAMINE (VARIOUS)

- **Uses:** heparin antagonist
- **Dose:** titrated on basis of coagulation test (e.g., ACT); protamine 1 mg neutralizes 90 units heparin (lung) or 115 units heparin (intestinal mucosa).
- **Site of clearance:** N/A
- $t^{1/2}$: 7.4 min
- **Interaction/toxicity:** Potentiates vasodilators; anaphylactic reactions especially in patients with fish allergy or diabetics treated with protamine-containing insulin solutions; complement-mediated pulmonary vasoconstriction.

PYRIDOSTIGMINE (REGONOL, MESTINON)

- **Uses:** anticholinesterase; myasthenia gravis
- **Dose:** (IV) 0.2 mg/kg. Note: Atropine sulfate 0.6–1.2 mg IV immediately prior to pyridostigmine minimizes dose effects.
- **Site of clearance:** renal, hepatic
- $t^{1/2}$: 1–2 h
- **Interaction/toxicity:** Bradycardia, salivation.

QUINIDINE GLUCONATE (VARIOUS) BBW

- **Uses:** antidysrhythmic
- **Dose:** (IV) 100–300 mg administer at rate <1 mL/min (16 mg/min) (dilute 10 mL [880 mg] in 50 mL D_5W).
- **Site of clearance:** hepatic
- $t^{1/2}$: adults 6–8 h, prolonged in elderly or with cirrhosis or CHF
- **Interaction/toxicity:** Reduced by hypokalemia (also increases risk of Torsades de Pointes). Verapamil, cimetidine, antacids enhance activity by increasing quinidine plasma concentration. Potentiates nondepolarizer neuromuscular blockers and succinylcholine.

RANITIDINE (ZANTAC)

- **Uses:** histamine antagonist (H_2)
- **Dose:** Adults: (PO) 150 mg q12h; (IV) 50 mg q6–8h (dilute in 100 mL NS or D_5W). Children 1 mo to 16 yr: (PO) 2–4 mg/kg/

day divided q12h, max 300 mg/day; (IV) 2–4 mg/kg/day divided q6–8h, max 150 mg/day.
- **Site of clearance:** hepatic, renal
- **t½:** PO 2.5–3 h, IV 2–2.5 h
- **Interaction/toxicity:** Bradycardia with IV administration.

REMIFENTANIL (ULTIVA)

- **Uses:** analgesia
- **Dose:** (IV) induction 0.5–1 mcg/kg/min (through intubation) over 30–60 sec, continuous infusion 0.1–2 mcg/kg/min.
   Monitored anesthesia care: (IV) 1 mcg/kg, continuous infusion 0.025–0.2 mcg/kg/min.
- **Site of clearance:** plasma and tissue esterases
- **t½:** 10 min
- **Interaction/toxicity:** Hypotension, respiratory depression, and nausea and pruritus. Potentiated by sedatives, hypnotics, tranquilizers. Decreases effects of diuretics in congestive heart failure. Contraindicated for use in epidural or intrathecal administration due to glycine in formulation.

RITODRINE (YUTOPAR)

- **Uses:** uterine relaxation
- **Dose:** (IV) 0.1–0.3 mg/min.
- **Site of clearance:** renal
- **t½:** 60–156 min
- **Interaction/toxicity:** CV effects (dysrhythmias and hypotension) seen with meperidine and general anesthetics. Concomitant use of corticosteroids may lead to pulmonary edema.

ROPIVACAINE (NAROPIN)

- **Uses:** local anesthetic
- **Dose:** infiltration 5–200 mg; peripheral nerve block 175–250 mg; lumbar epidural 75–150 mg; thoracic epidural 25–75 mg.
- **Site of clearance:** renal
- **t½:** epidural 5–7 h, IV 2–4 h
- **Interaction/toxicity:** Increased plasma ropivacaine levels seen with theophylline, imipramine, fluvoxamine, and verapamil. CV toxicity less than that of bupivacaine, otherwise similar.

SCOPOLAMINE (VARIOUS)

- **Uses:** anticholinergic; amnesia
- **Dose:** *Preoperative:* Adults: (IV, IM, SC) 0.2–0.4 mg, MR q4–6h. Children: (IM, SC) 6 mcg/kg, max 0.3 mg/dose.

- **Site of clearance:** renal
- **t½:** 9.5 h
- **Interaction/toxicity:** CNS excitation or sedation (central anticholinergic syndrome). Antihistamines, procainamide, sedatives, hypnotics, and opioids intensify effect. Amnesia, vertigo, and dry mouth.

SECOBARBITAL (SECONAL)

- **Uses:** hypnotic; premedication
- **Dose:** *Preoperative sedation:* Adults: (IV) 100–300 mg 1–2 h before procedure. Children: (IV) 2–6 mg/kg (max dose 100 mg) 1–2 h before procedure.
- **Site of clearance:** hepatic
- **t½:** 19–34 h
- **Interaction/toxicity:** Barbiturates decrease effects of theophylline. β-Adrenergic blockers, corticosteroids, tricyclic antidepressants, and MAOIs increase action.

SODIUM BICARBONATE (VARIOUS)

- **Uses:** correct metabolic acidosis
- **Dose:** Adults, children, and infants: (IV) dosage based on following formula if blood gases and pH measurements available: HCO_3 (mEq) = 0.3 × weight (kg) × base deficit (mEq/L). Administer half dose initially, then remaining half dose over the next 24 h. If acid-base status is not available dose for older children and adults, use 1–2 mEq/kg infusion over 4–8 h; subsequent doses should be based on acid-base status.
- **Site of clearance:** lungs
- **t½:** N/A
- **Interaction/toxicity:** Increase sodium retention, intracerebral bleed (neonates); urinary alkalinization increases duration of action of certain drugs.

SUCCINYLCHOLINE (ANECTINE) BBW

- **Uses:** depolarizing neuromuscular blocker
- **Dose:** Adults: (IV) 1–1.5 mg/kg, up to 150 mg total dose; continuous infusion 10–100 mcg/kg/min (dilute to concentration of 1–2 mg/mL in D_5W or NS). Children: (IV) initial 1–2 mg/kg, maintenance 0.3–0.6 mg/kg. Because of the risk of malignant hyperthermia, use of continuous infusions is not recommended in infants and children.
- **Site of clearance:** plasma cholinesterase enzyme
- **t½:** 1 min

■ **Interaction/toxicity:** Elevates serum potassium, especially in burn patients and patients with spinal cord injury or progressive neuromuscular disease; trigger for MH, causes increased IOP. Can cause bradycardia, especially with repeated administration at short intervals (<5 min). Cross-sensitivity in patients allergic to other muscular relaxants.

SUFENTANIL (SUFENTA)

■ **Uses:** analgesia
■ **Dose:** *Anesthetic adjunct:* Adults: (IV) 1–2 mcg/kg, maintenance 10–25 mcg prn (in obese, use lean body weight). Children: (IV) 0.5–2 mcg/kg, maintenance infusion 1–3 mcg/kg/h. *Main anesthetic:* (IV) 10–15 mcg/kg.
  Premedication: (intranasal) 2 mcg/kg.
■ **t½:** 158–164 min
■ **Site of clearance:** hepatic
■ **Interaction/toxicity:** Benzodiazepines potentiate hypotensive action; truncal muscle rigidity may be seen during induction and emergence. Bradycardia.

SUMATRIPTAN SUCCINATE (IMITREX)

■ **Uses:** migraine and cluster headaches
■ **Dose:** (SQ) 6 mg, second injection 60 min later, NTE 2 injections in 24 h; (nasal spray) 5–20 mg, MR after 2 h, max daily dose 40 mg; (PO) initial 25–100 mg at onset of headache, MR q2h, max daily dose 300 mg.
■ **Site of clearance:** enzymatic
■ **t½:** 2 h
■ **Interaction/toxicity:** Contraindicated in patients with CAD or coronary vasospasm and uncontrolled HTN, and in patients being treated with ergotamines. Administer with caution to patients with hepatic dysfunction.

TERBUTALINE (BRETHAIRE, BRICANYL)

■ **Uses:** bronchodilator; premature labor
■ **Dose:** *Premature labor:* Acute: (IV) 2.5–10 mcg/min, increase gradually q10–20min. Effective max dosages from 17.5–30 mcg/min have been used with caution. Duration of infusion is at least 12 h. Maintenance: (PO) 2.5–10 mg q4–6h for as long as necessary to prolong pregnancy depending on patient tolerance.
  Bronchoconstriction: Adults and children >15 yr: (PO) 5 mg q6h tid; if side effects occur reduce dose to 2.5 mg q6h, NTE

15 mg in 24 h; (SC) 0.25 mg repeated once in 15–30 min, NTE total dose of 0.5 mg within 4 h period. Children 12–15 yr: (PO) 2.5 mg q6h tid, NTE 7.5 mg/24 h. Children <12 yr: (PO) 0.05 mg/kg tid, increased gradually, max 0.15 mg/kg tid–qid or 5 mg/24 h; (SC) 0.005–0.01 mg/kg (max dose 0.3 mg) q15–20 min for 3 doses.
- **Site of clearance:** hepatic
- **t½:** 11–26 h
- **Interaction/toxicity:** Potentiates MAOIs; halogenated anesthetics sensitize (especially halothane) myocardium to sympathomimetic effects (dysrhythmias).

TETRACAINE (PONTOCAINE)

- **Uses:** regional/topical anesthesia
- **Dose:** spinal 4–15 mg; topical 80 mg.
- **Site of clearance:** plasma cholinesterase, hepatic
- **t½:** N/A
- **Interaction/toxicity:** Beta-blockers decrease hepatic clearance; cimetidine increases serum level. Plasma concentration >8 mcg/mL may cause seizures, respiratory/cardiac depression.

THEOPHYLLINE (VARIOUS)

- **Uses:** bronchodilator
- **Dose:** Adults: (IV) loading 6 mg/kg over 20–30 min, then 0.5–1 mg/kg/h, NTE 25 mg/min; maintain serum levels at 10–20 mcg/mL; (PO) loading 5 mg/kg, then 4 mg/kg q6h. Children: (IV) 5 mg/kg, then 0.5–1 mg/kg/h; (PO) loading 5 mg/kg, then 3–4 mg q6h, max daily dose 18–24 mg/kg. Each 0.5 mg/kg administered as loading dose increases serum theophylline levels by 1 mcg/mL.
- **Site of clearance:** hepatic
- **t½:** highly variable and dependent on age, liver function, cardiac function, lung disease and smoking history.
- **Interaction/toxicity:** Contraindicated in patients with poorly controlled dysthymias, peptic ulcer disease, or uncontrolled seizure activity. May cause dysrhythmias with halogenated anesthetics and seizures with ketamine. The following can decrease theophylline levels: barbiturates, carbamazepine, sympathomimetics, phenytoin, and loop diuretics. The following can increase theophylline levels: beta-blockers, calcium channel blockers, antibiotics, steroids, cimetidine, and CHF. Antagonizes effects of hydantoins, lithium, and nondepolarizing muscle relaxants. Parenteral preparations may

contain alcohol or preservatives and should not be used in children.

THIOPENTAL (PENTOTHAL)

- ■ **Uses:** induction agent
- ■ **Dose:** *Induction anesthesia:* Adults: (IV) 3–5 mg/kg. Children 1–12 yr: (IV) 5–6 mg/kg. Infants: (IV) 5–8 mg/kg.
  Maintenance anesthesia: Adults: (IV) 25–100 mg prn. Children: (IV) 1 mg/kg prn.
  Increased intracranial pressure: Adults and children: (IV) 1.5–5 mg/kg, repeat prn to control intracranial pressure.
- ■ **Site of clearance:** hepatic
- ■ **t½:** 3–11.5 h, decreased in children
- ■ **Interaction/toxicity:** Releases histamine; may cause hypotension or respiratory depression; may trigger porphyria, allergic reaction.

TRAMADOL (ULTRAM)

- ■ **Uses:** analgesic
- ■ **Dose:** (PO) 50–100 mg tid, NTE 400 mg/day.
- ■ **Site of clearance:** renal
- ■ **t½:** 6 h
- ■ **Interaction/toxicity:** Carbamazepine increases tramadol metabolism. Quinidine increases plasma tramadol levels. Increased seizure risk with concomitant administration of SSRIs, tricyclic antidepressants, opioids, MAOIs, neuroleptics. Potentiate respiratory depression of anesthetics. Impaired renal function results in decreased clearance.

TRIMETHAPHAN (ARFONAD)

- ■ **Uses:** vasodilator (ganglionic blocker)
- ■ **Dose:** Adults: (IV) 2–4 mg/min (dilute 500 mg in 500 mL D_5W). Children: (IV) 50–150 mcg/kg/min.
- ■ **Site of clearance:** plasma cholinesterase
- ■ **t½:** N/A
- ■ **Interaction/toxicity:** Histamine release. Produces mydriasis, ileus, dilation, and respiratory depression.

d-TUBOCURARINE (VARIOUS)

- ■ **Uses:** nondepolarizing neuromuscular blocker
- ■ **Dose:** (IV) 0.3–0.5 mg/kg.

■ **Site of clearance:** renal
■ **t½:** 173 min
■ **Interaction/toxicity:** Potentiated by volatile anesthetics, hypokalemia, antibiotics (aminoglycosides), lithium, magnesium, local anesthetics, procainamide, quinidine, monoamine oxidase inhibitors, trimethaphan, and propranolol. Prolongation of neuromuscular blockade may occur in patients with renal and/or hepatic disease. Releases histamine.

VANCOMYCIN (VARIOUS)

■ **Uses:** antibiotic
■ **Dose:** (IV) 1 g q12h, max daily dose 4 g.
   Pseudomembranous colitis produced by Clostridium difficile: Adults: (PO) 125 mg q6h, max daily dose 2 g. Children: (IV) 40 mg/kg/day divided q6–8h, max daily dose 2 g. Dosing intervals should be extended in patients with renal impairment.
■ **Site of clearance:** renal
■ **t½:** adults 5–11 h, children (>3 yr) 2.2–3 h, ESRD 200–250 h.
■ **Interaction/toxicity:** Reduce dose in renal dysfunction or with patients receiving nephrotoxic or ototoxic drugs. Administer as infusion over 60 min. Rapid IV infusion associated with "red man syndrome" (hypotension with vasodilation due to histamine release). Potentiates nondepolarizing neuromuscular blockers and histamine release of anesthetic drugs.

VASOPRESSIN (PITRESSIN)

■ **Uses:** vasoconstrictor, neurogenic diabetes insipidus
■ **Dose:** *Vasodilatory shock/septic shock:* (IV) 0.01–0.04 units/min. Doses >0.05 units/min may have more cardiovascular side effects.
   Cardiac arrest: (IV): 40 units IV push may be given via ETT one time.
   Abdominal distention: (IM) 5 units stat, 10 units q3–4h.
   Diabetes insipidus: Adults: (IM, SC) 5–10 units bid–qid prn. Children: (IM, SC) 2.5–10 units bid–qid prn. Adults and children: (IV) 0.0005 unit/kg/h continuous infusion, double dosage prn q30min to max of 0.01 unit/kg/h.
■ **Site of clearance:** hepatic, renal
■ **t½:** 10–20 min
■ **Interaction/toxicity:** Coronary artery vasoconstriction, allergic reactions, HTN.

VECURONIUM (NORCURON) BBW

▦ **Uses:** nondepolarizing neuromuscular blocker
▦ **Dose:** *Surgery:* Adults and children >1 yr: (IV) loading 0.08–0.1 mg/kg or 0.04–0.06 mg/kg after initial dose of succinylcholine for intubation; maintenance 0.01–0.015 mg/kg 25–40 min after initial dose, then 0.01–0.015 mg/kg q12–15 min, may be administered as a continuous infusion at 0.8–2 mcg/kg/min. Infants >7 wk to 1 yr: (IV) loading 0.08–0.1 mg/kg, maintenance 0.05–0.1 mg/kg q60min prn.

ICU: (IV) 0.05–0.1 mg/kg bolus followed by 0.8–1.7 mcg/kg/min once initial recovery from bolus observed or 0.1–0.2 mg/kg q1h.
▦ **Site of clearance:** hepatic, renal
▦ **t½:** 51–80 min
▦ **Interaction/toxicity:** Potentiated by volatile anesthetics, hypokalemia, antibiotics (aminoglycosides), magnesium, local anesthetics, procainamide, quinidine. Conditions associated with increased volume of distribution (e.g., slower circulation time, edematous states, and old age) may be associated with delay in onset. Prolongation of neuromuscular blockade may occur in patients with renal and/or hepatic disease. Theophylline and phenytoin decrease effects. Bradycardia may occur with rapid administration in patients receiving opioids.

VERAPAMIL (CALAN, ISOPTIN)

▦ **Uses:** antidysrhythmic, antihypertensive
▦ **Dose:** *Dysrhythmia (SVT):* Adults: (IV) 2.5–5 mg over 2 min, second dose of 5–10 mg (~0.15 mg/kg) may be given 15–30 min after the initial dose if patient tolerates but does not respond to initial dose; max total dose 20 mg. Children <1 yr: (IV) 0.1–0.2 mg/kg over 2 min, MR q30min prn. Children 1–15 yr: 0.1–0.3 mg/kg (max 5 mg) over 2 min, MR in 15 min if adequate response not achieved, max for second dose 10 mg.

Angina: (PO) initial 80–120 mg bid (elderly or small stature 40 mg bid), range 240–480 mg/day tid–qid.

HTN: (PO) immediate release 80 mg tid, usual dose range 80–320 mg/day divided bid; sustained release 240 mg/day, usual dose range 120–360 mg/day qd or divided bid (120 mg/day in elderly or small patients). No evidence of additional benefit in doses >360 mg/day.
▦ **Site of clearance:** renal
▦ **t½:** Adults single dose 2–8 h, multiple doses up to 12 h.

■ **Interaction/toxicity:** Potentiates beta-blockers, theophylline; increases digoxin levels. Barbiturates may decrease bioavailability. Cimetidine increases bioavailability.

WARFARIN (COUMADIN) `BBW`

■ **Uses:** anticoagulant
■ **Dose:** (PO) 5–10 mg. Adjust dose for prothrombin time 1.5–2 times control.
■ **Site of clearance:** hepatic
■ **t½:** 20–60 h
■ **Interaction/toxicity:** Platelet aggregation inhibitors (e.g., salicylates, dipyridamole, indomethacin), procoagulant inhibition factors (e.g., quinidine) increase risk of hemorrhage. Decreased effect with enzyme inducers (e.g., barbiturates, phenytoin).

APPENDIX H ■ HERBAL MEDICATIONS

The authors and publisher have exerted every effort to ensure that the drug selection and dosage set forth in this appendix are in accord with current recommendations and practice at the time of publication. However, in view of ongoing research, changes in government regulations, and the constant flow of information relating to drug therapy and drug reactions, the reader is urged to check the package insert for each drug for any change in indications and dosage and for added warnings and precautions. This is particularly important when the recommended agent is a new or infrequently used drug.

The editors wish to acknowledge the contribution of Stella A. Haddadin, BSc, PharmD, Yale–New Haven Hospital, Department of Pharmacy Services, in the preparation of this appendix.

ALFALFA
Uses: Diuretic, kidney, bladder and prostate conditions, hyperglycemia, asthma, arthritis, indigestion
Interaction/toxicity: Excessive use may interfere with anticoagulant therapy, potentiate drug-induced photosensitivity, and interfere with hormone therapy.

ANGELICA ROOT
Uses: Gastrointestinal spasm, loss of appetite, feeling of fullness, and flatulence
Interaction/toxicity: Can cause photodermatitis, claims to increase stomach acid, therefore, interferes with antacids, sucralfate, H2 antagonists, and proton pump inhibitors. Potentiates the effects and adverse effects of anticoagulants and antiplatelet drugs.

ANISE
Uses: Dyspepsia and as a pediatric antiflatulent and expectorant
Interaction/toxicity: Excessive doses can prolong coagulation, increasing PT/INR because of coumarin contained in anise. An interaction exists with anticoagulant therapy, MAOIs, and hormone therapy. Catecholamine activity might increase blood pressure readings and increase heart rate.

ARNICA FLOWER
Uses: Antiphlogistic, antiseptic, anti-inflammatory, analgesic
Interaction/toxicity: Potentiates anticoagulant and antiplatelet effect of drugs and possibly increases risk of bleeding.

ASAFOETIDA
Uses: Chronic bronchitis, asthma, pertussis, hoarseness, hysteria, flatulent colic, chronic gastric, dyspepsia, irritable colon, and convulsions
Interaction/toxicity: Might increase the risk of bleeding, and excessive doses might interfere with blood pressure control. Can irritate GI tract and is contraindicated in patients with infectious or inflammatory GI conditions.

BILBERRY
Uses: Peripheral vascular disease, diabetes, ophthalmologic diseases, peptic ulcer disease and scleroderma.
Interaction/toxicity: Excessive use may interfere with coagulation and inhibit platelet aggregation; alters glucose regulation.

BOGBEAN
Uses: Rheumatism, loss of appetite, dyspepsia
Interaction/toxicity: Potentiates anticoagulant and antiplatelet drugs and possibly increases risk of bleeding.

BROMELAIN
Uses: Acute postoperative and posttraumatic conditions of swelling, especially of the nasal and paranasal sinuses, osteoarthritis
Interaction/toxicity: Potentiates anticoagulant and antiplatelet drugs and possibly increases risk of bleeding. Increases plasma and urine tetracycline level.

CAYENNE
Uses: Muscle spasms, chronic pain
Interaction/toxicity: Overdose may cause hypothermia. May cause skin blisters.

CELERY
Uses: Rheumatism, gout, hysteria, nervousness, weight loss as a result of malnutrition, loss of appetite, exhaustion, sedative, mild diuretic, urinary antiseptic, digestive aid, antiflatulent, blood purification
Interaction/toxicity: Potentiates anticoagulant and antiplatelet drugs and possibly increases risk of bleeding. There is an additive effect with drugs with sedative properties and may cause increase

in phototoxic response to psoralen plus ultraviolet light A (PUVA) therapy because of its psoralen content.

CHAMOMILE
Uses: Flatulence, nervous diarrhea, restlessness, insomnia, antispasmodic
Interaction/toxicity: Concomitant use with benzodiazepines might cause additive effects and side effects. Potentiates anticoagulant and antiplatelet drugs and possibly increases risk of bleeding. Is an inhibitor of the cytochrome P450 3A4 enzyme system.

CLOVE
Uses: Flatulence, nausea, and vomiting
Interaction/toxicity: Potentiates anticoagulant and antiplatelet drugs and possibly increases risk of bleeding.

DANDELION
Uses: Diuretic, GI disorders and anti-inflammatory effect.
Interaction/toxicity: Excessive use may interfere with coagulation and inhibit platelet aggregation; alters glucose regulation. Do not use in the presence of biliary obstruction. Interactions with digoxin, lithium, insulin, oral hypoglycemics, cytochrome P450, ciprofloxacin, disulfram and metronidazole.

DANSHEN
Uses: Circulation problems, cardiovascular diseases, chronic hepatitis, abdominal masses, insomnia because of palpitations and tight chest, acne, psoriasis, eczema, aids in wound healing
Interaction/toxicity: Potentiates anticoagulant and antiplatelet drugs and possibly increases risk of bleeding. Increases the cardiovascular effects and side effects of digoxin.

DEVIL'S CLAW
Uses: Osteoarthritis, rheumatoid arthritis, gout, myalgia, fibrositis
Interaction/toxicity: Can affect heart rate, contractility of heart, and blood pressure. Might decrease blood glucose levels and have additive effects with medications used for diabetes. May cause an increase in gastric acid secretions.

DONG QUAI
Uses: Gynecologic ailments, menopausal symptoms
Interaction/toxicity: Potentiates anticoagulant and antiplatelet drugs and possibly increases risk of bleeding.

ECHINACEA

Uses: Common colds, urinary tract infections
Interaction/toxicity: May cause hepatotoxicity especially with other concomitant hepatotoxins. Antagonizes steroids and immunosuppressants. May possess immunosuppressive activity after long-term use.

EPHEDRA

Uses: Diet aid, bacteriostatic, antitussive
Interaction/toxicity: May cause arrhythmias with inhalation anesthetics and cardiac glycosides. Life-threatening reaction with MAOIs. May cause depletion of catecholamines and lead to perioperative hemodynamic instability. Can cause death.

FENUGREEK

Uses: Lower blood sugar in diabetics
Interaction/toxicity: Potentiates anticoagulant and antiplatelet drugs and possibly increases risk of bleeding. Inhibits corticosteroid drug activity, interferes with hormone therapy, can alter blood glucose control, and potentiate effect of MAOIs.

FEVERFEW

Uses: Migraine prophylaxis, antipyretic
Interaction/toxicity: Inhibit platelet activity. Potentiates anticoagulants. Abrupt withdrawal may cause rebound headaches. Uterine stimulant. Associated with serotonin syndrome.

FISH OIL

Uses: Cardiovascular disease, colon cancer, psychiatric disorders, diabetes, inflammatory disease, inflammatory bowel diseases, premenstrual syndrome and scleroderma.
Interaction/toxicity: Excessive use may interfere with coagulation and inhibit platelet aggregation; alters glucose regulation; potentiates anti-hypertensive drugs.

FLAXSEED OIL

Uses: Cardiovascular disease, colon cancer, psychiatric disorders, diabetes, inflammatory disease, inflammatory bowel diseases, breast cancer and depression.
Interaction/toxicity: Excessive use may interfere with coagulation and inhibit platelet aggregation; alters glucose regulation.

GARLIC (PERTAINS TO SUPPLEMENT PRODUCT)

Uses: Lower lipids, antihypertensive, antiplatelet, antioxidant, antithrombolytic

Interaction/toxicity: Potentiates anticoagulants, especially in the presence of drugs that inhibit platelet function. Potentiates vasodilator drugs and antihypertensives. May decrease blood glucose levels as a result of increased serum insulin levels.

GINGER (PERTAINS TO SUPPLEMENT PRODUCT)
Uses: Antinauseant, antispasmodic
Interaction/toxicity: Inhibits thromboxane synthetase. Potentiates anticoagulants. May alter effects of calcium channel blockers.

GINKGO
Uses: Circulatory stimulant, inhibit platelets
Interaction/toxicity: Potentiates anticoagulants, especially in the presence of aspirin, NSAIDs, heparin, and warfarin.

GINSENG
Uses: Antioxidant
Interaction/toxicity: Antagonize anticoagulants. Avoid use of sympathetic stimulants, which may result in tachycardia or hypertension. Possesses hypoglycemic effects. Potentiates digoxin and MAOIs.

GOLDENSEAL
Uses: Diuretic, anti-inflammatory, hemostatic
Interaction/toxicity: May worsen edema and hypertension. Oxytocic possesses activity.

GRAPE SEED
Uses: Anti-oxidant, cardiovascular disorders, peripheral circulatory disorders, multiple sclerosis, Parkinson's disease.
Interaction/toxicity: Excessive use may interfere with coagulation and inhibit platelet aggregation; may inhibit xanthine oxidase.

GREEN TEA
Uses: Improves cognitive performance, lowers cholesterol and triglycerides, aids in the prevention of breast, bladder, esophageal, and pancreatic cancers. Decreased risk of Parkinson's disease, gingivitis, obesity
Interaction/toxicity: Concomitant use might inhibit effect of adenosine and antagonize effect of warfarin. Because of the caffeine content, there is an increase in cardiac inotropic effects of beta-adrenergic agonist drugs, an increase in the effects and toxicity of clozapine, and an increased risk of agitation, tremors, and insomnia in combination with ephedrine. It might precipitate

hypertensive crisis with MAOIs as well. Might reduce sedative effects of benzodiazepines.

HORSE CHESTNUT
Uses: Scleroderma, peripheral vascular disorders, varicose veins and relieving pain, tiredness, tension, swelling in legs, itching, and edema.
Interaction/toxicity: Excessive use may interfere with coagulation and inhibit platelet aggregation; phosphodiesterase inhibitor and alters glucose regulation. Potentiates anticoagulant and antiplatelet drugs and possibly increases risk of bleeding, hypoglycemic effects, might interfere with binding of protein binding drugs.

KAVA-KAVA
Uses: Anxiolytic, analgesic
Interaction/toxicity: Potentiates barbiturates, opioids, and benzodiazepines.

LICORICE
Uses: Heal gastric and duodenal ulcers
Interaction/toxicity: May cause hypertension, hypokalemia, and edema.

LOVAGE ROOT
Uses: Used for inflammation of the lower urinary tract and prevention of kidney gravel; in "irrigation therapy," it is used as a mild diuretic
Interaction/toxicity: Might increase sodium retention and interfere with diuretic therapy.

MEADOWSWEET
Uses: Supportive therapy for colds
Interaction/toxicity: Can potentiate narcotic effects. Contains a salicylate constituent.

ONIONS
Uses: Loss of appetite, preventing atherosclerosis, dyspepsia, fever, colds, cough, tendency toward infection, and inflammation of the mouth and pharynx
Interaction/toxicity: May enhance antidiabetic drug effects and alter blood sugar control. Might enhance antiplatelet drug activity and increase bleeding risk.

PAPAIN
Uses: Inflammation and swelling in patient with pharyngitis
Interaction/toxicity: Concomitant use with anticoagulant and antiplatelet drugs may increase risk of bleeding.

PARSLEY
Uses: Breath freshener, urinary tract infections, and kidney or bladder stones
Interaction/toxicity: Might interfere with oral anticoagulant therapy because of the Vitamin K contained in parsley. May interfere with diuretic therapy by enhancing sodium retention. Might potentiate MAOI drug therapy.

PASSION FLOWER
Uses: Generalized anxiety disorder
Interaction/toxicity: Concomitant use with barbiturates can increase drug-induced sleep time; can potentiate the effects of sedatives and tranquilizers, including sedative effects of antihistamines.

QUASSIA
Uses: Anorexia, indigestion, fever, mouthwash, as an anthelmintic for thread worms, nematodes, and ascaris
Interaction/toxicity: Stimulates gastric acid and might oppose effect of antacids and H2 antagonists. Excessive doses might have additive effects with anticoagulant therapy with Coumadin. Concomitant use of potassium-depleting diuretics or stimulant laxative abuse might increase risk of cardiac glycoside toxicity as a result of potassium loss.

RED CLOVER
Uses: Hot flashes
Interaction/toxicity: Can increase the anticoagulant effects and bleeding risk because of its coumarin content. May interfere with hormone replacement therapy or oral contraceptives, and may interfere with tamoxifen because of its potential estrogenic effects. Can inhibit cytochrome P450 (cyp450) 3A4.

SAW PALMETTO
Uses: Benign prostatic hypertrophy, antiandrogenic
Interaction/toxicity: Potentiates birth control pills and estrogens. May cause hypertension.

ST. JOHN'S WORT
Uses: Depression, anxiety
Interaction/toxicity: Possible interaction/toxicity with MAOIs and meperidine. May prolong anesthetic effects. Potentiates digoxin. May decrease effects of warfarin, steroids, and possibly benzodiazepines and calcium channel blockers.

SWEET CLOVER
Uses: Chronic venous insufficiency, including leg pain and heaviness, night-time leg cramps, itching and swelling, for supportive treatment of thrombophlebitis, lymphatic congestion, postthrombotic syndromes, and hemorrhoids
Interaction/toxicity: Use with hepatotoxic drugs might increase risk of hepatotoxicity. Concomitant use with anticoagulant and antiplatelet drugs may increase risk of bleeding.

TUMERIC
Uses: Dyspepsia, jaundice, hepatitis, flatulence, abdominal bloating
Interaction/toxicity: Concomitant use with anticoagulant and antiplatelet drugs may increase risk of bleeding.

VALERIAN
Uses: Sedative, anxiolytic
Interaction/toxicity: Potentiates barbiturates and anesthetics. May blunt symptoms of benzodiazepine withdrawal.

VITAMIN E
Uses: Vitamin E deficiency, heart disease
Interaction/toxicity: Concomitant use with anticoagulant and antiplatelet drugs may increase risk of bleeding. Might prevent tolerance to nitrates.

WILLOW BARK
Uses: Lower back pain, fever, rheumatic ailments, headache
Interaction/toxicity: Enough salicylate is present in willow bark to cause drug interactions common to salicylates or aspirin. Can impair effectiveness of beta-adrenergic blockers, probenecid, and sulfinpyrazone. Can increase effects, side effects, or toxicity of alcohol, anticoagulants, carbonic anhydrase inhibitors, heparin, methotrexate, NSAIDs, sulfonylureas, and valproic acid.

Page numbers followed by t and f indicate tables and figures, respectively.